Atlas of Cutaneous Laser Surgery

Atlas of Cutaneous Laser Surgery

Editor

David B. Apfelberg, M.D.
Atherton Plastic Surgery Center
Atherton, California
Assistant Clinical Professor of Plastic Surgery
Stanford University Medical Center
Stanford, California

Raven Press ❦ New York

Raven Press, 1185 Avenue of the Americas, New York, New York 10036

© 1992 by Raven Press, Ltd. All rights reserved. This book is protected by copyright. No part of it may be reproduced, stored in a retrieval system, or transmitted, in any form or by any means, electronic, mechanical, photocopying, or recording, or otherwise, without the prior written permission of the publisher.

Printed and bound in Hong Kong

Library of Congress Cataloging-in-Publication Data

Atlas of cutaneous laser surgery / editor, David B. Apfelberg.
    p.   cm.
  Includes bibliographical references and index.
  ISBN 0-88167-764-7
  1. Lasers—Therapeutic use—Atlases. 2. Skin—Surgery—Atlases.
I. Apfelberg, David B.
  [DNLM: 1. Laser Surgery—atlases. 2. Skin—surgery—atlases. WR
17 A8816]
RL120.L37A85   1992
617.4'77059—dc20
DNLM/DLC
for Library of Congress   90-9239

  The material contained in this volume was submitted as previously unpublished material, except in the instances in which some of the illustrative material was derived.
  Great care has been taken to maintain the accuracy of the information contained in the volume. However, neither Raven Press nor the editor can be held responsible for errors or for any consequences arising from the use of the information contained herein.

9 8 7 6 5 4 3 2 1

Contents

	PREFACE	vii
	ACKNOWLEDGMENTS	viii
	CONTRIBUTORS	ix
1	THE PHYSICAL PRINCIPLES OF LASERS	1
2	LASER SAFETY	13
3	EYE SAFETY DURING LASER EYELID TREATMENT	21
4	CARBON DIOXIDE LASER	23

Vascular and Related Lesions, *25*; Malignant and Premalignant Lesions, *33*; Inflammatory/Infectious Lesions, *51*; Tattoo, *78*; Miscellaneous, *91*; Surgical Procedures, *162*

5	ARGON LASER	209

Vascular and Related Lesions, *210*; Inflammatory/Infectious Lesions, *259*; Tattoo, *260*; Miscellaneous, *266*; Surgical Procedures, *287*

6	YAG LASER	291

Vascular and Related Lesions, *292*; Malignant and Premalignant Lesions, *312*; Tattoo, *314*; Miscellaneous, *316*; Surgical Procedures, *320*

7	TUNABLE DYE LASER	341

Vascular Malformations, *342*

8	NEW TECHNOLOGIES	401

Vascular and Related Lesions, *402*; Malignant and Premalignant Lesions, *428*; Tattoo, *436*; Miscellaneous, *445*

	REFERENCES	459
	GLOSSARY	461
	BIBLIOGRAPHY	463
	INDEX	475

Preface

This atlas is intended to show "how to" do a certain procedure. Neophytes can refer to the atlas before beginning a laser surgery. Veteran laser users, who are already familiar with one or two laser wavelengths, may wish to learn how a procedure is done by someone else or with a different laser. This atlas will allow patients to see how their laser procedure is going to be performed and what type of results they might expect. Support personnel in the office or operating room will gain a clearer idea about set-up and assistance.

The material is presented in case summary form. Each author has selected one or more lesions that are amenable to treatment by various lasers. The author then provides a brief review of the case and describes why a particular laser was chosen for such a case. Laser power and exposure settings are also included. The figure captions are designed to demonstrate exactly how the laser procedure was performed from the initial untreated lesion to the final completed result. In most cases, all significant interim steps are illustrated and described. Various tips about the procedure, precautions, or things to watch out for are detailed in the Additional Information section. Finally, post-treatment care instructions are provided.

A glossary has been compiled for the reader's reference. And, a comprehensive bibliography of laser usage in the field of cutaneous lesion surgery is included.

David B. Apfelberg

Acknowledgments

I am grateful to my colleagues who have contributed such excellent case summaries. This international group of laser experts and thought-leaders have dedicated themselves to the promotion and teaching of safe, effective, and often innovative uses of lasers.

Contributors

Bruce M. Achauer, M.D.
Director, Plastic Surgery Division, Beckman Laser Institute and Medical Center, Associate Adjunct Professor, Department of Surgery, Division of Plastic Surgery, University of California, Irvine Medical Center, 101 City Drive South, Orange, California 92668

David B. Apfelberg, M.D.
Atherton Plastic Surgery Center, Suite 201, 3351 El Camino Real, Atherton, California 94027; and Assistant Clinical Professor of Plastic Surgery, Stanford University Medical Center, Stanford, California

Kenneth A. Arndt, M.D.
Professor of Dermatology, Harvard Medical School, Dermatologist-in-Chief, Department of Dermatology, Beth Israel Hospital, 330 Brookline Avenue, Boston, Massachusetts 02215

Billie L. Aronoff, M.D.
Clinical Professor of Surgery, Department of Surgery, University of Southwestern Medical School; and 3600 Gaston Avenue, Dallas, Texas 75246

Philip L. Bailin, M.D., F.A.C.P.
Chairman, Department of Dermatology and Head, Section of Dermatologic Surgery and Oncology, Cleveland Clinic Foundation, One Clinic Center, 9500 Euclid Avenue, Cleveland, Ohio 44195-5032

David W. Becker, Jr., M.D.
Department of Plastic and Reconstructive Surgery, Twin Falls Clinic and Hospital, 666 Shoshone Street East, Twin Falls, Idaho 83301

Gary J. Brauner, M.D.
Clinical Associate Professor of Dermatology, Department of Dermatology, New York Medical College; and 125 East 63rd Street, New York, New York 10021

J. M. Brunetaud, M.D.
Professor of Medicine, Department of Laser Research, Hôpital Claude Huriez, Place de Verdun, 59037 Lille Cedex, France

J. A. S. Carruth, F.R.C.S.
Consultant Otolaryngologist, Royal South Hants Hospital, Lyon Street, Southampton S09 4PE, United Kingdom

Dan J. Castro, M.D.
Assistant Professor of Surgery, Department of Surgery/ Division of Head and Neck, University of California, Los Angeles, School of Medicine; and 10833 Le Conte Avenue, Los Angeles, California 90024

Jack A. Coleman, Jr., M.D.
Instructor, Department of Otolaryngology, Vanderbilt University Medical Center, Nashville, Tennessee 37232-2559

Thomas J. Dougherty, Ph.D.
Head, Division of Radiation Biology, Roswell Park Cancer Institute, Elm and Carlton Streets, Buffalo, New York 14263-0001

Richard E. Fitzpatrick, M.D.
Assistant Clinical Professor, Department of Medicine/ Dermatology at University of California San Diego; and Dermatology Associates of San Diego County, 477 El Camino Real, Suite B303, Encinitas, California 92024

Jerome M. Garden, M.D.
Director of Laser Surgery, Divisions of Dermatology and Plastic Surgery, Children's Memorial Hospital, 2300 Children's Plaza, Chicago, Illinois 60614

David J. Goldberg, M.D.
Chief of Dermatologic Surgery, New Jersey Medical School, Newark, New Jersey, and, Director, Skin Laser Center, Department of Dermatology, Pascack Valley Hospital; and 400 Old Hook Road, Westwood, New Jersey 07675

Mitchel P. Goldman, M.D.
Assistant Clinical Professor of Dermatology/Medicine, University of California, San Diego; and Dermatology Associates of San Diego, Incorporated, 850 Prospect Street, La Jolla, California 92037

John N. Graber, M.D.
Clinical Instructor in Surgery, Chairman of Laser Committee, Abbott Northwestern Hospital, University of Minnesota, 2545 Chicago Avenue South, #600, Minneapolis, Minnesota 55404

Geoffrey G. Hallock, M.D.
Division of Plastic Surgery, The Allentown Hospital-Lehigh Valley Hospital Center; and 1230 South Cedar Crest Boulevard, Suite 306, Allentown, Pennsylvania 18103

Elaine Harrison-Khanwilkar, B.S.N.
Clinical Coordinator, Endoscopic and Laser Surgery, University of Utah Hospital, 50 North Medical Drive Room 3A210, Salt Lake City, Utah 84132

Darrell L. Henderson, M.D.
Plastic Surgery Associates, Suite 400, 1101 South College Road, Lafayette, Louisiana 70503

H. Raul Herrera, M.D.
Associate Clinical Professor, University of Rochester, Chief of Plastic Surgery, Rochester General Hospital, Department of Surgery (Plastics), University of Rochester/Rochester General Hosptial, 1445 Portland Avenue, Rochester, New York 14621

Lovic W. Hobby, M.D.
Chief, Plastic Surgery Service, Director, Laser Treatment Center, Piedmont Hospital; and 35 Collier Road NW, Suite 485, Atlanta, Georgia 30309

J. P. Hulsbergen Henning, M.D.
Department of Dermatology, St. Joseph Hospital, Dommelstraat Zuid 40, P.O. Box 7777, 5500 MB Veldhoven, The Netherlands

Jyri J. Hukki, M.D., Ph.D.
Consultant Plastic Surgeon, Division of Plastic Surgery, Helsinki University Central Hospital, Töölö Hospital, Topeliuksenkatu 5, SF-00260 Helsinki, Finland

Gregory S. Keller, M.D.
Western Institute for Laser Treatment, 2323 DeLaVina #105, Santa Barbara, California 93105

Ronald Allen Kirschner, D.O.
Professor and Chairman, Department of Otorhinolaryngology and Facial Plastic Surgery, Philadelphia College of Osteopathic Medicine; and Plaza 13, Two Bala Plaza, Bala Cynwood, Pennsylvania 19004

Raymond J. Lanzafame, M.D., F.A.C.S.
Assistant Professor of Surgery, Director, Laser Center, Department of Surgery, University of Rochester, Rochester General Hospital, 1445 Portland Avenue #G06, Rochester, New York 14621

Barry Leshin, M.D.
Assistant Professor of Dermatology and Otolaryngology, Bowman Gray School of Medicine of Wake Forest University, 300 South Hawthorne Road, Winston-Salem, North Carolina 27103

Thomas S. Mang, Ph.D.
Director, Photodynamic Therapy Center, Assistant Professor of Biophysics, Department of Radiation Biology, Roswell Park Cancer Institute, Elm and Carlton Streets, Buffalo, New York 14263

Morton Richard Maser, M.D.
Assistant Clinical Professor of Surgery, Department of Plastic Surgery, Stanford University Hospital; and Palo Alto Medical Foundation, 300 Homer Avenue, Palo Alto, California 94301

James S. McCaughan, Jr., M.D.
Director, Laser Medical Research, Foundation and Grant Laser Center, 323 East Town Street, Columbus, Ohio 43215

David H. McDaniel, M.D.
Laser Center of Virginia, 1815 Colonial Medical Court, Virginia Beach, Virginia 23454

S. Teri McGillis, M.D.
Department of Dermatology, Section of Mohs Micrographic Surgery and Oncology, Cleveland Clinic Foundation, 9500 Euclid Avenue, Cleveland, Ohio 44195-5032

Thomas O. McMeekin, M.D.
Clinical Associate Professor, University of Rochester School of Medicine; and 300 White Spruce Boulevard, Rochester, New York 14623

Iain D. Miller, M.D.
University of Strathclyde and Derma-Lase Ltd., Schaw Medical Centre, Bearsden, Glasgow, Scotland

Leo J. Miserendino, D.D.S., M.S.
Assistant Clinical Professor, Department of Endodontics, Marquette University Dental School; and 2504 Washington Street, Waukegan, Illinois 60085

Harry Mittelman, M.D.
Associate Clinical Professor, Facial Plastic Surgery, Department of Head and Neck Surgery, Stanford University Medical Center; and 770 Welch Road, Palo Alto, California 94304

Muneo Miyasaka, M.D.
Instructor of Plastic and Reconstructive Surgery, Department of Plastic and Reconstructive Surgery, Tokai University School of Medicine, Isehara City, Kanagawa, Japan 259-11

Serge Mordon, Ph.D.
Research Physicist, Unité 279, Institut National de la Sante, et de La Recherche Medicale, (Inserm), 1 Rue du Professeur Calmette, 59019 Lille Cedex, France

Taichin Morita, M.D.
Instructor of Plastic and Reconstructive Surgery, Department of Plastic and Reconstructive Surgery, Tokai University School of Medicine, Bohseidai, Isehara City, Kanagawa Prefecture 259-11, Japan

Michael J. Murphy, Ph.D.
University of Strathclyde/Derma-Lase Limited, Schaw Medical Centre, 69 Schaw Drive, Bearsden, Glasgow, Scotland, United Kingdom

Christine C. Nelson, M.D.
Assistant Professor of Ophthalmology, Co-Director of Eye Plastic and Orbital Surgery, Department of Ophthalmology, University of Michigan, Kellogg Eye Center, 1000 Wall Street, Ann Arbor, Michigan 48105

J. Stuart Nelson, M.D., Ph.D.
Associate Director, Beckman Laser Institute and Medical Clinic, University of California at Irvine, 1002 Health Sciences Road East, Irvine, California 92715

Joel Mark Noe, M.D.
Assistant Clinical Professor of Surgery, Department of Plastic Surgery, Harvard Medical School, Boston, Harvard Medical School/Beth Israel Hospital, 575 Boylston Street, Newton, Massachusetts 02159

Arie Orenstein, M.D.
Department of Plastic Surgery, Chaim Sheba Medical Center, Tel-Hashomer, Israel

Mitsuhiro Osada, M.D.
Professor of Plastic and Reconstructive Surgery, Department of Plastic and Reconstructive Surgery, Tokai University School of Medicine, Ohseidai, Isehara City, Kanagawa Ken, 259-11, Japan

Robert H. Ossoff, D.M.D., M.D., F.A.C.S.
Guy M. Manness Professor and Chairman, Department of Otolaryngology, Medical Center North S-2100, Vanderbilt University Medical Center, Nashville, Tennessee 37232-2559

Krystyna A. Pasyk, M.D., Ph.D.
Assistant Research Scientist, Plastic and Reconstructive Surgery Section, University of Michigan, 1500 East Medical Center Drive, Ann Arbor, Michigan 48109-0340

Robert M. Pick, D.D.S., M.S., F.A.C.D.
Associate Clinical Professor of Periodontics, Department of Periodontics, Northwestern University Dental School and Northwestern Memorial Hosptial, 240 East Huron, Chicago, Illinois 60611

John Louis Ratz, M.D., F.A.C.P.
Director, Center for Dermatologic, Cosmetic and Laser Surgery, and Associate Professor of Dermatology, Rush-Presbyterian-St. Luke's Medical Center, Department of Dermatology; and 4050 Health Way Drive, Suite 220, Aurora, Illinois 60504

Syrus Rayhan, M.D.
Associate Clinical Professor, Department of Dermatology, University of California at Irvine; and 17822 Beach Boulevard, Huntingdon Beach, California 92647

William H. Reid, M.B., Ch.B., F.R.C.S. (EDINBURGH, GLASGOW, ENGLAND)
West Scotland Plastic Surgery Unit, Canniesburn Hospital, Glasgow, Scotland

David C. Rice, P.E.
Director, Microsurgery/Laser Laboratory, Department of Microsurgery/Laser Laboratory, The Allentown Hospital-Lehigh Valley Hospital Center, 1200 South Cedar Crest Boulevard, Allentown, Pennsylvania 18103

Wm. Russell Ries, M.D., F.A.C.S.
Assistant Professor, Department of Otolaryngology, Vanderbilt University Medical Center, S-2100 Medical Center North, Nashville, Tennessee 37232-2559

Randall K. Roenigk, M.D.
Associate Professor and Consultant, Department of Dermatology, Mayo Clinic, 200 First Street, SW, Rochester, Minnesota 55905

Harold L. Rosenfeld, M.D.
Clinical Assistant Professor of Surgery, Department of Surgery; Plastic Surgery Division; and 39 Congress Street, Suite 301, Pasadena, California 91105

Timothy J. Rosio, M.D.
Director: Mohs and Laser Surgery, Department of Dermatology and Cutaneous Surgery, Marshfield Clinic, 1000 North Oak Avenue (4K-5), Marshfield, Wisconsin 54449

Elston Rothermel, D.P.M.
Clinical Assistant Professor, Department of Dermatology/Podiatry, Stanford University School of Medicine; and Podiatrist, Comprehensive Laser Center, Palo Alto Medical Foundation, 300 Homer Avenue, Palo Alto, California 94301

Guy Rotteleur, M.D.
Department of Dermatology and Laser Center, Hospital Claude Huriez, Place de Verdun, 59037 Lille Cedex, France

Javier Ruiz-Esparza, M.D.
Dermatology Associates of San Diego County, Inc., 477 North El Camino Real, Suite B-303, Encinitas, California 92024

Alan Schliftman, M.D.
Assistant Clinical Professor of Dermatology, New York Medical College, Department of Dermatology, Westchester County Medical Center, Valhalla, New York 10595

Tom Schröder, M.D., Ph.D.
Professor of Surgery, Department of Surgery, Laserklinikka, Gyldenintie 2A, 00200 Helsinki, Finland

Leonard S. Schultz, M.D.
Clinical Assistant Professor of Surgery, University of Minnesota/Abbott, Northwestern Hospital, Suite 600, 2545 Chicago Avenue, Minneapolis, Minnesota 55404

Karen A. Sherwood, M.D.
Children's Hospital of Los Angeles, 4650 Sunset Boulevard, Los Angeles, California 90027

Lester Silver, M.D.
Chief, Division of Plastic Surgery, The Mount Sinai Medical Center, One Gustave Levy Place, (Box 1262), New York, New York 10029

Teruko Smith, R.N., P.A.-C.
Department of Plastic Surgery, Palo Alto Medical Foundation, Comprehensive Laser Center, 300 Homer Avenue, Palo Alto, California 94301

Patricia Z. Spector, R.N. MHS, P.A.-C.
Clinical Instructor, Department of Family Medicine, Stanford University Medical Center; and Comprehensive Laser Center, Palo Alto Medical Foundation, 300 Homer Avenue, Palo Alto, California 94301

Ryuzaburo Tanino, M.D.
Associate Professor of Plastic and Reconstructive Surgery, Department of Plastic and Reconstructive Surgery, Tokai University School of Medicine, Bohseidai, Isehara City, Kanagawa, Japan 259-11

Mark B. Taylor, M.D.
Clinical Instructor, Department of Dermatology, University of Utah, 50 North Medical Drive, Salt Lake City, Utah 84103

Victoria M. Vander Kam, R.N.
Department of Surgery, Division of Plastic Surgery, Beckman Laser Institute, University of California at Irvine, 1002 Health Sciences Road East, Irvine, California 92175

Tom D. Wang, M.D.
Consultant, Department of Otorhinolaryngology, Mayo Clinic, 200 First Street S.W., Rochester, Minnesota 55905

Ronald G. Wheeland, M.D., F.A.C.P.
Associate Professor and Chairman, Department of Dermatology, University of California, Davis; and 1605 Alhambra Boulevard, Suite 2300, Sacramento, California 95816

Duane C. Whitaker, M.D.
Associate Professor, Department of Dermatology, University of Iowa Hospitals and Clinics, Iowa City, Iowa 52242

Brummitte D. Wilson, M.D.
Roswell Park Cancer Institute, Departments of Dermatology and Radiation Biology, Elm and Carlton Streets, Buffalo, New York 14263

Hiroto Yamada, M.D.
Department of Plastic Surgery, Tokai University Hospital, Boseidai, Isehara City, Kanagawa Prefecture 259-11, Japan

1

THE PHYSICAL PRINCIPLES OF LASERS

Dan J. Castro

HISTORICAL PERSPECTIVES

Laser is the acronym for *l*ight *a*mplification by *s*timulated *e*mission of *r*adiation (Fig. 1-A). A laser is capable of generating an intense, almost parallel beam of electromagnetic energy of a given wavelength or color (Fig. 1-B). These characteristics make the laser a unique device for many medical and surgical applications. The principles necessary for formulation of the concept of the laser were firmly established early in the twentieth century with the advent of Bohr's theory and optical resonators. Planck in 1908 and Einstein (1) in 1917 proposed the concept of stimulated emission or the quantum theory, thus laying the foundation for Schawlow and Townes (1954) and Prokhorov and Basov to independently describe the physical principles of the maser (*m*icrowave *a*mplification by *s*timulated *e*mission of *r*adiation). The first successful application of stimulated emission of microwaves was made by Gordon et al. (2) in 1955. In 1960 Maiman (3) first observed stimulated emission in the visible portion of the spectrum by exciting a ruby rod with intense pulses of light from a flash lamp, generating the first laser beam. In 1961 Javan et al. (4) developed the first gas laser and demonstrated the first continuously operating laser, using a mixture of helium and neon. Also that year, using a neodymium-doped yttrium-aluminum-garnet (Nd:YAG) rod, Johnson (5) developed a laser that emitted energy in the near infrared portion of the spectrum. The argon laser, emitting energy in the blue-green portion of the spectrum, was developed by Bennett et al. (6) in 1962. The carbon dioxide laser emitting spectral energy in the mid-infrared portion was developed in 1964 by Patel et al. (7).

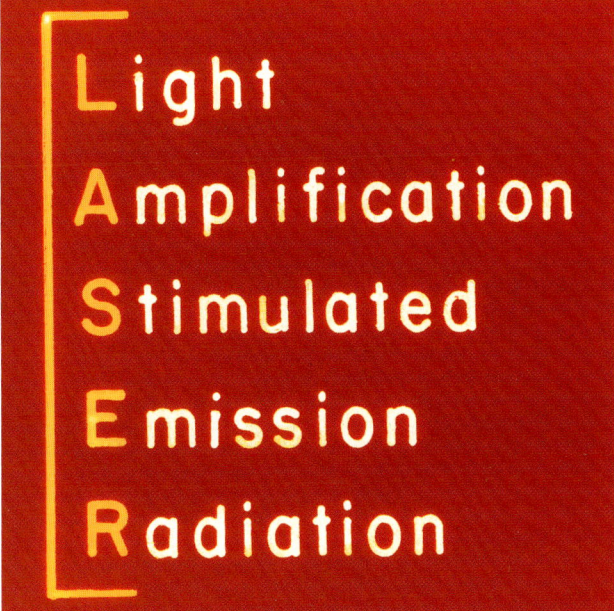

FIG. 1-A. Acronym for Laser.

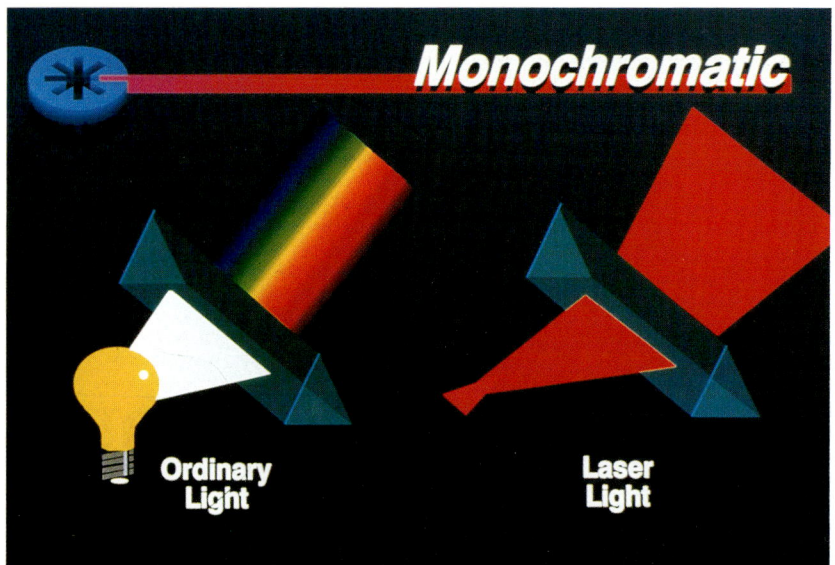

FIG. 1-B. Ordinary versus laser light. Monochromaticity of laser light.

BASIC CONCEPTS OF A LASER

The basic concept of spontaneous emission of radiation states that some electrons of atomic or molecular systems can be in at least two different energy states. The normal or basal energy state is referred to as the ground state (Fig. 1-C). With the addition of thermal, electrical, chemical, plasma, nuclear, or radiation energy stimulation, higher energy levels or excited states are attained (Fig. 1-C). After energy is absorbed, the excited electrons of these atoms spontaneously return to lower energy levels and liberate the quantum of absorbed energy in the form of photons at characteristic transition frequencies. This process is referred to as spontaneous or incoherent emission of radiation. From this spontaneous emission a stimulated emission process will be initiated. Atoms in the upper energy level will begin making stimulated transitions or "jumps" downward in energy (Fig. 1-D). Each such downward transition emits a photon which stimulates other atoms to emit. This process is termed stimulated emission of radiation (Fig. 1-D).

For laser action to occur, the energy pumping process must produce a condition in which more atoms are excited into some higher quantum energy level than in some lower energy level in the laser medium. This condition of "population inversion" may be obtained in many ways and with a wide variety of laser materials (Fig. 1-E).

To create a laser oscillator, a feedback process is formed using a resonant optical cavity (Fig. 1-C). A mirror is placed at each end of the laser cavity so that

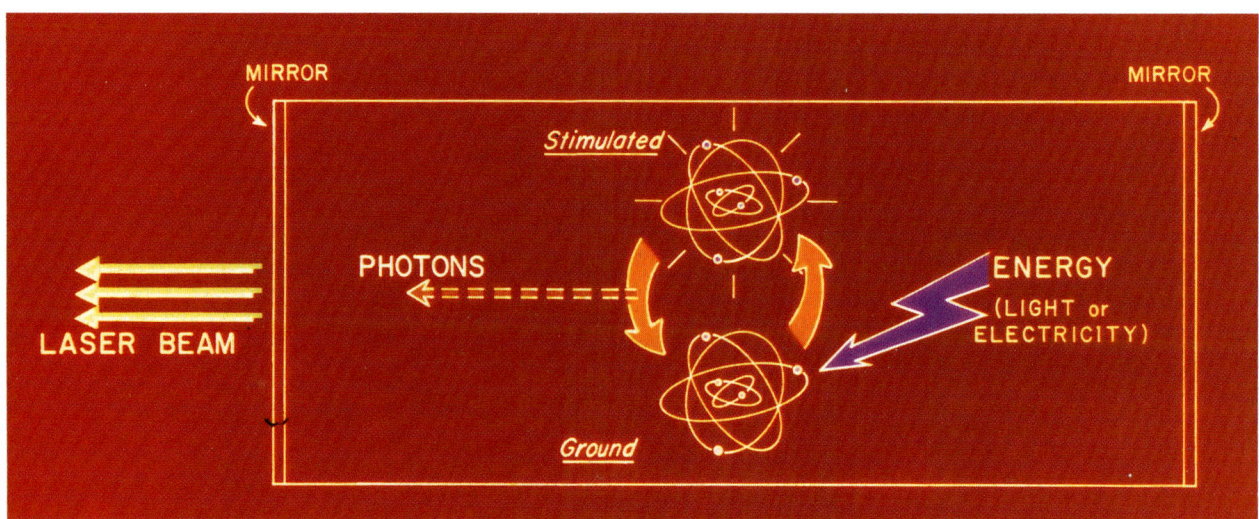

FIG. 1-C. Concept of spontaneous emission of radiation and generation of a laser beam.

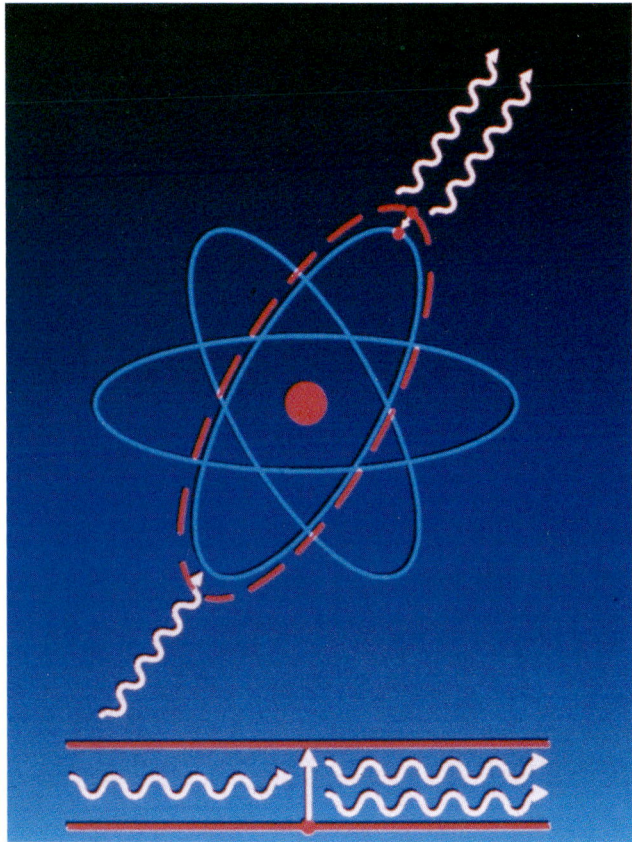

FIG. 1-D. Concept of stimulated emission of radiation.

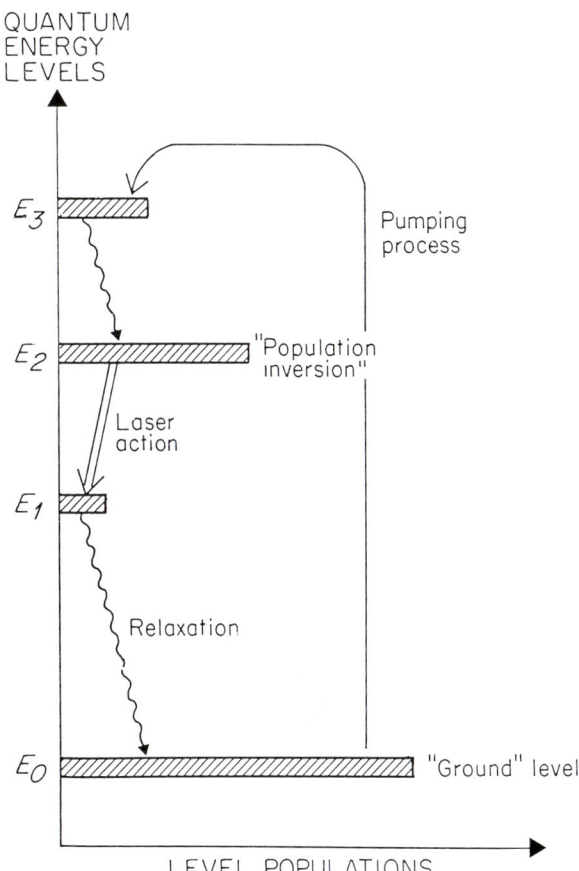

FIG. 1-E. Formation of a population inversion in a four-level laser.

a beam of light may be reflected from one mirror to the other. When photons reach the end of the laser cavity they are reflected by the end mirror back into the material where the chain reaction continues and the number of photons is increased. When the photons arrive at a partially reflecting mirror, a portion will be reflected back into the cavity and the rest will emerge as a laser beam.

CATEGORIES OF LASERS

Lasers are identified by the type of material in the optical cavity, most emit at a single color or wavelength (Fig. 1-F). Among the gas lasers, argon employs a pure gas emitting energy in the visible blue-green spectrum, the gold vapor and the carbon dioxide (CO_2) lasers employ a mixture of gases emitting in the visible (628 nm) and mid-infrared range, respectively, and the excimer lasers emit in the ultraviolet spectrum of light. Liquid lasers, such as the argon-pumped rhodamines or coumarin lasers employ an active organic dye in a solution or suspension (Fig. 1-F). These dye lasers may be tunable in the visible spectrum of light (Fig. 1-F). Semiconductor lasers such as gallium-arsenide employ n-type and P-type semiconducting elements. Among the solid state lasers, the neodymium-doped yttrium-aluminum garnet (Nd:YAG) is a crystal laser which emits an intense electromagnetic beam of photons in the near-infrared spectrum at 1.06 μm and the KTP-532 (potassium titanyl phosphate) laser emits in the visible spectrum of 532 nm (Fig. 1-F).

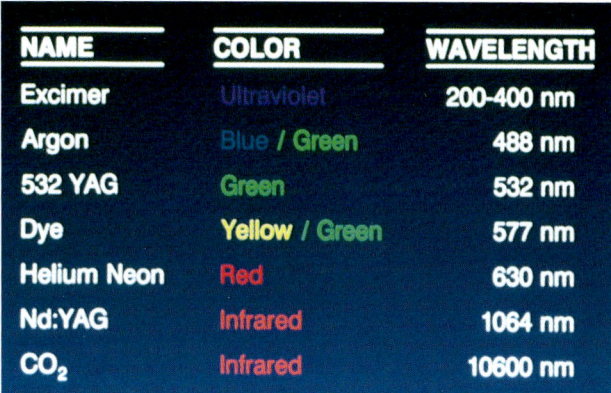

FIG. 1-F. Laser types.

NAME	COLOR	WAVELENGTH
Excimer	Ultraviolet	200-400 nm
Argon	Blue / Green	488 nm
532 YAG	Green	532 nm
Dye	Yellow / Green	577 nm
Helium Neon	Red	630 nm
Nd:YAG	Infrared	1064 nm
CO_2	Infrared	10600 nm

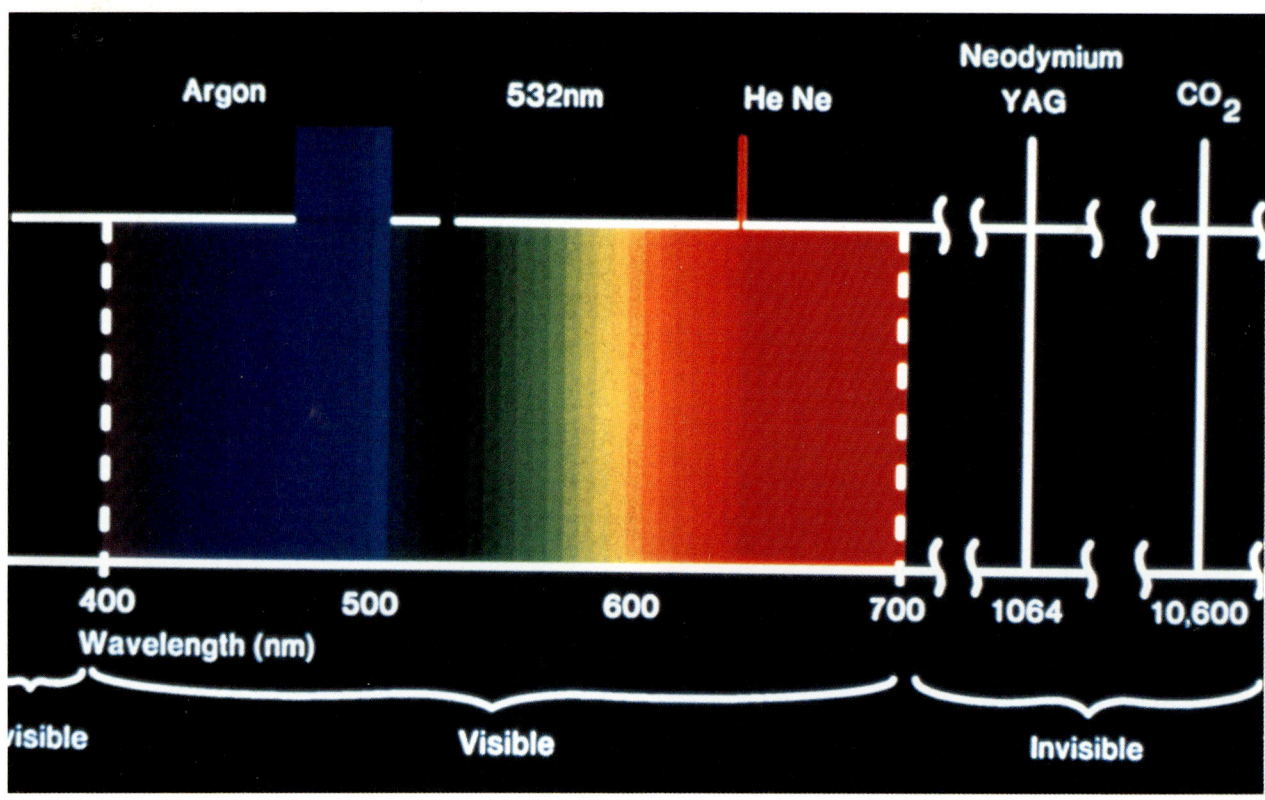

FIG. 1-G. The electromagnetic spectrum and different laser wavelengths.

PHYSICAL PROPERTIES

The laser beam has three unique physical properties:

(i) Generation of monochromatic, parallel, and coherent light (Fig. 1-B). A monochromatic beam emits at a single wavelength or color and is defined as a pure light. With an incandescent or polychromatic light, all the wavelengths in the visible spectrum will appear when using a prism (Fig. 1-B). The electromagnetic spectrum of light expands from 10^{-4} angstroms to 10^{11} meters (Fig. 1-G). Among the most common surgical lasers, the argon and KTP-532 lasers emit in the visible blue-green range, the Nd:YAG laser emits in the near-infrared range of 1.06 μm and the CO_2 laser emits in the mid-infrared range of 10.6 μm (Fig. 1-G).

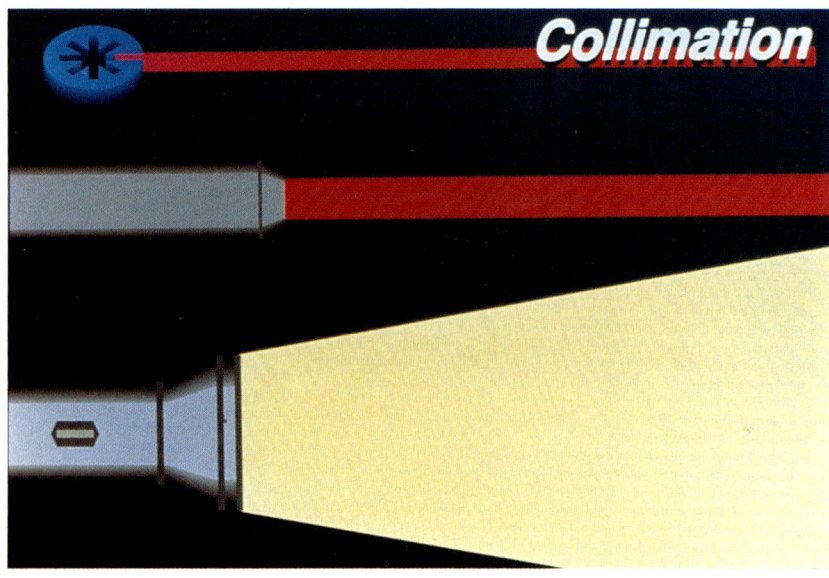

FIG. 1-H. Collimation of a laser beam versus a normal light source.

PHYSICAL PRINCIPLES OF LASERS

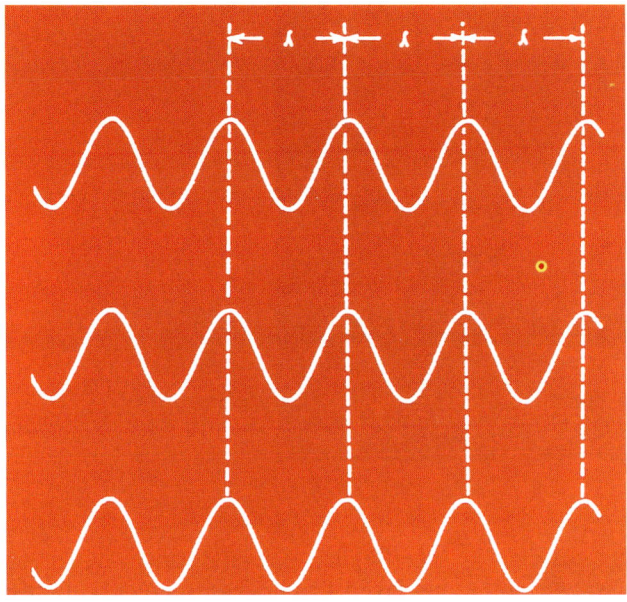

FIG. 1-I. Beam coherence.

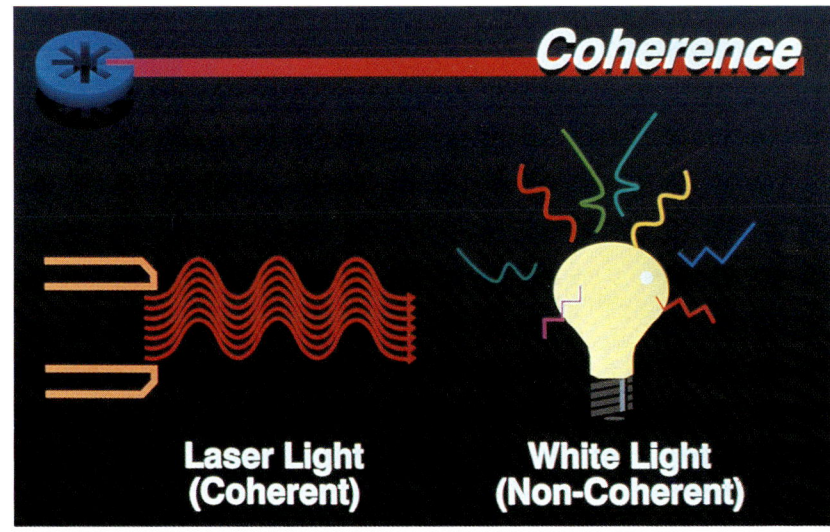

FIG. 1-J. Coherence of a laser light versus a non-coherent white light.

(ii) Collimation or parallelism of light (Fig. 1-H). This is true when a laser beam is emitted from its source. Since beams are now transmitted via different hand-pieces or waveguides, the collimation can be lost due to the nature of the various lenses placed at the tips of these optic devices (Fig. 1-H).

(iii) Coherence of light (Fig. 1-I). This term refers to a relationship between one signal at one point in space and time (Fig. 1-I), with the same or another signal at other points in space and time. A group of well drilled marching soldiers illustrates a coherent light. The soldiers walk a given distance abreast in parallel rows which is the spatial coherence; they also march in step with the same stride, which is the temporal coherence. The photons from an incandescent bulb are quite incoherent in both respects, more or less like a dismissed soldier, since the lamp emits different wavelengths in different directions, therefore lacking temporal and spatial coherence (Fig. 1-J).

DELIVERY SYSTEMS

The versatility of lasers make them a unique tool in medicine. Beams can be delivered to their target in numerous imaginative ways. Laser fiberoptics have allowed clinicians to see and treat diseases previously treated with open surgical procedures. Sapphire-tips or Sharplase-shaped fibers used in contact laser surgery control the pattern of energy delivery to tissues.

PHYSICAL PRINCIPLES OF LASERS 5

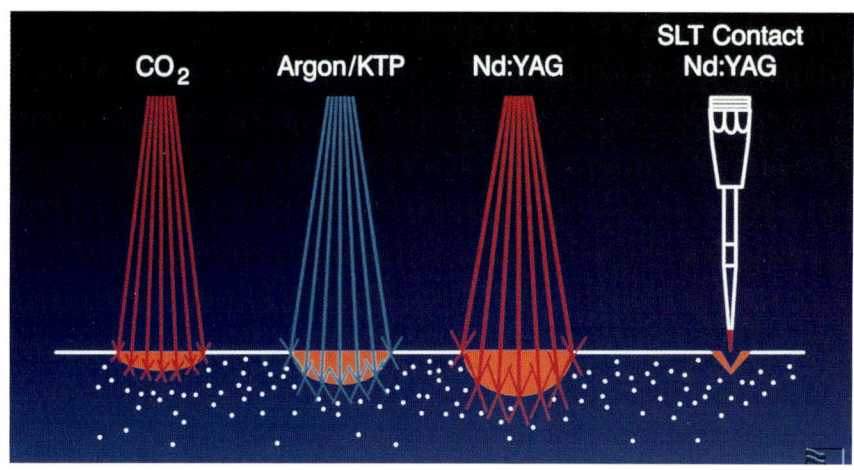

FIG. 1-K. Comparative thermal effects and tissue interactions.

They limit the depth of penetration and enhance cutting and coagulation (Fig. 1-K). In the future, interstitial laser therapy with magnetic resonance imaging guided laser fiberoptics may become a noninvasive technique for the treatment of deep and unreachable tumors. And, advances in three-dimensional magnetic resonance imaging may allow us to visualize tumors, calculate volumes, and help guide laser fiberoptics. Beams transmitted through microscopes would provide the nontraumatic and precise modality required when treating delicate organs such as the brain or vocal cords.

RATE OF DELIVERY

The rate at which energy is delivered defines the laser's temporal modes of operation (Fig. 1-L). In a continuous wave (CW) laser the peak power is equal to the average power output and the beam irradiance is constant with time (Fig. 1-L). Pulsed or superpulsed lasers produce repetitive pulses. Lasers are available with pulse repetition frequencies as high as several hundreds or thousands of pulses per second. A pulsed laser's peak power is much higher than that typically achieved from a continuous wave device (Fig. 1-L). Q-switched lasers are capable of delivering very high peak powers. A shutter is placed in the optical cavity between the mirrors. The shutter enables the accumulation of a very large population inversion, which is released in an extremely short pulse when it is turned off (Fig. 1-L).

TEMPORAL MODE OF OPERATION

A wave pattern across the direction of propagation is characteristic of all beam geometries. These wave patterns across the beam are identified with transverse electromagnetic wave mode notation or TEM. A laser operating in a TEM_{00} or single mode has a Gaussian profile (Fig. 1-M). Lasers can also operate in multiple complex modes. To generate such high power output most lasers operate in complex modes, which render the measurements of beam profiles difficult. Since Nd:YAG and CO_2 lasers produce light at wavelengths of 1.06 and 10.6 μm, respectively, in the near- and mid-infrared portion of the electromagnetic spectrum the

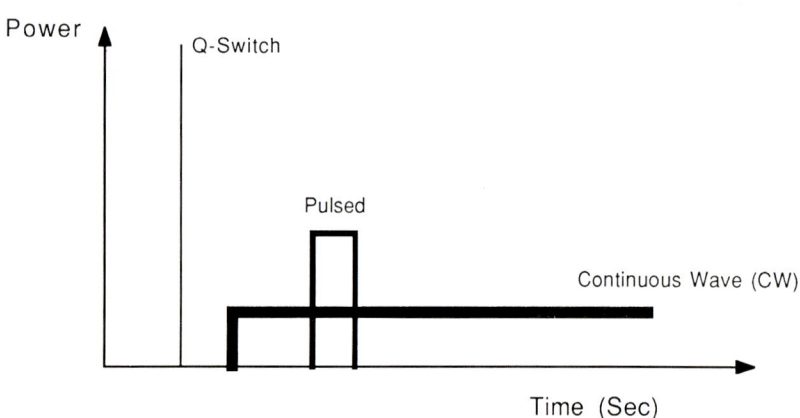

FIG. 1-L. Different modes of lasers.

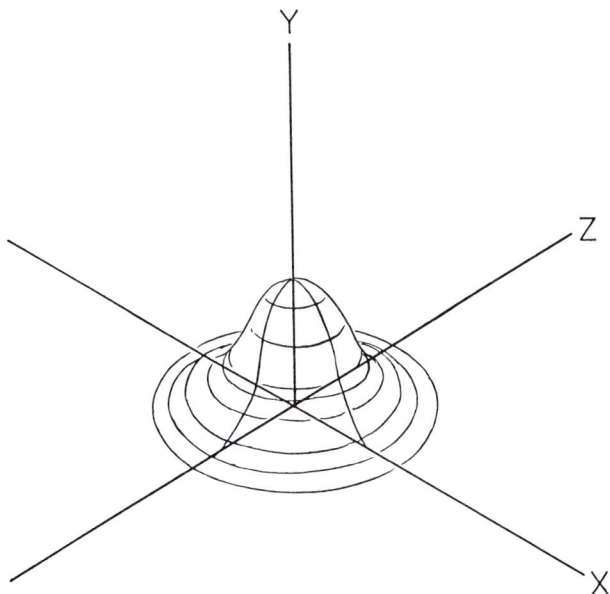

FIG. 1-M. Gaussian beam profile.

TABLE 1. *Comparison between CO₂ and Nd:YAG lasers*

Property	CO₂	Nd:YAG
Wavelengths	10.6 μm	1.06 μm
Absorption (water)	Heavy	Poor
Tissue scattering	Poor	Heavy
Tissue penetration	Shallow	Deep
Vascular	Poor	Good
Coagulation	0.5 mm	2–3 mm

beams are invisible (Fig. 1-G). Most Nd:YAG and CO_2 lasers employ a visible beam as an aiming device. This beam appears as a red dot when helium-neon is used and in other colors with other gas mixtures or with different filters. It indicates where the invisible Nd:YAG or CO_2 lasers beam will strike the tissue.

LASER-TISSUE INTERACTIONS

When a beam is directed onto an operative site, the laser may react on the tissue in four different ways (Fig. 1-N): (i) Absorption by target tissue; (ii) Scattering, which refers to the wide diffusion of the beam's energy within the tissue; (iii) Reflection, which could be caused by the nature, density, and color of the tissue, and by a shiny surgical instrument that is accidently hit by the laser beam; and (iv) Transmission, which occurs when the laser beam passes through tissue with little or no effect to the tissue (Fig. 1-N).

Since lasers emit at different colors or wavelengths their effect on tissues will vary. When a laser beam with sufficient incident energy density is heavily absorbed by tissue with a temperature beyond 100°C, tissue vaporization occurs with the production of stream and tissue debris. The surgical result of this insult is an incision with a shallow zone of coagulation necrosis (Fig. 1-O). High-power pulsed lasers, particularly excimer or Q-switched lasers, are capable of producing intense pressure waves that can tear tissues or fragment stones. Low intensity laser beam can be used to excite fluorescent dyes for tumor localization or tumor destruction as defined by the concept of photodynamic therapy. The CO_2 laser beam, which emits in the mid-infrared range of 10.6 μm, is heavily absorbed by water and poorly scattered in tissues resulting in a small zone of coagulation necrosis or tissue evaporation making it an efficient scalpel (Table 1). However, it is a relatively poor coagulator when the beam is defocused, since it is capable of coagulating vessels up to 0.5 mm in diameter. The 1.06 μm of the Nd:YAG laser is poorly absorbed by water, but heavily scattered and diffused by tissue inhomogeneities that result in deep tissue penetration (Table 1). It can be used effectively to thermally coagulate vessels up to

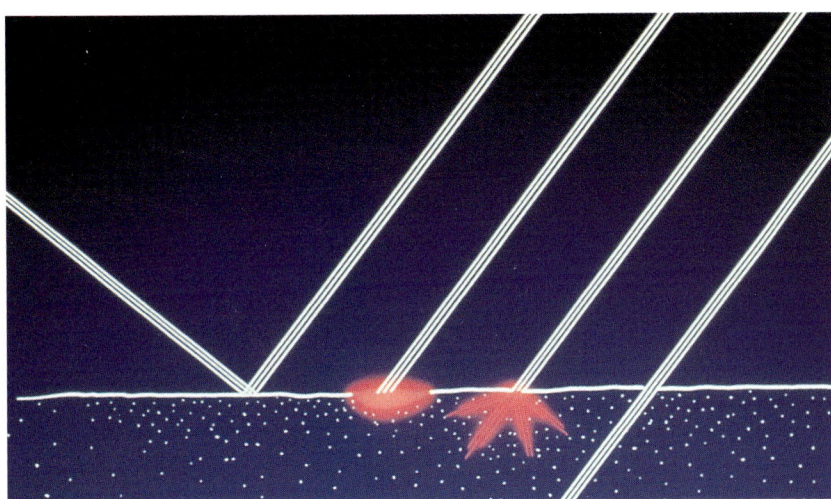

FIG. 1-N. Light–tissue interactions.

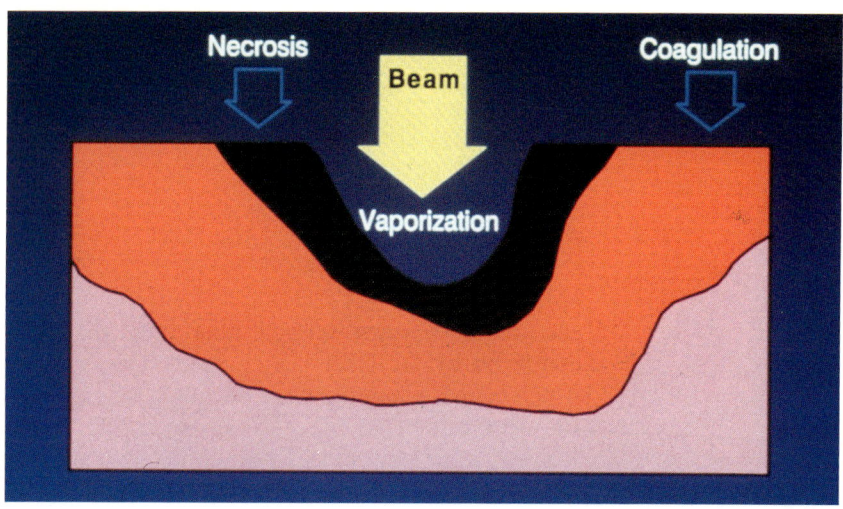

FIG. 1-O. Zones of tissue effect.

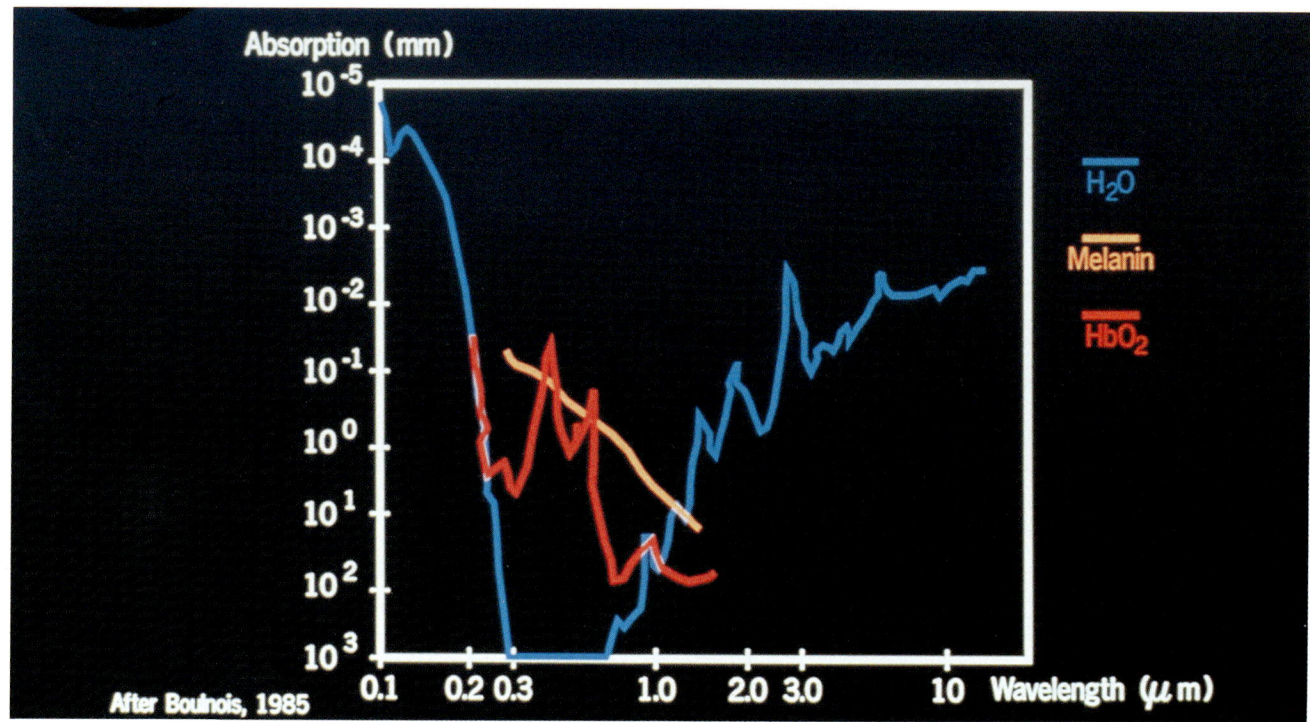

FIG. 1-P. Optical absorption depth versus wavelength.

2–3 mm in diameter. If the Nd:YAG laser beam is applied long enough tissue evaporation will occur, but with a surrounding capsule of coagulation and tissue damage far greater in thickness than with the CO_2 laser.

Since the introduction of contact probes and shaped fibers the Nd:YAG laser became an efficient cutting tool with minimal surrounding tissue damage. Contact probes are made of synthetic ceramic material, with different sizes and shapes for various cutting and coagulation properties. The Sharplase-shaped fibers are silica optical fibers and have a tip shape similar to contact probes (Fig. 1-K). The argon and KTP-532 wavelengths have high affinities for chromogens, melanins, and hemoglobin. They are poorly absorbed by water and have a spectrum of tissue effects between the CO_2 and Nd:YAG lasers (Fig. 1-P).

DOSIMETRY

In all medical and surgical applications of lasers it is crucial to know the amount of absorbed laser energy, for accurate interpretation and duplication of biological responses in tissues. To describe the effects of radiant energy upon tissues, most investigators are using

- SURFACE - GAUSSIAN BEAM - $S = \pi r^2 \, (cm^2)$

- INTENSITY - $I = \dfrac{POWER}{SURFACE} = \dfrac{WATTS}{cm^2}$

- ENERGY DENSITY - $E = \dfrac{POWER \times TIME}{SURFACE} = \dfrac{JOULES}{cm^2}$

FIG. 1-Q. Parameters for laser dosimetry.

the term energy density, or energy per surface area, equal to the amount of power of the laser, multiplied by the time of exposure and divided by the beam's surface area. These results are given in joules per square centimeter (Fig. 1-Q). Another common term is power density or intensity, which is the amount of power of the laser beam divided by the surface area, given in watts per square centimeter (Fig. 1-Q). Most lasers have a built-in time shutter for accurate control of time of exposure, and also have power and energy readouts on the consoles. The readouts do not reflect the amount of *absorbed* laser energy by the tissue, but rather the total amount of energy produced by the machine. Another complicating factor is how to measure the spot diameter of the CO_2 or Nd:YAG laser on the target tissue since they are invisible. Various spot sizes can generate different energy densities and subsequent biological effects in tissues. Previous investigators have measured either the diameter of the burned laser spot, or the diameter of the co-axial helium-neon beam. However, these measurements are false, since a burned laser spot varies in size greatly with time of exposure, and since the helium-neon beam has a different wavelength, which results in a different target spot size. Beam profiles can now be measured using a computerized photo-electric sensor slit. From these recorded beams, the actual spot diameter of the CO_2 or Nd:YAG laser can be derived at 50%, 37%, and 14% of the peak intensity or power density of the laser. Actual power of the laser at the target can be measured with a power meter, and subsequent power density and energy densities can be derived, and should be documented. The ultimate goal is to develop the basic unit of dosimetry of laser energy, termed LAD for laser absorptive dose, comparable to the RAD in radiation therapy (Fig. 1-R).

TYPES OF LASERS

The Nd:YAG Laser

The working medium of this laser is a crystal. The crystal is yttrium aluminum garnet (YAG) which is similar to the synthetic manufactured diamond. Embedded in the lattice are dopant neodymium (Nd) ions. The Nd:YAG crystal is a cylindrical rod, about 100 mm long and 6 mm in diameter. The light source which provides the excitation energy is typically a high-power krypton arc lamp, which has an output spectrum well matched to the absorption bands of neodymium. The rod and arc lamp are usually placed parallel and close together (Fig. 1-S), with an elliptical mirror wrapped efficiently into the crystal rod. The laser transition derives from excited states of the Nd ions. The lower level is short-lived because of interactions with the solid crystal lattice.

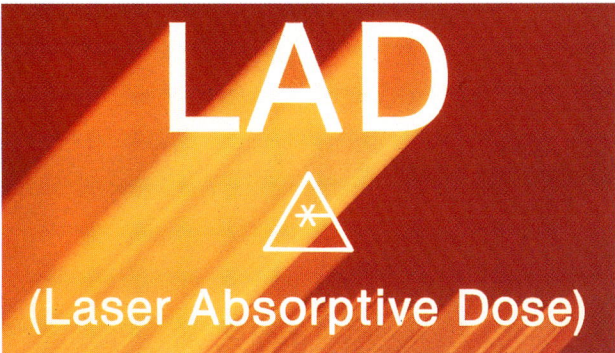

FIG. 1-R. Unit for laser dosimetry.

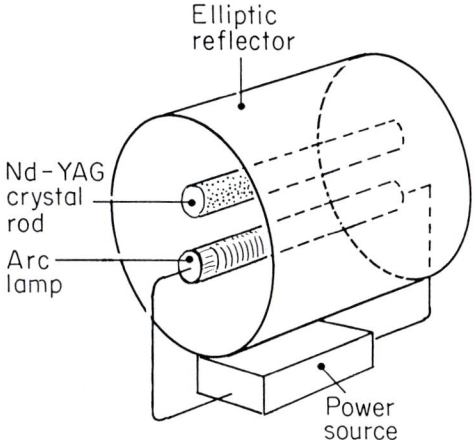

FIG. 1-S. Schematic diagram of an Nd:YAG laser.

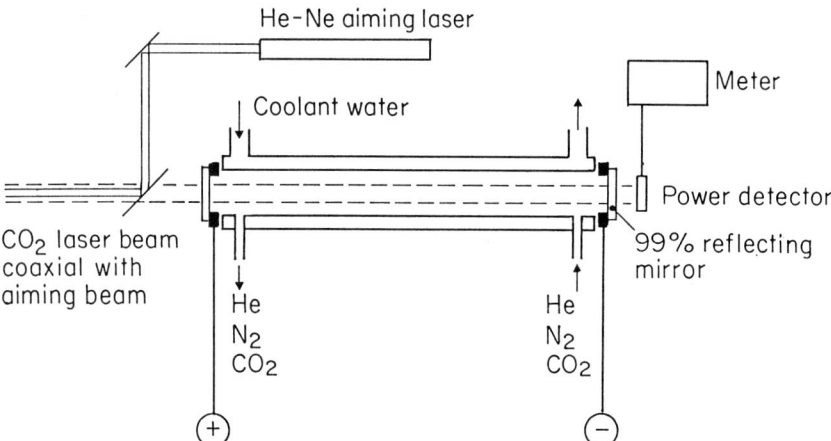

FIG. 1-T. Schematic diagram of a CO_2 laser.

Most Nd:YAG lasers operate in that continuous wave (CW) mode and can produce power outputs up to 100 watts. However, some are superpulsed or Q-switched.

Since Nd:YAG lasers produce light at a wavelength of 1.06 μm, in the near-infrared portion of the electromagnetic spectrum, the beam is invisible. Most Nd:YAG lasers employ a visible beam as an aiming device. This beam appears as a red dot when helium-neon is used, and appears in other colors with other gas mixtures or with different filters. It indicates where the invisible Nd:YAG laser beam will strike the tissue.

The CO_2 Laser

The working medium of this laser is a mixture of three gases CO_2 (5%), nitrogen (13%), and helium (82%). The gas of the CO_2 laser is generally supplied ready-mixed in cylinders. These have to be replaced periodically, because the gas in the discharge tube must flow constantly to avoid the build-up of unwanted chemical species such as carbon monoxide. Closed-cycle cooling systems are built around the laser tube, to assist the helium to cool the discharge (Fig. 1-T).

The CO_2 molecule is the one vibrating in the lasing process. The CO_2 molecule can vibrate in three independent ways. In the asymmetric stretch mode it has a relatively long lifetime, which allows the population of molecules in this site to build up. The constitution of a population inversion is a necessary characteristic for the 10.6 μm infrared laser transition. CO_2 molecules in the "ground" level collide either with fast moving electrons (electrical stimulation) or with excited nitrogen molecules. In either case, energy is transferred to the CO_2 molecules causing the molecules to vibrate. It so happens that the vibrational energy levels of nitrogen coincide with the energy of the asymmetric stretch mode of CO_2, which eases the transfer of energy. To shorten the lifetime of the "lower" level of energy, helium gas was added. Since helium is a light atomic gas, it conducts energy from the lower state and transfers it quickly to the tube walls. It also keeps the discharge temperature relatively low, preventing the build-up of CO_2 molecules in the lower laser level. The 10.6 μ of the CO_2 laser is invisible, therefore, helium-neon light is used. No efficient flexible fiberoptics are yet available for the transmission of the CO_2 laser beam to the operative site. However, some are undergoing clinical testing.

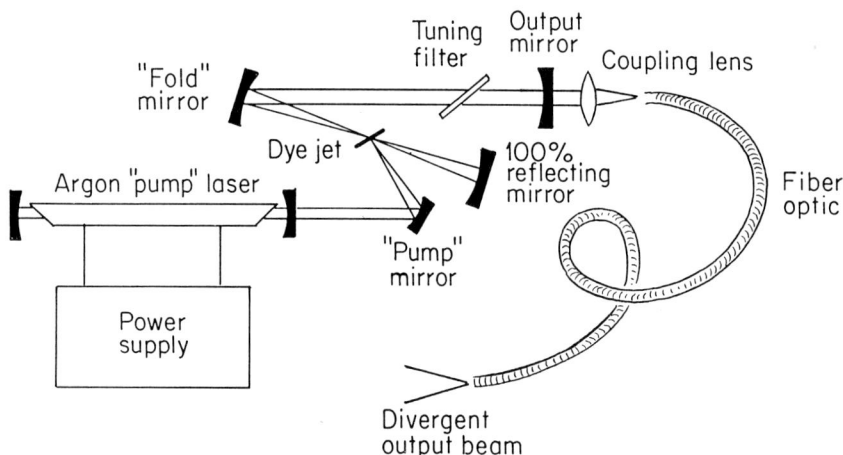

FIG. 1-U. Schematic diagram of an argon laser.

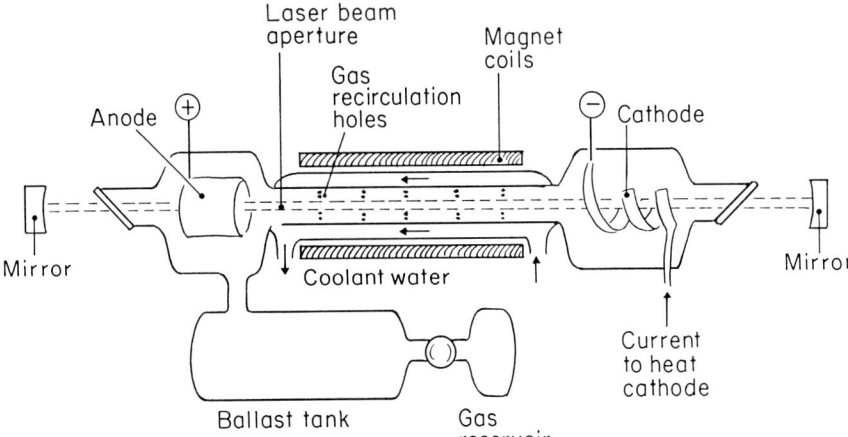

FIG. 1-V. Schematic diagram of a dye laser.

Argon Laser

The argon laser is a noble gas ion laser, action occurs between highly excited energy levels in either singly or doubly ionized atoms. The principal excitation mechanism is electron impact in high current discharges (Fig. 1-U). Atoms are ionized in one collison, and subsequent excitation to a highly excited state occurs via subsequent collisions. The ions then relax, cascading to lower states with many possible relaxation routes between 457.9 nm to 528.7 nm (visible, blue-green). The majority of the lasing transitions of the noble gas lasers have low gains. The main exception is the blue argon line at 488 nm. The laser transition at this wavelength is one order of magnitude higher than any other ions laser transition. Single line selection is usually achieved by placement of an intracavitary prism, which makes it more convenient for all medical applications. The natural lifetime of the upper level is 5 nanoseconds. The populations of the lower laser levels rapidly decay to the ground state. The ground state ions rapidly recombine to form neutral atoms. The rapid repopulation of the lower laser levels minimize the competition between different laser transitions.

Dye Lasers

The principle feature of dye lasers is that it can be tuned to lase at any wavelength in the visible, near-infrared, and near-ultraviolet spectrum. This facility arises because dyes are organic molecules comprising of many atoms, which can vibrate in many independent modes. The energy to excite the dye molecules is provided by an external light source. Since high intensity light is required to achieve the level of energy needed to excite the organic molecules, an argon laser is usually used to pump the energy (Fig. 1-V). To avoid a temperature rise of the dye, it is circulated. The dye is usually squirted through a nozzle forming a fine jet, which can then be illuminated by the pumping argon laser beam. This jet is then caught, and the dye is returned to the reservoir. The wavelengths of these lasers can easily be transmitted via flexible and other optic devices. The difficulties with dye lasers are mainly in trying to achieve stable power outputs and laser wavelengths. They are optically more complicated than other clinical lasers and require frequent realignments.

ACKNOWLEDGMENTS

This study was supported by the Division of Head and Neck Surgery and the CICR grant from the Jonsson Cancer Center, UCLA School of Medicine; American Academy of Otolaryngology-Head and Neck Surgery grant H870812 and NIH grant NS 01298.

REFERENCES

1. Einstein A. Zur Quantenthorie der Strahlung. *Physiolog Z* 1917; 18:121–128.
2. Gordon JP, Ziegler HJ, Townes CH. The maser-new type of amplifier, frequency standard and spectrometer. *Physiol Rev* 1955; 99:1264–1274.
3. Maiman TH. Stimulated optical radiation in ruby. *Nature* 1960; 187:493–494.
4. Javan A, Bennett WR Jr, Herriott DR. Population inversion and continuous optical maser oscillation in a gas discharge containing a HeNe mixture [letter]. *Physiol Rev* 1961; 6:106–110.
5. Johnson LF. Optical maser characteristics of rare-earth ions in crystals. *J Appl Physiol* 1961; 34:897–909.
6. Bennett WR Jr, Faust WL, McFarlane RA, et al. Dissociative excitation transfer and optical maser oscillation in NeO_2 and ArO_2 rf discharges [letter]. *Physiol Rev* 1962; 8:470–473.
7. Patel CKN, McFarlane RA, Faust WL. Selective excitation through vibrational energy transfer and optical maser action in N_2-CO_2. *Physiol Rev* 1964; 13:617–619.

2

LASER SAFETY

Elaine Harrison-Khanwilkar

In the 1990s we continue to be challenged to maintain our knowledge and expertise on the various laser wavelengths available to treat cutaneous skin lesions. As this technology becomes more complex and sophisticated, the demand for well educated personnel to operate and maintain this equipment will increase. Safety issues for each wavelength can vary. In order to provide maximum protection for the patient and staff, it is necessary to have an educated physician and laser operator in the room whenever a laser is being used.

This chapter reviews several of the different regulatory agencies that influence various aspects of medical lasers, the four types of laser classification, documentation for laser safety, ophthalmic injury and types of protective eyewear, environmental safety, administrative controls, physician education, maintenance of laser equipment, the laser safety officer, and some safety policies for lasers.

LASER SAFETY GUIDELINES

There are many articles published on the subject of laser safety, but at this time there is no current national laser safety standard. In 1988 the American National Standards Institute (ANSI) revised its guideline, *For the Safe Use of Lasers in Health Care Facilities*, known as ANSI Z136.3. This document serves as an excellent guide for establishing standards for a laser program and reviews all aspects of a medical laser program, from laser safety and training programs to hazard evaluation and classification.

The ANSI Z136.3 document was written to be a guideline for health care institutions that have or plan to have a laser program. The Laser Safety Committee (see section on Administrative Controls) is responsible for interpreting these guidelines and making recommendations to the institution regarding the standards of practice when lasers are used. The key words in the document are "should" and "shall". These words will assist the Laser Safety Committee in determining the priorities for the laser program.

The Joint Commission for Accreditation of Health Care Organizations (JCAHO) has general standards for lasers but expects each facility to provide specific standards for their laser program. In order for the health care facility to be accredited, the standards need to be implemented and monitored to verify that the standards are followed. JCAHO is very interested in the physician credentialing process for using lasers. When JCAHO came to the University of Utah Laser Surgery Unit, we were asked specific questions regarding the physician laser privilege list, education requirements for physicians using lasers, and specific policies for laser safety. The quality assurance safety audits to verify that safety protocols are followed were also reviewed.

Effective May 1988, the Occupational Safety and Health Administration's (OSHA) Hazard Communication Standard, or more commonly known as the Employee Right to Know Act, became law. This defines certain rights employees have when working around hazardous chemicals. Dye lasers that require dye changes must have a Material Safety Data Sheet on each type of dye employees will be using and exposed to. Even the possible hazardous compounds from the smoke plume produced during laser surgical procedures should be reviewed with employees before exposure to laser procedures.

The Food and Drug Administration (FDA) approves laser devices and procedures these devices can be used in. The lists of approved wavelengths and applications are frequently published, making this information easily accessible to any health care facility involved with a laser program.

The U.S. Food and Drug Administration's Center for Devices and Radiological Health (CDRH) has mandatory standards for the manufacturer of lasers and laser systems. The manufacturer will certify that their products meet these standards and specify which of the classes the device is in. This pertains only to the manufacturing process, not training or control measures.

The Association of Operating Room Nurses (AORN) have developed the following guidelines for laser use: *1990 Standards and Recommended Practices for Perioperative Nursing* and *Recommended Practice for Laser Safety in the Practice Setting*. These recommended practices address a variety of issues from eye protection to developing policies and procedures. It is also an excellent resource for standards of practice.

HAZARD EVALUATION AND CLASSIFICATION

All lasers have a classification of I, II, III, or IV based on four types of criteria. "The capability of the radiant energy of the laser system to injure health care personnel or the patient's body area other than the intended treatment sites, the environment in which the laser system is used, the personnel who may use, or be exposed to, laser radiation, and the non-emission hazard associated with the laser" (1).

Class I lasers are considered the least hazardous, incapable of producing hazardous emissions, for example grocery store scanners. Class II lasers applies to visible lasers that may be viewed directly for short periods of time, for example a laser pointer. Class III lasers may be hazardous under direct viewing, for example laser light shows. Class IV lasers are hazardous to the eye from the direct beam and diffuse reflections. Most surgical lasers are class IV lasers because of the potential skin and fire hazards (2).

SAFETY DOCUMENTATION

It is important for the nursing staff to ensure environmental safety before and during the use of the laser. In order to maintain consistency with standards of practice, a checklist of safety aspects can be easily incorporated into laser documentation. This checklist reviews pre-, intra-, and post-operative safety protocols and can include troubleshooting information. The Pre-operative Checklists should review the following: laser power, water (if applicable), signs and wavelength-specific goggles on doors, presence of accessory equipment such as a smoke evacuator, windows covered, whether or not there is enough protective eyewear for the staff and patient, and test firing of the laser to ensure it is in proper working order. The intra-operative checklist should review: wavelength-specificity of eyewear placed on the patient and given to all personnel before the laser is placed into operate mode, turning the laser on and setting the power and pulse duration per physician request, ensuring the laser foot pedal is not next to any other foot pedals, initiation of documentation, water present on back table, and having the laser operator standing next to the laser to place the laser in standby mode when it is not in use. The Post-operative Checklist should review the disassembly of the laser and accessories, gathering of eyewear and signs to ensure proper storage, removal of window coverings, and completion of documentation.

The documentation of laser utilization is very important during any laser involved procedure. Each facility's documentation standard will determine the format and implementation of the laser use record. For example, a separate laser log can be maintained, or a separate laser form may be used in addition to the current nursing notes or incorporated into existing nursing forms. It is essential to document which laser was used, the power setting, time used, any accessories used, and utilization of the safety checklist.

EYE INJURY

Laser wavelengths are capable of producing retinal or corneal damage depending on the particular wavelength of the laser. For example, the argon wavelength (488–514 nm) is able to produce retinal damage (Fig. 2-A); and the CO_2 wavelength (10,600 nm) is capable

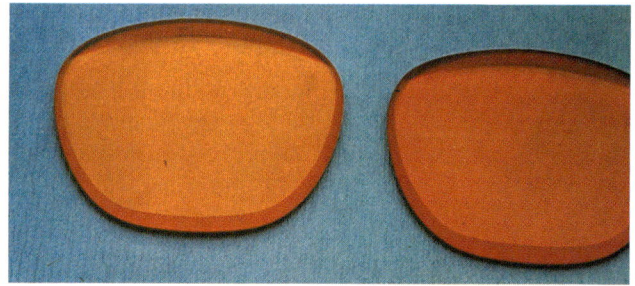

FIG. 2-A. Wavelength specific eye shields for 488–514 nm. These can be taped directly over the patient's eyes.

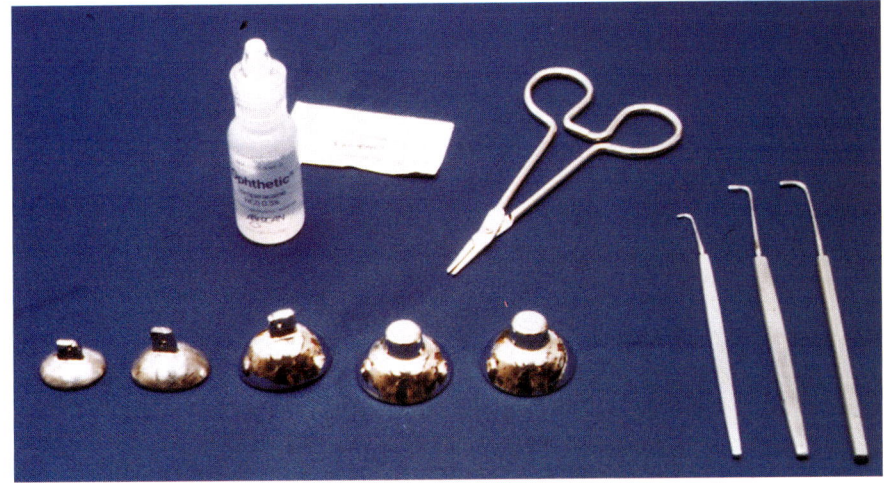

FIG. 2-B. Lead eye shields which can be inserted directly on the eye, providing protection during laser treatment of the eyelid or near the eye.

of producing corneal burns. This type of injury is serious, and the eye protection policy for patients and personnel must be followed. All personnel exposed to the laser environment should be educated about the necessary precautions to take to avoid injury. Unfortunately when a laser warning sign and a pair of goggles are hanging on a door, people entering the room do not always put the protective eyewear on! All personnel who work with lasers should have eye exams upon employment and when they leave. This exam should include an eye history and photographs of the fundus to be kept in the staff member's file. This is valuable information to have in case an eye injury occurs.

PATIENT EYE PROTECTION

The type of eye protection used on the patient will depend on a number of factors; the area to be treated by the laser, the type of laser which will be used, or whether the patient will be awake or asleep. If the patient is awake or asleep and the treatment area is not around the eyes, a pair of wavelength-specific goggles will be sufficient. If the treatment area is around or on the eye and the patient is awake, there are eye shields available to insert into an anesthetized and lubricated eye. Plastic eye shields are available, but do not use them if an argon laser is used because of the possibility of melting. Lead shields can be used for the argon and Nd:YAG wavelengths (Fig. 2-B). If the patient is receiving general anesthesia, the eyes can be covered with wet gauze or eye pads and wavelength-specific lenses or aluminum foil that can be taped in place if the treatment area is not near the eye. If the treatment area is around the eye, then eye shields should be used.

PERSONNEL EYE PROTECTION

Protective eyewear must be provided to all personnel who are in the room when a laser is being used (Fig. 2-C). This eyewear must provide protection for the entire eye. "The following factors shall be consid-

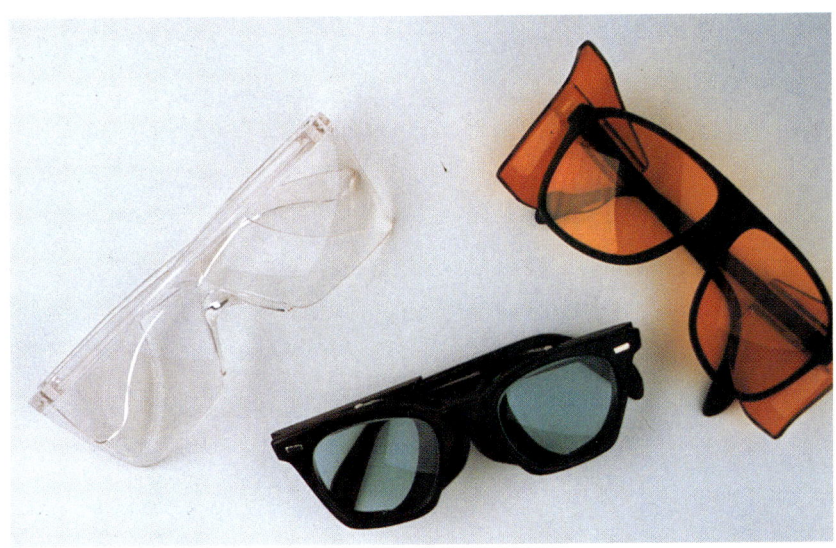

FIG. 2-C. Types of protective eyewear for staff. Verify that each pair of glasses or goggles is labeled with the wavelength it has been made to filter.

ered in determining the appropriate protective eyewear to be used:

1. Wavelength of laser output;
2. Potential for multi-wavelength operation;
3. Radiant exposure or irradiance;
4. Maximum permissible exposure;
5. Optical density of eyewear at laser output wavelength;
6. Visible light transmission requirement;
7. Peripheral vision requirement;
8. Radiant exposure or irradiance and the corresponding time factors at which laser safety eyewear damage (penetration) occurs, including transient bleaching;
9. Need for prescription glasses;
10. Comfort and fit;
11. Degradation of absorbing media, such as photobleaching;
12. Strength of materials (resistance to shock); and
13. Capability of the front surface to produce specular reflection''(3).

Each pair of glasses or goggles should have the specific wavelength and optical density written on the goggles/glasses. All personnel should verify that the eyewear is going to provide protection for the specific laser wavelength they will be exposed to. This is especially important in the case of tunable dye lasers. The eyewear can not be identified by color, due to the changing technology in the manufacturing of eyewear. For example, the Nd:YAG wavelength glasses have progressed from dark green to almost clear. This clear type of eyewear is not a hindrance during the procedure like the dark green eyewear was.

Education of staff is important for the care and storage of this eyewear. Wash the goggles/glasses with mild soap and warm water. Store the glasses in cases and place goggles in soft cloth cases or drawers to prevent damage to the lenses, which could possibly allow the eye to be burned due to inadvertent beam exposure. All eyewear should be routinely inspected for cracks, discoloration, and overall intactness. Contact lenses are not able to provide adequate eye protection during laser procedures.

ENVIRONMENTAL SAFETY

Warning Signs

"Sign dimensions, letter size, color, etc. shall be in accordance with American National Standard Specification for Accident Prevention Signs, ANSI Z35.1" (4). This document specifies the requirements for laser warning signs. The signs can be purchased from various companies. It is important to educate personnel about the sign requirements so that a paper sign saying "Laser in Use" is not used. Warning signs for Class IV lasers will have the word "Danger" on the upper panel, and specify which laser wavelength is being used. A pair of protective glasses/goggles should accompany the sign when it is on the door during the time a laser is in use (Fig. 2-D).

Window Coverings

All windows need to be covered during laser use to avoid accidental beam exposure to people who may look in the window (Fig. 2-E). The CO_2 laser wavelength will be absorbed by the glass in the window; therefore, when the CO_2 laseer is used, no window coverings are required. The types of window covering should be a material that is difficult to ignite. Generally plastic is the preferred window covering because it is relatively inexpensive and comes in a variety of colors.

Spectators

Rooms that are designated for lasers should have limited traffic when the lasers are in use. This reduces

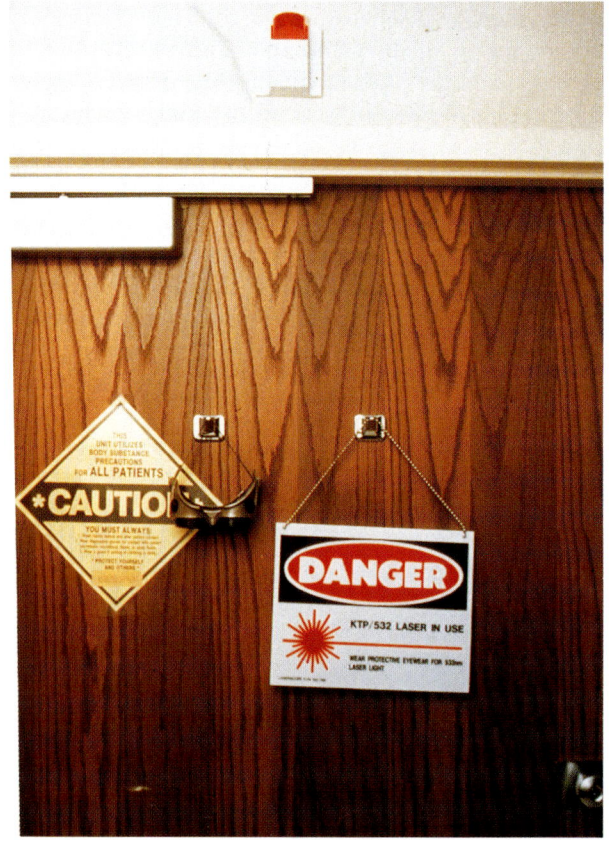

FIG. 2-D. A laser warning sign and a pair of wavelength-specific goggles on the door into an operating room using a laser. The red light above the door is turned on when a laser is in use.

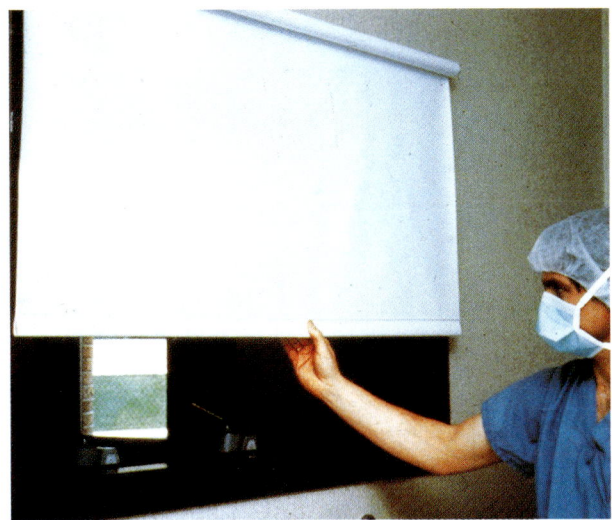

FIG. 2-E. Window covering for the operating room must be used to protect staff from accidental laser beam exposure.

the risk of accidental beam exposure. In teaching facilties, there may be more students in the room than staff and it is imperative to educate the students about the hazards of lasers and precautions to take when they are in a laser environment.

Designated Laser Operators

One person—a nurse, technician, or bioengineer should be designated as the laser operator during the procedure. This should not be the circulating nurse because he/she is not able to always be near the laser during the procedure. If one person operates the laser, and the laser is placed into standby when not in use, the risk of accidental fires decreases significantly. The laser operator should attend a laser course that reviews the various laser wavelengths, physics, safety, standards, and should have supervised hands-on with various lasers. They should also complete an orientation and preceptor program in the specific facility where they are employed. This does have a significant impact on staffing and cost of the procedure but the benefits of prevention outweigh the cost of training.

Electrical Safety

All hospitals have electrical safety programs for employees and when working with lasers the same precautions will apply. The power requirements to run a laser are much greater; therefore, an electrical shock could be fatal. It is important that employees follow electrical safety guidelines and that all laser preventive maintenance is done according to the manufacturers specifications. Water used for cooling the laser tube increases the electrical hazard (Fig. 2-F). Do not plug the laser in if the floor or personnel's feet are wet. Inspect the water hoses for leaks and use quick disconnect hose connectors to avoid water leaks. The heavy foot pedals can cause stress on the cord wires to the laser and is frequently a site where broken fibers will result in the malfunction of the laser.

Fire Prevention

Lasers can cause fires if the safety guidelines are not followed. Reviewing a safety checklist prior to the start of the laser procedure will significantly decrease the chances of a fire. Having water or saline on or near the operative field and/or using a wet towel or gauze around the operative site will provide maximum protection for the patient from a stray laser beam. There are flame retardant drapes available, but some of these do not prevent the laser beam from going through the drape and burning whatever is directly under the drape. When you are evaluating the type of drape pro-

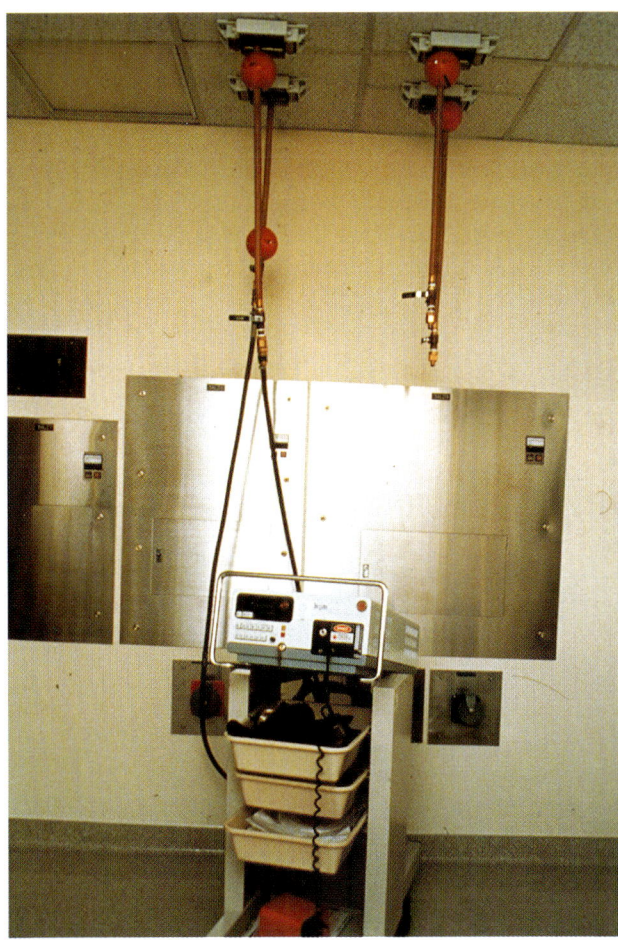

FIG. 2-F. Each operating suite has power outlets for the laser and water hoses to cool the laser. Electrical safety is mandatory when connecting the laser.

tection you want to use, test the product with a CO_2 laser to see what will actually happen before you decide on which type to purchase. If the operative site is around the hair, you can wet the hair; but this will not guarantee that the hair will not burn. When the CO_2 laser is used, verify the aiming beam and laser beam alignment prior to the start of the procedure. If you have a fiberoptic, ensure that the laser is in standby mode if it is placed on a towel, and that the laser operator places the laser in standby mode whenever it is not in use. Educate employees about what to do if a laser-caused fire does occur. Have standards of practice on personnel responsibilities during a laser-caused fire and review this annually. Define the role of the laser operator, circulating nurse, and physician. Each facility should have a standard that can be integrated easily into the existing fire or emergency standard. This will protect the patient, staff, and the facility if these standards are established and followed.

Another potential fire hazard is related to the type of atmospheric gas that the laser beam may be exposed to. For example, if the patient needs oxygen and the lesion is near the nose, how can the treatment be done? It will depend on the circumstances, but you could turn the oxygen off for short periods of time (if the patient can tolerate this) while treating the nasal area or turn the oxygen as low as possible and place a piece of foil or plastic inside a wet folded wash cloth and use this as a barrier between the laser beam and oxygen. It may require some creativity to protect the patient; but as long as the staff use their knowledge of laser safety to provide a safe environment for the patient, the goal will be achieved.

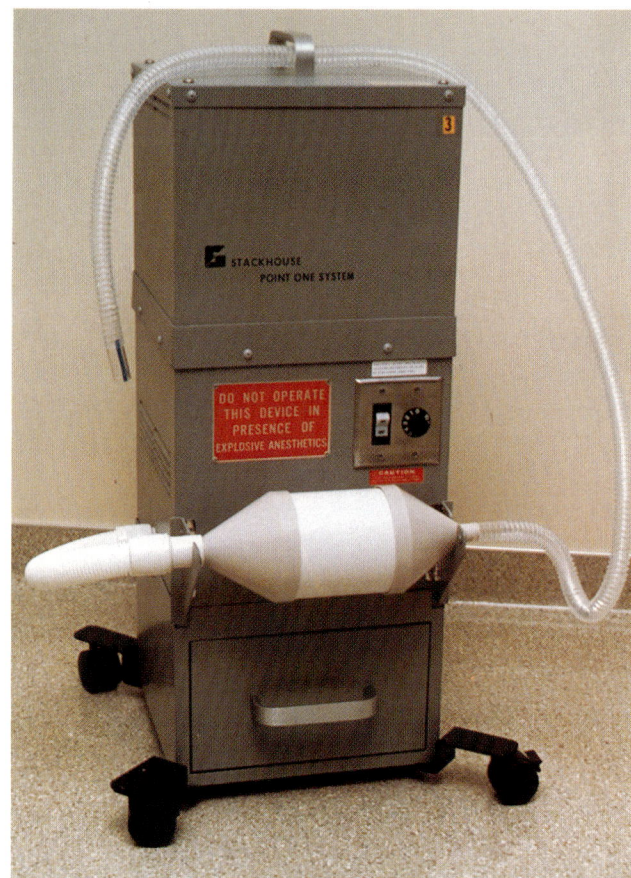

FIG. 2-G. One type of smoke evacuation available. The filter and hose are disposable.

Low Reflective Instruments

There are low-reflective instruments available to prevent specular reflection. Make sure they are available before the procedure begins. Shiny instruments can cause inadvertent beam reflection and possible burns to the patient and/or staff.

Smoke Evacuation

A smoke evacuation system should be used for all laser procedures that generate smoke (Fig. 2-G). The smoke plume may contain hazardous particles; and until there is conclusive evidence about the exact contents, it is necessary to properly evacuate the smoke and protect the patient and staff from having direct skin contact with the plume. The smoke also decreases the physician's ability to see the operative site, has an unpleasant odor, and will damage the unfiltered vacuum system of the facility.

Currently, there are many types of smoke evacuation systems available. A large smoke evacuator with disposable filters will provide excellent evacuation of smoke. The staff need to follow the manufacturers recommendations when changing the filter and tubing. Canisters with built in filters are also available. These canisters can also hold fluid; and if there is a possibility that fluid will be suctioned during the procedure, it may be the evacuator of choice. There are also in-line filters that can be connected directly into the suction tubing. These cannot handle a large amount of smoke but can be used when the smoke volume will be small. When holding the nozzle of the smoke evacuator, the optimum distance from the operative site is one to two inches. Wear a protective mask and gloves during smoke evacuation to prevent any direct skin contact with the smoke plume. Do not forget to provide this protection for the patient.

ADMINISTRATIVE CONTROLS

Laser Safety Committee

Each health care facility should have a laser safety committee to make recommendations and assist in standard development for the laser program. The members of this committee could be a chairman, representatives from each subspecialty that will be using lasers, head nurse of the patient care area(s) that will utilize lasers, a bioengineering staff member (if they are going to be responsible for laser maintenance), an administrator over the program, and a laser safety officer. The committee's responsibility is to:

1. Define criteria for physician's credentialing for laser privileges.
2. Establish facility laser safety standards.
3. Establish education requirements for staff who work in the areas where lasers will be used.
4. Establish a preventative maintenance program and documentation requirements.
5. Develop a job description for the laser safety officer.
6. Assist with any design of new laser facilities and purchases of laser equipment.
7. Assist in developing patient teaching brochures or pamphlets.

The activity of this committee will vary according to the institution needs. Once the laser program is established, the committee will meet less frequently.

PHYSICIAN EDUCATION

Currently, there is no national standard for educational requirements that physicians must meet before using lasers. The American Society for Laser Medicine and Surgery has established guidelines that hospitals can utilize for physicians who would like laser privileges. The ANSI Z136.3 document has also incorporated these guidelines:

> Suggested Standards of Practice for the Use of Lasers in Medicine and Surgery; Hospital privileges are, and must remain the responsibility of the hospital governing board. The following laser training and experience is recommended:
>
> 1. The applicant shall review the pertinent literature and audio-visual aids and shall attend training courses devoted to teaching of laser principles and safety. These courses shall include basic laser physics, laser tissue interaction, discussions of the clinical specialty field and hands-on experience with lasers. Such courses should entail a minimum of eight to ten hours.
> 2. The individual shall consult with an experienced operator in the specialty area involved. Such consultation may consist of several brief visits or a more prolonged stay, with a minimum of six to eight hours of observation and hands-on involvement. It is essential that the individual observe and document actual clinical application of the laser in the outpatient or hospital setting, as appropriate to the procedures in which the training is conducted (5).

The suggested standards of practice is longer and readers are encouraged to obtain a copy from the Laser Institute of America. It is evident that specific recommendations are made to assist a laser safety committee in establishing their own institutional standard.

A physician privilege list should contain the names of each physician and the wavelengths they have been approved to use. This list should be kept in an area where the lasers are scheduled and where the nursing staff are able to verify current approved physician users. If the medical director or laser safety officer are responsible to approve the physician applications, they should sign and date this list whenever a change has been made.

MAINTENANCE OF LASER EQUIPMENT

The bioengineering department generally does not assume responsibility for the repair and maintenance of lasers. If your facility feels this would be more cost effective, most laser companies will train an engineer to repair and maintain their laser.

All preventive maintenance and repairs done on lasers need to be documented and kept in a log. This should be readily available if there is any malfunction of the equipment so that the history of the laser can be reviewed.

If your institution has a maintenance or service contract with a laser manufacturer, it is important that the laser coordinator knows what this contract specifies regarding the number of preventive maintenance checks that will be done on an annual basis and that each preventive maintenance check is documented.

LASER SAFETY OFFICER

Each institution that has a laser program should have a laser safety officer (LSO). This person can be a physician, nurse, engineer, or administrator; a choice that will be up to each institution based on their needs. The laser safety officer is responsible for the safe use of lasers. This position needs to have a job description, and the LSO must have the authority to ensure lasers are used in accordance with the institutions standards of practice. If these standards are not followed, a written plan should be in place to assist the LSO in correcting this problem. Some of the expectations of the LSO are:

1. Ensure that all personnel working in a laser environment are educated about lasers.
2. Ensure that laser standards of practice have been written and implemented.
3. Ensure that the staff comply with the standards during a laser procedure.
4. Evaluate the laser environment for any hazards.
5. Assist the staff with purchasing accessory equipment or new lasers.
6. Make recommendations for new policies if the need arises.
7. Ensure that the lasers and accessories have been maintained as per manufacturers recommendations.
8. Assist quality assurance personnel in monitoring and evaluating the laser program.

The ANSI Z136.3 document reviews what responsibilities should be given to the LSO.

SAFETY POLICIES FOR LASERS

Each institution should write their own standards of practice for laser safety to meet their own needs and address the same general safety issues that are common to all lasers. For example:

1. Eye protection for personnel
2. Eye protection for patients
3. Environmental safety
4. Physician privileges for laser use
5. Fire prevention
6. Education of staff on laser safety
7. Maintenance logs
8. Documentation requirement
9. Emergency shut down criteria
10. Scheduling of lasers
11. Equipment operation and accessories for each laser
12. Smoke evacuation
13. Patient education.

SUMMARY

In summary, the ANSI Z136.3 document is an excellent resource for your laser program and all staff members who work with lasers should be familiar with the contents. There are also many other excellent books, periodicals, and articles to assist you with your laser program. The key to a successful program is education; not just for the physicians, but for nursing or technical staff that will be responsible for the operation and maintenance of laser equipment and accessories. Call other health care facilities and inquire about their laser program and if possible, obtain copies of their standards of practice. Attend laser conferences to keep up-to-date on all of the changes in the laser field. If your laser program has an established documentation format for lasers and has implemented laser specific standards of practice, the chances of having an undesirable medical-legal issue will be significantly decreased.

REFERENCES

1. American National Standards Institute. *For the safe use of lasers in health care facilities,* ANSI No. Z136.3. New York: American Standards Institute; 1988, p. 6, sec. 3.1.
2. Ibid.
3. Ibid., p. 11, sec. 4.6, 2.2.
4. Ibid, p. 12, sec. 4.7.1.
5. Ibid, p. 53, appendix C.

3

EYE SAFETY DURING LASER EYELID TREATMENT

Christine C. Nelson and Krystyna A. Pasyk

Eye safety is of the utmost importance when using a laser because the lens of the eye has the ability to focus the laser beam which may cause a dangerous concentration of its energy on the retina. Thermal and photochemical injury of the fovea centralis (retinal location of best vision) permanently decreases visual acuity. There is no pain or discomfort during retinal laser burns, therefore damage to the retina can only be found on dilated ophthalmic examination.

The risk to the retina is from all types of lasers producing visible light and near-infrared energy. Visible light transmits easily through the clear media (cornea, aqueous humor, lens, and vitreous body). Damage occurs when this light is absorbed by the retinal pigment epithelium and surrounding tissues. It is manifest by a vapor bubble or an "explosion" when the temperature in the retina, due to light absorption, is raised 10–20°C (1).

The risk to the cornea is from the CO_2 laser, producing far-infrared energy at 10,600 nm. The light is absorbed by the epithelium of the cornea causing thermal injury resulting in scarring and opacification, thereby decreasing the patient's vision.

Treatment of vascular and nonvascular skin lesions on the eyelids and orbital areas is considered the domain of several specialties such as dermatology, plastic surgery, ophthalmology, otolaryngology, and oncology. Surgeons must always be aware of the potential hazards when using this "light tool." Surgeons, operating room personnel, and patients require specialized eye goggle protection for each laser type during laser treatment of the areas distant from the ocular adnexa. These goggles will protect eyes in case of an accidental laser light exposure during an operation.

Detailed guidelines for medical laser safety eyewear were developed by the American National Standards Institute (ANSI) and the Laser Institute of America (LIA) (2,3). Many improved eye goggles currently exist on the market to protect the patient's and medical personnel's eyes from damage from reflected or direct laser light. It is important for the goggles to fit well and not allow unfiltered light access to the eye. Surprisingly, little has been written about protection of the patient's eyes in situations where the standard goggles are too large, for example in a child or when the eyelid and orbital areas under the goggles also need treatment. In these instances eye shields which fit under the eyelids are necessary during laser treatment for maximum protection. The use of moistened gauze covered with tape to protect the eye and eyelid is dangerous since both the tape and the gauze may burn if hit by the laser beam.

New safety eye products are continuously being added to the market. The Dermacare Laser Safety System[1] is a new product which reportedly provides

---
[1] DermaCare, a Division of PSC Corporation, 7651 National Turnpike, Louisville, KY 40214.

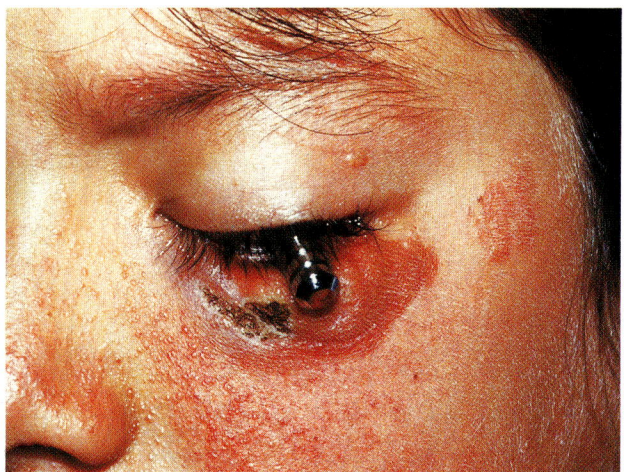

FIG. 3-A. Stefanovsky Laser Protective Eye Shield inserted under the eyelids of a patient with tuberous sclerosis with multiple lesions of the face. Fibromatous plaque during treatment with the argon laser. Note interference of treatment due to the downward position of the handle.

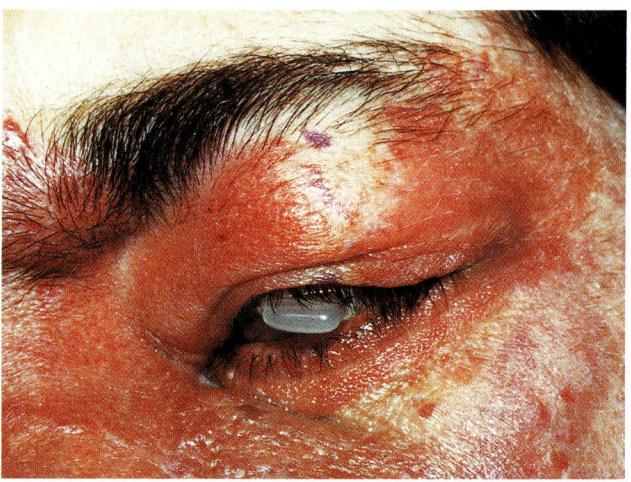

FIG. 3-B. New laser eye shield on a patient with port wine stain of the eyelid. Note there is no interference of the eyelid position.

protection at normal power limits with the most widely used lasers. It is made of a nonflammable matte-surfaced aluminum foil and the binocular eye shield fits securely over the eyelids and periorbital area. During clinical experiments on this device there was enough specular reflection to burn paper adjacent to the test site. We therefore urge great care to avoid any direct laser hit to this device as it may prove hazardous to operating room personnel due to reflection from the surface.

There are a few eye shields available on the market which fit under the eyelid and allow surgery to the eyelids. The protective plastic (methylmethacrylate) shields originally designed for eyelid surgery protect the eye from the scalpel (Smith Evaginated Corneal Protection Shield[2] and Hornblass Ocular Protection Shield[2] are dangerous during laser surgery because they absorb and transmit laser light. This may cause corneal or retinal damage (4–6). The metallic shields (Stefanovsky Laser Protective Eye Shields[3]) which were specifically developed for laser light protection are thick and heavy. They cause distortion of the lids and sink slowly into the inferior fornix during treatment. The knurled ball grip often interferes with lower lid treatment (Fig. 3-A). Furthermore, because these eyeshields are made of high grade highly polished stainless steel, the operating room personnel are subject to the risk of specular reflection during laser surgery.

---

[2] Mager and Gougelman, Inc., 120 East 56th Street, New York, NY 10022.

[3] Stefanosky and Associates, 30150 Royalview, Willowick, OH 44094.

A new patient laser eye shield has been developed to protect the patient's eye during eyelid treatment with the laser (7). This new device consists of a sandwich of polymethylmethacrylate and metallic foil. This eye shield is sturdy, light weight, resistant to heat build-up, and allows no harmful specular reflection. The clear polymethylmethacrylate allows the laser light to be diffusely reflected off the dull foil layer rather than be absorbed. It was tested with argon, dye, neodymium YAG, and CO_2 lasers. This new laser eye shield is safe, easy to clean and use for the surgeon, and is comfortable for the patient (Fig. 3-B). Currently, a patent application is pending and clinical testing is in progress.

Eye safety of both the patient and all operating personnel is critical during laser treatments. Proper use of the correct safety device is imperative.

REFERENCES

1. Weiter J. Phototoxic changes in the retina. Miller D, ed. In: Clinical light damage to the eye. New York: Springer-Verlag, 1987, 79–125.
2. Laser Institute of America: ANSI Z136.1. *Safe use of laser*. Orlando, FL: Laser Institute of America. 1986.
3. Laser Institute of America. *Laser Safety Guide*. 6th ed. Orlando, FL: Laser Institute of America, 1989.
4. Goldman L. Laser skin surgery. In: Epstein E, Epstein E Jr, eds. Skin surgery. Springfield, IL: Charles C Thomas, 1982, 1143–1160.
5. Summers CG, Hordinsky MD. Argon laser treatment of periocular lesions. An experimental study. *Ophthalmic Surg*, 1987; 18:100.
6. Wheeland RG, Bailin PL, Ratz JL, Schreffler DE. Use of scleral eye shields for periorbital laser surgery. *J Dermatol Surg Oncol* 1987; 13:156.
7. Nelson CC, Pasyk KA, Dootz GL. Eye shield for patients undergoing laser treatment. *Am J Ophthalmol*. 1990; 110(1):39–43.

4

CARBON DIOXIDE LASER

VASCULAR AND RELATED LESIONS
4.1 Capillary/cavernous hemangioma of the nose and forehead
4.2 Capillary/cavernous hemangioma of the forehead
4.3 Hemangiolymphangioma of the chest wall
4.4 Lymphangiohemangioma of the tongue

MALIGNANT AND PREMALIGNANT LESIONS
4.5 Early squamous cell carcinoma and severe diffuse actinic cheilitis of the lower lip
4.6 Actinic cheilitis of the lower lip
4.7 Actinic cheilitis with epithelial dysplasia
4.8 Actinic cheilitis and in situ squamous cell carcinoma
4.9 Basal cell carcinoma of the upper lip
4.10 Recurrent basal cell carcinoma
4.11 Superficial basal cell carcinoma
4.12 Squamous cell carcinoma in situ: Bowen's disease
4.13 Lentigo maligna

INFLAMMATORY/INFECTIOUS LESIONS
4.14 Condyloma acuminata
4.15 Penile condyloma
4.16 Condylomata acuminata
4.17 Perianal condyloma
4.18 Distal male urethral condyloma
4.19 Onychomycosis
4.20 Onychomycosis on the left great toe
4.21 Pyogenic granuloma
4.22 Pyogenic granulomas secondary to Sturge-Weber syndrome
4.23 Wart on the right index finger
4.24 Periungual wart
4.25 Periungual wart with invasion under the nail
4.26 Plantar warts, giant, and recalcitrant
4.27 Plantar wart
4.28 Plantar wart

TATTOO
4.29 Decorative tattoo
4.30 Decorative tattoo
4.31 Decorative tattoo
4.32 Decorative tattoo: Comparison of argon and CO_2 lasers
4.33 Homemade tattoo
4.34 Traumatic tattoo

MISCELLANEOUS
4.35 Chondrodermatitis nodularis chronica helicus
4.36 Comedones
4.37 Compound nevus
4.38 Adnexal neoplasm: cylindromas and eccrine spiradenoma
4.39 Digital myxoid cysts
4.40 Discoid lupus
4.41 Heterotopic gastric mucosa of the tongue
4.42 Irritation fibroma
4.43 Acne scarring and keloids
4.44 Keloid scars
4.45 Earlobe keloid
4.46 Keloid
4.47 Keloids
4.48 Multiple keloids
4.49 Lichen planus
4.50 Partial radical nail excision
4.51 Nevocellular nevus
4.52 Neurofibromatosis
4.53 Multiple cutaneous neurofibromata
4.54 Onychocryptosis
4.55 Painful red nose

MISCELLANEOUS (continued)
- 4.56 Periapical granuloma (oral)
- 4.57 Pincer nail deformity with onychocryptosis
- 4.58 Pilar cyst of the scalp
- 4.59 Post-thermal hypertrophic scar
- 4.60 Rhinophyma, large size
- 4.61 Rhinophyma, moderate size
- 4.62 Pigmented seborrheic keratosis
- 4.63 Facial syringomas
- 4.64 Syringoma
- 4.65 Trichoepithelioma
- 4.66 Xanthelasma on both lower eyelids

SURGICAL PROCEDURES
- 4.67 Basal cell carcinoma of the left parotid area
- 4.68 Blepharoplasty
- 4.69 Blepharopigmentation: eyeliner tattoo removal
- 4.70 Tattoo removal
- 4.71 Decorative tattoo [chemo-laser technique]
- 4.72 Chronic chest wall ulcer
- 4.73 De-epithelialization of skin flaps
- 4.74 Dupuytren's contracture of the right palm and ring finger
- 4.75 Fetal surgery [rat]
- 4.76 Excision of ganglion of the left foot
- 4.77 Bilateral heel ulcers
- 4.78 Right foot ischemic ulcer secondary to occlusive peripheral vascular disease
- 4.79 Laserabrasion of acne scars of the face
- 4.80 Lipoma excision of the anterior chest
- 4.81 Metastatic squamous cell carcinoma of the scalp
- 4.82 Xanthelasma palpebrarum
- 4.83 Mucous cyst of the DIP joint of the right middle finger
- 4.84 Excision of sebaceous cyst
- 4.85 Left preauricular invasive squamous cell carcinoma

CASE 4.1
Capillary/Cavernous Hemangioma of the Nose and Forehead

REVIEW OF CASE. This child presented with a rapidly growing capillary/cavernous hemangioma of the nose and forehead. Because the lesion was judged to be largely cavernous with a variable chance of spontaneous involution and was distorting normal adjacent tissue structures resection was deemed advisable. Resection was successfully accomplished with moderate blood loss.

CHOICE OF LASER: CARBON DIOXIDE. The CO_2 laser when finely focused cuts and coagulates very effectively. Thus it is indicated in the resection of vascular lesions such as hemangiomas. Flaps can also be dissected with this laser. Although large vessels still require identification, isolation, and ligation most smaller vessels are coagulated by the laser. 15–20 watts of continuous power with a 0.2–1 mm spot size was chosen.

ADDITIONAL INFORMATION. Adjacent skin areas must be draped with moist gauze for protection from stray beams. Protection for the patient's and operator's eyes must be provided as well. Approximately 1 mm of thermally damaged wound edge must be resected prior to closure to prevent wound healing or dehiscence problems if the skin is incised with the laser.

POST-TREATMENT CARE. The surgical wound is treated like any standard surgical wound, with a sterile compression dressing. Sutures may be left in place longer if delayed wound healing occurs.

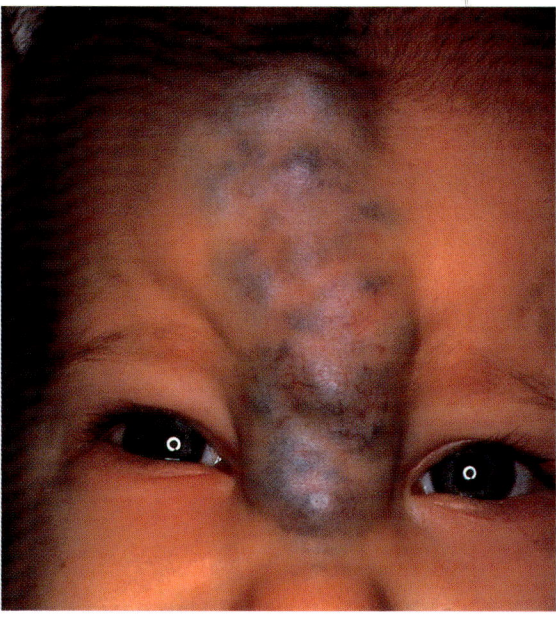

FIG. 4.1-A. Preoperative appearance of hemangioma of the nose and forehead from above.

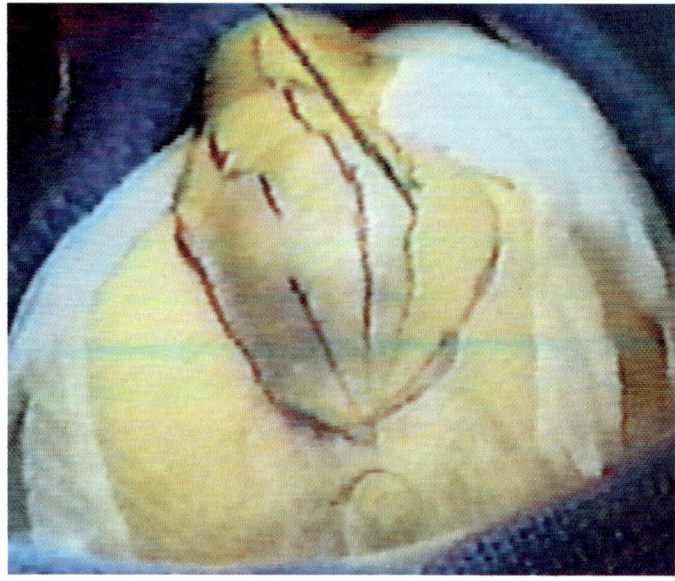

FIG. 4.1-B. Tissue marking of hemangioma and extra skin.

Case continues on following page.

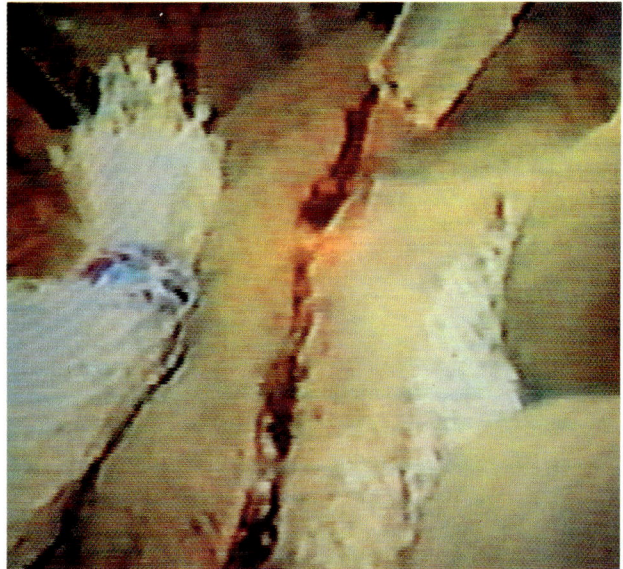

FIG. 4.1-C. Skin dissection using the CO_2 laser.

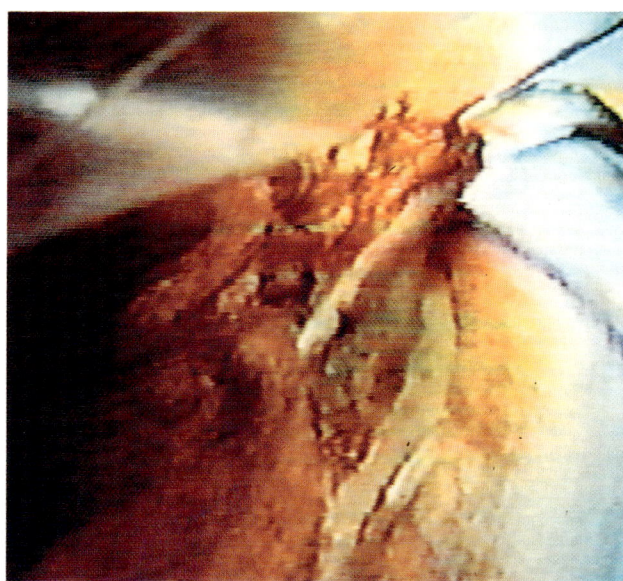

FIG. 4.1-D. Elevation of right flap using the CO_2 laser.

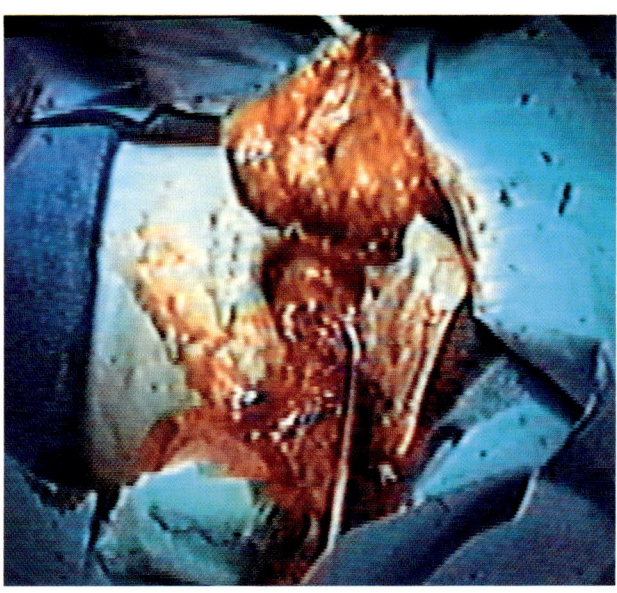

FIG. 4.1-E. Final dissection and removal of the hemangioma.

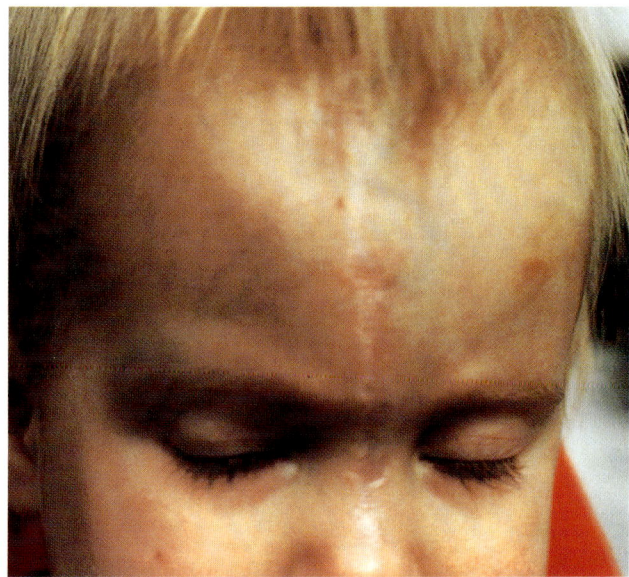

FIG. 4.1-F. Post-operative satisfactory cosmetic result after total hemangioma resection.

Case courtesy of *David B. Apfelberg*, M.D.

Reprinted with permission of Little, Brown and Company.
For literature pertaining to this case see References section.

CASE 4.2

Capillary/Cavernous Hemangioma of the Forehead

REVIEW OF CASE. This child presented with a rapidly growing capillary/cavernous hemangioma of the forehead above the left eyebrow. Because the lesion was judged to be largely cavernous with a variable chance of spontaneous involution and was distorting normal adjacent tissue structures resection was deemed advisable. Resection was accomplished successfully with moderate blood loss.

CHOICE OF LASER: CARBON DIOXIDE. The CO_2 laser when finely focused cuts and coagulates very effectively. Thus it is indicated in the resection of vascular lesions such as hemangiomas. Flaps can also be dissected with this laser. Although large vessels still require identification, isolation and ligation, most smaller vessels are coagulated by the laser. 15–20 watts of continuous power with a 0.2–1 mm spot size was chosen.

ADDITIONAL INFORMATION. Adjacent skin areas must be draped with moist gauze for protection from stray beams. Protection for the patient's and operator's eyes must be provided as well. Approximately 1 mm of thermally damaged wound edge must be resected prior to closure to prevent wound healing or dehiscence problems if the skin is incised with the laser.

POST-TREATMENT CARE. The surgical wound is treated like any standard surgical wound with a sterile compression dressing. Sutures may be left in place longer if delayed wound healing occurs.

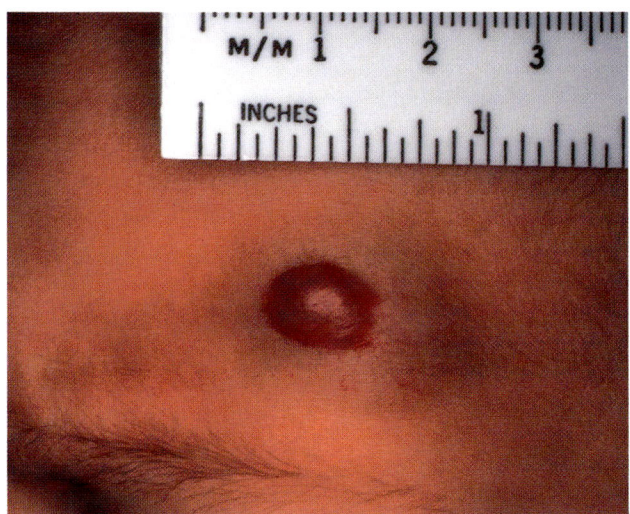

FIG. 4.2-A. Pre-operative appearance of hemangioma of the forehead. Note capillary hemangioma on the surface and deep blue cavernous hemangioma in the subcutaneous tissue.

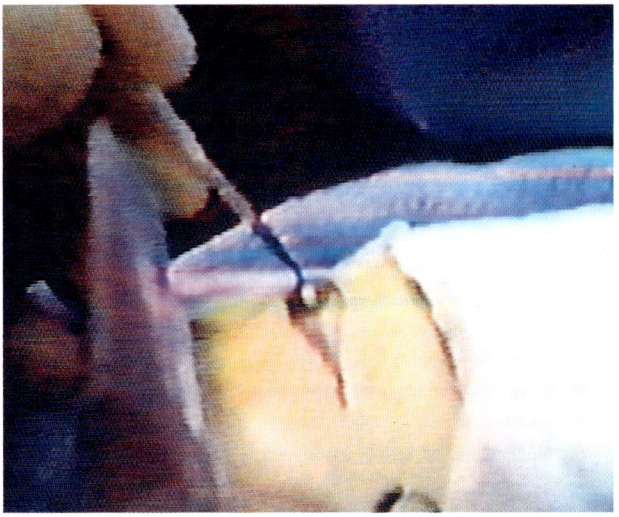

FIG. 4.2-B. Tissue marking of the hemangioma resection.

Case continues on following page.

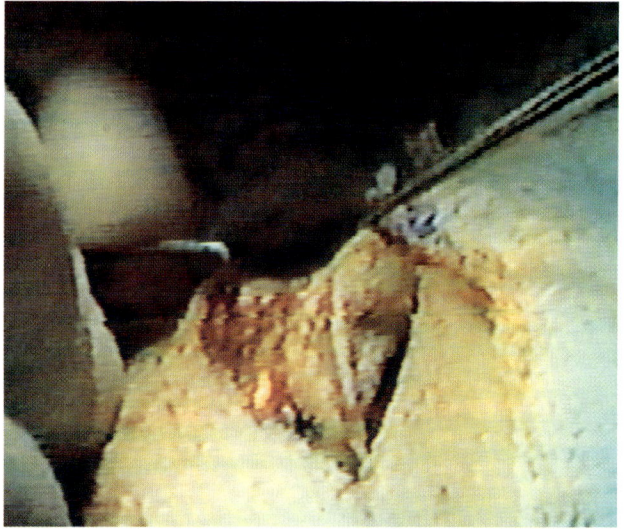

FIG. 4.2-C. Development of skin flaps superiorly and inferiorly using the CO_2 laser.

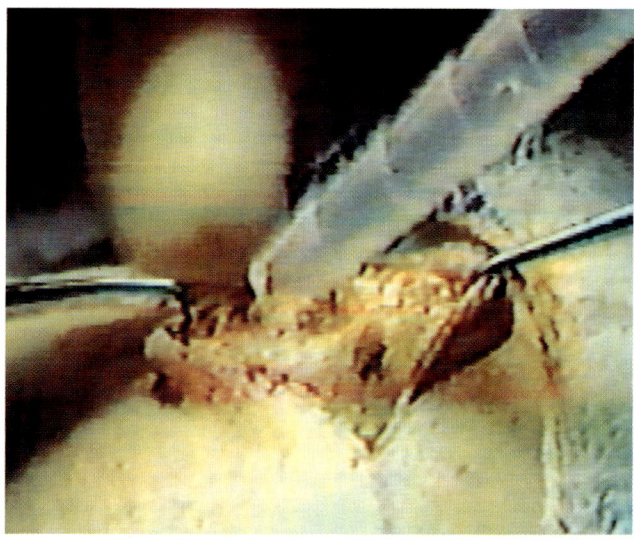

FIG. 4.2-D. Further development of skin flaps.

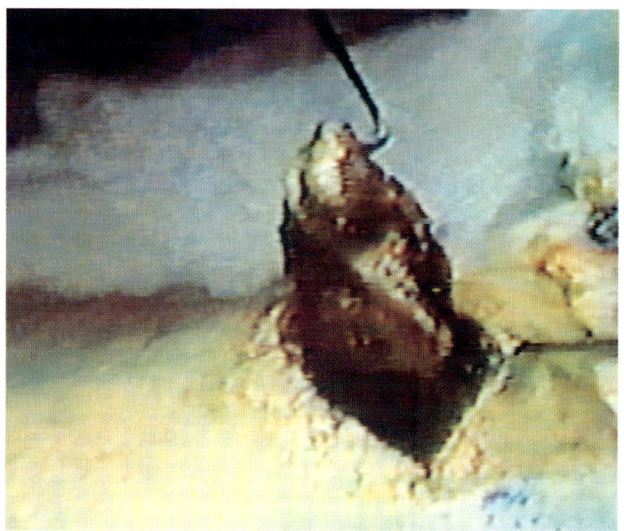

FIG. 4.2-E. Elevation and dissection of hemangioma after skin flaps have been developed.

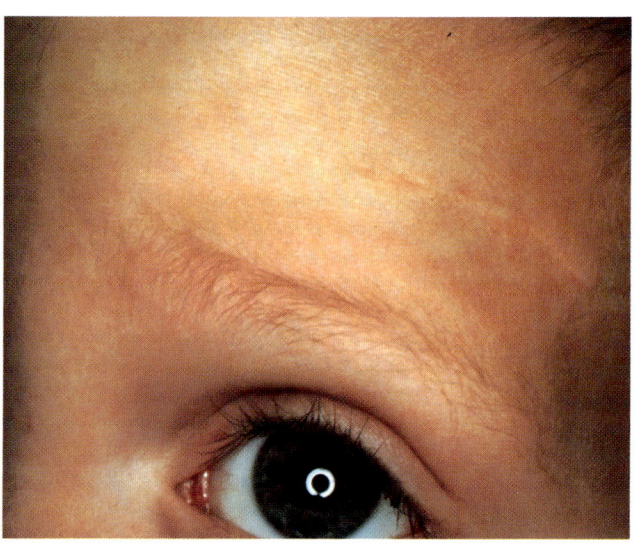

FIG. 4.2-F. Satisfactory cosmetic result six weeks after total hemangioma resection.

Case courtesy of *David B. Apfelberg*, M.D.

Reprinted with permission of Little, Brown and Company.
For literature pertaining to this case see References section.

CASE 4.3
Hemangiolymphangioma of the Chest Wall

REVIEW OF CASE. This patient presented with a history of chest wall lesion present since nine months of age. Thirteen previous procedures including multiple selective blood vessel ligations had been unsuccessful in its removal. The lesion was 20 cm in diameter, extending from the shoulder to the right costal margin and axilla almost to the midline. The lesion contained an A-V fistula as well. The CO_2 laser was used at 20 watts of focused power to resect the tumor including the subcutaneous tissue and muscle since there were no clear cleavage planes. Afferent vessels that required ligation varied between 3 and 12 mm and 2 units of blood replacement was required. The patient had a good result from this procedure without recurrence.

CHOICE OF LASER: CARBON DIOXIDE. The CO_2 laser was chosen because of its ability to provide excellent hemostasis during dissection and excision. Blood loss and problems of blood replacement had previously rendered this mass inoperable.

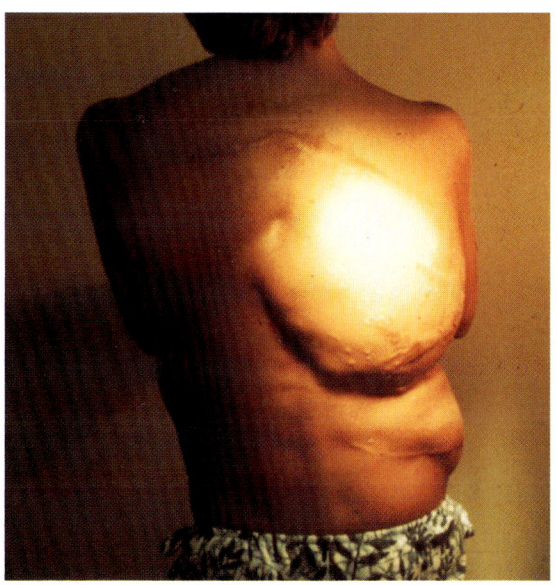

FIG. 4.3-A. Massive tumor growth on right chest wall. Tumor extends over the area of the costal margin with swelling of the mass occurring in the abdomen and retroperitoneal area distorting the right flank.

Case continues on following page.

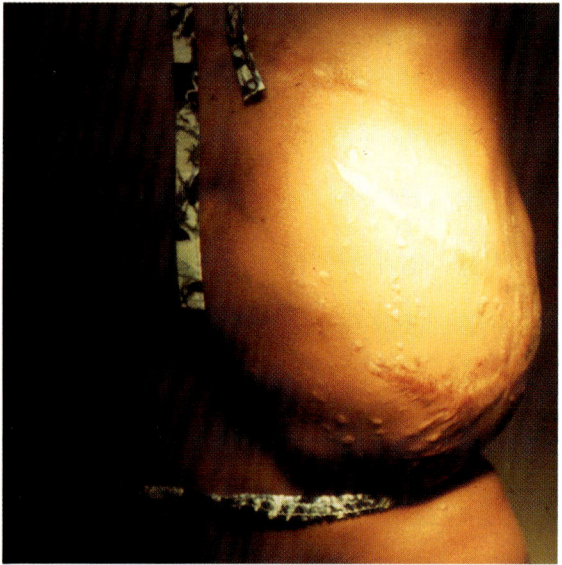

FIG. 4.3-B. Close-up of chest wall mass over the costal margin.

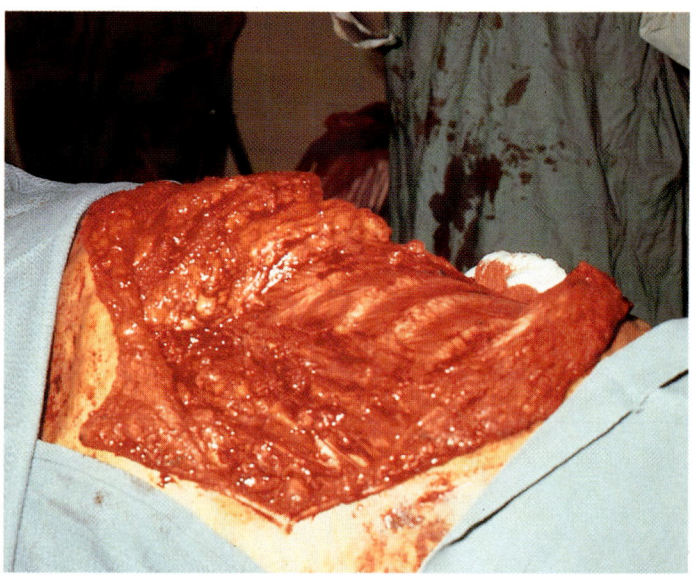

FIG. 4.3-C. Post-operative resection of the mass down to the ribs using a dry field.

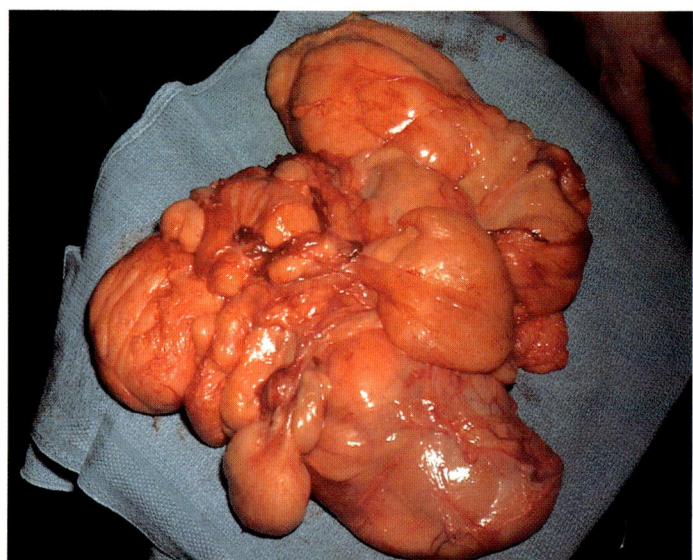

FIG. 4.3-D. Resection specimen.

Case courtesy of *Billie L. Aronoff*, M.D.

CASE 4.4
Lymphangiohemangioma of the Tongue

REVIEW OF CASE. This patient had onset at 3 years of age of submental and submandibular swellings later accompanied by numerous reddish-brown small lesions of the tongue dorsum. The tongue lesions were painful with easy bleeding and required periodic antibiotic therapy for recurrent pain, swelling, and infection. During the laser procedure, vaporization caused the individual lesions to swell and burst and decrease in size as the lymphatic fluid was exuded. Previous non-laser procedures had caused extensive swelling of the tongue necessitating inpatient hospitalization for several days, however, following the laser procedure the patient was able to comfortably eat a general diet and was discharged on the first post-operative day. Regression of most of the lesions has been permanent.

CHOICE OF LASER: CARBON DIOXIDE. The CO_2 laser was chosen because of its ability to clot lymphatic vessels. In a continuous defocused mode, the entire dorsum of the tongue was rapidly vaporized with 15 watts of power. Lymphatic fluid exuded as small lymphatics were ruptured and then sealed with the laser. This patient had practically no drainage from the wound with rapid healing occurring. Exophytic lesions at the angle of the mouth could be bloodlessly and directly excised as well.

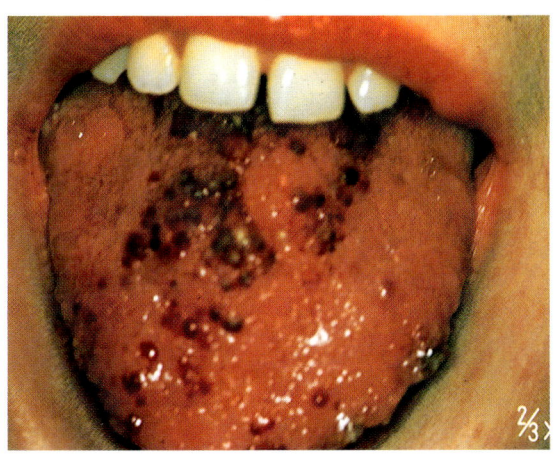

FIG. 4.4-A. Entire dorsum of the tongue showing various types of lymphangiohemangiomas, both exophytic and flat lesions are present.

Case continues on following page.

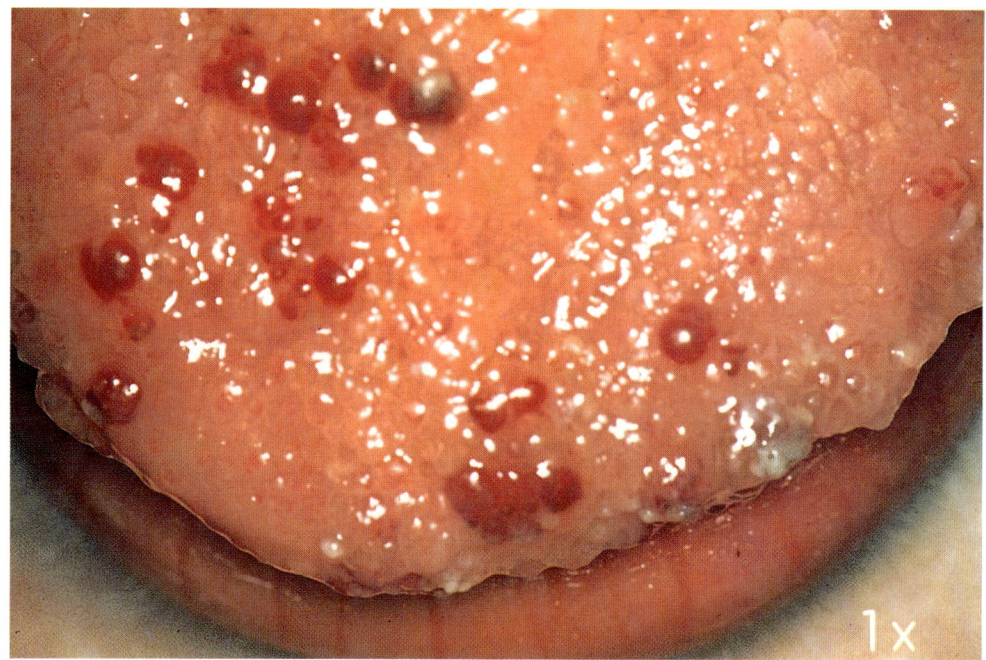

FIG. 4.4-B. Close-up of Fig. A shows the extent of the lesion.

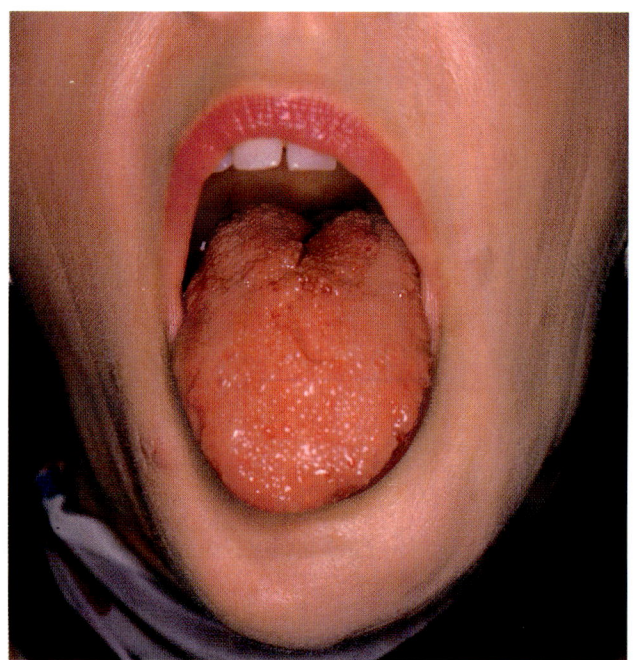

FIG. 4.4-C. The patient at present with no lymphangiomas and relatively normal tongue contour.

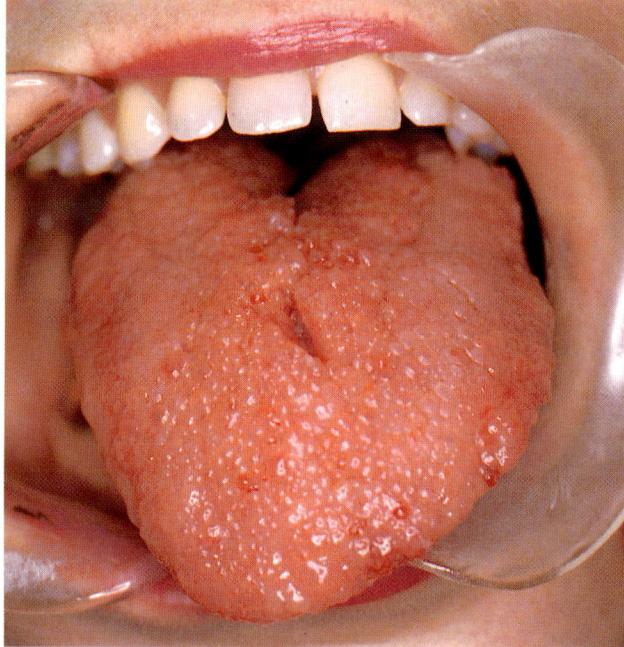

FIG. 4.4-D. Close-up of tongue demonstrating smooth surface without recurrence.

Case courtesy of *Billie L. Aronoff*, M.D.

CASE 4.5

Early Squamous Cell Carcinoma and Severe Diffuse Actinic Cheilitis of the Lower Lip

REVIEW OF CASE. This 73-year-old gentleman with a long history of chronic sun damage to the lower lip was referred by his dermatologist and dermatopathologist for possible carbon dioxide laser "lip shave" or vermilionectomy.

CHOICE OF LASER: CARBON DIOXIDE. Biopsy results showed that the superficial squamous cell cancer was completely excised, however, there was extensive surrounding actinic keratosis and dysplastic changes. It was felt that the carbon dioxide laser would produce less morbidity than traditional vermilionectomy. It is also a simpler procedure with reduced recovery time and reduced risks of complications.

ADDITIONAL INFORMATION. This procedure begins using a topical anesthetic "hurricane" and subsequent injection of 2% Xylocaine with epinephrine. Moistened, wet gauze is used behind the lip to carefully block the teeth to avoid accidental damage to the enamel.

The areas of severe actinic damage are identified first and vaporized with the carbon dioxide laser using continuous wave mode and a 1.0 mm spot with 10.0 watts defocused continuous painting technique and loupe-assisted vision. The treatment margins of the vermilion are then outlined both anteriorly and posteriorly. The posterior portion of the lip presents a fairly well demarcated zone of transition between damage and normal mucosa. The anterior margin should be carefully traced to conform with the actual vermilion border. The patient should be cautioned that the post-treatment color of the lower lip may be a brighter (more youthful) shade of red and will not match the upper lip. Lightly defocused airbrushing to "resurface" the upper lip can be performed if needed to match the upper and lower lip, especially in younger men and women.

Case continues on following page.

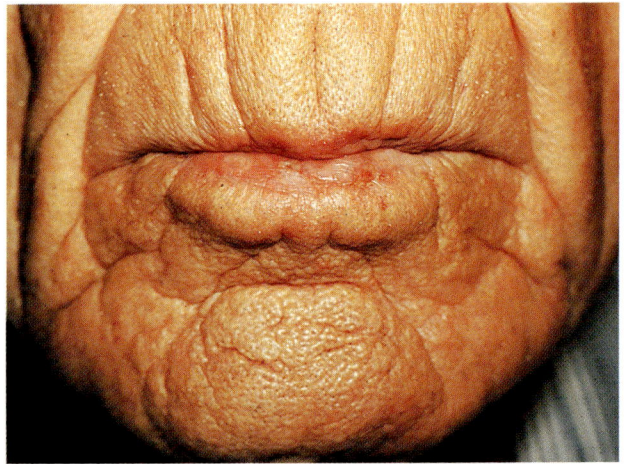

FIG. 4.5-A. Baseline pre-treatment photograph.

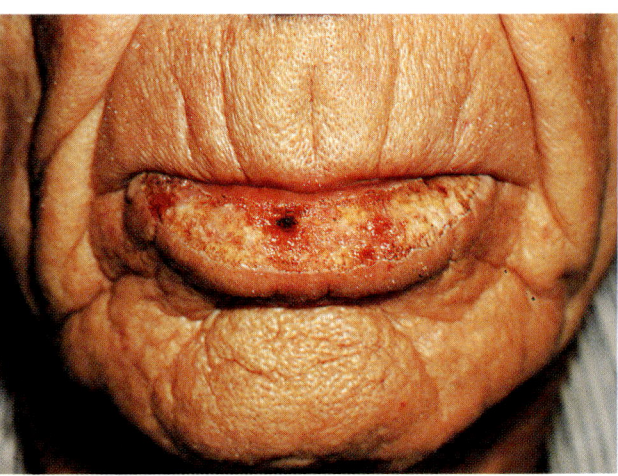

FIG. 4.5-B. Immediately post-treatment. Note that while some areas show focal deep vaporization, the majority of the lip shows a rather uniform appearance.

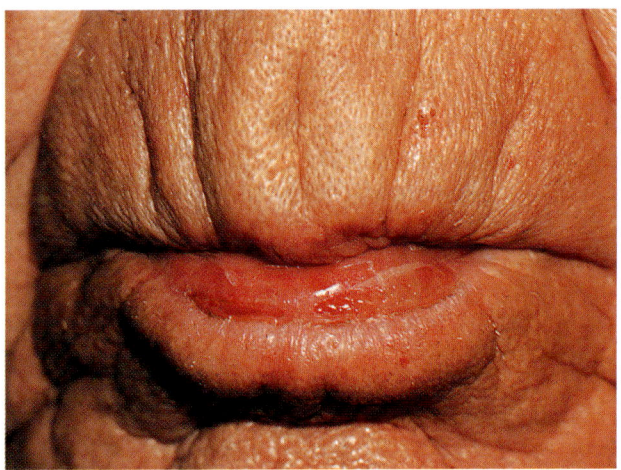

FIG. 4.5-C. Three weeks post-treatment. After care consists of topical antibiotics and saline or peroxide soaks. A flare-up of labial herpes should be treated immediately with Zovirax. Remarkably little interference with eating habits is generally encountered, weight loss is usually minimal, and pain is usually limited as well.

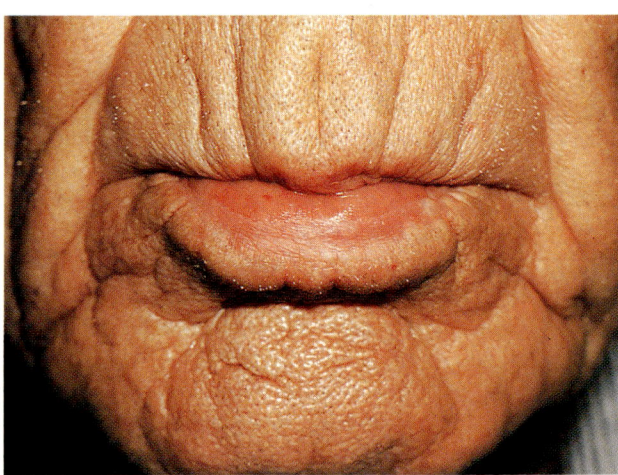

FIG. 4.5-D. Three and a half months post-treatment. Although no scarring is present in this case, small white fibrotic or stellate scars may rarely occur.

Case courtesy of *David H. McDaniel, M.D.*

CASE 4.6
Actinic Cheilitis of the Lower Lip

REVIEW OF CASE. This 57-year-old male with a history of extensive sun exposure presented with a two-year history of episodic scaling, crusting, and erosion of the lower lip. The patient had previously undergone multiple spot treatments with cryotherapy. Results of a punch biopsy ruled out squamous cell carcinoma and confirmed the diagnosis of actinic cheilitis.

CHOICE OF LASER: CARBON DIOXIDE. Electrosurgery and caustic methods of destruction have been employed in the treatment of actinic cheilitis as well as surgical excision and the use of topical 5-fluorouracil. The CO_2 laser is absorbed in the first few millimeters of tissue and does not cause a deep thermal burn or alter the very fine sensory perception of the lip. The histopathology of this disease is confined to the epidermis. Only the CO_2 laser allows the precise control necessary for an excellent cure with minimal post-operative morbidity. A lower power range of 3–6 watts is used in defocused mode with continuous power. Some operators may prefer a pulse duration of 0.5 seconds.

ADDITIONAL INFORMATION. It is important to use a lower power setting because excess destruction can cause scarring. One should start the laser at a low setting and increase only if there is a thickened keratotic lesion to remove. This is a vaporization procedure, *not* an excision technique. The oral cavity and tongue are easily protected by placing a moist cover over the teeth and upper lip. Anesthesia is easily obtained by either mental nerve blocks or local infiltration with an anesthetic.

POST-TREATMENT CARE. A bandage is not applied. Patients are instructed to clean the lip with hydrogen peroxide on cotton-tipped applicators 3 times daily following meals. A thin coating of Polysporin or bacitracin antibiotic ointment is then applied. Patients should avoid foods with abrasive surfaces (e.g., potato chips, crackers, dry toast). There are no other dietary instructions. Generally there is no need for analgesics. If anything is required, Tylenol should suffice. Follow-up visits are at two weeks and four weeks. Ninety percent of patients will be fully epithelialized by the second visit. Lip balm with a sunscreen should be started on a regular basis to prevent recurrence of disease.

Case continues on following page.

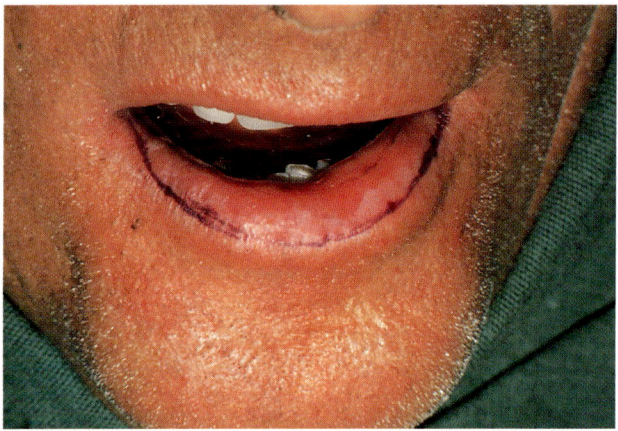

FIG. 4.6-A. Diffuse actinic cheilitis of the lower lip. The sun-exposed portion of the vermilion is outlined with tissue marker.

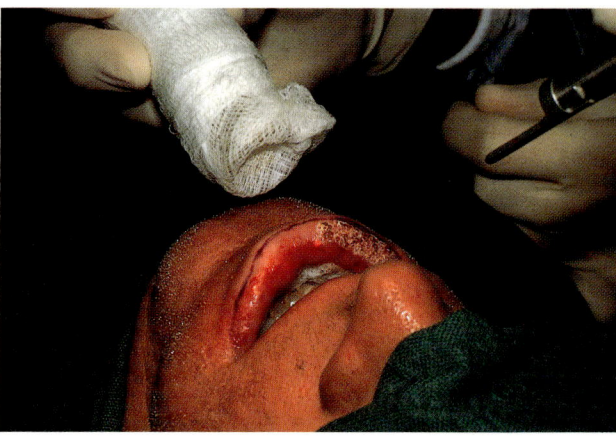

FIG. 4.6-B. After local anesthesia is obtained, treatment is begun with the CO_2 laser in defocused mode at a low power setting (3–6 watts).

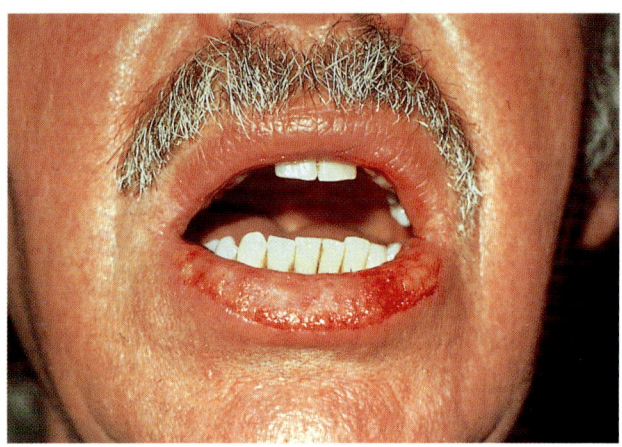

FIG. 4.6-C. Typical appearance of the lip following CO_2 laser ablation. No bandage is applied. Patients are instructed to cleanse the area and apply antibiotic ointment t.i.d.

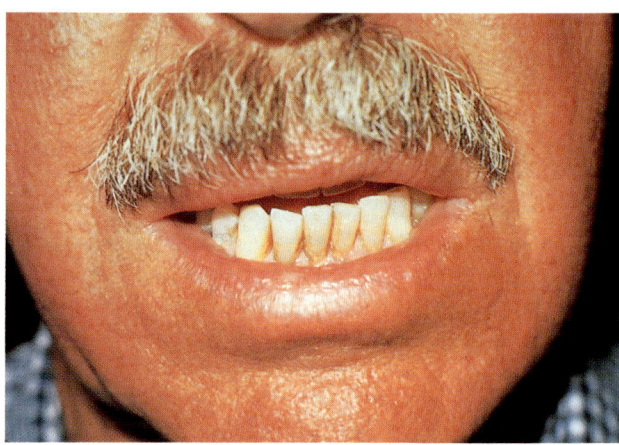

FIG. 4.6-D. Appearance of the lip at four weeks with complete healing after CO_2 laser ablation of the vermilion. There is no scarring or diminished sensation as may be seen in surgical vermilionectomy.

Case courtesy of *Duane C. Whitaker*, M.D.

CASE 4.7
Actinic Cheilitis with Epithelial Dysplasia

REVIEW OF CASE. This 68-year-old white male complained of painful fissures on his lower lip with occasional ulceration over the past year. A shave biopsy confirmed actinic cheilitis with epithelial dysplasia. There was no evidence of squamous cell carcinoma both histologically and clinically. The entire lower lip was treated with the CO_2 laser using a local anesthetic including a bilateral mental nerve block.

CHOICE OF LASER: CARBON DIOXIDE. Precision with the CO_2 laser makes this the treatment of choice for actinic cheilitis. Other treatment options include cryosurgery, retinoic acid, trichloroacetic acid, 5-fluorouracil, electrosurgery, and vermilionectomy. The cure rates for actinic cheilitis are the same as for vermilionectomy. However, vermilionectomy often results in significant minor complications including dysesthesia, excessive scarring, loss of lip plasticity, and an inward turning of the lower lip. CO_2 laser vaporization of the lip is a quick procedure that can be readily performed in an office setting. Using low power settings of 3 to 7 watts with a continuous beam in a defocused mode, one can cause enough denaturation of the epithelium to result in a dermal-epidermal junction split. This allows precise excision of the epithelium leaving the normal dermis intact. The denatured epithelium is then wiped clean with peroxide. Re-vaporization with a second pass is rarely necessary.

ADDITIONAL INFORMATION. Some physicians actually vaporize the lower lip causing the characteristic black char. I find that this results in slightly more scarring. Using a lower power setting or moving your hand more quickly across the lip causes the epithelium to turn white and blister. This bloodless procedure is superior technically and cosmetically than vermilionectomy in most cases. Decreased surgical time and the office setting makes this procedure less costly, despite the expense of the CO_2 laser.

POST-TREATMENT CARE. Standard second-intention wound healing with antibiotic ointment (2% erythromycin in petrolatum) and non-adherent gauze. Re-epithelialization normally takes three to four weeks. The patient can eat normally but must take smaller bites (i.e., not taking a big bite out of an apple, but rather cutting an apple into smaller pieces). Normal lip plasticity returns in approximately three months.

For literature pertaining to this case see References section.

Case continues on following page.

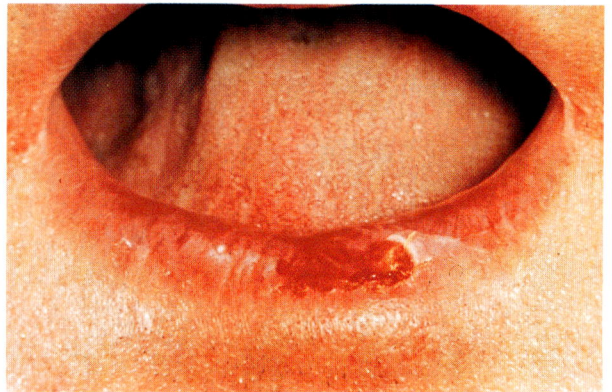

FIG. 4.7-A. Pre-operative actinic cheilitis.

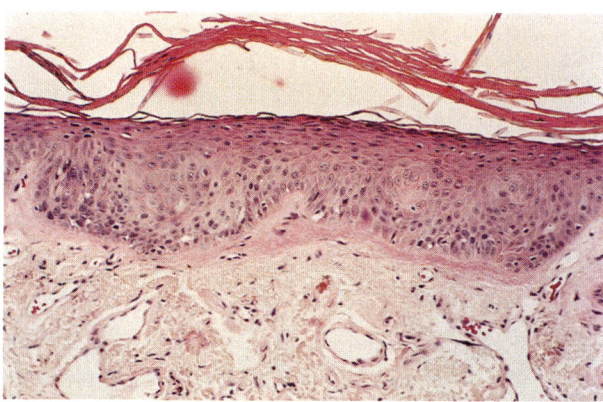

FIG. 4.7-B. Histology of intraepithelial squamous dysplasia (hematoxylin-eosin, × 40).

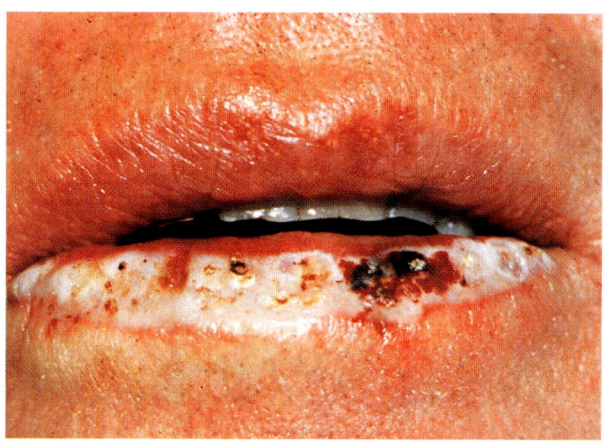

FIG. 4.7-C. Predominantly white denaturation of the epithelium immediately post-operation; small blisters bubble up intraoperatively as a result of the dermal-epithelial split.

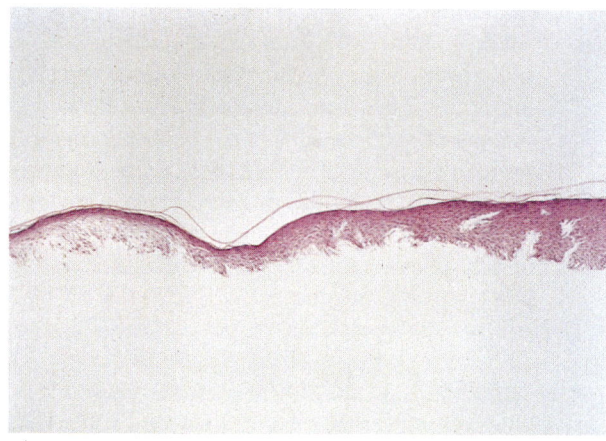

FIG. 4.7-D. Histology of the white coagulated epithelium shows the intact basal cell layer with separation from the dermis.

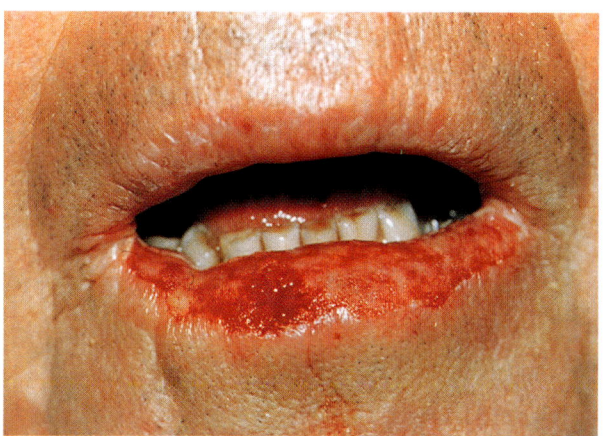

FIG. 4.7-E. Immediately post-operation; epithelium is wiped off.

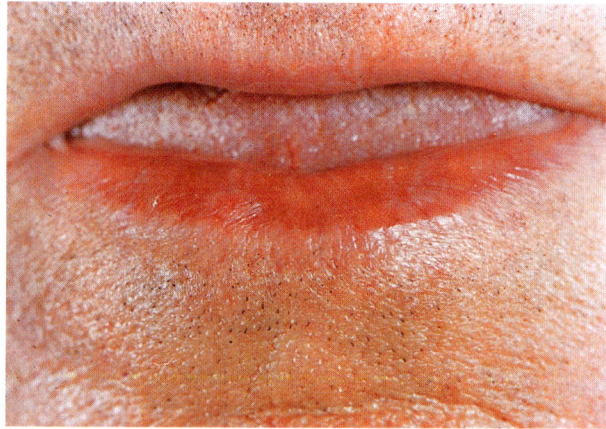

FIG. 4.7-F. Post-operatively at six weeks, the lip is completely re-epithelialized without scar and plasticity is returning to normal.

Case courtesy of **Randall K. Roenigk,** M.D.

CASE 4.8

Actinic Cheilitis and In Situ Squamous Cell Carcinoma

REVIEW OF CASE. This 70-year-old male with cheilitis of over 5 years in duration complained of burning, irritation, occasional crusting, and sensitivity of the lower vermilion. Careful visual examination and bidigital palpation of the lip revealed no induration or evidence of invasive disease. Palpation of regional nodes was also negative.

CHOICE OF LASER: CARBON DIOXIDE. The CO_2 laser was chosen to remove the dysplastic and in-situ anaplastic vermilion from the underlying tissue at a natural plane corresponding to the dermal (or sub-mucosal)-epithelial interface. Rapidly expanding steam from vaporization of tissue water beneath the basal cell layer separates the tissue layers more precisely than using scalpel or scissors.

Experience with laser vermilionectomy has shown superior cosmetic and functional results over cold steel surgery. Laser vermilionectomy maintains the normal depth of the lip (the second dimension). It also avoids the "pulled-in" lip appearance and stinging sensation occurring in males from the lower lip whiskers contacting the upper vermilion. Laser vermilionectomy also maintains the original thickness of the lip (the third dimension).

Two techniques may be utilized: (i) high-power pulse with a power setting of 20 watts, repeat pulse mode, pulse duration of 0.05 sec, and a spot size between 4 and 5 mm; and (ii) low-power continuous wave with a power setting of 3–6 watts, continuous wave mode, and a spot size between 2 and 5 mm.

ADDITIONAL INFORMATION. Marking of the vermilion with a pen, followed by submental nerve blocks, and then local Xylocaine infiltration ensures a smooth, even line and a comfortable patient. The additional local anesthetic smooths out any furrows in the epithelium and contributes a "heat sink" to further protect the underlying labial tissues from thermal injury.

Early cases of actinic cheilitis require only the briefest laser exposure signaled by opacification of the tissue accompanied by a blister. Slight charring with the pulse techniques is very acceptable since this layer will be completely removed. Gentle wiping with two moistened cotton applicators or gauze facilitates complete separation. More severe cases may require a second pass or spot vaporization. This will result in some charred tissue which should be wiped away.

Induration or nodularity or any indication of invasion warrants a biopsy prior to laser vermilionectomy (or perhaps an alternative approach such as Mohs' surgery or vermilionectomy with margin control and mucosal advancement flap).

POST-TREATMENT CARE. The major complaint by patients is discomfort from drying and cracking of the lip during re-epithelization. The problem of maintaining lubrication during the day is solved by the frequency of application of antibiotic ointment. The main problem occurs at night. I have largely solved this by having patients apply night-time ointment, then applying a template of vaseline-impregnated gauze twice as deep as the vermilion held in place by telfa and tape.

Case continues on following page.

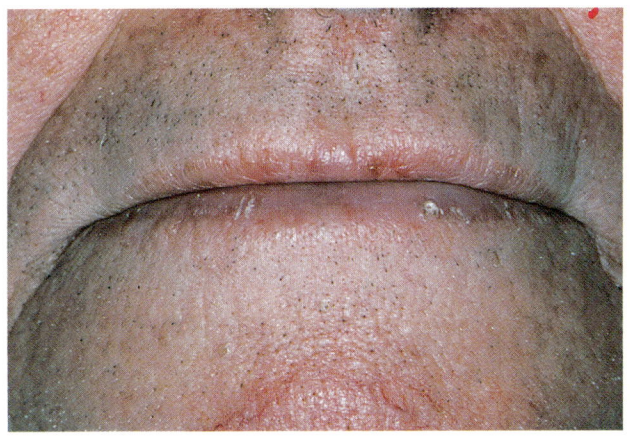

FIG. 4.8-A. Actinic Cheilitis.

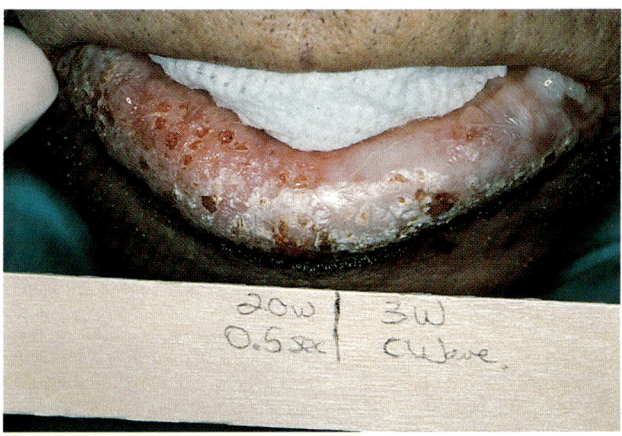

FIG. 4.8-B. Pulse mode versus continuous wave vermilionectomy. Early cases of actinic cheilitis require only the briefest laser exposure signaled by opacification of the tissue accompanied by a blister.

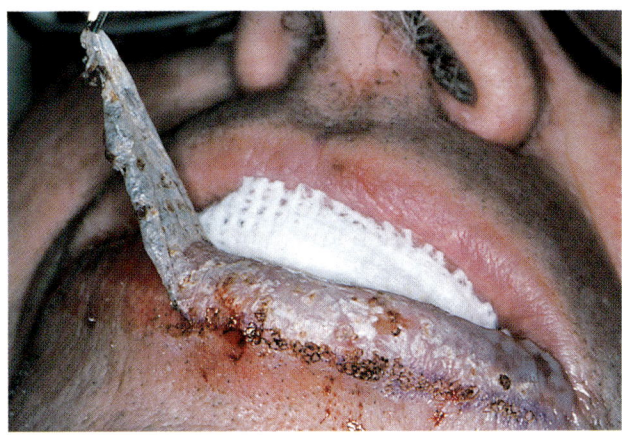

FIG. 4.8-C. Peeling off vermilion. Slight charring with the pulse technique is very acceptable since this layer will be completely removed. Gentle wiping with two moistened cotton applicators or gauze facilitates complete separation.

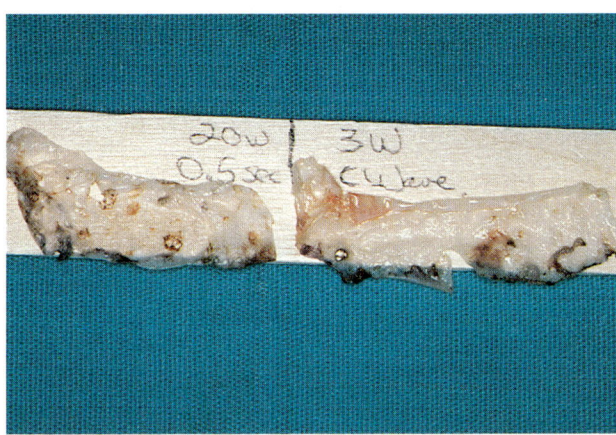

FIG. 4.8-D. Close-up of vermilion tissue; comparison of pulse (*left*) versus continuous wave (*right*) techniques (tongue blade for reference).

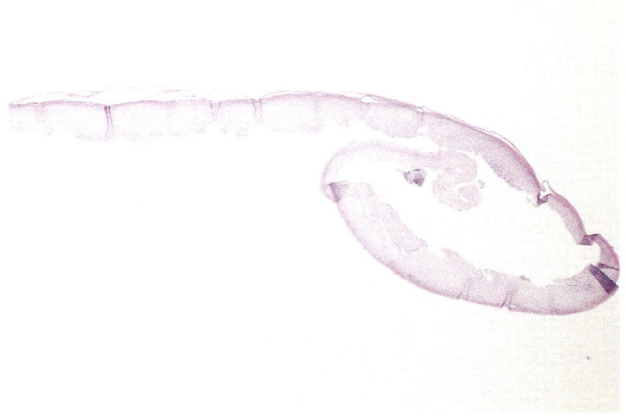

FIG. 4.8-E. Photomicrographs of vermilion removed with CO_2 laser.

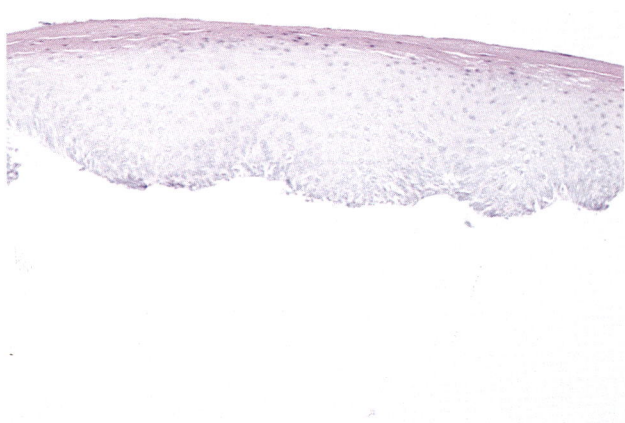

FIG. 4.8-F. Healed normal mucosa without distortion of dermis or epidermis. No recurrence noted.

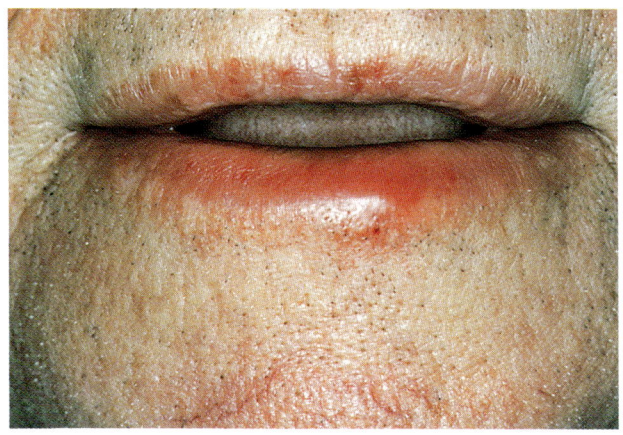

FIG. 4.8-G. Satisfactory cosmetic result six weeks after laser vermilionectomy.

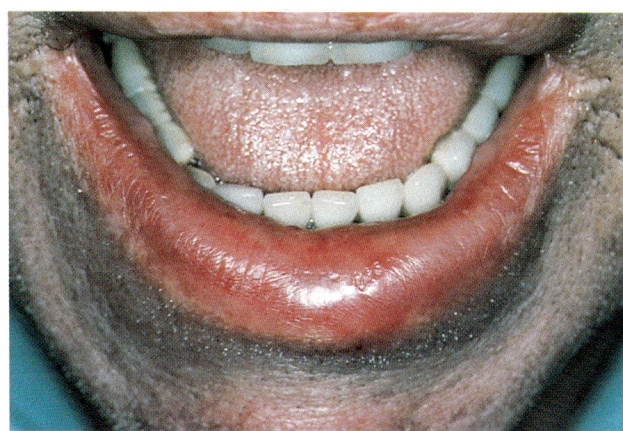

FIG. 4.8-H. Same as Fig. G.

Case courtesy of *Timothy J. Rosio*, M.D.

CASE 4.9
Basal Cell Carcinoma of the Upper Lip

REVIEW OF CASE. This patient presented with a slowly, enlarging lesion of the upper lip which had been present for several months and bled easily with trauma from shaving. The 2 cm lesion was deeply invasive with adjacent tissue destruction and submucosal extension.

CHOICE OF LASER: CARBON DIOXIDE. The CO_2 laser at 25 watts was the instrument of choice, with the option to use scalpel or electric cautery if necessary. The CO_2 laser was chosen for the following reasons: (i) rapid incision of skin with a good, clean incision line; (ii) coagulation and sealing of lymphatics; and (iii) superior hemostasis. It is important on tumors of this type to use multiple frozen sections for adequacy of margins. The CO_2 laser when finally focused and used with magnification can be used to take a lesser amount of tissue and preserve important structures.

ADDITIONAL INFORMATION. Incisions were made with the laser and the tumor was undermined and removed with frozen section confirmation of clear margins. Advancement alar flaps were developed using the laser. Blood loss was minimal, lymphatic drainage was sealed, and tumor seeding was controlled by the laser. Healing was rapid and the cosmetic result was satisfactory.

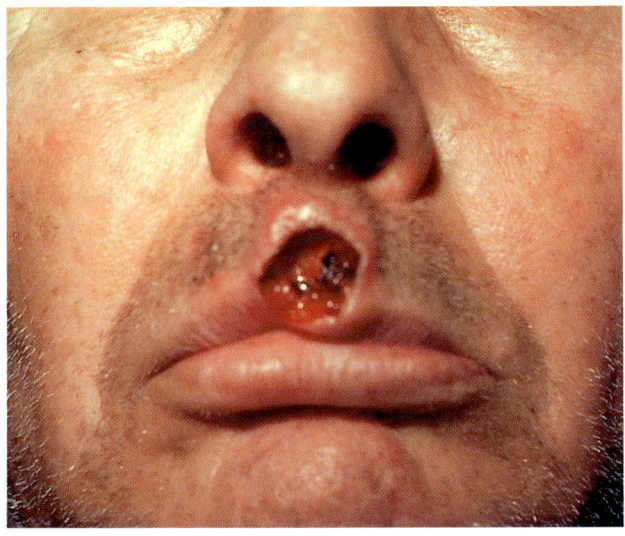

FIG. 4.9-A. Full face view showing basal cell carcinoma of the upper lip.

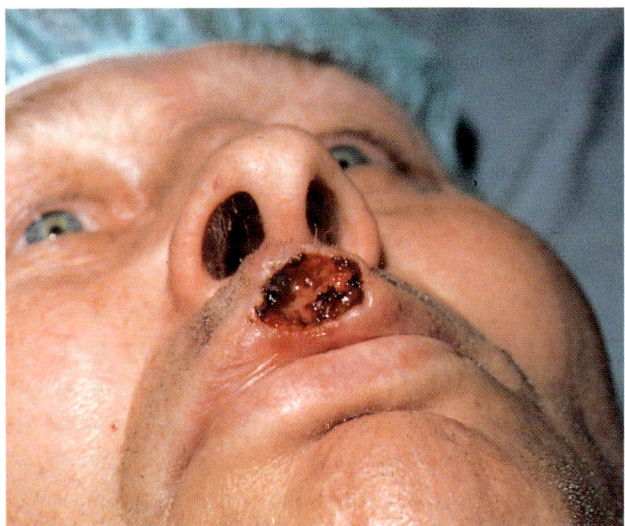

FIG. 4.9-B. Extent of the tumor on the mucosa.

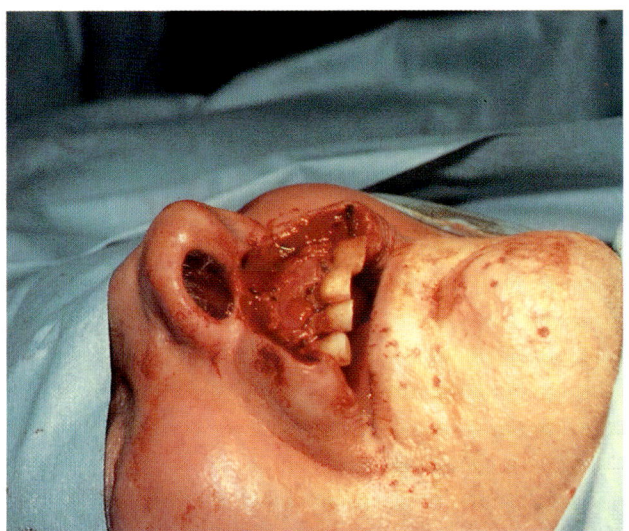

FIG. 4.9-C. The area has been excised and sent for frozen section.

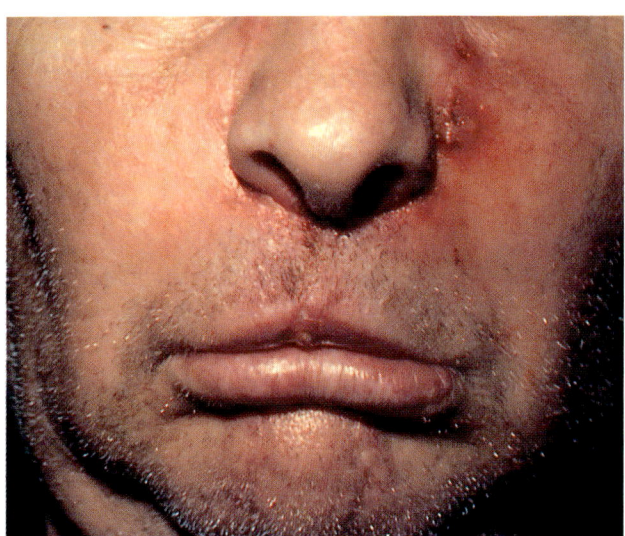

FIG. 4.9-D. Post-operative reconstruction ten days after surgery.

Case courtesy of *Billie L. Aronoff*, M.D.

CASE 4.10
Recurrent Basal Cell Carcinoma

REVIEW OF CASE. This patient is a 47-year-old white male with a recurrent basal cell carcinoma over the right temple. The primary tumor was treated four years previously with cryotumorectomy. The area apparently never healed completely and in fact had increased in size.

CHOICE OF LASER: CARBON DIOXIDE. Mohs' micrographic technique was indicated for treating this large recurrent tumor. The CO_2 laser was used in place of cold steel surgery to modify the technique because it was anticipated that the tumor extended into and around the rich vascular supply in the area. The laser provides excellent hemostasis in such cases. The power for incision was 20 watts with a continuous beam focused to 0.1 mm (This can be defocused to 2 mm for further hemostasis of larger vessels). Mohs' sections were obtained in the usual manner and evaluated until a tumor free plane was obtained. Tissue sections were easily interpreted due to minimal thermal effects. All bleeding was controlled with the laser. The wound was allowed to heal via second intention. The cosmetic result is a wide but flat and asymptomatic scar. There has been no further recurrence.

ADDITIONAL INFORMATION. The great versatility of the CO_2 laser is exemplified in this case where it has been used to modify Mohs' original technique. Advantages to using the laser as a scalpel are as follows:

(i) The laser routinely seals small blood vessels, allowing good intraoperative visibility with less post-operative bleeding and hematoma formation.
(ii) It is highly recommended for patients who are anticoagulated or functioning with a pacemaker.
(iii) The laser seals not only blood vessels but also lymphatics and may result in less edema and possibly less chance for tumor spread.
(iv) Post-operative pain, while highly subjective, appears to be less in laser-produced wounds and more likely from sealing of sensory nerves.
(v) The wound is sterile in that there is no actual contact with instruments, and the beam destroys bacteria as it cuts and vaporizes tissue.
(vi) Laser therapy delays the inflammatory response and is ideal for doing Mohs' surgery over a two-day period. Scalpel surgery and fixed tissue technique evoke a more immediate reaction which can obscure histologic tumor identification.

POST-TREATMENT CARE. The wound was allowed to granulate in by second intention. Antibiotic ointment and a nonstick dressing were used b.i.d. for approximately eight weeks.

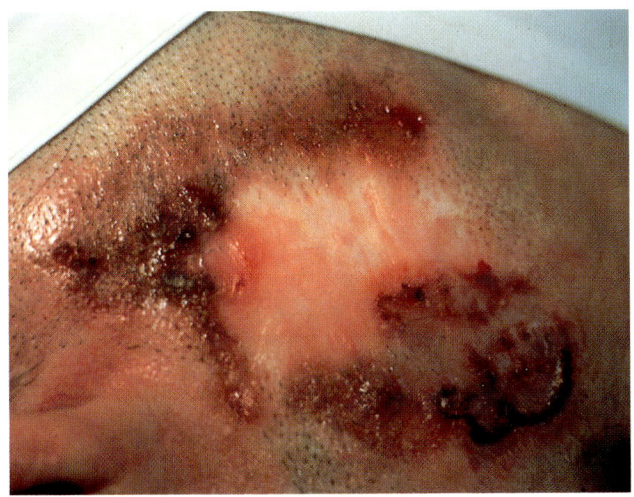

FIG. 4.10-A. Recurrent basal cell carcinoma of right temple. Tumor size: 5.8 × 4.6 cm.

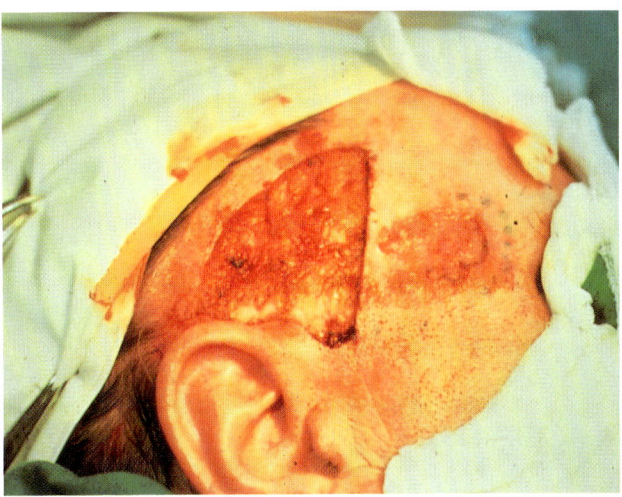

FIG. 4.10-B. Patient following removal of Mohs' section from first stage. Note precision removal with minimal bleeding.

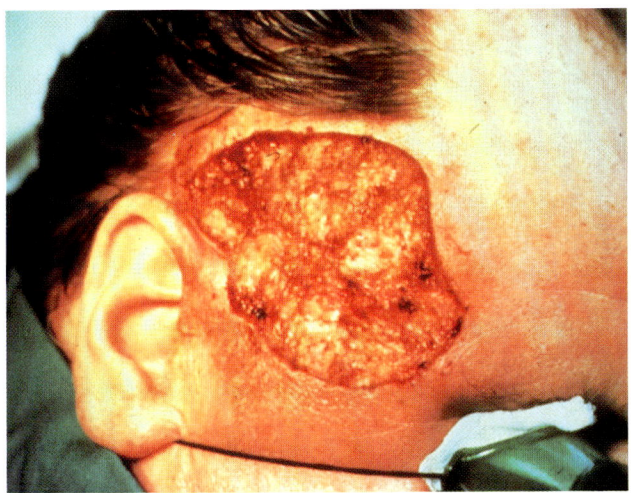

FIG. 4.10-C. Patient immediately post-operation at completion of Mohs' surgery.

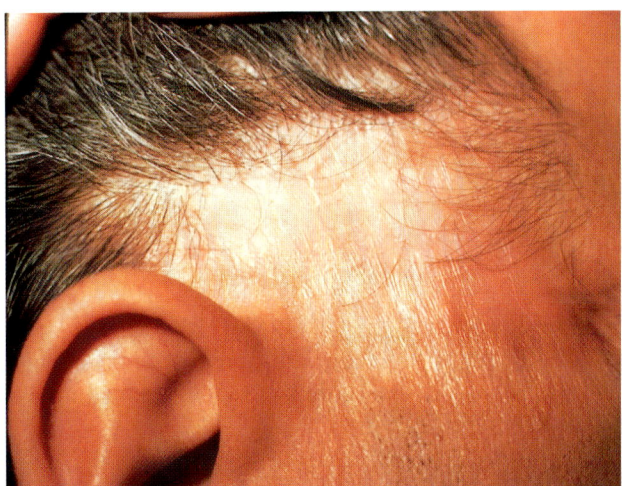

FIG. 4.10-D. Patient three months post-operation with very acceptable cosmetic result.

Case courtesy of *S. Teri McGillis,* M.D., and *Philip L. Bailin,* M.D.

CARBON DIOXIDE LASER

CASE 4.11
Superficial Basal Cell Carcinoma

REVIEW OF CASE. This 62-year-old white male had a long history of multiple skin cancers, all of which were superficial basal cell carcinoma and on the trunk. Treatment options in the past have included electrodesiccation and currettage and cryosurgery. Treatment with the CO_2 laser has resulted in diminished pain post-operatively and wound healing with minimal scarring.

CHOICE OF LASER: CARBON DIOXIDE. Non-selective, easily controlled superficial destruction with CO_2 laser vaporization is well-suited to treatment of superficial basal cell carcinoma. Like any superficial destructive technique there is a lack of pathologic margin control, a significant limitation. However, in our series of over 300 superficial basal cell carcinomas treated with the laser, none had recurred (1). Remember that there are over 15 histologic subtypes of basal cell carcinoma, and recurrence rates vary considerably. Recurrence rates of basal cell carcinoma are also dependent on the anatomic location of the tumor. Superficial basal cell carcinoma has a very low recurrence rate regardless of therapy, and when on the trunk makes recurrence even less likely (2). The choice of the CO_2 laser is based mainly on its ability to do very little damage to the remaining dermal tissue, providing a good matrix for cosmetically acceptable scar formation. Other standard options such as electrosurgery, cryosurgery, and excision would be equally curative. The CO_2 laser power settings are 15 watts for the first pass, decreasing to 7 to 10 watts for subsequent passes as needed, using a continuous defocused beam. Note that pockets of tumor (dermal nests of tumor) can be clearly delineated with this technique.

ADDITIONAL INFORMATION. For a tumor that is easily cured by standard methods, it is unethical to charge a differential fee for using the CO_2 laser to treat this condition. However, the cosmetic results are superior. This technique is especially helpful in patients with basal cell nevus syndrome.

POST-TREATMENT CARE. Standard second-intention wound dressing with antibiotic ointment (2% erythromycin in petrolatum), hydrogen peroxide cleansing, and nonadherent gauze dressing. Wound healing normally takes three to six weeks.

For literature pertaining to this case see References section.

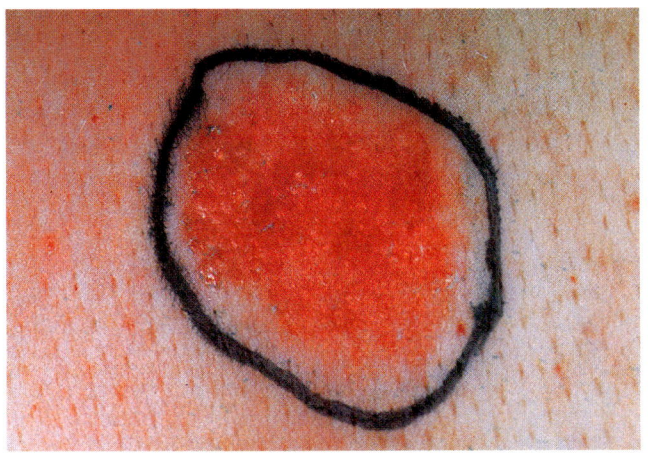

FIG. 4.11-A. Superficial basal cell carcinoma of the trunk.

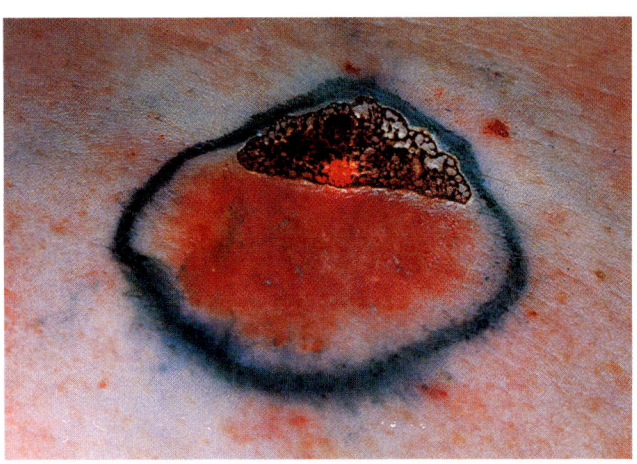

FIG. 4.11-B. CO_2 laser vaporization with a defocused beam.

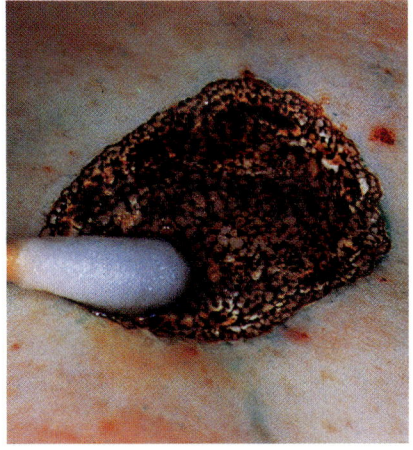

FIG. 4.11-C. The char is cleansed with hydrogen peroxide.

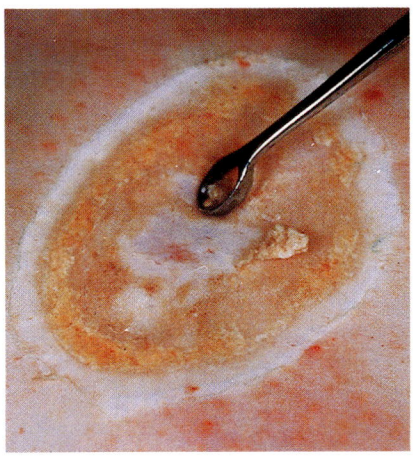

FIG. 4.11-D. Pockets of tumor are easily identified and removed with a dermal curet.

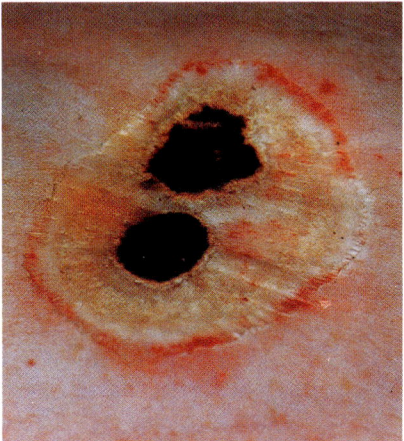

FIG. 4.11-E. Pockets of tumor treated a second time with the CO_2 laser.

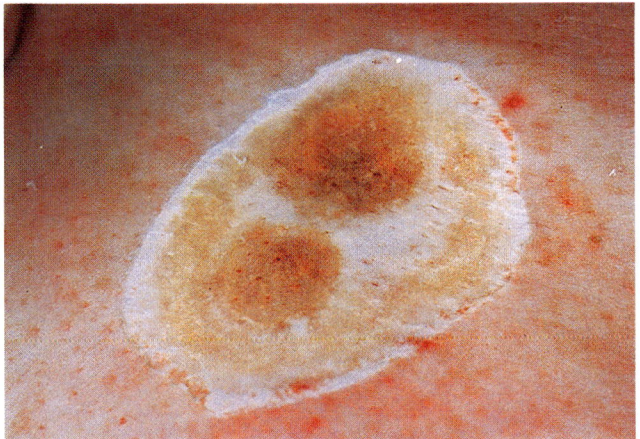

FIG. 4.11-F. Immediate post-operative result.

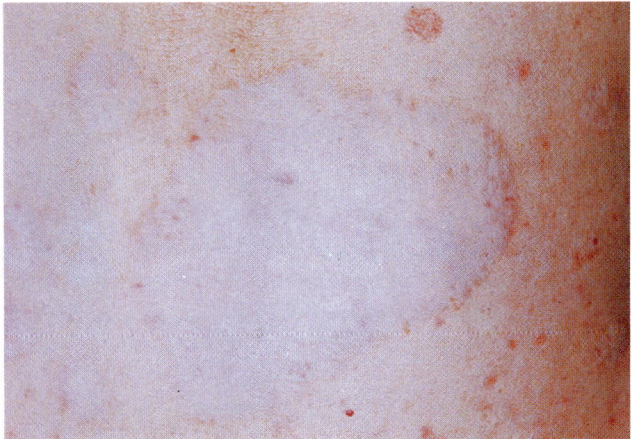

FIG. 4.11-G. Different patient from that in Fig. F. Result one year post-operation of a large and several small superficial basal cell carcinomas on the trunk treated using the CO_2 laser.

Case courtesy of *Randall K. Roenigk,* M.D., and *Ronald G. Wheeland,* M.D.

CASE 4.12
Squamous Cell Carcinoma In Situ
Bowen's Disease

REVIEW OF CASE. Case 1: This 71-year-old white male presented with an asymptomatic patch of biopsy-proven squamous cell carcinoma in situ on the left index finger that was present for 16 years and never previously treated. Since this lesion almost completely surrounded the digit, staged CO_2 laser vaporization was performed. The dorsal surface of the finger was vaporized using local anesthesia and the wound was allowed to heal and mature for six months prior to treating the ventral surface of the finger. Re-epithelialization was complete in six to eight weeks, however, it took several months for full range of motion of the digit to be normal. The ventral surface was then treated in a similar manner with equally good results.

Case 2: This 66-year-old white male presented with biopsy-proven squamous cell carcinoma in situ on the right fourth and fifth toe involving approximately 90% of the fifth toe circumferentially. The lesion was treated in two stages. The dorsal portion was completely re-epithelialized in eight weeks. The second stage was completed five months after the first.

CHOICE OF LASER: CARBON DIOXIDE. Squamous cell carcinoma in situ or Bowen's disease is considered a precancerous lesion but very often undergoes a chronic biologically benign course. Often, these lesions are on anatomically important sites. Surgical excision and reconstructive efforts might be quite extensive. Considering that these lesions are limited to the epidermis, CO_2 laser vaporization is a very reasonable approach to precisely treat the diseased skin while leaving a matrix of normal dermis behind. These lesions are treated much like actinic cheilitis, at lower power settings (10 watts) using a continuous defocused beam. When the lesion involves the circumferential digit, it seems best to perform the procedure in stages to avoid risk to the digit from vasoconstriction and tip necrosis due to the edematous stages of wound healing.

ADDITIONAL INFORMATION. A digital block with local anesthetic without epinephrine is used.

POST-TREATMENT CARE. Standard second-intention wound care with antibiotic ointment (2% erythromycin in petrolatum) and nonadherent gauze dressing. The wound is cleansed twice daily with hydrogen peroxide until re-epithelialization is complete. On functional digits such as the fingers, the patient is instructed to exercise regularly to maintain full range of motion.

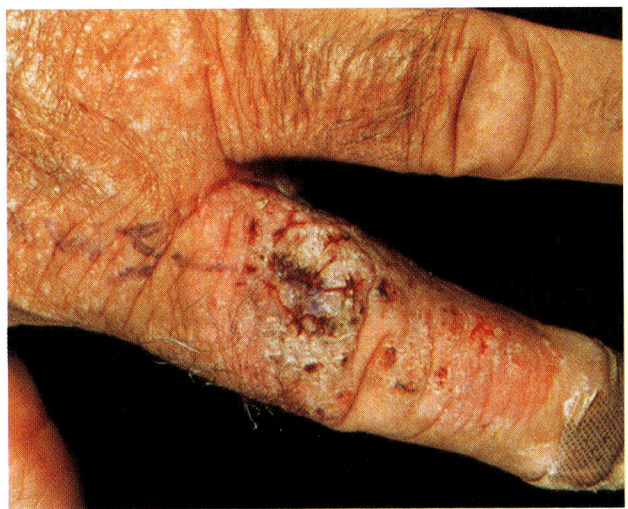

FIG. 4.12-A. Case 1: Pre-operation.

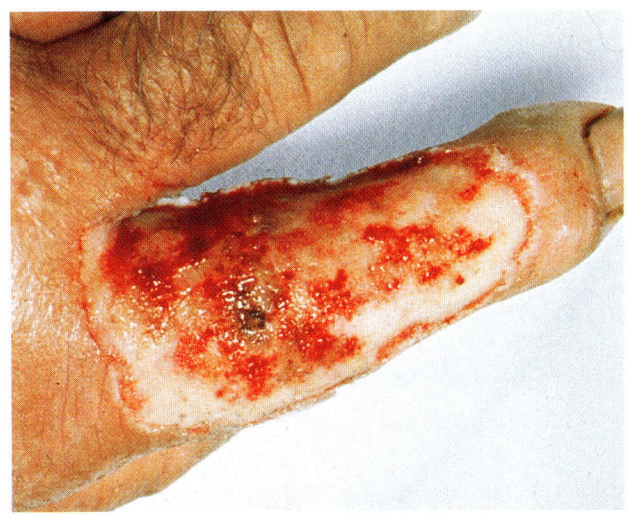

FIG. 4.12-B. Case 1: Immediately post-operation.

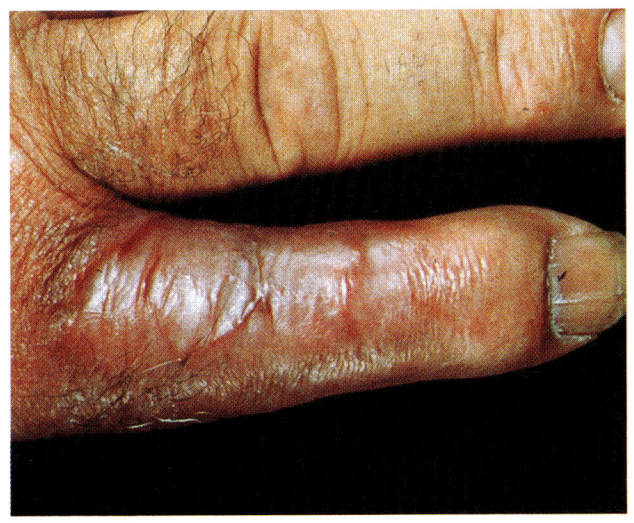

FIG. 4.12-C. Case 1: Seven months post-operation.

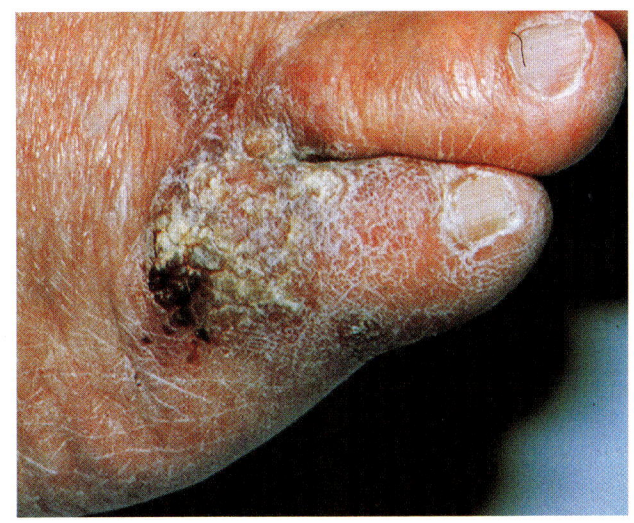

FIG. 4.12-D. Case 2: Pre-operation.

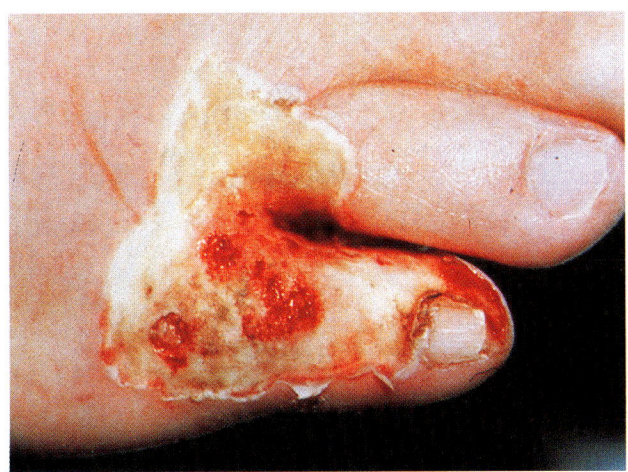

FIG. 4.12-E. Case 2: Immediately post-operation.

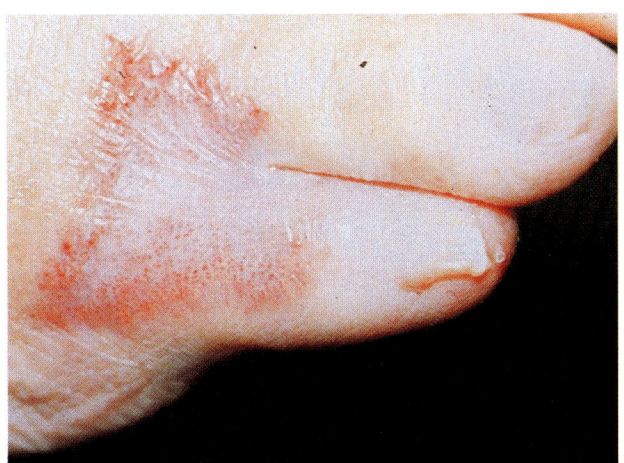

FIG. 4.12-F. Case 2: Six months post-operation.

Case courtesy of ***Randall K. Roenigk***, M.D.

CARBON DIOXIDE LASER

CASE 4.13
Lentigo Maligna

REVIEW OF CASE. This 79-year-old man presented with a verrugated, pigmented lesion of the right infra-auricular area that measured 4 × 3 cm in size and which had been present for over a year and seemed to be enlarging.

CHOICE OF LASER: CARBON DIOXIDE. The CO_2 laser was chosen because it is a very precise cutting tool that does not penetrate deeply into the surrounding tissues and provides adequate hemostasis for these types of lesions. The suprapulse mode causes less damage to the surrounding tissues. Because of these properties, the laser can be used to remove a lesion with little surrounding destruction, and also allows the pathologist to receive a specimen that will permit him to read the margins. It also facilitates the surgeon to use the laser to elevate skin flaps in a bloodless manner in order to reconstruct the defect easily and rapidly.

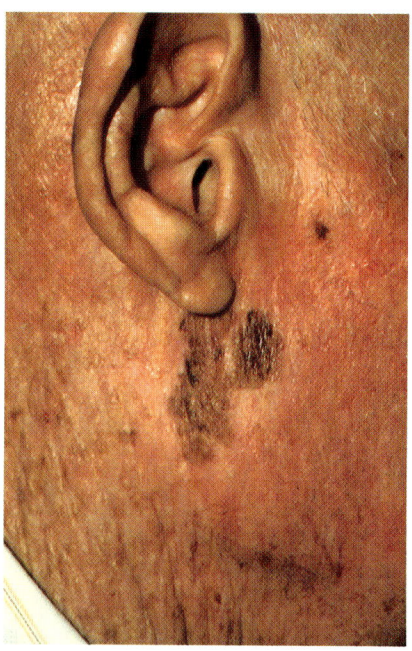

FIG. 4.13-A. Area of the lesion to be treated. Note the close proximity to, but non-involvement of, the lobe of the ear and rest of the auricle. Care must be taken not to damage these structures during treatment.

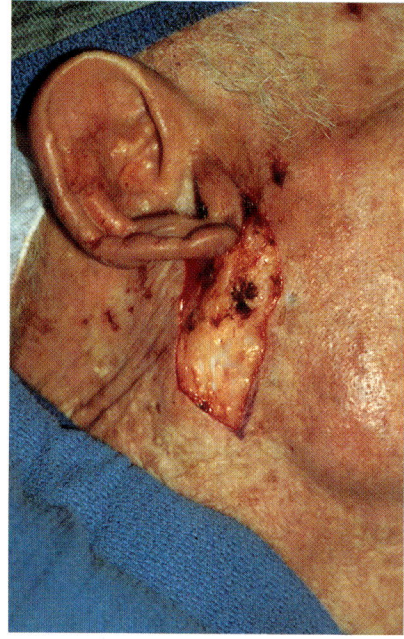

FIG. 4.13-B. The lesion has been excised and the flaps elevated using the laser at 10 watts, continuous, suprapulse mode. Note that most of the char has been removed with the exception of that caused by using the laser in a defocused mode to control bleeding vessels. Also, note the other lesions in the same area that have been treated.

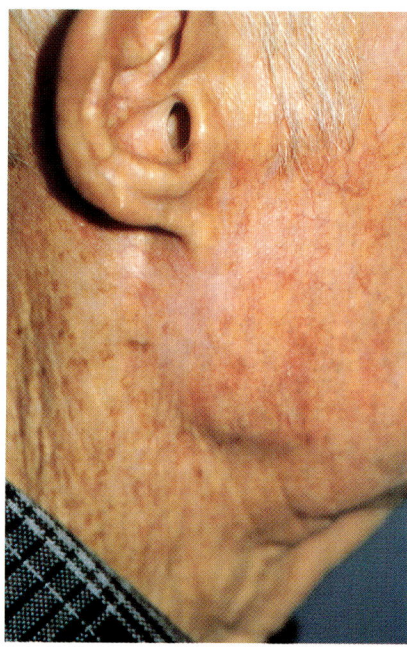

FIG. 4.13-C. One year after excision the area is well healed with no residual lesion and with minimal distortion of the lobule. Post-operative wound care consisted of local cleansing and antibiotic ointment.

Case courtesy of *Jack A. Coleman, Jr.*, M.D., *Robert H. Ossoff*, D.M.D., M.D., and *Wm. Russell Ries*, M.D.

CASE 4.14
Condyloma Acuminata

REVIEW OF CASE. This patient is a 19-year-old white female who is an insulin-dependent diabetic. She had condyloma on the labia majora, labia minora, vagina, and anal area that were painful to the touch. She had been treated unsuccessfully with podophyllum, liquid nitrogen, and dinitrochlorobenzene (DNCB). Because of the number of lesions, the high chance of recurrence was discussed with the patient. The pathology report on the biopsy obtained during the laser procedure confirmed the presence of warts. She had a few lesions which recurred after laser therapy, however this time she responded to liquid nitrogen therapy.

CHOICE OF LASER: CARBON DIOXIDE. CO_2 laser was chosen because the lesions could be vaporized with the defocus beam.

POST-TREATMENT CARE. The patient received IV antibiotic therapy during surgery and oral erythromycin after surgery. A large lymph node on her right groin gradually disappeared.

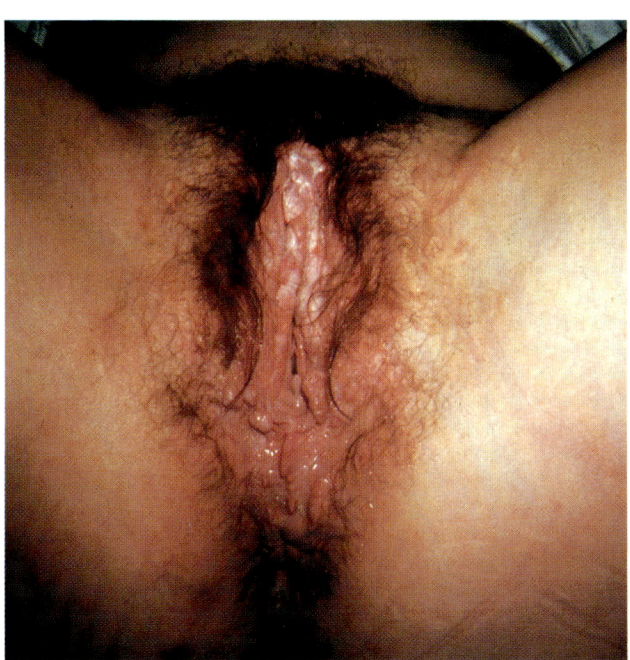

FIG. 4.14-A. Severe condyloma involving the labia majora, labia minora, and vagina.

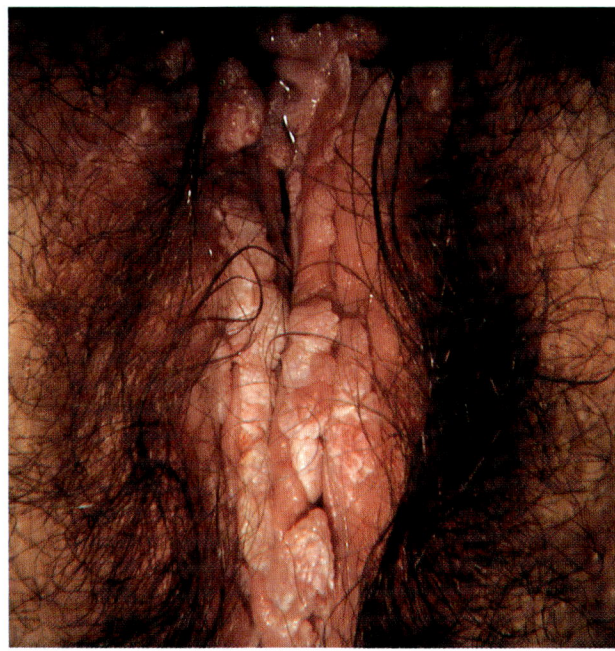

FIG. 4.14-B. Close-up of Fig. A.

Case continues on following page.

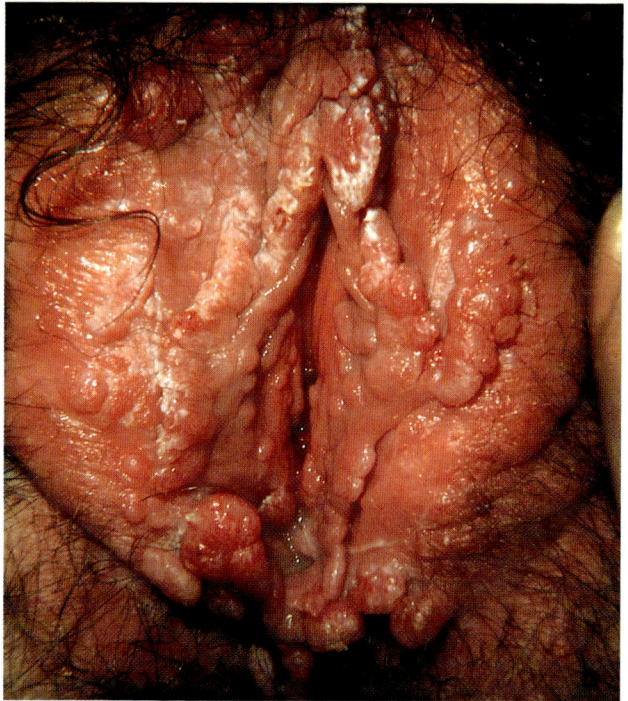

FIG. 4.14-C. Close-up of Fig. B. A biopsy was done to rule out the possibility of malignancy.

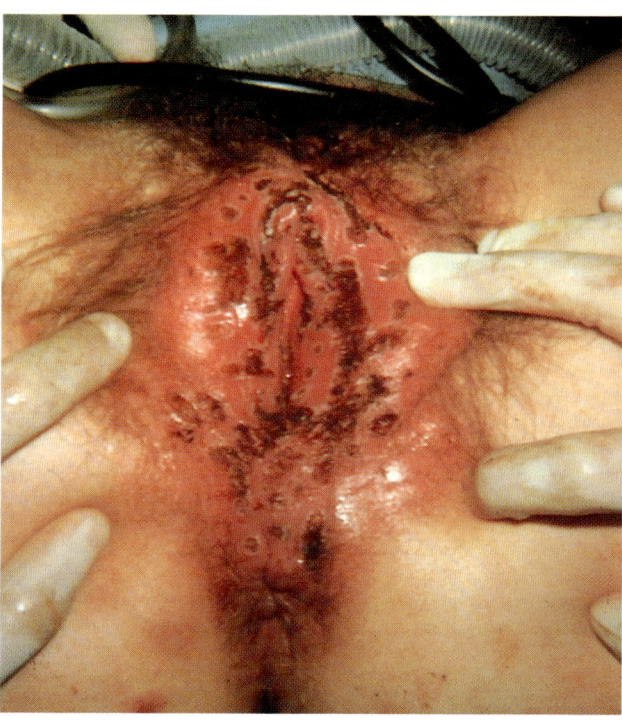

FIG. 4.14-D. The lesions were vaporized under general anesthesia with the CO_2 laser defocus beam, power of 10 watts.

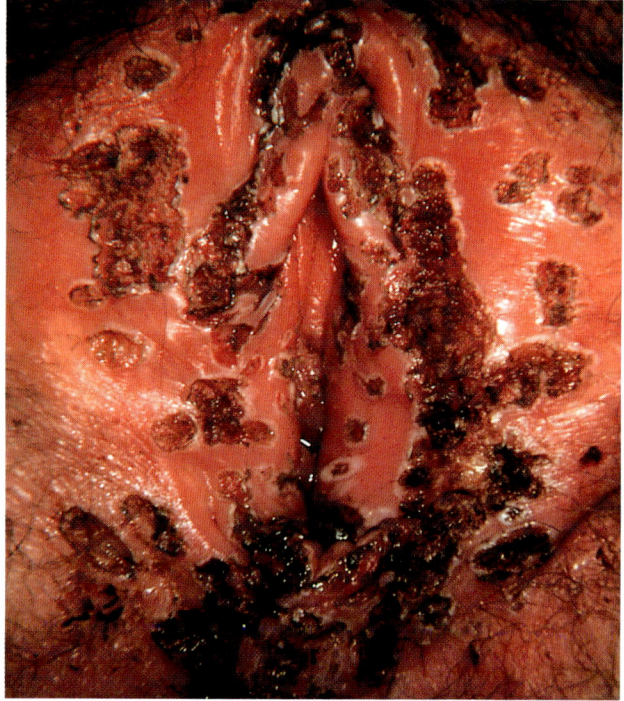

FIG. 4.14-E. Close-up of Fig. D. The area was cleaned with normal saline.

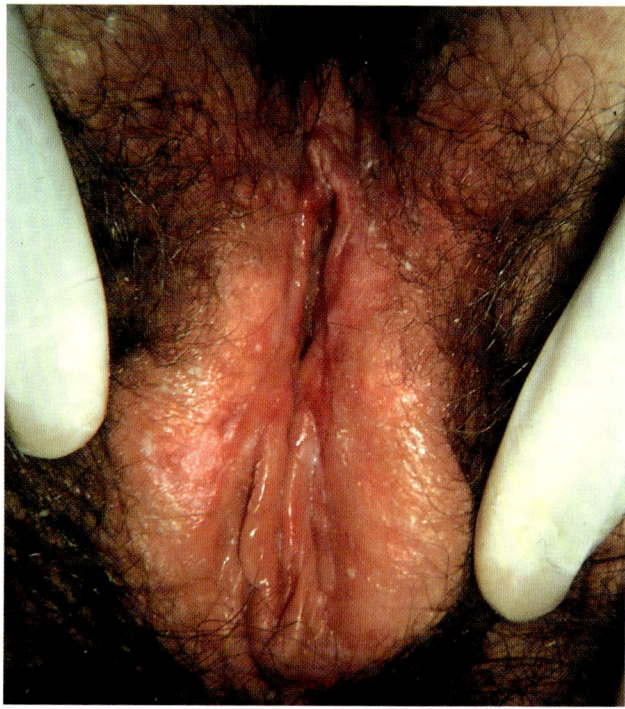

FIG. 4.14-F. Healed post-operative area without scarring or complications.

Case courtesy of **Syrus Rayhan,** M.D.

CASE 4.15
Penile Condyloma

REVIEW OF CASE. This 30-year-old male presented with a history of penile warts for over one year duration unsuccessfully treated with electrocautery, podophyllum, and liquid nitrogen. Microscopic examination after acetowhitening revealed some scattered smaller warts not visible without acetowhitening as well as the larger visible warts. The distal urethra, glans, scrotum, perineum, hands, and oral cavity were free of visible warts. A few small condyloma were also discovered in the rectal area. (This area should be examined even in heterosexual men since occasionally warts will be present and may have been missed by the referring physician.)

CHOICE OF LASER: CARBON DIOXIDE. The CO_2 laser was chosen because of the patient's history of treatment failure with standard techniques. HPV typing was not performed. Careful evacuation of the CO_2 laser plume should be observed on all condyloma cases with an attempt to keep the evacuation handpiece opening a maximum of 5 to 10 mm from the impact site of the CO_2 laser beam. All operating room personnel should wear a surgical mask (one of the types shown to be most effective for small articulate matter).

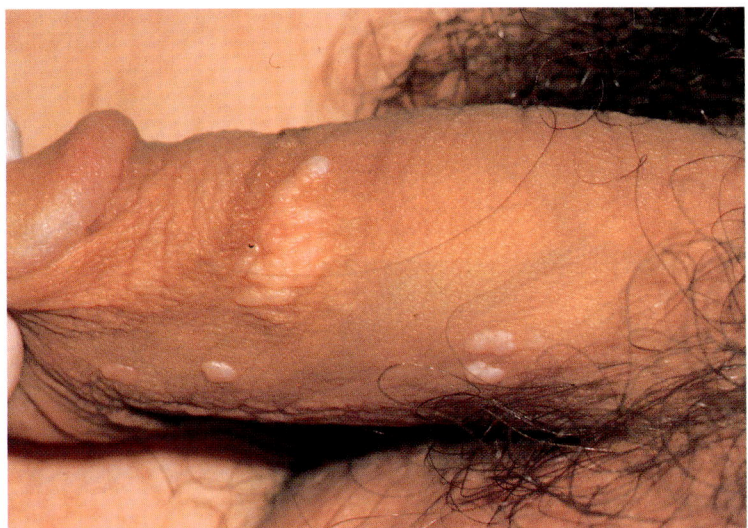

FIG. 4.15-A. Penile condyloma prior to surgery after 10 minutes acetowhitening with 5% acetic acid. Note that the lesions are more visible than the typical condyloma. Occasionally, warts will not acetowhiten. After five years experience with acetowhitening in many hundreds of patients, it is this authors opinion that acetowhitening should be mandatory for *all* male initial-excising treatments and follow-up checks.

Case continues on following page.

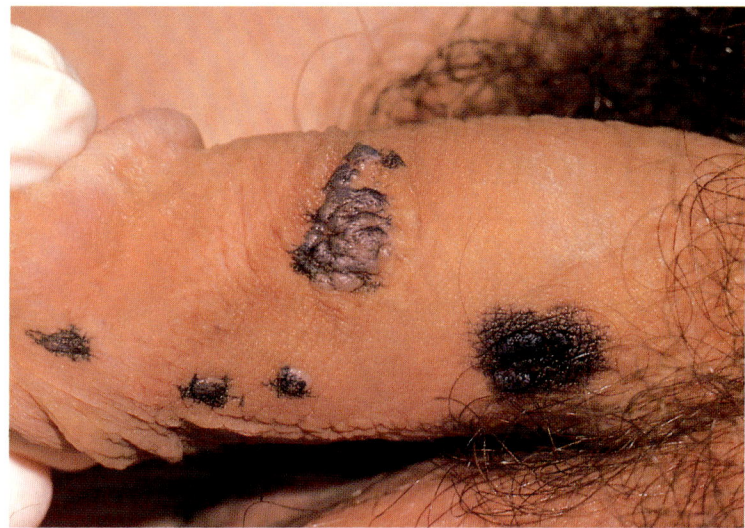

FIG. 4.15-B. The same areas as in Fig. A are marked with skin marking dye prior to surgery. This is performed when there are extensive lesions since the acetowhitening effect is rather transient and may not persist throughout the entire procedure.

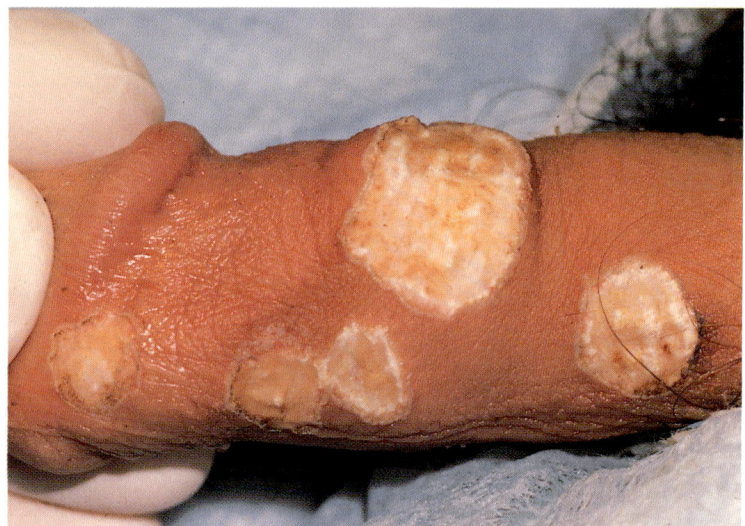

FIG. 4.15-C. Immediately post-treatment. A 1.0 mm spot, continuous wave defocused mode was used with ×10.0 and ×15.0 loupe-assisted vision and painting technique utilized. Note that a 5 mm border of skin surrounding the clinically visible wart margins has been superficially vaporized with the CO_2 laser in a severely defocused manner. The individual warts often become rather large confluent islands after treatment. It is also possible to apply either topically or intralesionally one of the interferons (1 to 5 million units) to perhaps enhance resolution of the lesions in difficult cases. Generally minimal systemic side effects are experienced at these close levels.

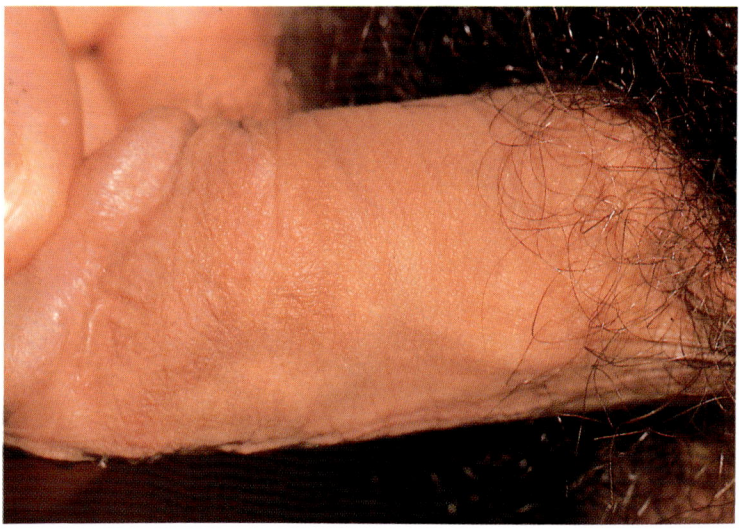

FIG. 4.15-D. Four and a half months post-treatment. Note the excellent healing. Sometimes hypopigmentation or hyperpigmentation or textural changes may be present but often these resolve. Even deeply pigmented skin is very forgiving and usually repigments within a year.

Case courtesy of *David H. McDaniel*, M.D.

CASE 4.16
Condylomata Acuminata

REVIEW OF CASE. This 36-year-old male had many unsuccessful treatments with podophyllum and liquid nitrogen and desired another treatment modality. After he received treatment with the CO_2 laser, however, he had several recurrences and was again treated using the CO_2 laser.

CHOICE OF LASER: CARBON DIOXIDE. The CO_2 laser was chosen because with the defocused beam, the lesions including a few millimeters of normal looking surrounding skin can be vaporized. The rate of success with one treatment is about 80% to 95%.

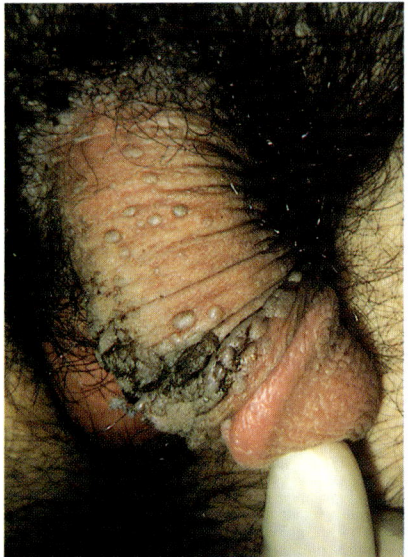

FIG. 4.16-A. Condylomata acuminata.

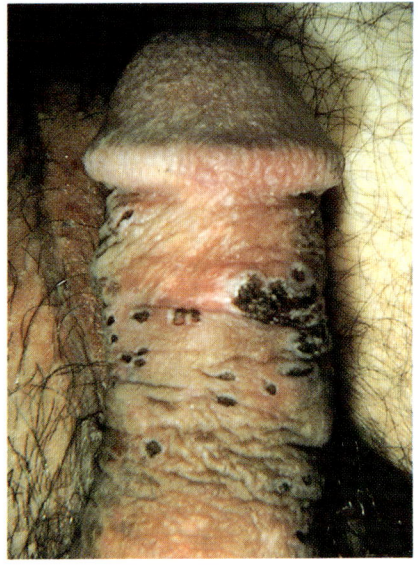

FIG. 4.16-B. Immediately post-treatment after vaporizing the lesions with the CO_2 laser. The treatment was performed under local anesthesia using a 5 watt defocused beam under magnification.

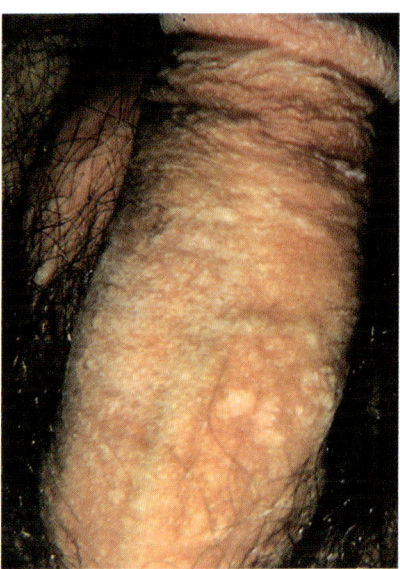

FIG. 4.16-C. Healed lesions with hypopigmentation.

Case courtesy of *Syrus Rayhan*, M.D.

CASE 4.17
Perianal Condyloma

REVIEW OF CASE. This patient is an 18-year-old male with large multiple condyloma in the perianal area and a wart on the left index finger. The patient has been treated with liquid nitrogen and podophyllum on several occasions unsuccessfully, and developed a severe reaction to podophyllum. His VDRL was nonreactive.

CHOICE OF LASER: CARBON DIOXIDE. The CO_2 laser was chosen to vaporize the lesions. It has been shown that lasers are able to treat wart lesions with a high rate of cure.

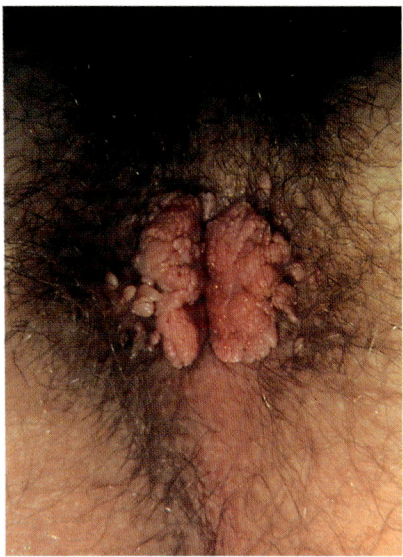

FIG. 4.17-A. Large perianal condyloma. Anoscopy revealed a wart inside of the anal area.

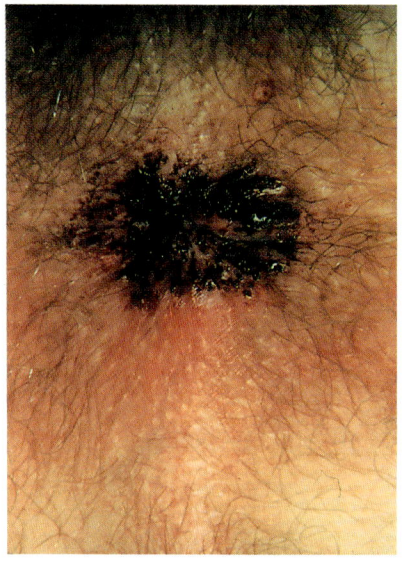

FIG. 4.17-B. CO_2 laser used to excise the lesion with a 5 watt focused beam and a spot size of 0.1 mm. The base of the lesion and inside anal wart was vaporized with a 5 watt defocused beam by applying several passes. The patient had five lesions recur which were treated with electrosurgery.

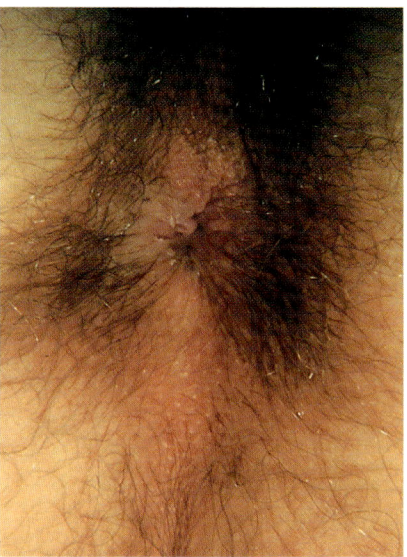

FIG. 4.17-C. Healed lesions without scarring.

Case courtesy of *Syrus Rayhan*, M.D.

CASE 4.18
Distal Male Urethral Condyloma

REVIEW OF CASE. This is a 28-year-old male with a history of condyloma three years previously "successfully" treated with podophyllum. He had no history of new lesions but routine examination by the author with micro-acetowhitening of the penis and distal urethra revealed the distal intraurethral warts visible in Fig. A.

CHOICE OF LASER: CARBON DIOXIDE. The CO_2 laser was chosen to vaporize these warts because of the reduced risk of edema and possible urethral obstruction post-operatively as well as the precision of treatment and the very distal location of the warts.

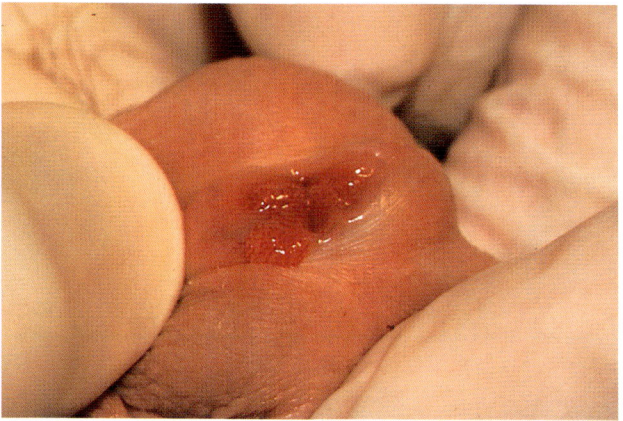

FIG. 4.18-A. Pre-treatment condyloma. Topical Xylocaine was used for anesthesia. It may be supplemented with a small amount of 2% Xylocaine by injection if needed.

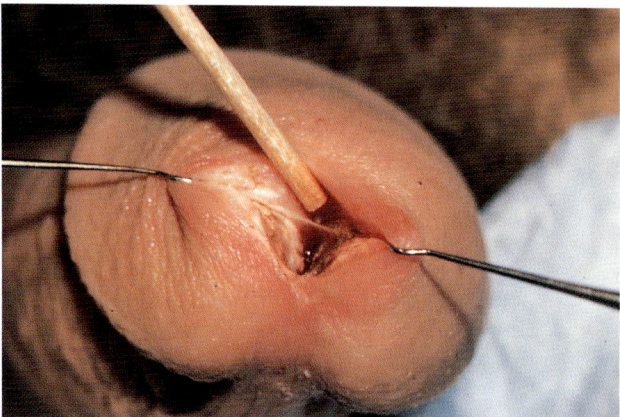

FIG. 4.18-B. Immediately post-treatment. The CO_2 laser was used with a 1.0 mm spot continuous wave defocused beam at 10 watts using loupe-assisted vision. The warts were vaporized and then superficially air brushed in a very defocused mode (to the extent possible) 5 mm in diameter around the clinically visible edge of the wart. Skin hooks or a pediatric nasal speculum are excellent for this procedure. (Caution needs to be exercised about specular reflection when using polished instruments.)

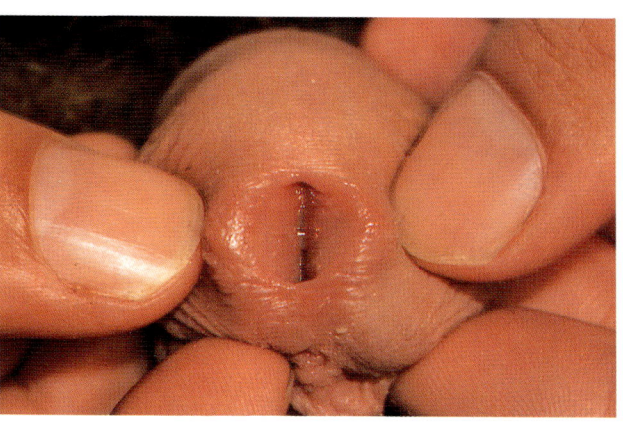

FIG. 4.18-C. Two weeks post-treatment. Note excellent healing. There is generally minimal discomfort except for some dysuria for the first few days. Such patients and their partners need to be carefully examined for condyloma elsewhere. Urethroscopy is probably warranted at this stage as well.

Case courtesy of *David H. McDaniel*, M.D.

CASE 4.19

Onychomycosis

REVIEW OF CASE. This is a 60-year-old male with a 20 year history of abnormal nail plates of the left foot. Pressure of the onychomycotic build-up of tissue beneath the nail plate produced chronic pain.

CHOICE OF LASER: CARBON DIOXIDE. The CO_2 laser was chosen to photovaporize the entire nail plate and the underlying hyperkeratotic tissue on the nail bed. The high heat of the laser destroys the mycotic organisms and allows the entire nail bed to be totally clean of underlying mycotic hyperkeratotic material. This allows the nail plate to grow out on a more normal nail bed to encourage proper reattachment of the nail plate.

POST-TREATMENT CARE. An antibacterial cream is applied to the treated nail bed. The patient can bathe the area in 24 hours and reapply an antibacterial cream using a bandaid until the area is healed. Care must be taken to not allow the hyperkeratosis to reoccur on the treated nail bed. If this begins to reform, it must be trimmed regularly.

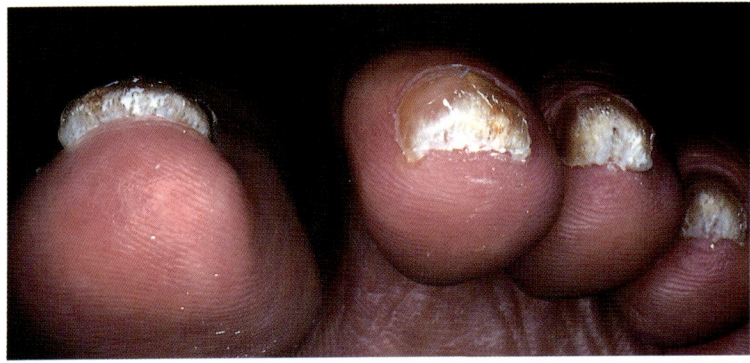

FIG. 4.19-A. Multiple onychomycotic nail plates.

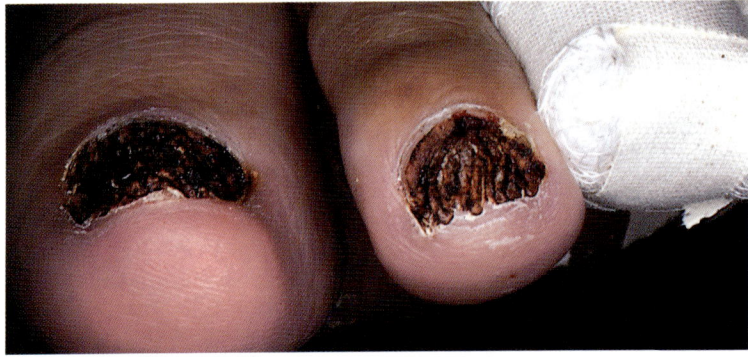

FIG. 4.19-B. Using a 15 watt focused 1 mm CO_2 laser beam the involved nail plate and underlying hyperkeratotic tissue is photovaporized. The involved nail plate may be avulsed before photovaporization is started to gain access directly to the involved nail bed material. This will speed up the treatment time.

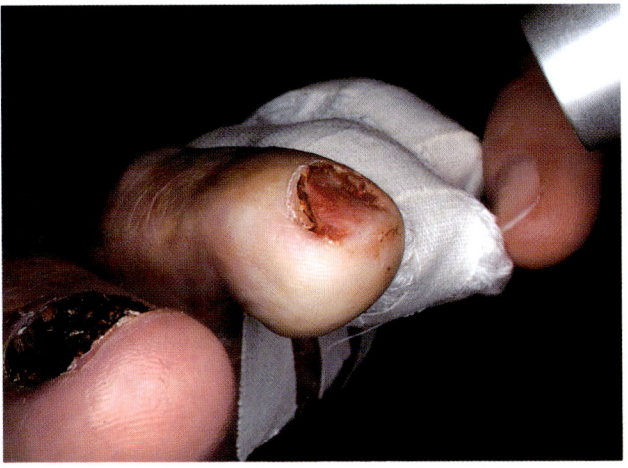

FIG. 4.19-C. The photovaporized tissue is then cureted down to the normal nail bed. If proper photovaporization is performed, the abnormal tissue will easily peel off the underlying normal nail bed.

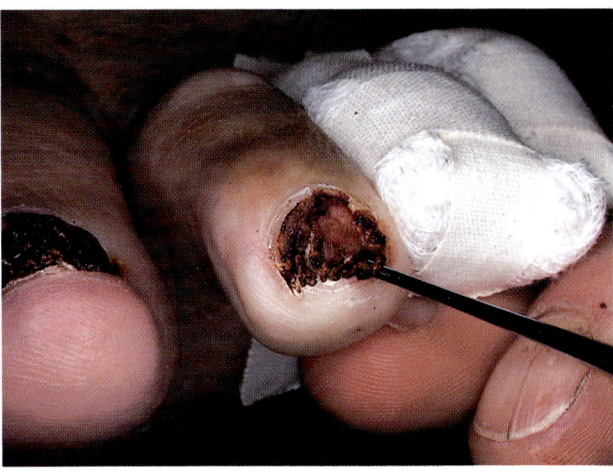

FIG. 4.19-D. If any abnormal tissue remains on the nail bed this can be vaporized with a defocused laser beam.

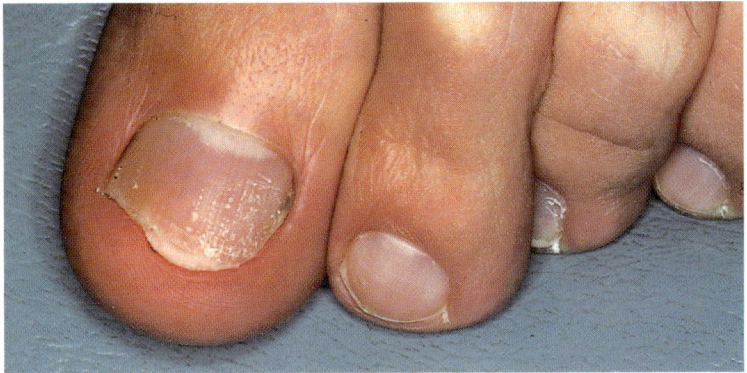

FIG. 4.19-E. Four years post-treatment. The nail plate has completely regrown and attached to the nail bed.

Case courtesy of *Elston Rothermel*, D.P.M.

CASE 4.20

Onychomycosis on the Left Great Toe

REVIEW OF CASE. This is a 56-year-old diabetic with a fungus infection on the left great toe. He was treated with oral griseofulvin by his family physician for about one year without any improvement. His initial fungus culture was negative but a culture done during laser therapy revealed dermatophyte. Since he did not want to continue taking griseofulvin, he insisted on laser therapy.

CHOICE OF LASER: CARBON DIOXIDE. Since removal of the infected area by laser may cure the lesion or reduce the course of griseofulvin therapy, the CO_2 laser was chosen. The lesion was vaporized using the CO_2 laser and combined with two months of oral griseofulvin therapy. The lesion cleared without recurrence since 1987. The CO_2 laser has an advantage in being able to work in tight locations such as the proximal nail fold.

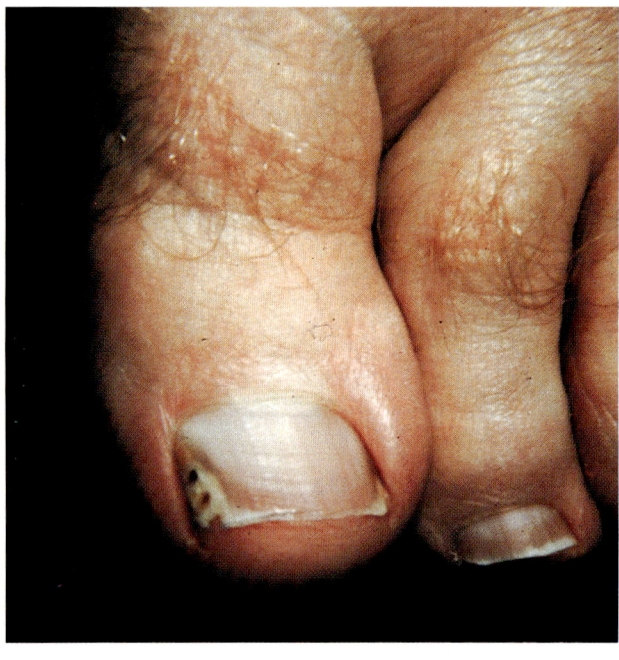

FIG. 4.20-A. Fungus infection, left great toe.

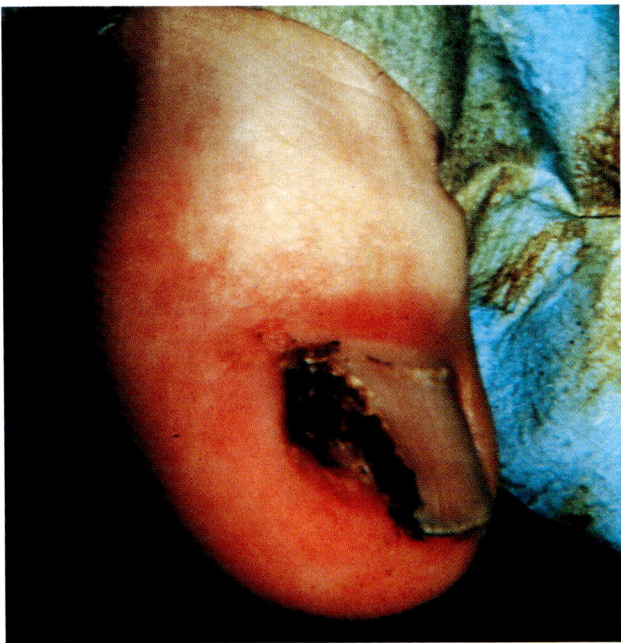

FIG. 4.20-B. Under local anesthesia, the area was cleaned with Betadine. The infected nail was cut with a nail clipper. Two cultures were done by scraping the keratin layer under the nail. The proximal nail fold was lifted and another fungus culture was done. The nail bed including the area under the proximal nail fold was vaporized with the CO_2 laser using a 5 watt defocused beam.

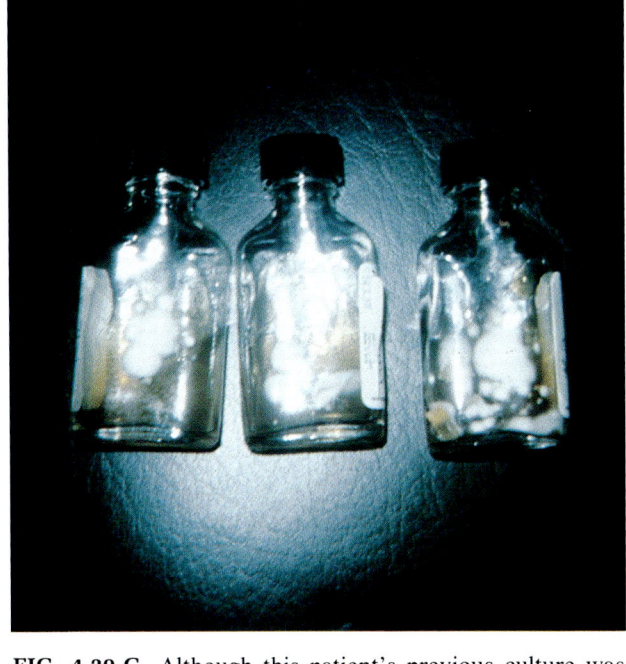

FIG. 4.20-C. Although this patient's previous culture was negative, and commonly cultures taken from the edge of the infected toe with fungi may show negative results, all three cultures taken from under the nail and from the proximal nail fold showed dermatophyte. Three cultures were done in order to find a positive one and also to determine the extent of involvement of the infection.

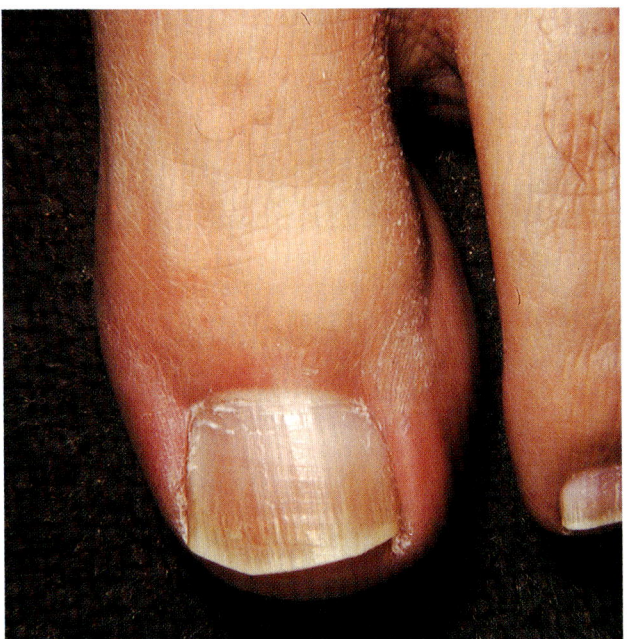

FIG. 4.20-D. Fungus infection cleared. Two years follow-up revealed no recurrence.

Case courtesy of *Syrus Rayhan,* M.D.

CASE 4.21
Pyogenic Granuloma

REVIEW OF CASE. This is a 20-year-old female who presented with a pyogenic granuloma involving the palmar surface of the left index finger of three weeks duration.

CHOICE OF LASER: TUNABLE DYE AND CARBON DIOXIDE. The patient was originally scheduled for dye laser treatment since the specificity of the yellow wavelengths for vascular lesions would provide the best results with the lowest risk and the lesion was thin enough to be treated with this modality.

However, the patient returned seven days later for the procedure and the lesion had increased in volume to 4 to 6 times its original size and was actively bleeding. Attempts to treat the lesion at this size (see Fig. A) is generally ineffective using the dye laser for a single treatment unless the energy is increased to ablative levels. An attempt was then made with 577 nm and 585 nm yellow dye laser light with a 1.0 mm spot using 0.60 watts continuous wave painting technique without success in penetrating to the deepest feeder vessels. Treatment of the patient was then switched to the CO_2 laser described in Fig. B. (A continuous wave argon laser could probably also have been used successfully.)

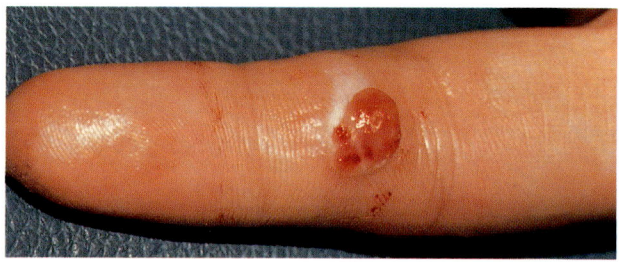

FIG. 4.21-A. Pre-treatment pyogenic granuloma.

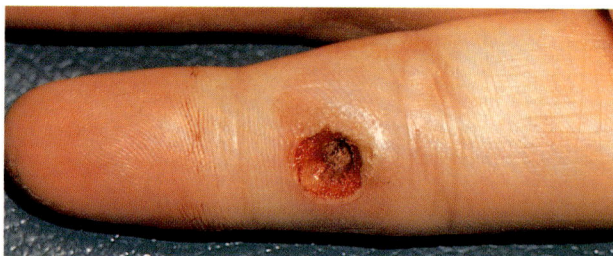

FIG. 4.21-B. Immediately after using the CO_2 laser. The lesion was excised using a 1.0 mm spot continuous wave focused CO_2 laser beam at 15 watts with loupe-assisted vision. Subsequently, vaporization and sculpting of the base was performed until the feeder vessel was sealed off using the same parameters but in a defocused mode.

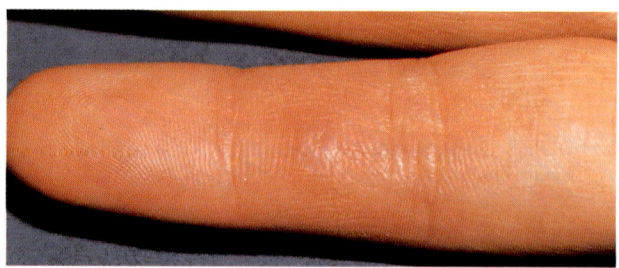

FIG. 4.21-C. The same site three weeks post-treatment.

Case courtesy of *David H. McDaniel,* M.D.

CASE 4.22
Pyogenic Granulomas Secondary to Sturge-Weber Syndrome

REVIEW OF CASE. This patient is a 32-year-old white female with Sturge-Weber sydrome. The patient's chief complaint was that of intraoral lesions, specifically a lesion located midline between her maxillary central incisors. This midline lesion kept the patient from smiling and opening her mouth in public. The patient states that the lesions appeared during a prior pregnancy. Intraoral lesions only appeared on the patient's left side; the side consistent with her port wine stain.

CHOICE OF LASER: CARBON DIOXIDE. A CO_2 laser was chosen to be used for the biopsy of her lesion and for the ablation of the rest of her lesions. The CO_2 laser has been shown to be the laser of choice for intraoral soft tissue lesions. Advantages of the laser over conventional scalpel surgery are: (i) decreased to absent surgical and post-surgical bleeding, (ii) little chance for mechanical trauma to the tissues, (iii) sterilization of the wound site, (iv) minimal swelling and scarring, and (v) probably from the patient's point of view minimal to absent post-operative pain in the majority of cases. In addition, due to the vascular nature of this type of case, hemorrhage was kept to a minimum as the patient lost less than 3 cc's of blood. Due to this type of case however, the patient was still cross-matched for blood.

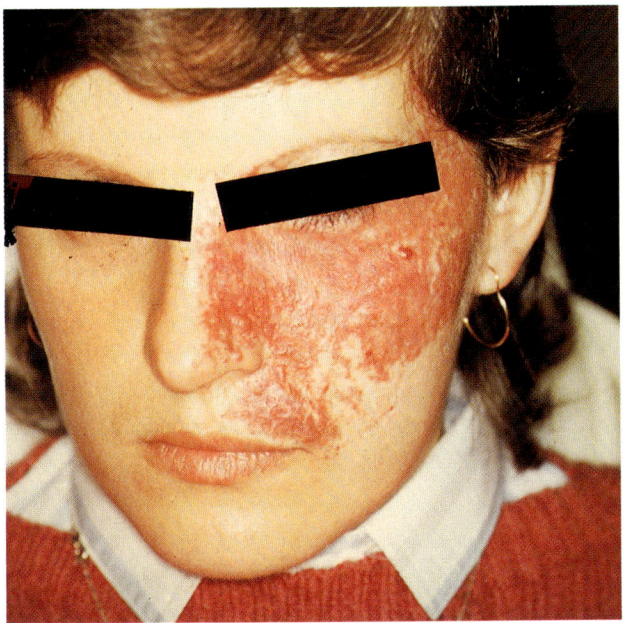

FIG. 4.22-A. A patient presenting with Sturge-Weber syndrome with intraoral involvement. Note the port wine stain following the maxillary branch of the trigeminal nerve (V2). Also, note the somber appearance on the patient's face. She would not smile due to the intraoral lesion.

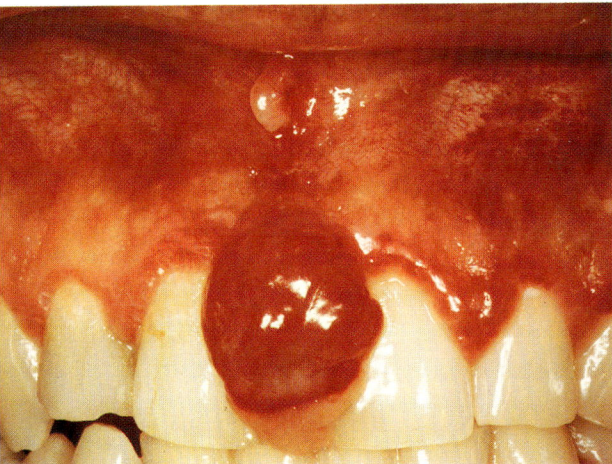

FIG. 4.22-B. Intraoral lesion present between the maxillary central incisors. Note the size and the vascular appearance of the lesion. An excisional laser biopsy was performed on this particular lesion using 10 watts of power and a focused beam. Normal margins were excised with the lesion. Biopsy showed the lesion to be a pyogenic granuloma.

Case continues on following page.

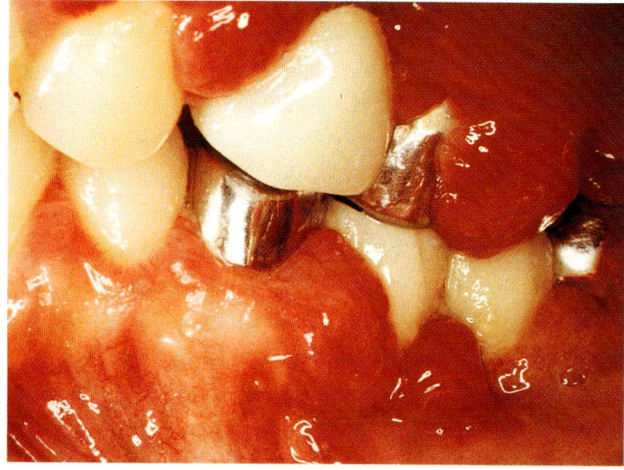

FIG. 4.22-C. Note the pyogenic masses on the buccal surfaces covering the majority of the restorations.

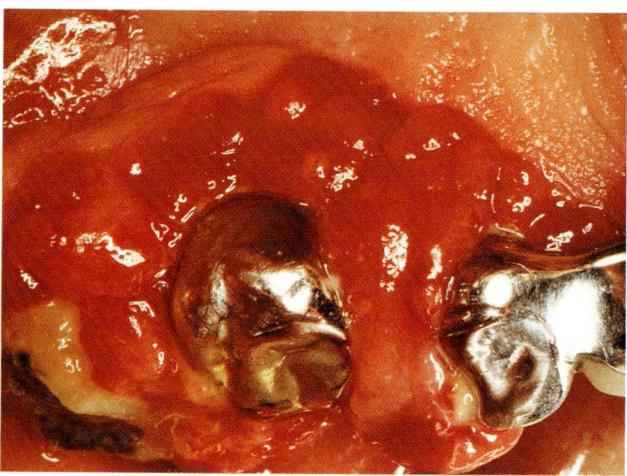

FIG. 4.22-D. An impressive pyogenic mass on the palate.

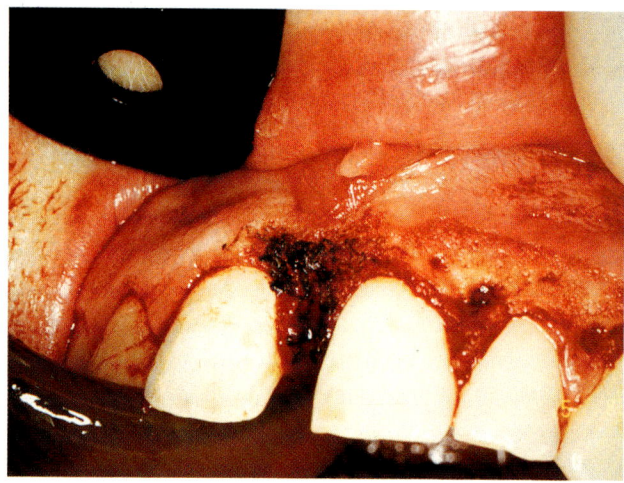

FIG. 4.22-E. Appearance of area after excisional biopsy. Using a defocused mode at 10 watts, the area is then lased to create a "char layer" to ensure a hemorrhage-free postoperative course.

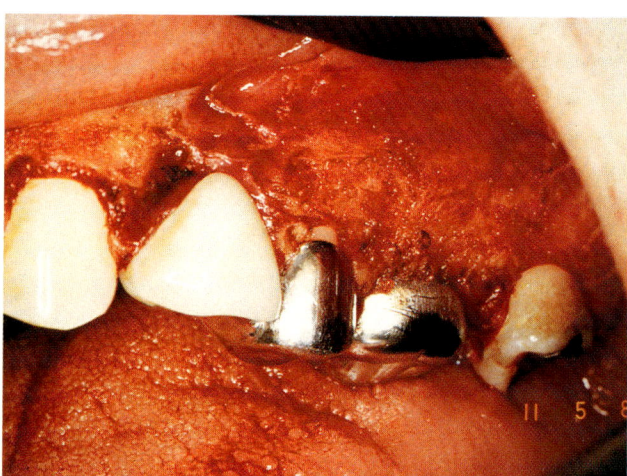

FIG. 4.22-F. Removal of the lesion from the maxillary buccal mucosa. Through this area the lesion was vaporized using 10 watts and a defocused mode. After lasing, the char layer can be wiped down to expose the underlying tissue to ensure that all of the lesion is removed. If not, further lasing and charring can be accomplished, hence a "lasing and wipedown." Removing this char layer can result in the breaking of already sealed vessels thus yielding hemorrhage. Because of this, the char layer is always placed as a final step to ensure a maximum hemorrhage-free wound. This shows the area before the final char layer is placed.

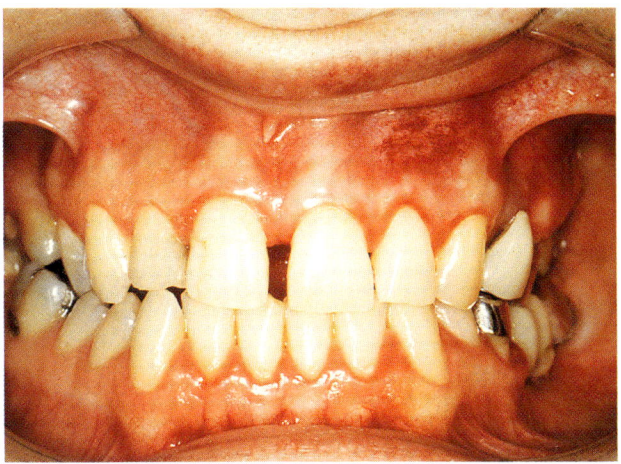

FIG. 4.22-G. The patient four months after laser surgery—maxillary incisor region.

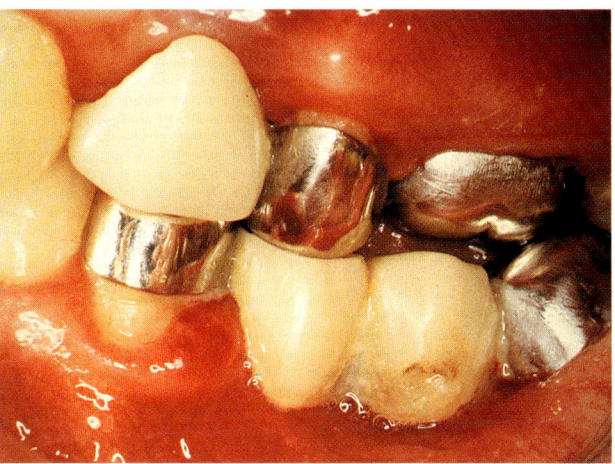

FIG. 4.22-H. The patient four months after laser surgery—maxillary and mandibular buccal region.

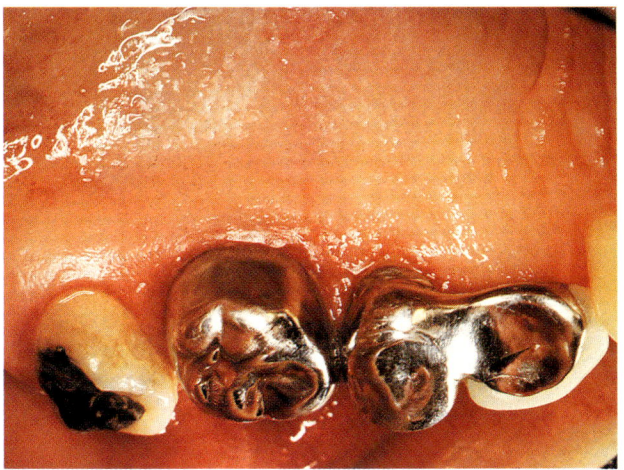

FIG. 4.22-I. The patient four months after laser surgery—maxillary palate.

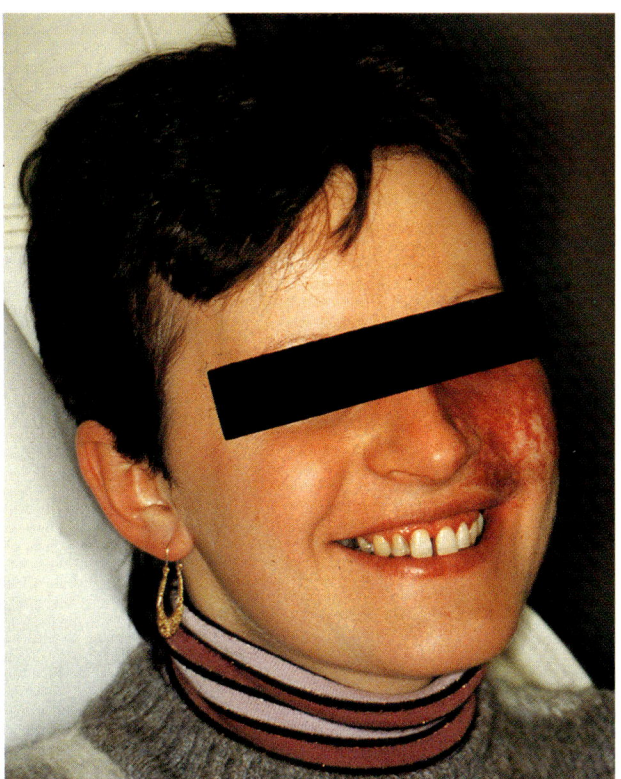

FIG. 4.22-J. The patient four months after laser surgery. Note that the patient is now willing to smile.

Case courtesy of *Robert M. Pick*, D.D.S.

CASE 4.23

Wart on the Right Index Finger

REVIEW OF CASE. This is a 32-year-old male meat cutter with a wart on his right index finger. The wart has been present for several years. The lesion has been treated several times previously with liquid nitrogen without success.

CHOICE OF LASER: CARBON DIOXIDE. The CO_2 laser was chosen to excise the wart because the combination of excision of the lesion and vaporization of the base of the lesion plus the surrounding normal looking epidermis can be accomplished successfully with this laser.

The CO_2 handpiece is held from the skin at a greater distance of focal lengths of the lens to produce the defocused beam. Before therapy, focal point or focal length can be tested on a piece of wet tongue blade by gradually withdrawing the handpiece from the wet tongue blade. Regular glasses are used for the patient and staff for eye protection and to avoid accidental burning of the cornea. A wet towel is placed around the lesion to also avoid accidental burning. Surgical gloves and mask should be used. The lesion should be marked to include a few millimeters of normal looking skin surrounding it. A defocused beam is used mostly for thin lesions and a power of 5–10 watts is usually sufficient. By holding the smoke evacuator about 2 cm from the lesion, vaporization can begin. Using a magnifier can be helpful. The char should be wiped with normal saline and a sterile cotton tip applicator. Several passes may be necessary to remove the wart. It may, at times, be difficult to decide the end points of lasering. One of the reported criteria for the determination of end points is usually to see tissue contraction, however, seeing contraction means injury to the dermis while increasing the possibility of scarring. If using this criteria, the laser should be stopped at the point where minimum contraction is seen under magnification. Most of the time after trying one or two passes on the surface of the wart, because of the heat, the lesion separates itself from the dermis and then the keratin layer or epidermis can be easily removed by using scissors or a curet. If there is a remaining wart, it is easily visible and it can be vaporized.

ADDITIONAL INFORMATION. For thick or large lesions, the excisional method is more commonly used. Making an incision around recalcitrant warts with the CO_2 laser and then peeling them off from the dermal-epidermal junction causes less scarring than with laser vaporization. I call this method "epidermal excision with peeling" or the EEP method. This technique results in much less plume emissions, is quicker to perform, and diminishes the chances of penetrating the cutaneous and subcutaneous tissue. It permits the preservation of tissue for pathologic confirmation to rule out the possibility of malignancy. Most of the time, the separated tissue guides you to the level of the invasion of the lesion. If the lesion were vaporized instead, there is a higher chance of not getting the whole lesion or that the laser may reach the fat level, especially in the case of the above patient. Figure E shows a very thin dermis at the base. Remember that the wart is in the epidermis and that it is not necessary to damage the dermis.

The edge of the separated wart shows the thick epidermis is very light purple but the dermis is more purple in color. This helps to identify the dermal-epidermal junction. Sometimes because of multiple previous therapy and previous scarring, separation of the wart is not easy. In such cases, the vaporization technique can be used.

Case courtesy of *Syrus Rayhan,* M.D.

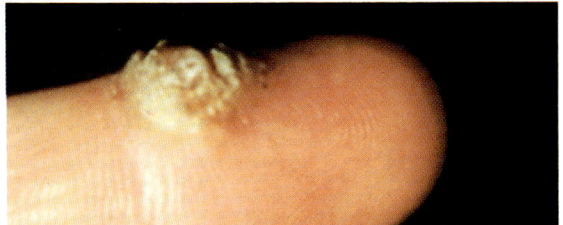

FIG. 4.23-A. Wart on the right index finger present for several years. It had been treated unsuccessfully before with liquid nitrogen and chemicals.

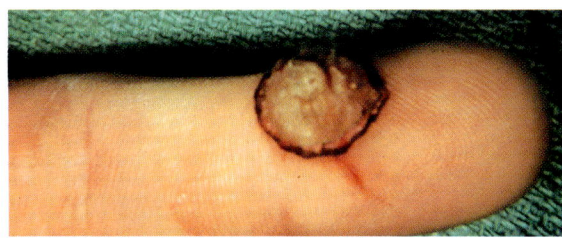

FIG. 4.23-B. 1% Xylocaine with adrenalin was injected with a dermajet with 1% Xylocaine with adrenalin in a syringe then injected for further infiltration of the base of the lesion. The border of the lesion was marked with a marker pen. Using a Sharplan 1020 unit with a 5 watts focused beam and a spot size of 0.22 mm, an incision was made around the lesion. A baby tourniquet with a clamp was used at the base of the finger to control bleeding. Note: Local anesthetic containing adrenalin should be used cautiously in areas of the body supplied by end arteries.

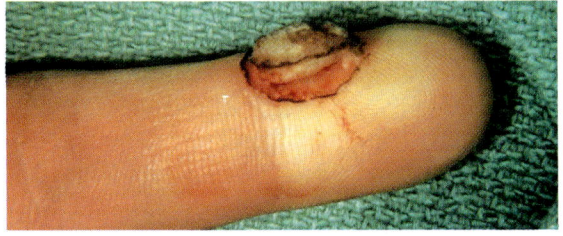

FIG. 4.23-C. With the help of 4 × 4 gauze or by using fingers, the lesion is starting to separate from the dermal-epidermal junction. Notice there is no bleeding.

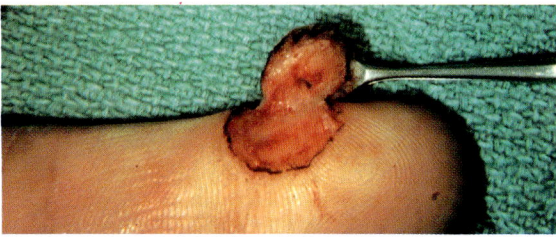

FIG. 4.23-D. The lesion is further separated from the dermal-epidermal junction with the help of forceps and gentle pulling. Notice there is no bleeding.

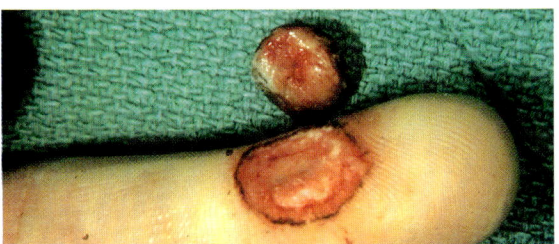

FIG. 4.23-E. Entire lesion separated from the dermal-epidermal level. There is no bleeding because of the 1% Xylocaine with adrenalin injection and the use of a tourniquet at the base of the finger. Notice the lesion has been growing inward, similar to a plantar wart. There is an atrophic thin dermis at the base. A blood vessel is seen in the middle of the dermis. The specimen was submitted to pathology for evaluation.

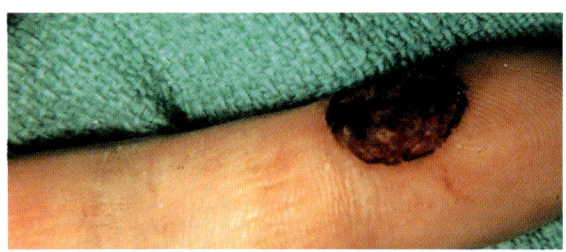

FIG. 4.23-F. The base of the lesion, which is the superficial layer of the dermis, with a few mm of normal looking epidermis surrounding the base was vaporized with a 5 watt defocused beam in order to reduce the chance of recurrence.

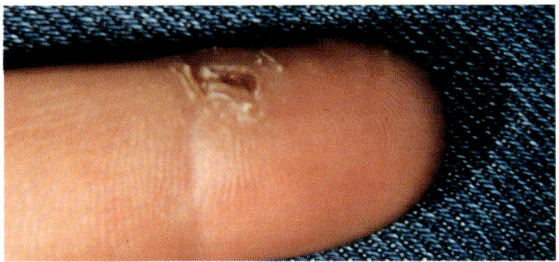

FIG. 4.23-G. Wound healing without infection or complications.

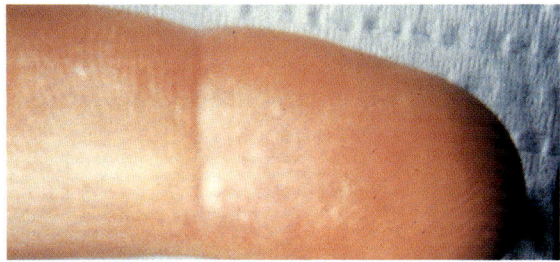

FIG. 4.23-H. Wound healed without scarring. One year follow-up shows no recurrence.

CASE 4.24
Periungual Wart

REVIEW OF CASE. This is a 24-year-old white female with a history of Hodgkin's disease, and splenectomy in December, 1985 with radiation therapy. She complained of painful periungual warts on most of her fingers. Treatment was initiated using the CO_2 with laser with a digital block. Since the patient could not tolerate local anesthesia, she was treated under general anesthesia in January, 1987. She was last examined by her oncologist during 1989 and had no sign of recurrence.

CHOICE OF LASER: CARBON DIOXIDE. A CO_2 laser was chosen because the lesions could be excised from the dermal-epidermal junction and then peeled off. Then the base of the lesion with a few millimeters of normal looking epidermis surrounding the lesion can be vaporized.

ADDITIONAL INFORMATION. A vacuum must be used for the protection of the patient and staff since it has been shown that smoke by itself may be harmful to the lungs, and there is suspicion that the smoke may contain viral particles.

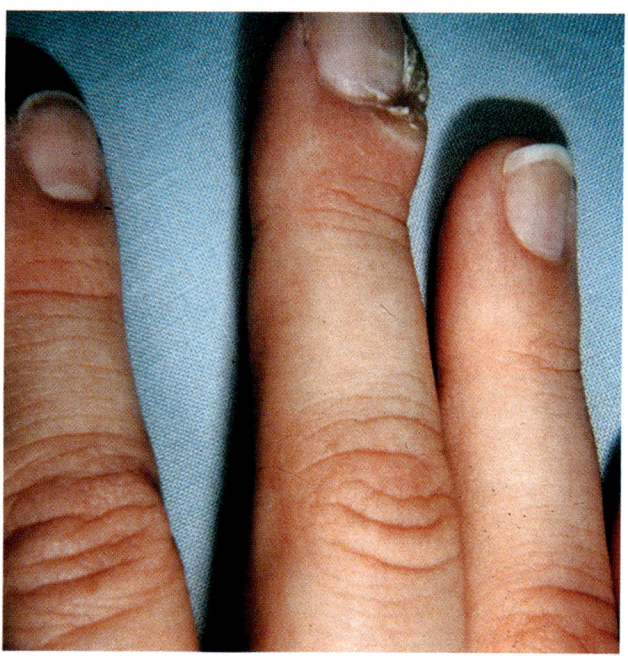

FIG. 4.24-A. Painful periungual warts involving most of the fingers.

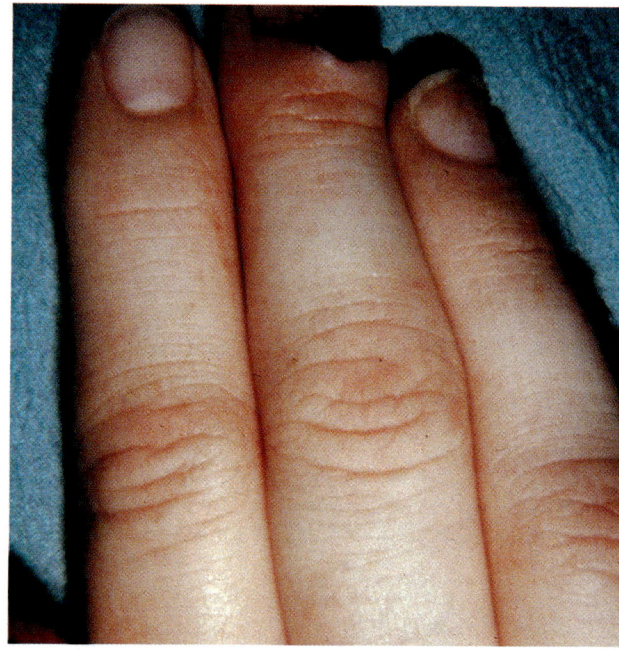

FIG. 4.24-B. Immediately after laser excision and vaporization.

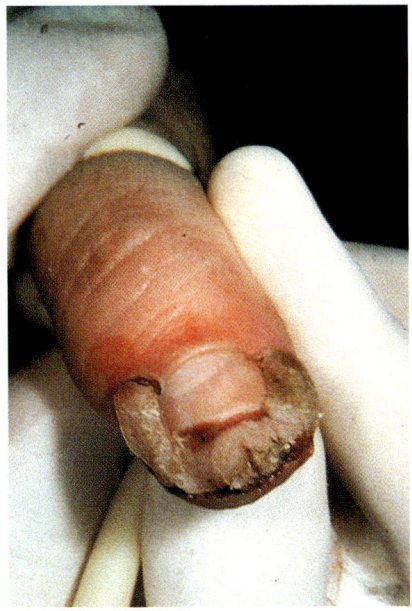

FIG. 4.24-C. Painful periungual warts on the thumb. Nail clipping was done to visualize the extent of involvement. Note that a baby tourniquet was applied on the base of the thumb with some pressure to control bleeding.

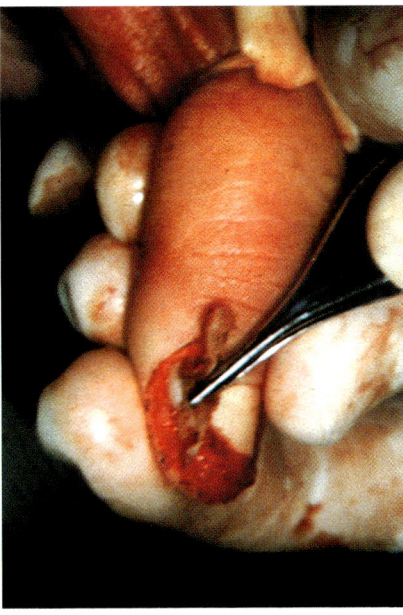

FIG. 4.24-D. An incision was made around the lesion using the CO_2 laser with a 5 watt focused beam. The wart was separated or peeled off from the dermal-epidermal level. The lesion was invading under the nail. Note excision of the lesion end point with scissors.

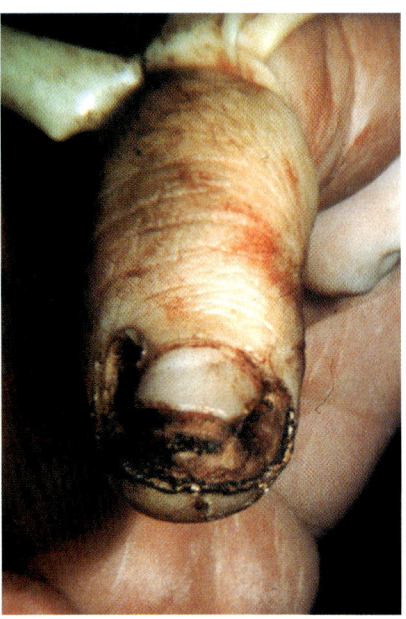

FIG. 4.24-E. The CO_2 laser was applied at the base of the lesion including a few millimeters of tissue surrounding the epidermis using a 5 watt defocused beam.

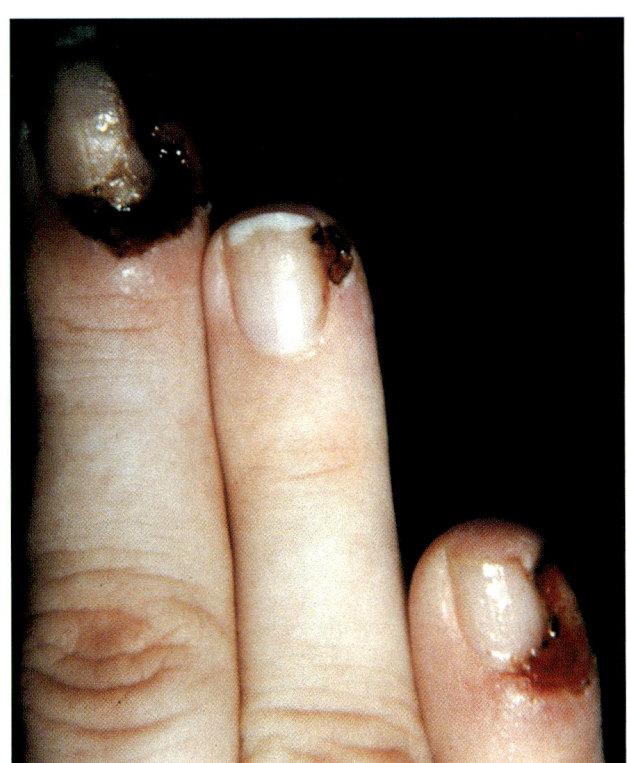

FIG. 4.24-F. Immediately following CO_2 laser excision using a 5 watt focused beam and a 0.1 mm spot size, and CO_2 laser vaporization using 8 watts.

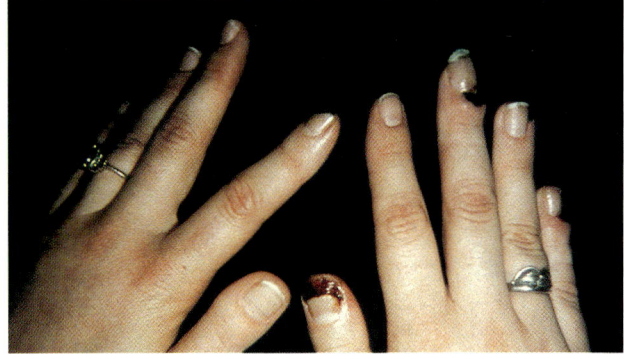

FIG. 4.24-G. One week post-operation.

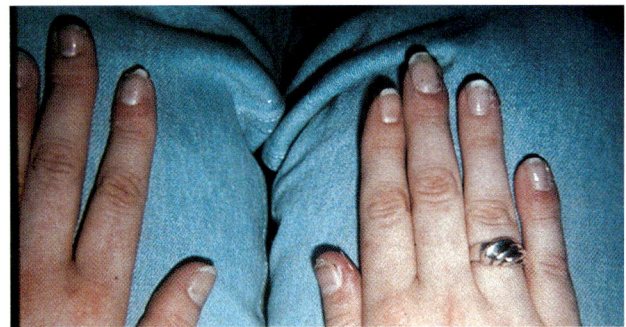

FIG. 4.24-H. Four weeks post-operation. The patient has healed without scarring and with no evidence of recurrence with up to two years of follow-up.

Case courtesy of **Syrus Rayhan,** M.D.

CASE 4.25

Periungual Wart with Invasion Under the Nail

REVIEW OF CASE. This is a 59-year-old female who was examined in June, 1987 with a five year history of a painful periungual wart with several other lesions on the fingers. The periungual lesion had been biopsied and treated five times previously with liquid nitrogen without success.

CHOICE OF LASER: CARBON DIOXIDE. The CO_2 laser was chosen because the CO_2 excision or vaporization method can be used and the rate of cure with one treatment is reported to be 80% to 95%.

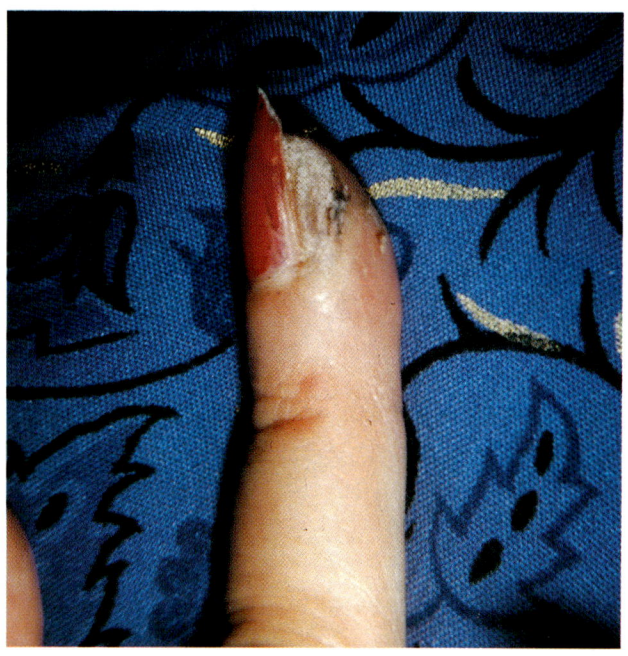

FIG. 4.25-A. Painful periungual wart on the left middle finger for five years duration. The patient had been treated unsuccessfully 5 times in the past with liquid nitrogen.

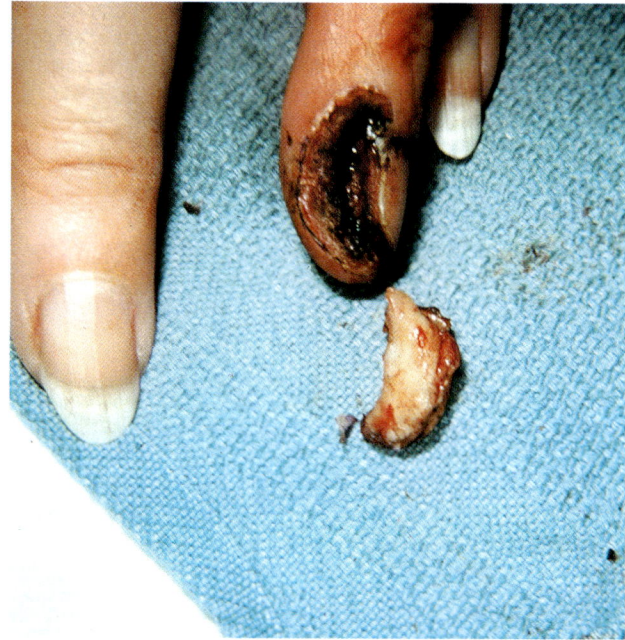

FIG. 4.25-B. A portion of the nail was removed to visualize the wart. A CO_2 laser with a 3 watt focused beam and a spot size 0.1 mm was used to make an incision around the lesion. Then with the help of 4 × 4 gauze and slight pressure, the lesion was separated from the dermal-epidermal level. The base of the lesion, which is the superficial layer of the dermis, including a few millimeters of normal looking epidermis surrounding the lesion was vaporized using the CO_2 laser with a 5 watt defocused beam in order to reduce the possibility of recurrence and to stop bleeding. A baby tourniquet with a clamp was used at the base of the finger to control bleeding. The entire lesion was submitted to pathology for evaluation.

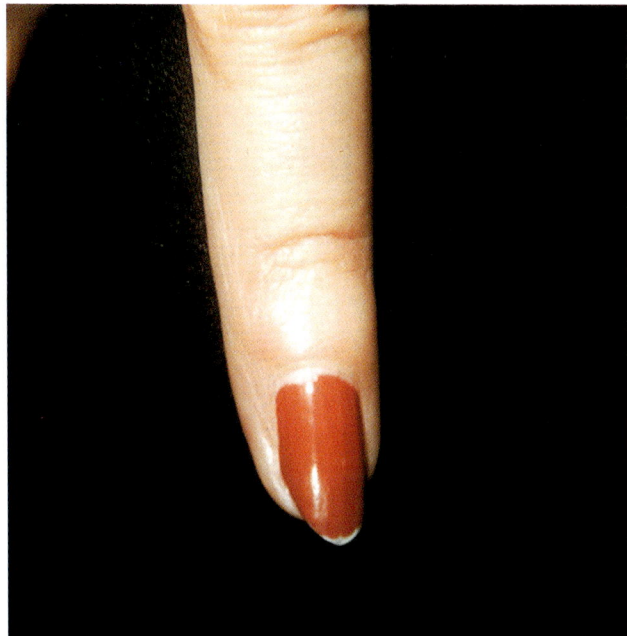

FIG. 4.25-C. The finger is completely healed without scarring and without recurrence for three years to date.

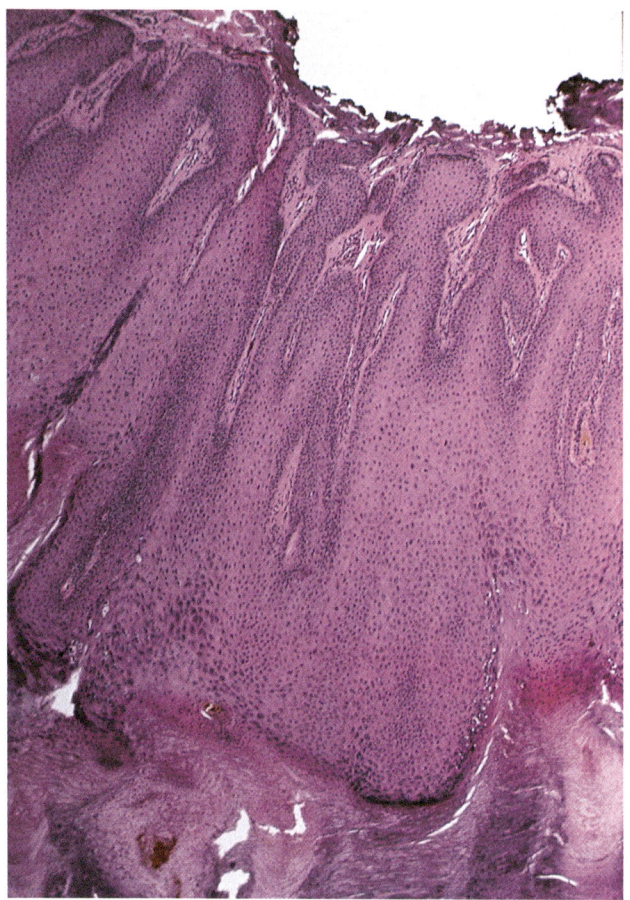

FIG. 4.25-D. Histology is preserved. There is hyperkeratosis with severe acanthosis. No change toward malignancy. The lesion has been separated from the dermal-epidermal junction with a very thin collagen layer. With this technique, the patient has minimal injury to the dermis, therefore, the chance of scarring is very small to none.

Case courtesy of *Syrus Rayhan, M.D.*

CASE 4.26
Plantar Warts, Giant, and Recalcitrant

REVIEW OF CASE. This 39-year-old white female had warts on the plantar surface of her feet for over 25 years. She had been to many physicians and had been treated by all standard and many "experimental" therapies. Immunological workup was normal, and diagnosis was confirmed by histology. Because of the size of these warts, her feet were always foul-smelling, she had diminished sensation, and wore shoes two sizes larger than normal.

CHOICE OF LASER: CARBON DIOXIDE. The CO_2 laser is a very precise method to physically destroy superficial lesions regardless of their thickness. The "end point" of treatment, a clinically wart-free plane, is more easily delineated with the bloodless field that results after CO_2 laser vaporization. Because of the thickness of her warts, a combination of CO_2 laser excision and vaporization was used. Also, because of the size of her warts, the treatment was performed in stages, using local anesthesia. CO_2 laser vaporization left a matrix of normal dermis that allowed re-epithelialization by second intention to be excellent cosmetically and functionally. Despite undergoing a total of six staged CO_2 laser procedures in separate areas, only once was there a recurrence in a previously treated site. The power setting was 25 watts using a continuous defocused beam. A focused beam (0.1 mm) was used in some areas to excise larger nodules. During the last pass, the power setting was decreased to 15 watts to minimize damage to the remaining normal dermis.

ADDITIONAL INFORMATION. The use of a posterior tibial nerve block to treat plantar warts allows a small amount of anesthetic to safely block almost the entire plantar surface. This is a much less painful injection and easily provides anesthesia for office/outpatient procedures.

To avoid excessive exposure to the potentially contaminated CO_2 laser plume, and in addition to using gloves, masks, and smoke evacuators, a combination of laser and surgical debulking is helpful. After the first pass at a high power setting, a large percentage of the wart can be debulked with a blunt curet, scissors, and forceps. This may cause a lot of capillary bleeding; a sign that wart is present. Then use the laser to vaporize more deeply. The bleeding stops once the wart is gone.

POST-TREATMENT CARE. These wounds are allowed to heal by second intention, which require antibiotic ointment (2% erythromycin in petrolatum) and a nonadherent gauze bandage. Re-epithelialization often takes six weeks and sometimes longer for larger wounds. The infection rate is low, but pain may be significant. Pain normally does not begin until three to seven days post-operatively and lasts for one to two weeks on average. Significant pain can be treated by bedrest and leg elevation, while topical anesthetics and occasionally oral analgesics such as acetaminophen with codeine are required. The amount of pain is highly variable, but patients need to be warned so that physical activity post-operatively can be appropriately planned. Recurrences of wart occur and must be monitored up to one year post-operatively, but are less common than after other surgical methods.

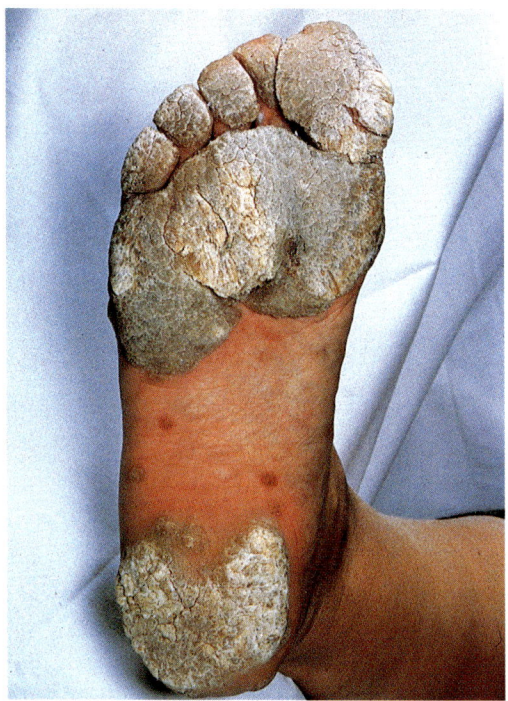

FIG. 4.26-A. Right foot pre-operation.

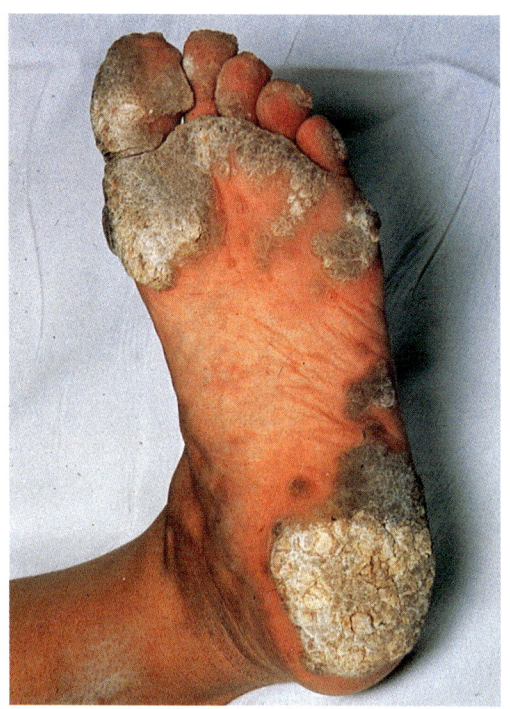

FIG. 4.26-B. Left foot pre-operation.

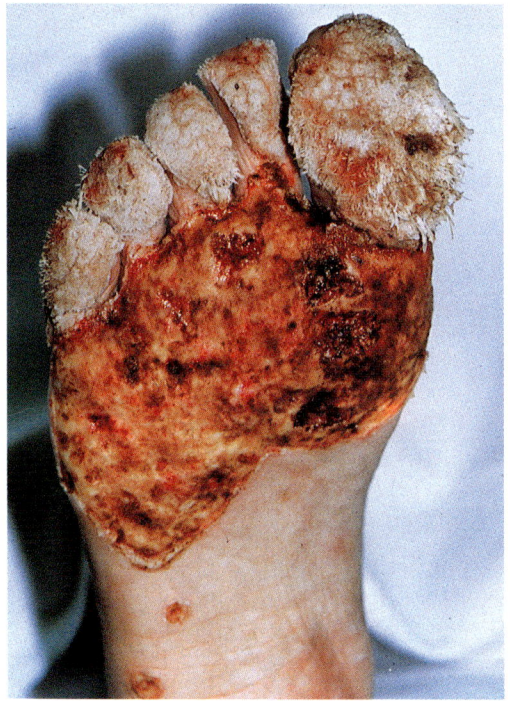

FIG. 4.26-C. Immediately postoperation; staged vaporization right metatarsal area.

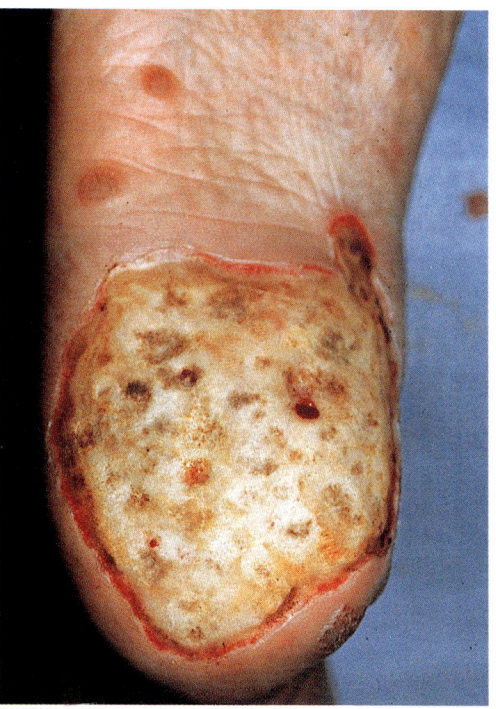

FIG. 4.26-D. Immediately postoperation; staged vaporization. Note bloodless field on right heel.

Case continues on following page.

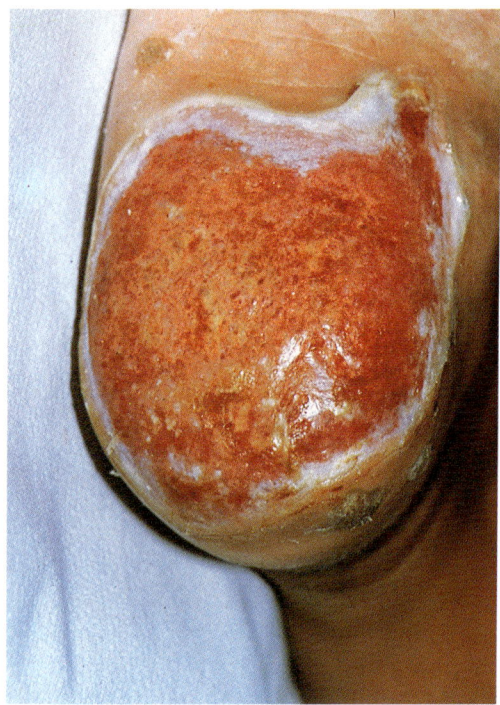

FIG. 4.26-E. Right heel 5 weeks post-operation. Granulation is complete and re-epithelialization is progressing.

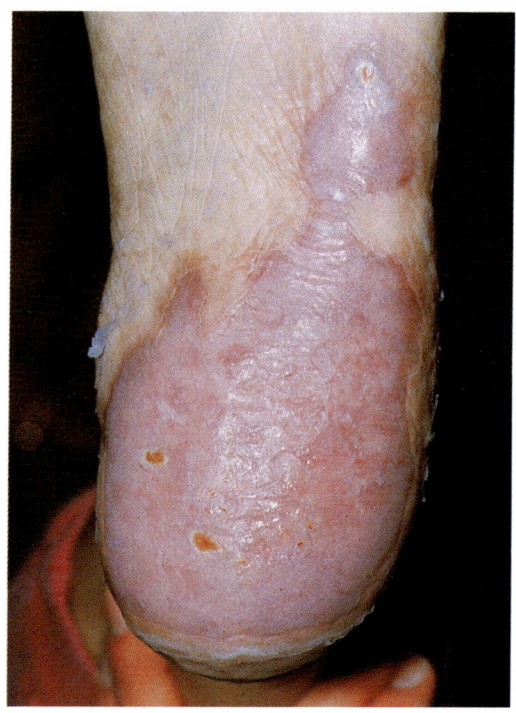

FIG. 4.26-F. Left heel 2 months post-operation; epithelialization complete but the epidermis is thin and fragile.

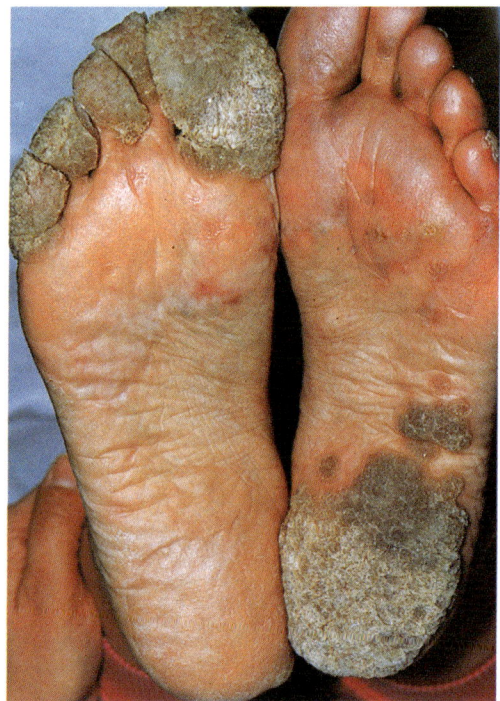

FIG. 4.26-G. Mature wound healing on right and left metatarsal area, right heel, and toes on the left foot. Scarring is imperceptible and the skin is pliable with normal function and sensation. One focus of recurrence is noted on the left proximal metatarsal area. Treatment of the left heel and toes of the right foot took two more stages with equally good results and no further recurrence to date.

Case courtesy of ***Randall K. Roenigk***, M.D.

CASE 4.27

Plantar Wart

REVIEW OF CASE. This is a 34-year-old female with a three year history of painful plantar wart. This lesion had been treated 3 times previously with liquid nitrogen and electrocautery without success. The patient was having difficulty wearing shoes comfortably and had chronic drainage from the warts.

CHOICE OF LASER: CARBON DIOXIDE. The CO_2 was chosen to photovaporize this plantar wart. It has been shown that the laser is able to successfully treat intractable plantar warts that have been unsuccessfully treated by other methods of treatment. The high heat of the laser sterilizes the viral particles and prevents recurrence. The fact that the CO_2 laser seals small lymphatics and nerve endings also provides more comfortable wound healing with less pain and edema and patients are able to walk more comfortably in a short period of time.

POST-TREATMENT CARE. A mild compression dressing is applied to the treatment area. Use a nonadherent dressing material with an antibacterial cream. Keep dressing in place 24 hours before patient reapplies a similar dressing daily until healed. Instruct patient to keep the dressing off at night as soon as minimal drainage is present. This allows faster healing to occur by allowing the wound to dry.

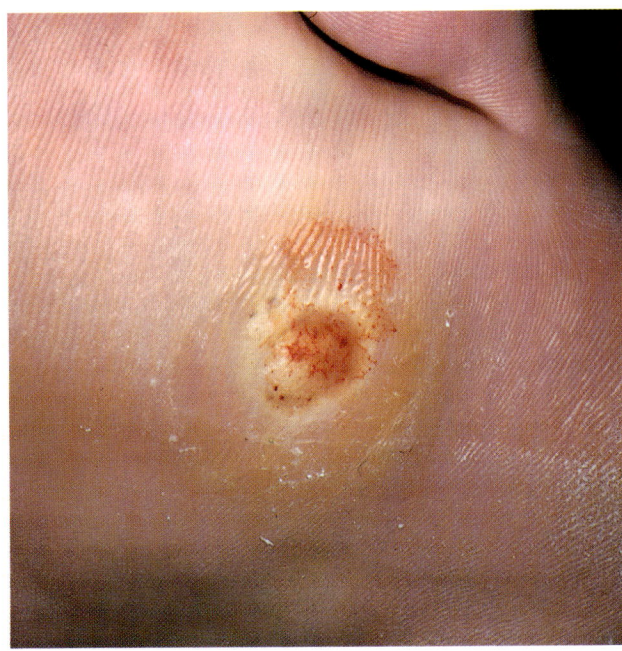

FIG. 4.27-A. Chronic non-healing plantar wart that is draining and has been treated 3 times unsuccessfully in the past with liquid nitrogen and cautery.

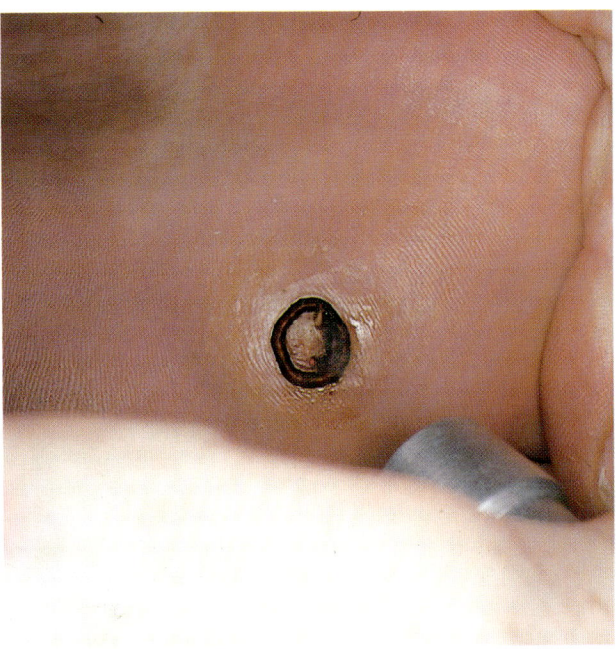

FIG. 4.27-B. Using a 10 watt focused 1 mm CO_2 laser beam, 2 to 3 mm around the wart of normal skin is circumscribed.

Case continues on following page.

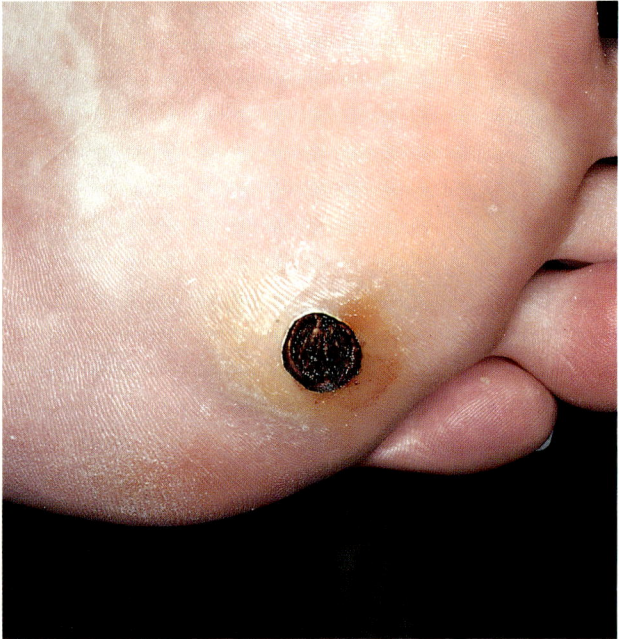

FIG. 4.27-C. The entire wart tissue is then photovaporized using a focused laser beam and a circular movement used from the periphery to center of the wart. This produces a constant depth of tissue destruction by using the laser beam with a constant speed.

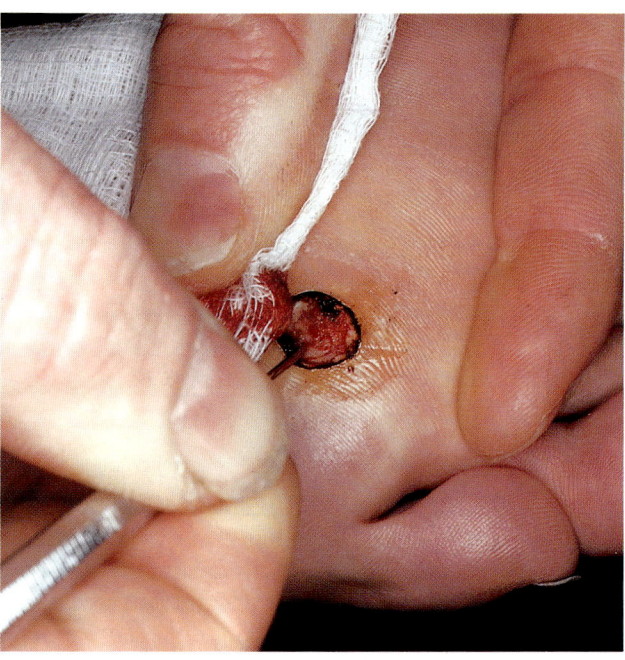

FIG. 4.27-D. All charred debris is gently removed with a curet. Any further gritty granular or bubbly material is further photovaporized with the defocused laser. Curet down to the superficial fascia which is easily identified just deep to the capsule of the wart. There is no need to extend into the subcutaneous fat. If the subcutaneous fat is exposed this will lead to potential scar formation.

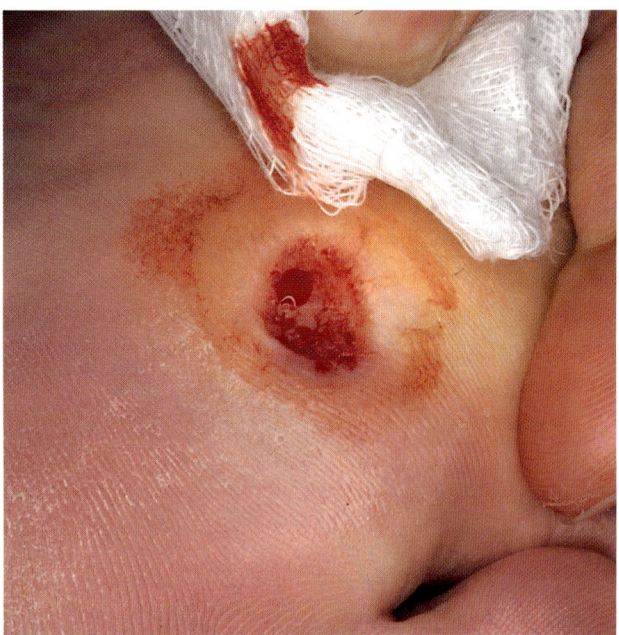

FIG. 4.27-E. At the conclusion of the procedure, there is a clear clean superficial fascia and no residual wart tissue. A central vessel may bleed a little and this can be cauterized by a defocused laser.

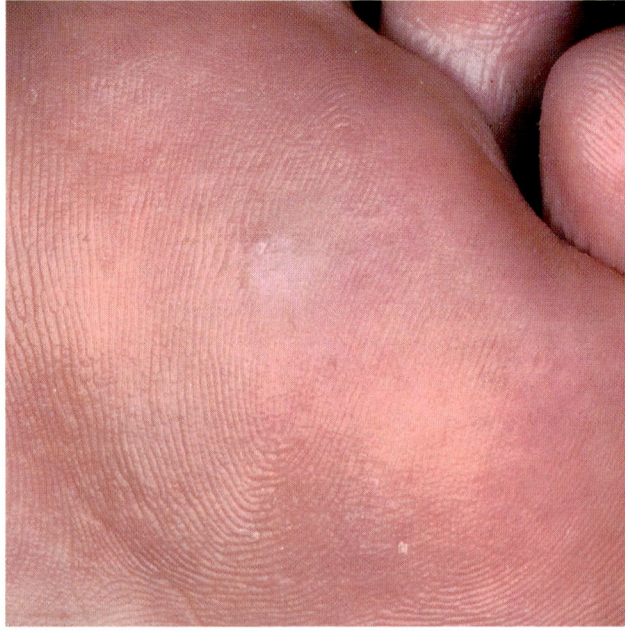

FIG. 4.27-F. The foot is completely healed after six months without scarring and without evidence of residual wart.

Case courtesy of *Elston Rothermel*, D.P.M.

CASE 4.28
Plantar Wart

REVIEW OF CASE. This patient is a 43-year-old male with a 20 year history of painful plantar warts on a large area of his left foot. The lesions had been treated in the past with drugs, liquid nitrogen, and dry ice without success. The pain was so severe that the patient had difficulty wearing shoes.

CHOICE OF LASER: CARBON DIOXIDE. This patient received other treatments for a long time without any success. Treatment using the CO_2 laser proved successful. The CO_2 laser has excellent vaporizing and hemostatic effects, and the high heat of the laser sterilizes the virus effectively and prevents recurrence. Post-operative swelling and pain are minimal. After treatment, the patient was able to put on shoes and walk more comfortably.

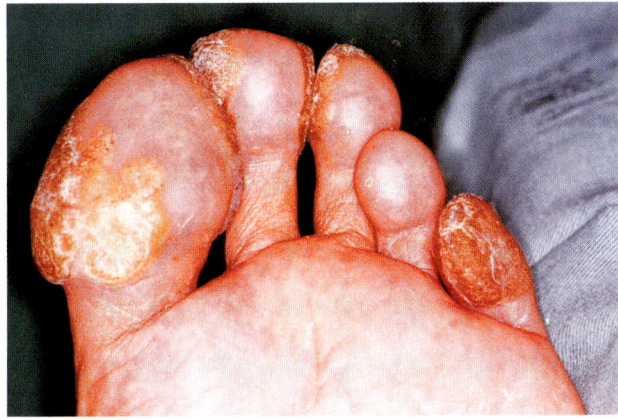

FIG. 4.28-A. Extremely painful warts are seen covering a wide area on the left foot, and on the first, second, third, and fifth toes.

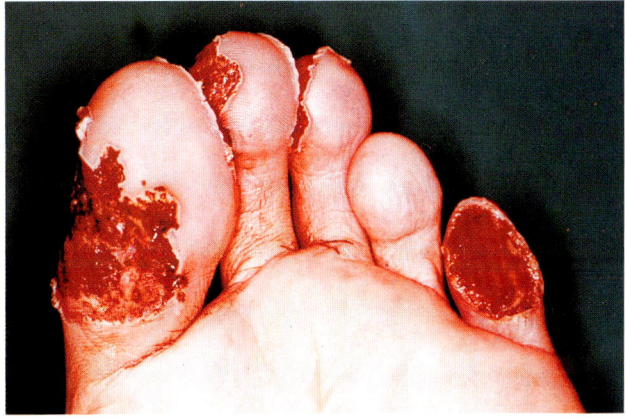

FIG. 4.28-B. Immediately after CO_2 laser treatment.

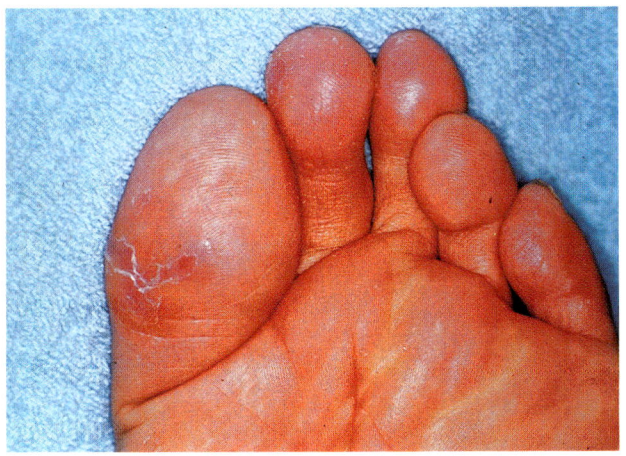

FIG. 4.28-C. Six months after CO_2 laser irradiation. The foot is healed completely, and the scars are barely noticeable.

Case courtesy of *Hiroto Yamada*, M.D., *Taichin Morita*, M.D., *Muneo Miyasaka*, M.D., *Ryuzaburo Tanino*, M.D., *and Mitsuhiro Osada*, M.D.

CASE 4.29

Decorative Tattoo

REVIEW OF CASE. This is a 28-year-old white female with several professional tattoos on her upper back. The tattoo in question was multi-colored and had been present for approximately ten years. The patient sought consultation regarding tattoo removal.

CHOICE OF LASER: CARBON DIOXIDE. The CO_2 laser vaporization was chosen to treat this tattoo. Laser vaporization permits complete pigment removal in a single session, based on optimal pigment visualization due to the blood-free field produced by laser therapy. The CO_2 laser not only seals blood vessels but also small lymphatics and nerve endings, giving a more comfortable wound as compared to more traditional methods such as dermabrasion or salabrasion.

Tattoo removal is achieved using either continuous emission or superpulsed settings in a vaporizational mode. The superpulsed technique was used in this case. High peak powers of short exposure duration are produced which theoretically provide less nonspecific thermal injury and the potential for less scarring. We used an average power of 5 watts with a pulse width of 300 microseconds and a repetition rate of 100 Hertz. The spot size was 2 mm. Charred tissue is removed after each pass with hydrogen peroxide. This tattoo required six passes to achieve a pigment-free field. The cosmetic result is a flat non-tender scar that is very acceptable, especially in areas under tension where other techniques may give a symptomatic stretched or hypertrophic scar.

POST-TREATMENT CARE. The patient is instructed to cleanse the wound twice daily to avoid crust formation with 3% hydrogen peroxide followed by application of a thin layer of antibiotic ointment and a non-stick dressing. Avoidance of sun exposure is stressed. The patient is seen one week post-operatively. Complete healing occurs in approximately six to eight weeks.

ADDITIONAL INFORMATION. If a tattoo has a distinctive shape or name, removal must include blending and contouring of the margins so that the scar won't duplicate the tattoo. Similarly, it is important to remove pigment from the "side walls" of the wound bed to prevent shadowing of the tattoo. Small individual flecks of pigment that are left in the base of the wound bed will be extruded during the inflammatory phase of healing.

All tattoo removal procedures leave scars and this needs to be stressed during the consultation as many patients have misconceptions regarding laser therapy.

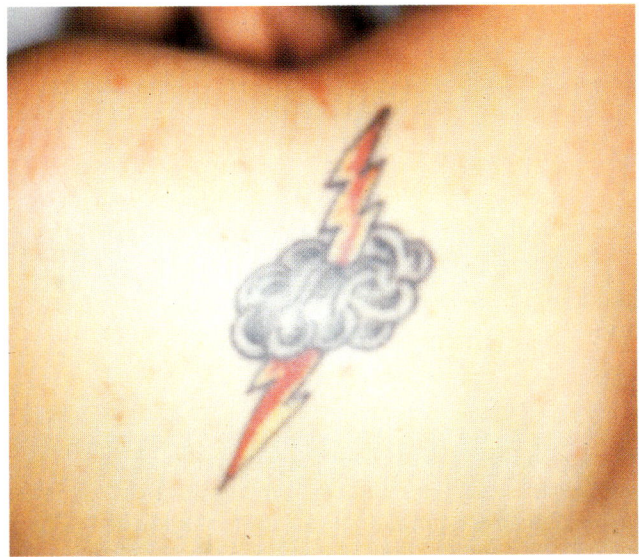

FIG. 4.29-A. Tattoo prior to removal.

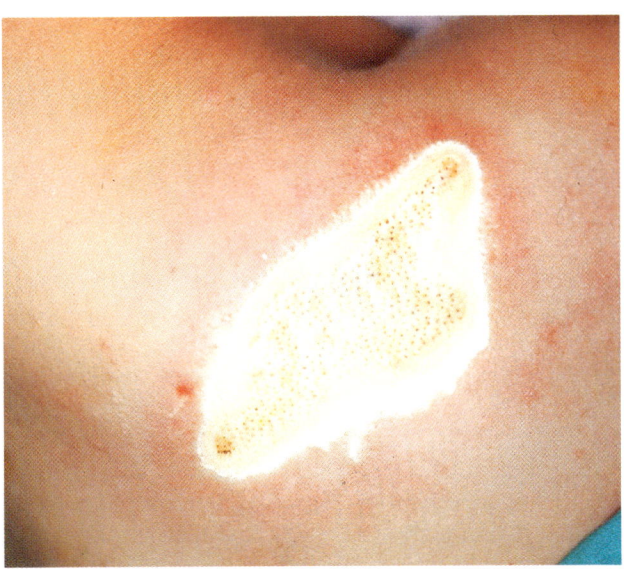

FIG. 4.29-B. Wound bed shown immediately post-vaporization. Essentially all pigment is removed. Darker tattoo pigment was at deeper dermal plane as seen.

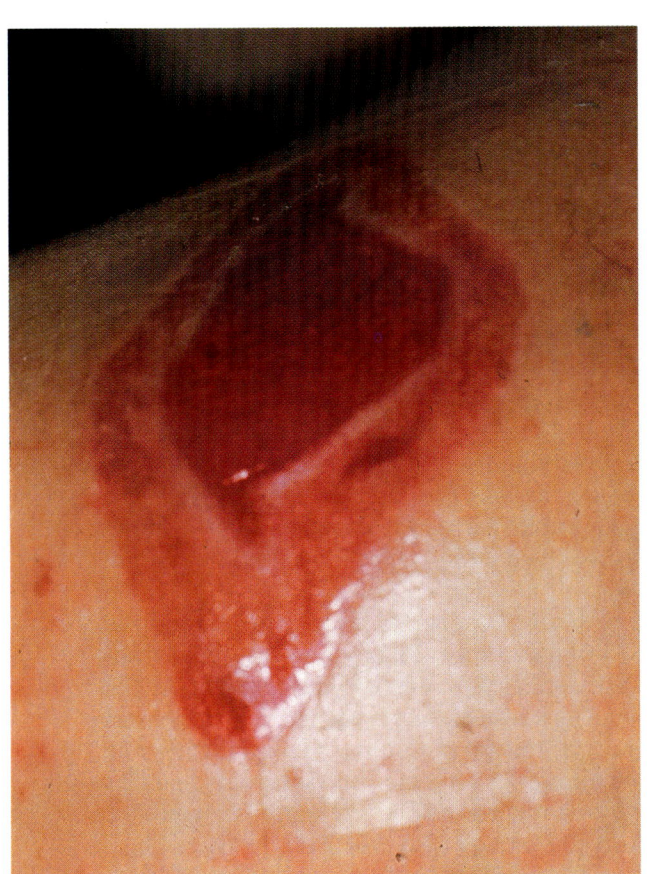

FIG. 4.29-C. Lesion seen at one month following vaporization. Note the clean, flat granulation tissue.

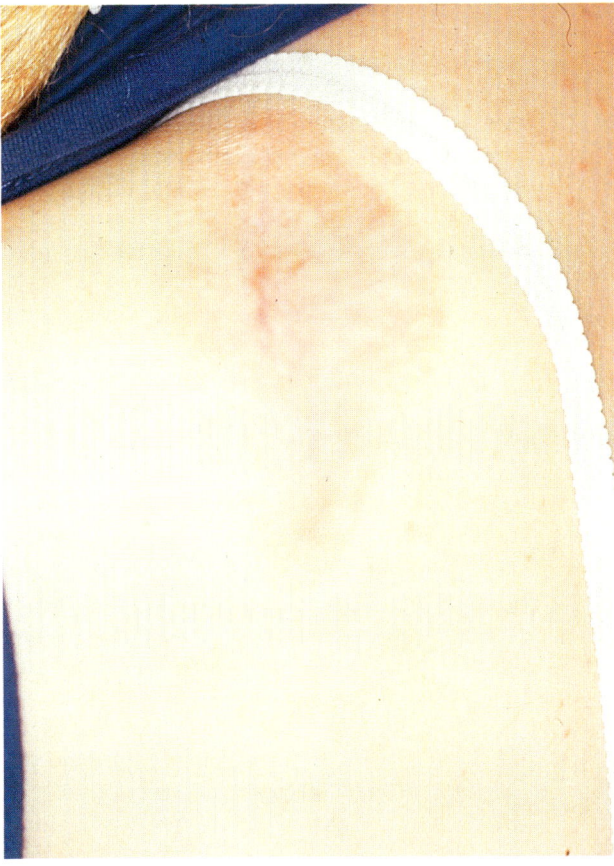

FIG. 4.29-D. Resultant scar seen six months post-operation. Scar remains flat with no residual pigment.

Case courtesy of **S. Teri McGillis,** M.D., and **Philip L. Bailin,** M.D.

CARBON DIOXIDE LASER

CASE 4.30
Decorative Tattoo

REVIEW OF CASE. This 32-year-old female had multiple professional tattoos of a long-standing duration. It was stressed pre-operatively that the tattoo would be traded for a scar and the resulting scar could possibly be markedly disfiguring.

CHOICE OF LASER: CARBON DIOXIDE. While many different types of lasers may be used in treatment of decorative tattoos and poor to excellent results can be obtained from any of them, I prefer the CO_2 laser and feel it is consistently easier and more predictable in its use and the results are usually better than with other lasers. The goal of treatment should be to have absolutely no residual pigment (ghosting) and a minimum amount of scar. The CO_2 laser can be more precisely utilized and the control of heat made with more certainty. It allows more dermis to be left behind between the spots of pigmentation than any of the other lasers.

ADDITIONAL INFORMATION. Unwanted heat is the most frequent side affect of this surgery and the major cause for hypertrophic and undesirable scars. The entire area should be iced with crushed ice in a sterile plastic bag for at least ten minutes prior to treatment. Only a small area should be treated and then immediately re-iced. While the initial area is being cooled, a secondary area can be treated. It is easy for the surgeon to be overly concerned with the laser treatment of the tattoo and forget the importance of icing the area. Because of this, the scrub nurse or assistant is informed beforehand to remind the surgeon frequently to move out of the way to allow the area to be iced.

Anesthesia may be local anesthesia, regional block, or general anesthesia depending on the location.

The operating microscope is always used. This allows the surgeon to use his intrinsic muscles, as opposed to the large muscles of the forearm, thereby giving marked improvement of control. It allows magnification, thereby increasing precision and it gives absolute control of the spot size and resultant power density for more predictable results.

A 2 mm spot size is selected with a power window varying from 16 to 28 watts depending on the location on the body and the water content of the tissue. The laser is initially used in a continuous mode, airbrushing over the involved tattooed area in a very fast manner, lasering both the tattooed area and the non-tattooed area to end up in a "feathering" appearance. It is important not to simply create just a ghost image of the tattoo.

After the tattoo is vaporized, it should be wiped with a wet sponge to remove the carbonized tissue. The power setting should be adjusted so that it takes approximately five episodes of airbrushing the tissue with the laser and wiping it with a wet gauze to end up with removal of 60% of the pigment. Once approximately 60% of the pigment has been removed, individual pigment dots will be seen in the tissue. It is usually appropriate at this point to turn the magnification up so as to appreciate the normal untattooed dermis remaining between the very small tiny spicules of pigment. The laser should then be turned down to the minimum spot size (approximately 0.2 to 0.4 mm). Because of the increased power density the power also will have to be reduced markedly. Continuous mode should be discontinued at this point and intermittent impulses of laser energy beamed at each individual spicule of pigment. The goal at this point is to totally eliminate all the tiny spots of pigment while allowing every possible bit of dermis between the spicules to remain. Extreme control of unwanted heat is important at this stage to avoid damaging the tiny dermal appendages between the points of laser impaction. Superpulse, if available, will decrease the overall heat generated.

At the end of the procedure, the area is treated with an antibiotic ointment such as gentamicin and the patient is instructed to keep the wound meticulously clean.

The final results are dependent on absolute control of unwanted heat, as well as the tissue that is left behind. If all of the dermis is removed uniformly, the result is usually too deep an injury in the skin and a bad scar will result. The usual result is a scar with pigmentation and texture with a variation from normal, but not a hypertrophic scar.

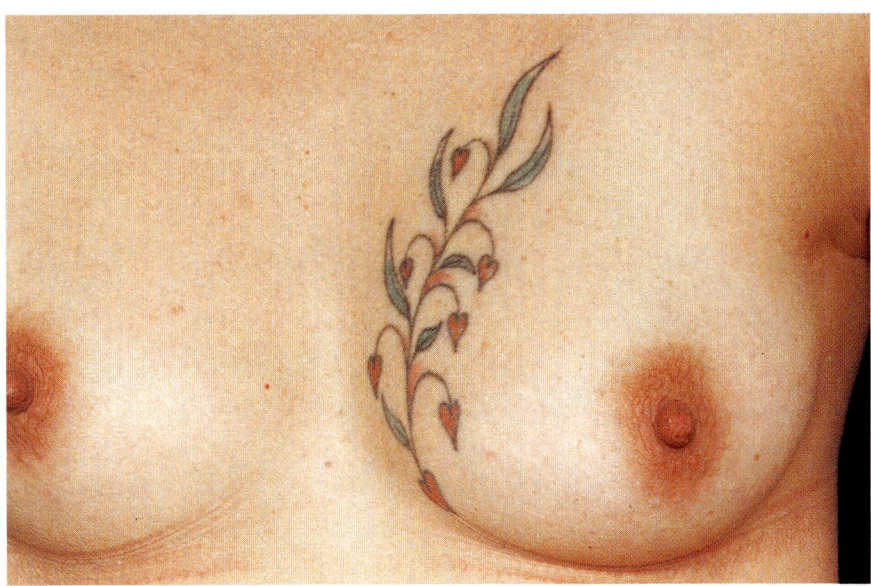

FIG. 4.30-A. Note the professional tattoo on the medial upper aspect of the left breast, an area well known for the development of hypertrophic scars.

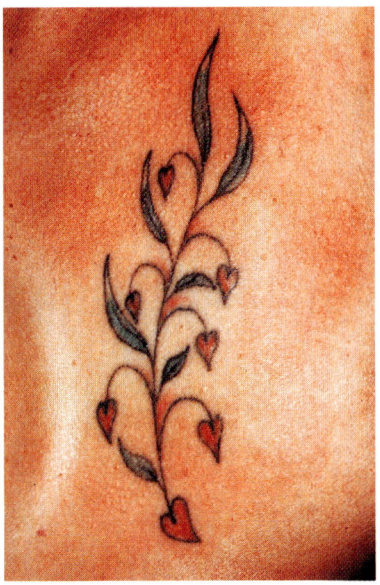

FIG. 4.30-B. Note the red erythema of the skin after ten minutes of cooling with ice bags immediately prior to surgery.

Case continues on following page.

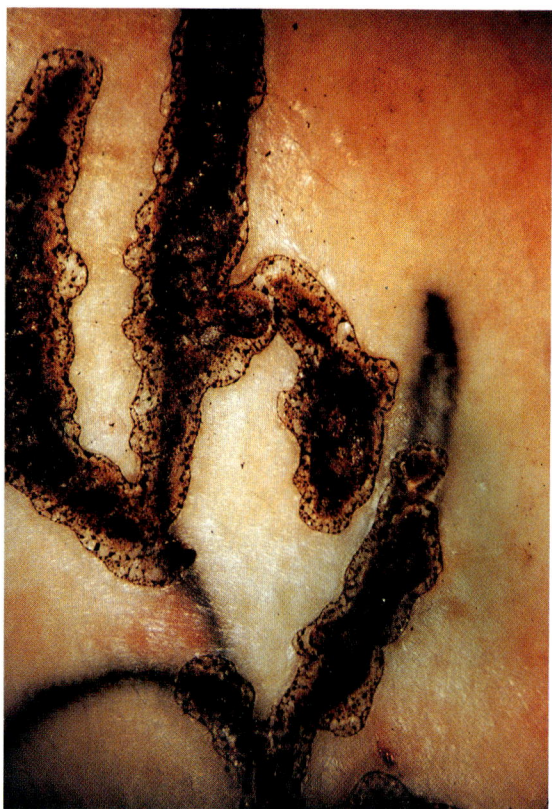

FIG. 4.30-C. This is a magnified image of the carbonization after the entire tattoo has been lasered.

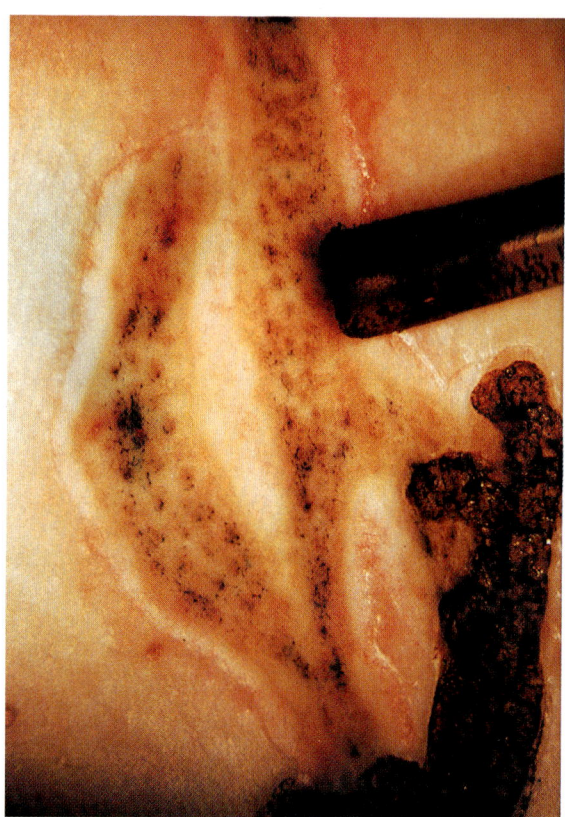

FIG. 4.30-D. Approximately 60% of the pigmentation has been removed. High power magnification shows the tiny spicules of pigment with totally normal dermis remaining between the spicules of pigment.

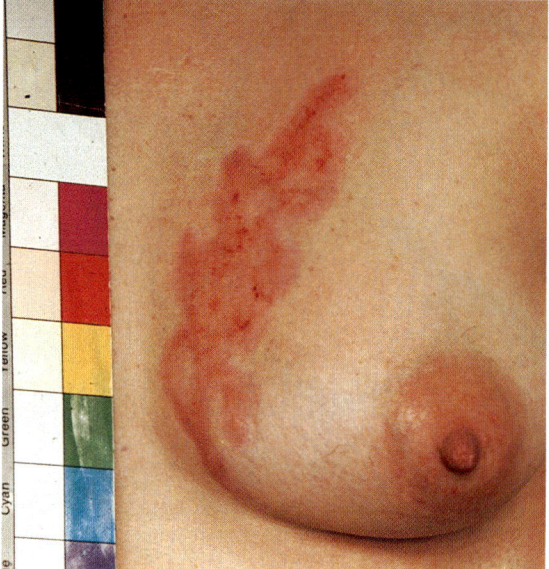

FIG. 4.30-E. Two months after surgery, erythema, and slight scar hypertrophy can be seen.

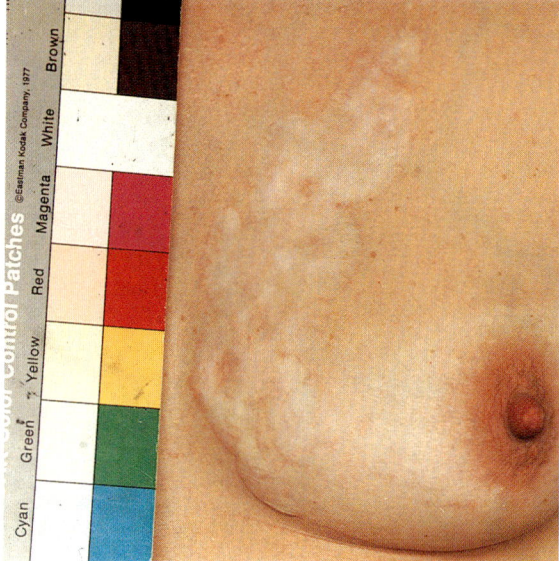

FIG. 4.30-F. One and a half years later, there is residual hypopigmentation and texture change but no evidence of scar contracture, ghosting of the original tattoo or scar hypertrophy. While some tattoo scars may be virtually invisible, this is the more routine type of post-operative scar.

Case courtesy of *Darrell L. Henderson*, M.D.

CASE 4.31
Decorative Tattoo

REVIEW OF CASE. This 26-year-old female desired removal of a home-made india ink tattoo of the left deltoid area.

CHOICE OF LASER: CARBON DIOXIDE. The CO_2 laser has no color specificity and is absorbed nonselectively by pigmented and non-pigmented tissue with a high water content such as skin which is composed of 80% to 95% water. With each successive pass of the laser over the area, a selective layer by layer removal of a 30–100 μm segment is accomplished. The high heat of the laser (70–100°C) changes the water in the cells to steam causing ejection of the solid component and consequent tissue vaporization with virtually no damage to surrounding tissue. Mechanical debridement of each char layer with a saline or hydrogen peroxide soaked gauze or applicator removes each layer until all pigment is removed down to the upper layers of the dermis. The result is a re-epithelialization with removal of tattoo pigment and preservation of near-normal skin color and texture. The laser is used in a continuous mode with 10–20 watts of defocused power in a rapid "paint brush" manner.

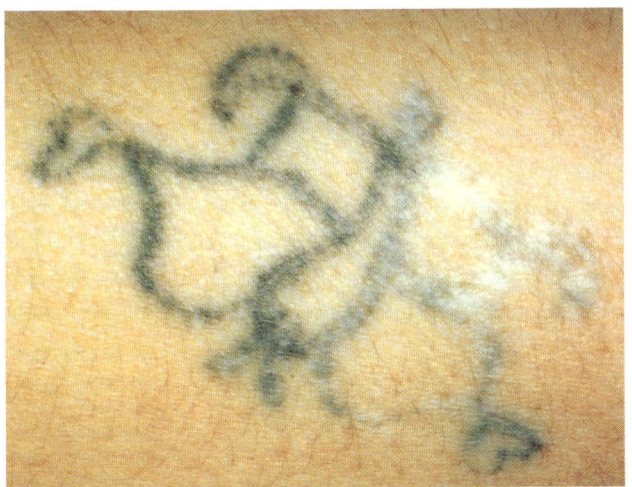

FIG. 4.31-A. Home-made tattoo of forearm prior to treatment.

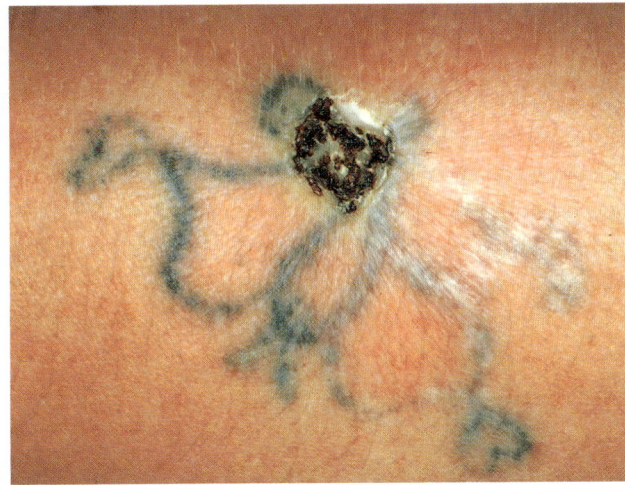

FIG. 4.31-B. Test patch of superior portion.

Case continues on following page.

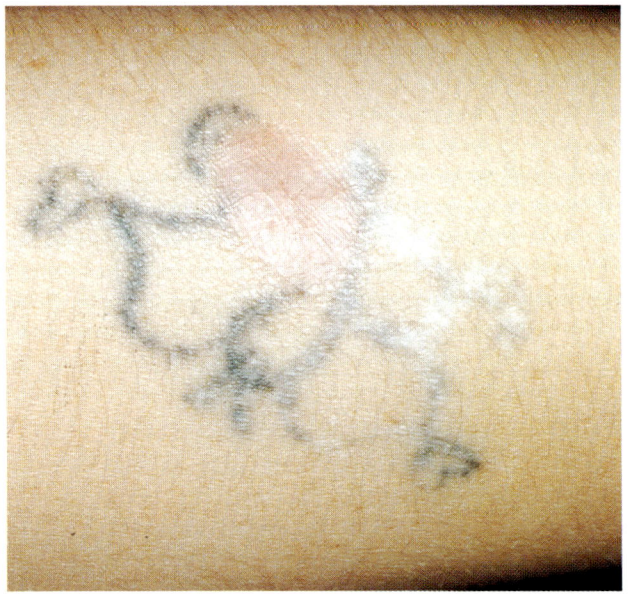

FIG. 4.31-C. Satisfactory healing of test area after ten weeks with pigment removal and no hypertrophic scarring.

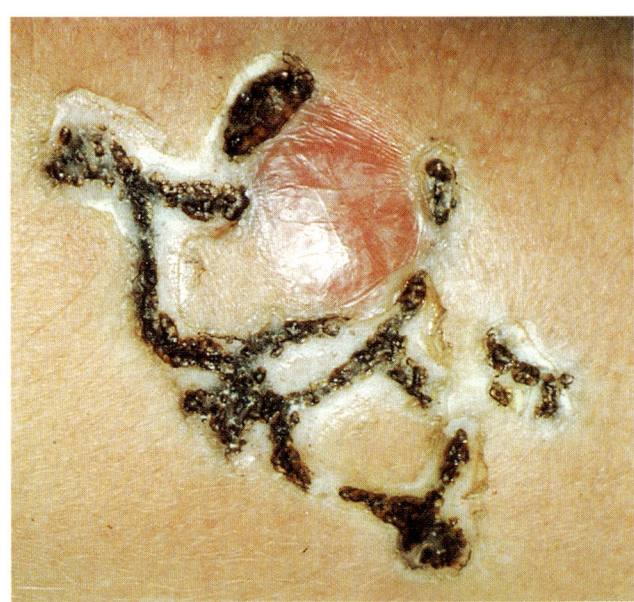

FIG. 4.31-D. Remainder of tattoo is treated.

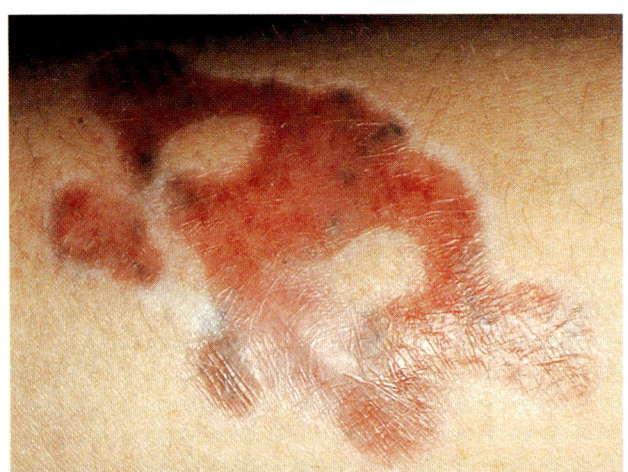

FIG. 4.31-E. Result after eight weeks.

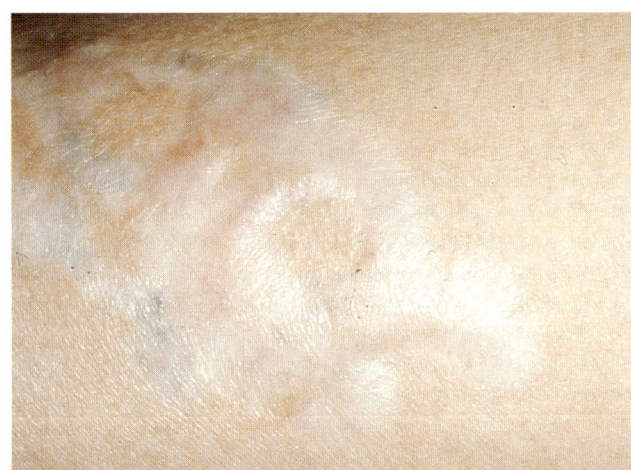

FIG. 4.31-F. Final result after six months with good result of healing, absence of almost all pigment, but permanent residual skin texture and color change.

Case courtesy of *David B. Apfelberg*, M.D.

CASE 4.32
Decorative Tattoo

Comparison of Argon and CO₂ Lasers

REVIEW OF CASE. This 34-year-old male desired removal of a home-made india ink tattoo of the left deltoid area.

CHOICE OF LASER: CARBON DIOXIDE. The CO_2 laser has no color specificity and is absorbed nonselectively by pigmented and non-pigmented tissue with a high water content such as skin which is composed of 80% to 95% water. With each successive pass of the laser over the area, a selective layer by layer removal of a 30–100 μm segment is accomplished. The high heat of the laser (70–100°C) changes the water in the cells to steam causing ejection of the solid component and consequent tissue vaporization with virtually no damage to surrounding tissue. Mechanical debridement of each char layer with a saline or hydrogen peroxide moistened gauze or applicator removes each layer until all pigment is removed down to the upper layers of the dermis. The result is a re-epithelialization with removal of tattoo pigment and preservation of near-normal skin color and texture. The laser is used in a continuous mode with 10–20 watts of defocused power in a rapid "paint brush" manner.

ADDITIONAL INFORMATION. The laser is passed over the skin in a defocused manner with a rapid "paint brush" manner. With each successive pass, the charred skin layer with its enclosed tattoo pigment is mechanically wiped away. After the first pass which removes the overlying epidermis, the tattoo pigment is revealed even more brilliantly. Each subsequent application removes progressively more tattoo pigment. Care must be taken not to penetrate completely through the dermis producing a full thickness wound which would result in a hypertrophic or keloid scar.

POST-TREATMENT CARE. The wound is treated as an open partial-thickness injury wound. The patient is instructed to shower daily and apply either antibiotic ointment or aloe vera gel. A bandage is worn in areas where there could be trauma or underclothes.

Reprinted with permission of Little, Brown and Company.
For literature pertaining to this case see References section.

Case continues on following page.

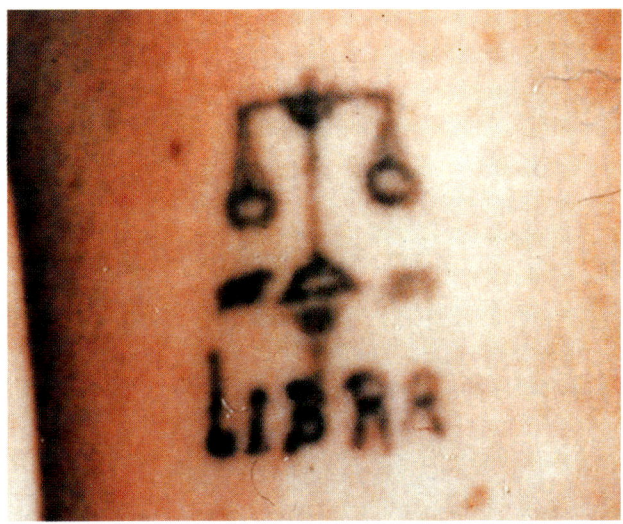

FIG. 4.32-A. Pre-operative view of decorative tattoo on left deltoid area.

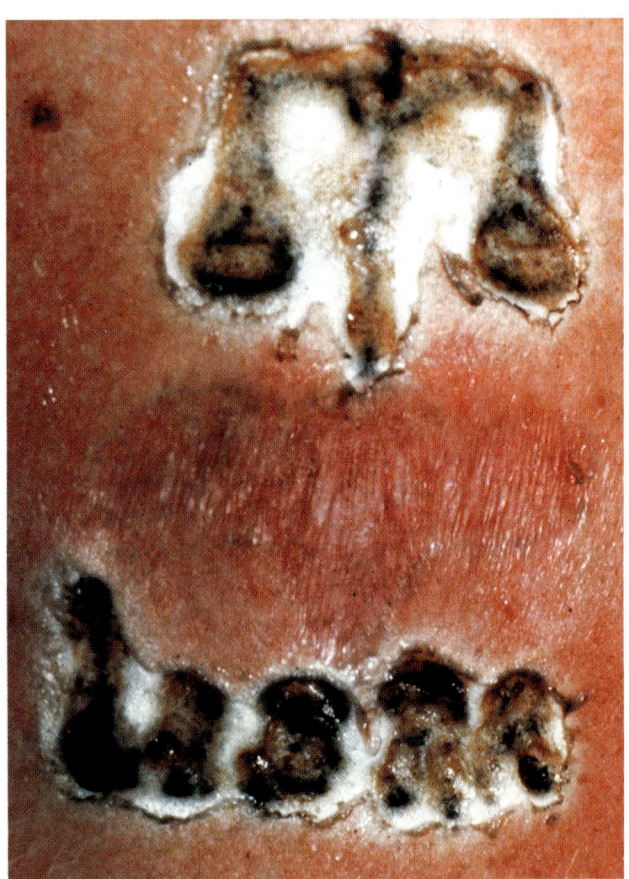

FIG. 4.32-B. Central portion has been treated with the argon laser with excellent result. Superior and inferior areas have been photovaporized by multiple passes with the CO_2 laser.

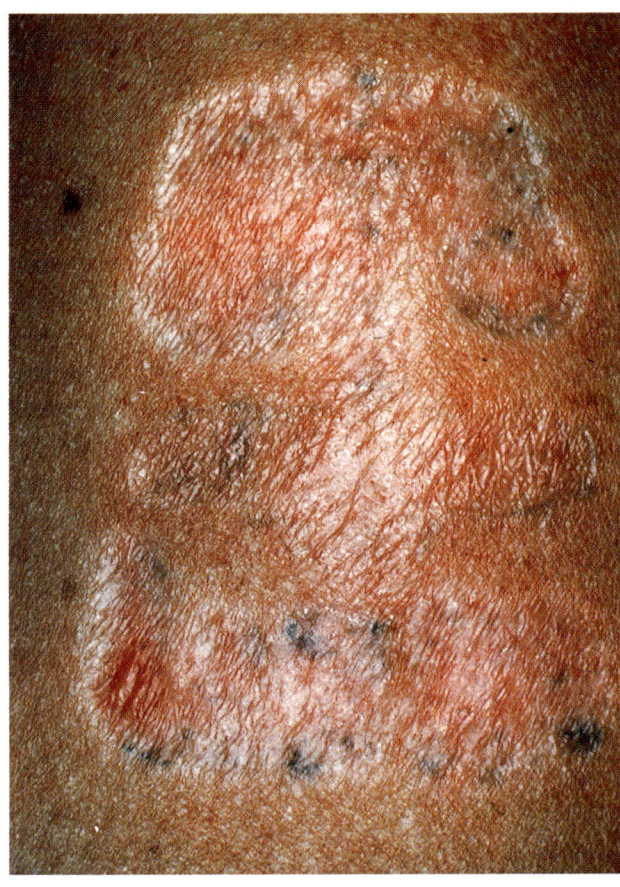

FIG. 4.32-C. Final result of obliteration of tattoo pigment in all areas by both lasers. Clinical result is equivalent between the two lasers.

Case courtesy of *David B. Apfelberg,* M.D.

CASE 4.33

Homemade Tattoo

REVIEW OF CASE. This is a 17-year-old female with an amateur "name" tattoo on the left arm. Tattoo dimensions were 10 cm × 3 cm, and it had been present for three years. The patient and family believed the tattoo would interfere with an improving self image, future relationships, and employment opportunities.

CHOICE OF LASER: CARBON DIOXIDE. The CO_2 laser was chosen to vaporize tattoo pigment from the dermal tissue. Highly efficient absorption of CO_2 laser radiation in water-rich cutaneous tissues reduces nonspecific thermal injury and scarring in adjacent tissues. The large size, shape, and location of the tattoo on the arm would not allow cosmetically acceptable full-thickness excision and closure with sutures. Dermabrasion with or without salabrasion is an alternative procedure with poorer visualization due to bleeding intraoperatively; it therefore frequently leaves behind residual pigment or risks greater scarring from penetration to deep dermis and fat.

Physiology and mechanisms include efficient vaporization of water-rich dermal tissue and macrophages containing tattoo pigment. Dermabrasion or laser removal techniques require removal of the majority of the pigment at the time of surgery. Small amounts of residual pigment may be shed by exudation and the removal of devitalized tissue during re-epithelization. Greater pigment depth is associated with more difficult removal and greater risk of scarring. Experience has shown older tattoos and those applied by amateurs to contain deeper pigment depots than recent or commercially applied tattoos.

ADDITIONAL INFORMATION. Initial power settings are between 10 and 20 watts using the continuous wave technique with a spot size of 3–4 mm. Removal of the majority of pigment is accomplished with rapid, barely overlapping, carefully controlled circular movements of the hand and wrist (airbrush technique). The tattoo shape or figure is traced with repeated passes, layer by layer. Fastidious removal of charred tissue is performed after each pass employing damp gauze wiping and/or various sized curets.

Focal, deep pigment depots will be evident once the majority of superficial-to-mid depth tattoo pigment is removed with the airbrush technique. Focal pigment is spot vaporized with 0.05 second pulses. The small spot size (0.5–2.0 mm) and pulse duration minimizes peripheral tissue damage. The very small full-thickness defects and intact surrounding dermal framework helps prevent contraction and hypertrophic scarring. Magnifying loupes may be useful in this step (Fig. B).

The third step is softening edges of letters/component figures of the tattoo. Airbrush technique with 5–15 watts and a 2–3 mm spot size is commonly employed. Elevated (non-tattooed) tissue within the tattoo area is vaporized down to an intermediate depth. Blunting or softening figures avoids recognizable patterns or shapes. The overall outline shape of the tattoo is converted commonly to an oval or rounded corner rectangle shape.

The final step is feathering or blending the periphery of the tattoo removal area into surrounding skin. Airbrush technique at 20 watts, 3–4 mm spot size is applied in overlapping layers of increasing radius. For example each of several passes may extend the periphery an additional 5 mm. The transition is transformed from a canyon to a gradually sloping valley that is less noticeable.

The careful combination of the above techniques addresses the criticism of early CO_2 laser tattoo removal technique which left a scar with obvious outlines of the original tattoo.

Case continues on following page.

POST-TREATMENT CARE. Moist healing dressings are maintained and changed once daily until re-epithelization is completed. Antibiotic ointments and nonadherent dressings are applied. Tap water alone or four parts water to one part hydrogen peroxide may be used to loosen and cleanse adherent dressings or crust from the wound. Observation for any early signs of hypertrophic scar formation in the six weeks after re-epithelization allows treatment with intralesional steroids.

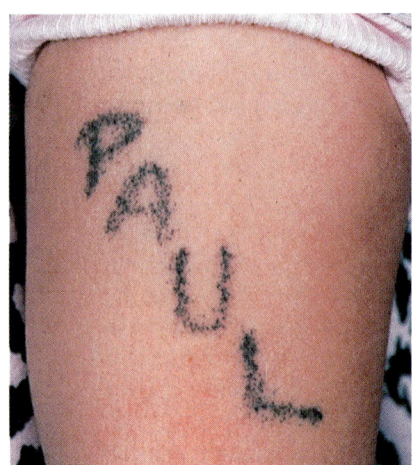

FIG. 4.33-A. Home-made tattoo.

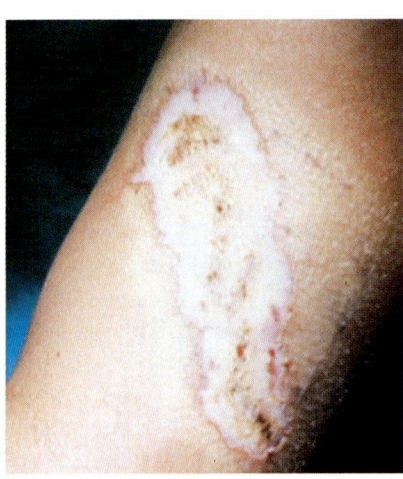

FIG. 4.33-B. Pigment depots spot vaporized and layered feathering.

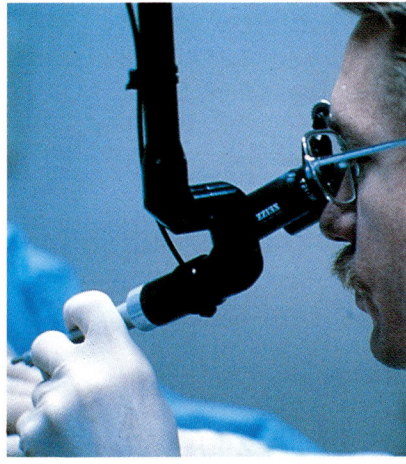

FIG. 4.33-C. Use of magnifying loupes to spot vaporized pigment depots with a 1 mm spot size.

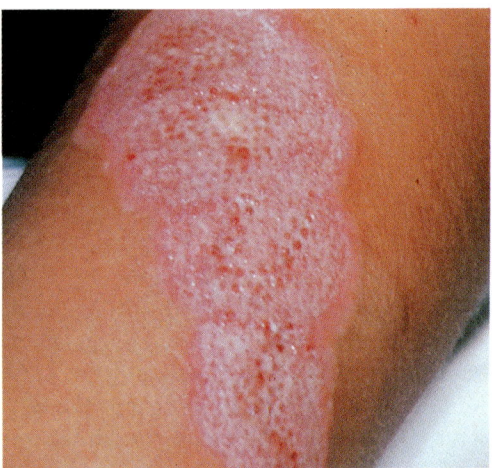

FIG. 4.33-D. Re-epithelialization at 10–14 days post-operation.

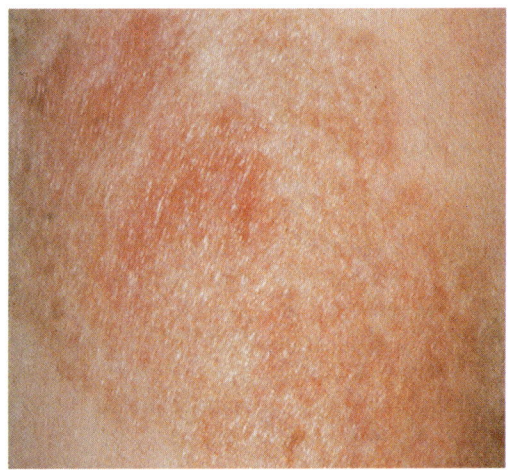

FIG. 4.33-E. Six months after surgery.

Case courtesy of *Timothy J. Rosio*, M.D.

CASE 4.34
Traumatic Tattoo

REVIEW OF CASE. This 28-year-old male sustained a traumatic tattoo with petroleum foreign body particles when a machine blew up in his face. Pigment was present on the forehead, eyelids, nose, and cheeks.

CHOICE OF LASER: CARBON DIOXIDE. The CO_2 laser has the ability to vaporize small foreign body particles out of the skin and dermis. The high heat of the laser (70–100°C) changes the water in the cells to steam causing ejection of the solid component which is vaporized as well. Surrounding tissue is virtually undamaged and subsequent heating and re-epithelialization is good. The laser is used with short bursts of either focused or defocused power of 10–20 watts in a laserbrasion manner.

ADDITIONAL INFORMATION. Each individual pigment deposit is photovaporized out of the skin by a short burst of defocused laser pulse. The area is gently debrided with an applicator of saline or hydrogen peroxide until all pigment is removed.

POST-TREATMENT CARE. The wound is treated as an open partial-thickness injury wound. The patient is instructed to shower daily and apply either antibiotic ointment or aloe vera gel. A bandage is worn in areas where there could be trauma or underclothes.

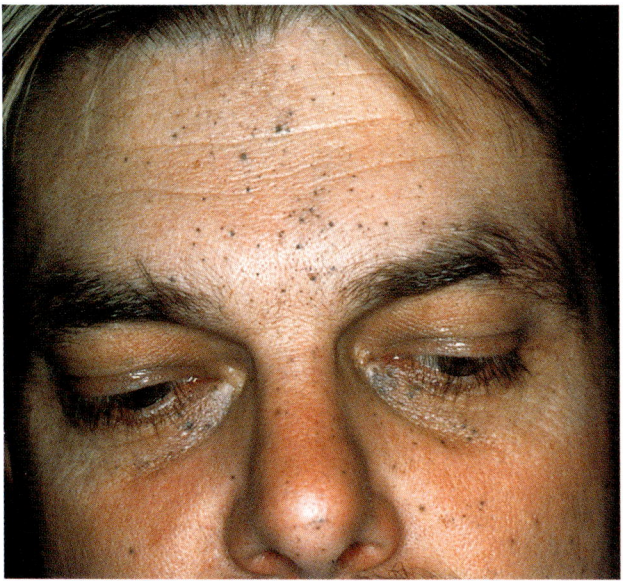

FIG. 4.34-A. Pre-operative appearance of 28-year-old male with embedded foreign body particles of petroleum following explosion of machine.

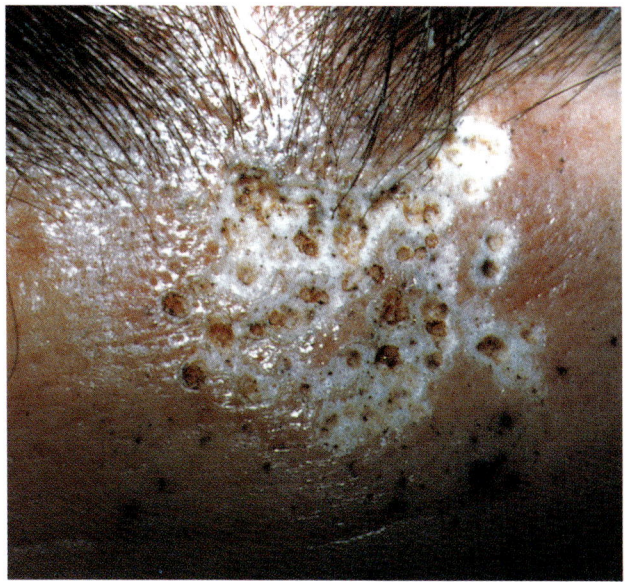

FIG. 4.34-B. Demonstration of appearance after CO_2 laser photovaporization plus debridement with hydrogen peroxide.

Case continues on following page.

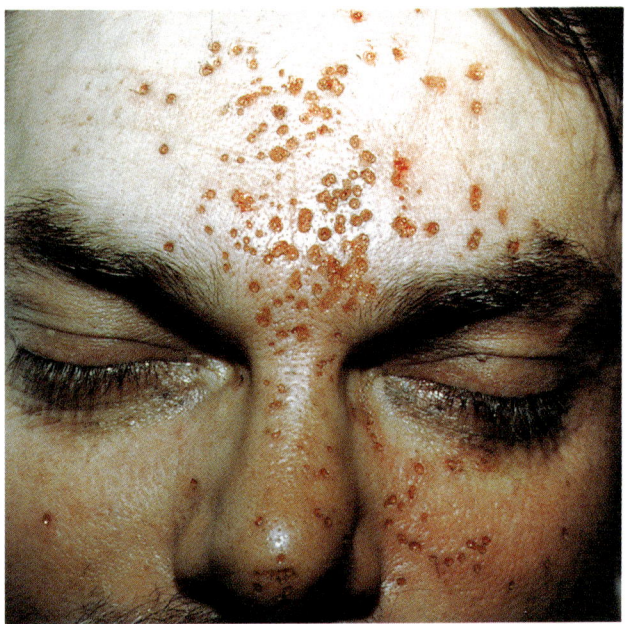

FIG. 4.34-C. Appearance immediately following laser vaporization of individual particles of pigment from forehead, nose, and eyebrows.

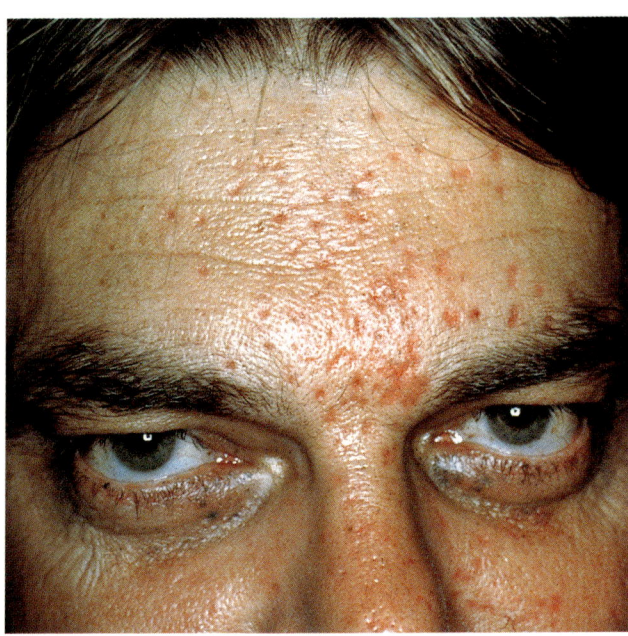

FIG. 4.34-D. Appearance of lesions one week after treatment.

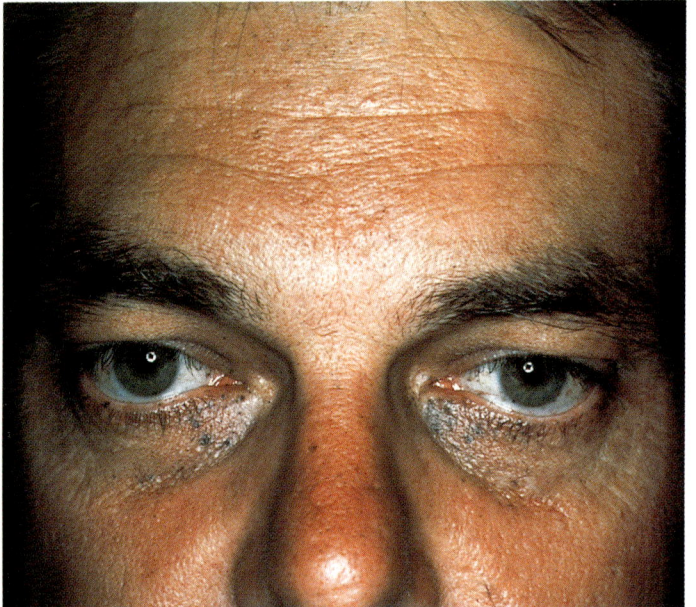

FIG. 4.34-E. Final result demonstrating complete removal of all pigment without significant scarring or texture change.

Case courtesy of *David B. Apfelberg*, M.D.

Reprinted with permission of Wiley-Liss, a division of John Wiley and Sons, Inc., copyright © 1990.
For literature pertaining to this case see References section.

CASE 4.35
Chondrodermatitis Nodularis Chronica Helicus

REVIEW OF CASE. This patient complained about a persistent painful lesion on his right ear. He was unable to sleep on the right side because of pain. He had been treated with topical and intralesional steroids without success.

CHOICE OF LASER: CARBON DIOXIDE. The CO_2 laser has the ability to very accurately vaporize this lesion while leaving adjacent tissue intact. Chondrodermatitis nodularis chronica helicus is notorious for recurrence after one or more traditional treatments including injection of corticosteroids and excision. CO_2 laser vaporization offers an excellent treatment of this lesion with a high success rate and few complications. Pain relief is immediate following laser treatment.

ADDITIONAL INFORMATION. After local anesthesia, the visible nodule is removed to the level of the cartilage with a curved, double-edged razor blade and this specimen is sent to pathology for histologic confirmation of the diagnosis. The adjacent skin and partial thickness of cartilage is then carefully vaporized using 5–10 watts of power, 5 ms pulses, and a focused 1 mm spot size. Inflamed tissues can be removed without excessive thermal necrosis and the defect can be laterally contoured to give a cosmetically appealing final result.

POST-TREATMENT CARE. Topical and systemic antibiotics are administered post-operatively and the wound is covered with a sterile bandage. Gentle daily cleansing of the wound with hydrogen peroxide and reapplication of the topical antibiotic are repeated until a dry eschar appears. Usually the wound can be left open in a clean environment after three to four days. Healing is complete within three to four weeks in most cases.

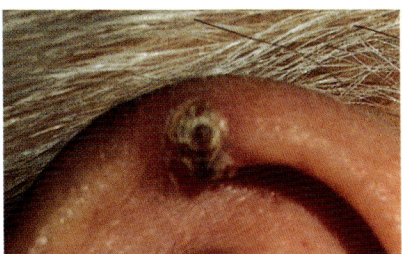

FIG. 4.35-A. Chondrodermatitis nodularis chronica helicus pre-operation.

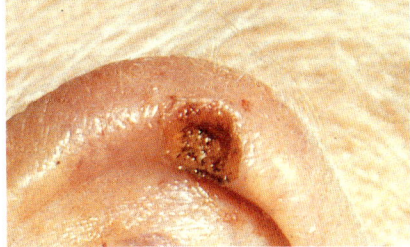

FIG. 4.35-B. Immediately post-operative. Entire lesion is vaporized down to underlying cartilage. The resultant defect is allowed to granulate and epithelialize by second intention.

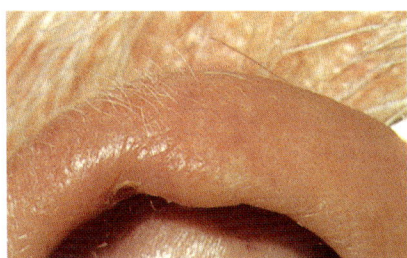

FIG. 4.35-C. Five weeks post-operation.

Case courtesy of *Mark B. Taylor*, M.D.

CASE 4.36

Comedones

REVIEW OF CASE. This elderly gentleman complained about numerous unsightly comedones. Previous non-surgical topical treatments had proven unsuccessful. Comedones did not respond to acne surgery with incision application of a comedone extractor. Bruising of fragile periorbital skin and inability to extract the cyst contents mandated an alternative therapy. Lengthy topical treatments were deemed to be less satisfactory than more rapid surgical evacuation.

CHOICE OF LASER: CARBON DIOXIDE. The CO_2 laser has the ability to very accurately penetrate the top of the cyst without damage to adjacent tissue structures. Following cyst evacuation, it is not necessary to surgically excise the cyst sac because vaporization eradicates this structure so recurrence is prevented. This treatment method is very useful in the treatment of multiple cysts and comedones of Maladie de Favre et Racouchot and comedones that do not respond to traditional acne surgery.

ADDITIONAL INFORMATION. Using a focused beam, a 0.3 to 1.0 mm spot and 250 ms pulses, a small laser hole is made in the roof of the comedones and cysts. Small cysts less than 1 mm in diameter are vaporized through this single step procedure. Larger cysts are then expressed through the laser hole using a Schamberg Comedone Extractor. As the cyst contents are evaginated the cyst sac is exposed which can then be vaporized with a second laser application. Treating the sac will tend to prevent recurrence of the cyst in an empty sac. This procedure can be tolerated by the patient without anesthesia.

POST-TREATMENT CARE. Topical antibiotic ointment is applied post-operatively. The patient is allowed to wash the face daily. Healing is usually complete within 14 days.

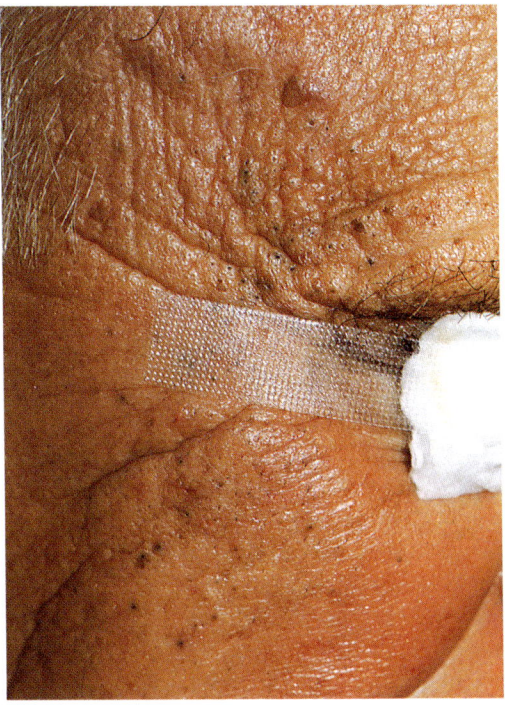

FIG. 4.36-A. Maladie de Favre et Racouchot pre-operation.

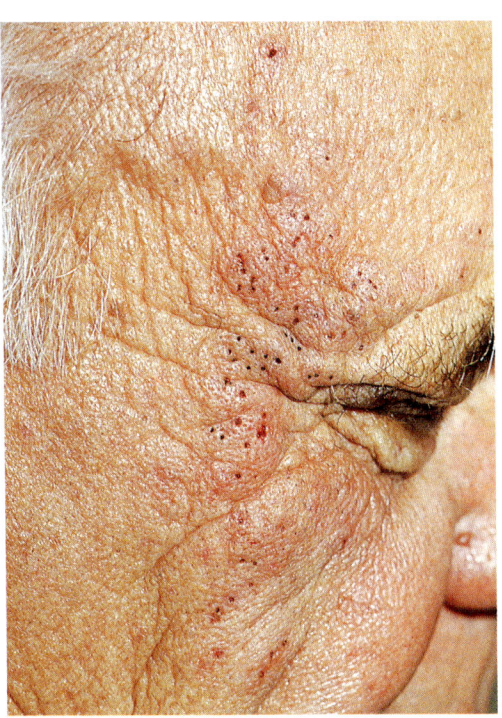

FIG. 4.36-B. Immediately post-operation. Small cysts are vaporized, larger ones are opened, the contents evacuated, and the sac is evaginated and vaporized.

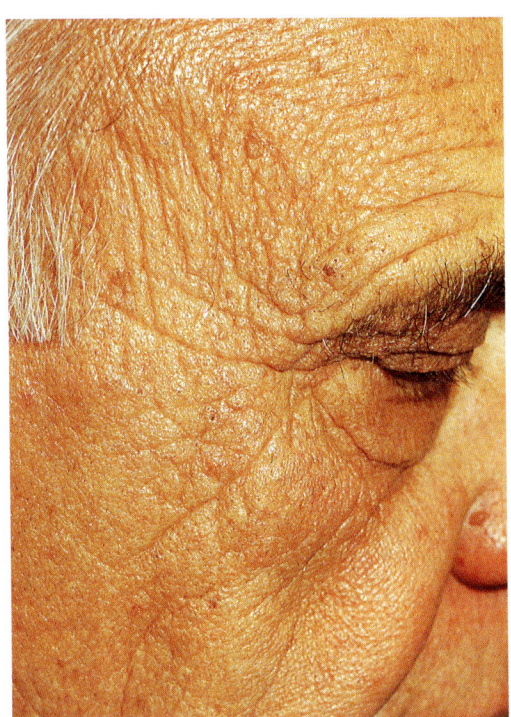

FIG. 4.36-C. One month post-operation.

Case courtesy of *Mark B. Taylor,* M.D.

CASE 4.37

Compound Nevus

REVIEW OF CASE. This is a 39-year-old female with several large compound nevi present on the left chin and the left cheek. The patient desires removal for cosmetic purposes.

CHOICE OF LASER: CARBON DIOXIDE. The CO_2 laser is able to photovaporize pigmented lesions of the skin. Using a defocused "paint brush" technique one can remove layer by layer of these nevi until the upper dermis is present and the base of the nevus is removed. The lesion is photovaporized and smoke evacuation of the plume is very important. The CO_2 laser is selectively absorbed by the water in the cells of the nevus and as this water is converted to steam the cells explode, producing the laser plume. Adjacent skin is not affected.

ADDITIONAL INFORMATION. It is very important to biopsy any lesion, especially a pigmented lesion, which is photo destroyed by the laser. One would not want to photovaporize a pigmented basal cell carcinoma or melanoma inadvertently. Therefore, it is recommended that a small incisional biopsy be removed before destroying any pigmented lesion. It is important not to completely penetrate through the dermis as this would produce a full-thickness injury and subsequent hypertrophic scar.

POST-TREATMENT CARE. The patient is instructed to apply aloe vera ointment or antibiotic ointment and is allowed to shower normally. No bandage is required.

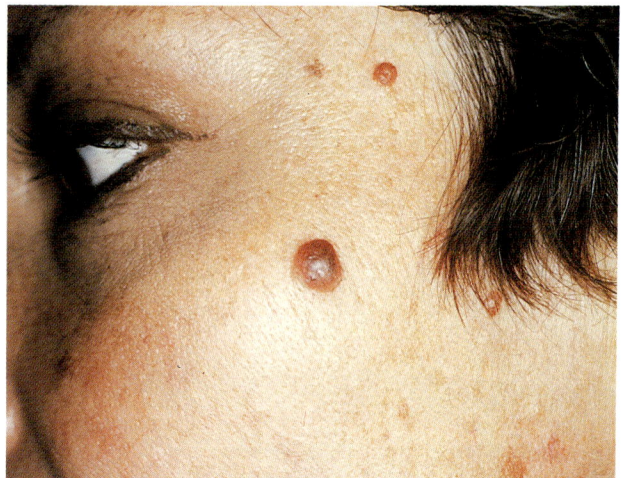

FIG. 4.37-A. Pre-operative appearance of compound nevus of left cheek and malar area.

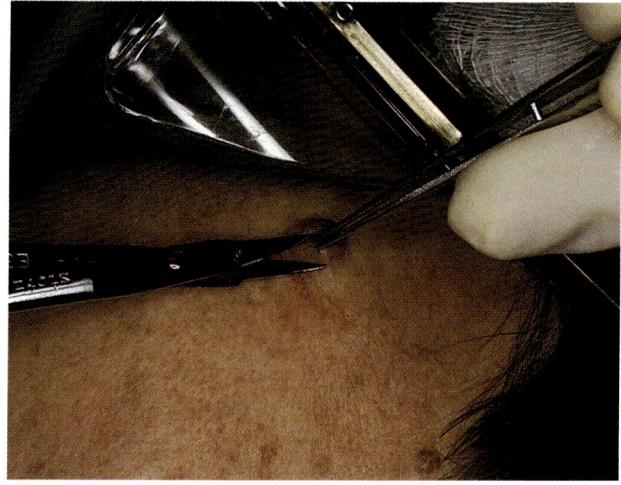

FIG. 4.37-B. Illustration of biopsy technique.

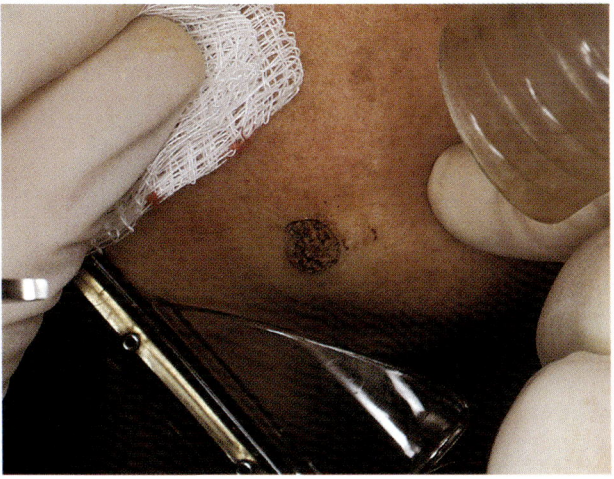

FIG. 4.37-C. Photovaporization of the lesion.

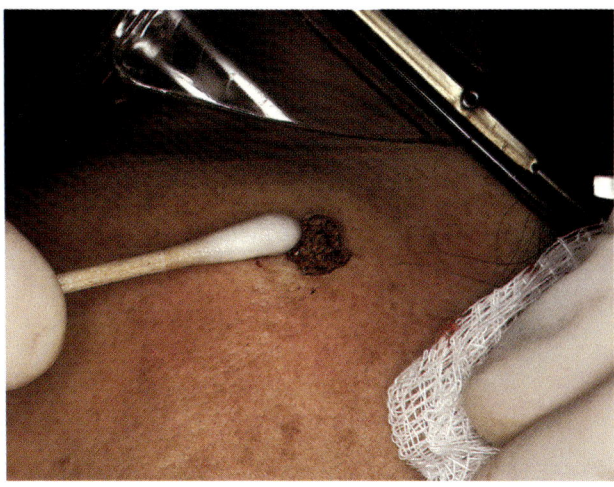

FIG. 4.37-D. The charred area is wiped with a saline antibiotic solution and any residual nevus is examined.

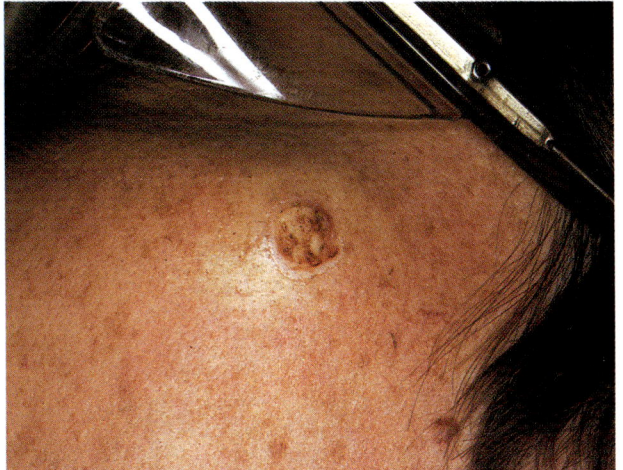

FIG. 4.37-E. Some nevus tissue remains in the base of the wound.

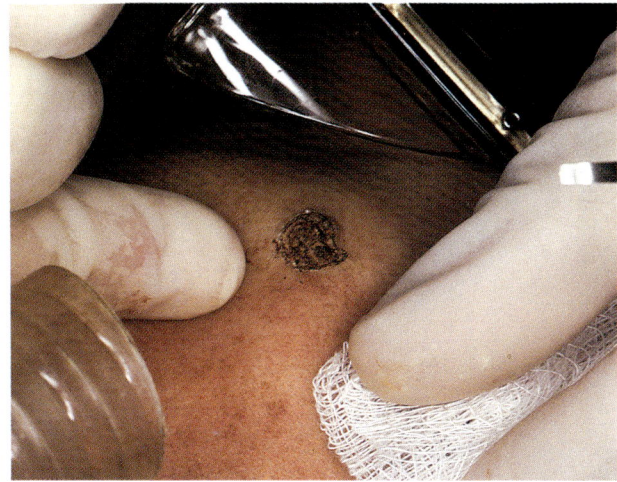

FIG. 4.37-F. The area is re-lasered using a defocused paint brush motion.

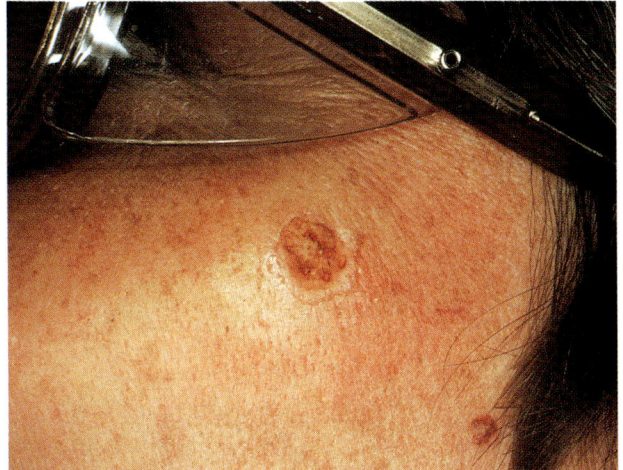

FIG. 4.37-G. Final result showing that the base of the lesion is completely removed down to but not through the upper dermis.

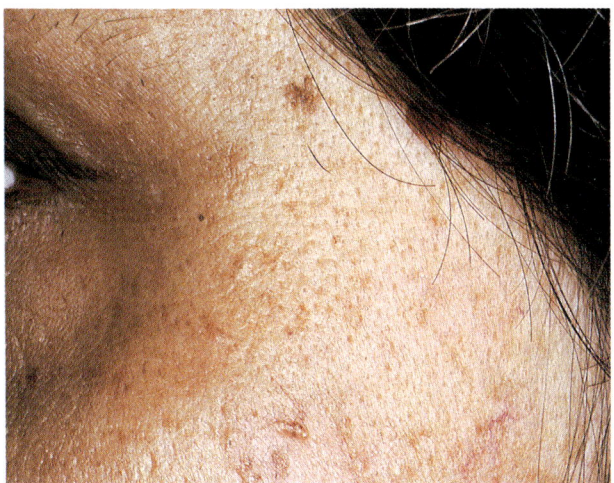

FIG. 4.37-H. Completed result eight weeks following treatment with minimal residual cosmetic deformity of the face.

Case courtesy of *David B. Apfelberg*, M.D.

CASE 4.38

Adnexal Neoplasm

Cylindromas and Eccrine Spiradenoma

REVIEW OF CASE. This is a 58-year-old woman with a 30 year history of cylindromas and eccrine spiradenomas on her face. The lesions around the ear had become so numerous as to begin to obstruct her hearing. They had been unresponsive to cryosurgery and electrocautery.

CHOICE OF LASER: CARBON DIOXIDE. The CO_2 laser was chosen to vaporize many lesions at one time. This laser has been shown to be very successful in the treatment of patients with multiple cutaneous adnexal neoplasms. The fact that the CO_2 laser seals small lymphatics and nerve endings provides a more comfortable wound healing, less pain, and a fairly good cosmetic result.

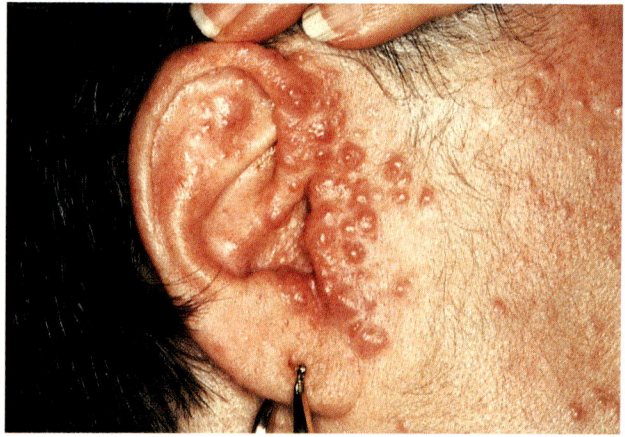

FIG. 4.38-A. Multiple cylindromas and eccrine spiradenomas around the ear.

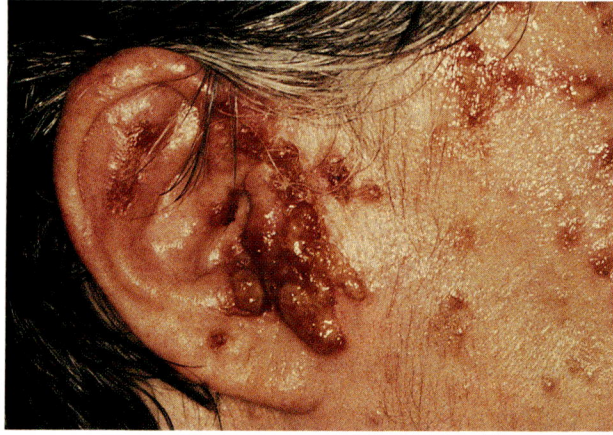

FIG. 4.38-B. Four days following CO_2 laser vaporization. Many lesions were removed using a 6 watt defocused CO_2 laser beam with a 2 mm spot size.

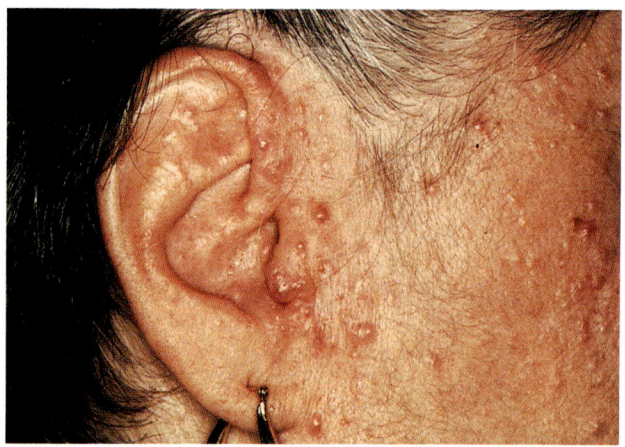

FIG. 4.38-C. One year following CO_2 laser vaporization. Some lesions have recurred, but innumerable lesions have not returned and a fairly good cosmetic result is apparent.

Case courtesy of *David J. Goldberg*, M.D.

CASE 4.39
Digital Myxoid Cysts

REVIEW OF CASE. This patient presented with a painful, tense cystic mass proximal to the nail bed. Excisional surgery was declined by the patient.

CHOICE OF LASER: CARBON DIOXIDE. The CO_2 laser has the ability to open and evacuate the myxoid cyst. The tract or base of the cyst which connects to the dorsal joint capsule must be obliterated to prevent recurrence of the cyst. Digital myxoid cysts have a high recurrence rate after excision or injection with corticosteroids. CO_2 laser vaporization of these cysts is often successful when traditional methods of treatment have failed.

ADDITIONAL INFORMATION. The digit is blocked with a local anesthetic. Using a scalpel or sterile razor blade the roof of the cyst is removed with a shave biopsy procedure and sent for pathologic examination. A clear gelatinous material in the cyst is clinical confirmation of the diagnosis. Drysol (20% aluminum chloride [hexahydrate]) is applied to the biopsy site to provide hemostasis. Using a Pfizer portable CO_2 laser at a setting of 5 watts of power, 5 to 10 ms pulses, and focused with a 1 mm spot size, the mucinous matrix lining of the cyst is vaporized, being careful not to penetrate the periosteum or nail matrix.

POST-TREATMENT CARE. Topical antibiotic ointment is applied to the resultant wound. Patients are instructed to gently cleanse the wound once or twice a day with hydrogen peroxide followed by an application of antibiotic ointment and a sterile adhesive bandage. Systemic antibiotics are administered by mouth for ten days. Patients are instructed to avoid potential contamination of the wound. After 3–4 days the wound may be left open at night to encourage the formation of a dry eschar. Healing is usually complete within three weeks. Occasional recurrences can be retreated successfully by repeating the procedure.

Case continues on following page.

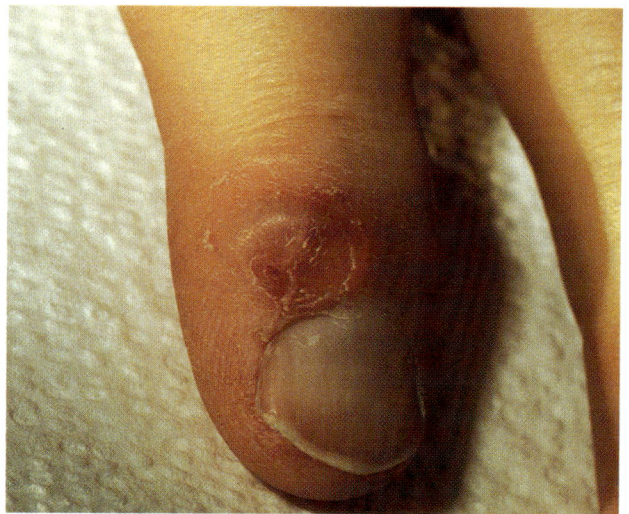

FIG. 4.39-A. Digital myxoid cyst pre-operation.

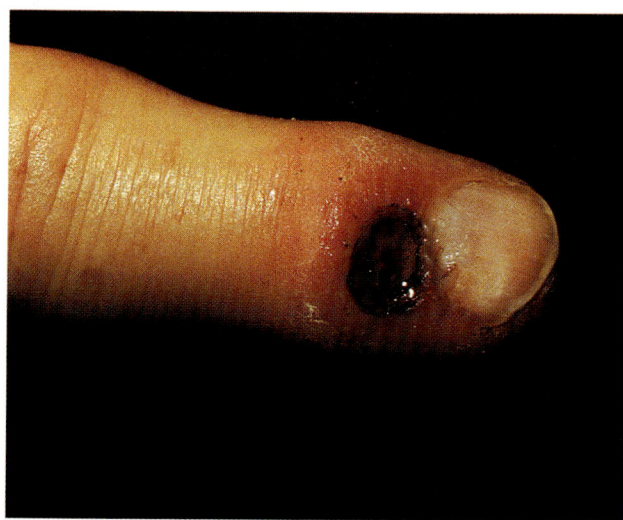

FIG. 4.39-B. Four days post-operation. The top of the cyst is first penetrated by the laser, the mucoid content is evacuated, and then the base and tract is vaporized.

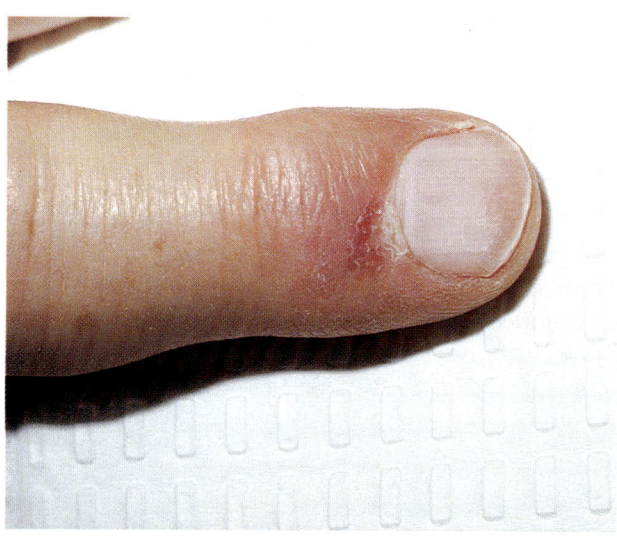

FIG. 4.39-C. Two months post-operation.

Case courtesy of *Mark B. Taylor*, M.D.

CASE 4.40
Discoid Lupus

REVIEW OF CASE. This patient developed discoid lupus erythematosis at age 23 in 1969. She had been treated in the past with topical steroids and intralesional triamcinolone, as well as antimalarial drugs with hydroxychloroquine. She developed some resolution of her lupus but continued to get net lesions histologically demonstrative of discoid lupus erythematosis, in spite of the use of sunscreens. Sun exposure caused an exacerbation of her condition. She had marked disfigurement on her face.

CHOICE OF LASER: CARBON DIOXIDE. The CO_2 laser was chosen in this case, in as much as it is a good instrument for dermabrading the skin. It is well known that ultraviolet light causes discoid lupus to exacerbate. It was therefore thought that since the light emitted by the CO_2 laser is infrared, at the opposite end of the spectrum; it might possibly cause an improvement and resolution of discoid lupus.

ADDITIONAL INFORMATION. This patient had a test area dermabraded with a standard Stryker dermabrader and another area dermabraded with the CO_2 laser. A lasting effect was found in the area laser dermabraded but only a temporary improvement was found in the mechanically dermabraded area.

Accordingly, in 1982, all of the areas of discoid lupus were dermabraded with the CO_2 laser with dramatic improvement. She developed some recurrence in areas that were not dermabraded deep enough with the laser. This was repeated again. Repeat biopsies of the skin failed to reveal any residual discoid lupus and her skin is no longer sensitive to ultraviolet light from the sun.

A test laser dermabrasion is essential in treating this condition. We have found that approximately 75% of patients with discoid lupus respond exceedingly well with laser dermabrasion but some simply do not respond. Because of the significant depth that is required in the laser dermabrasion, there always is hypopigmentation as a result of the treatment, although many times, this is already present because of the discoid lupus. While we haven't encountered a case of significant hypertrophic scar, as related to the laser, this is a very distinct possibility in view of the large amount of tissue that must be dermabraded and the depth. The patient should understand this in detail. It is important to take histological biopsies before and after the treatment.

Case continues on following page.

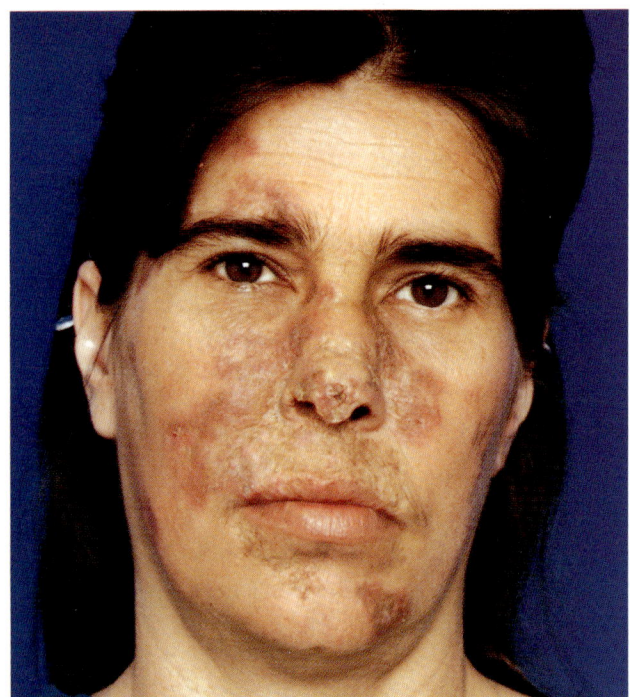

FIG. 4.40-A. Pre-operative appearance in 1982. Note marked changes in the patient's skin and the active lesions still present.

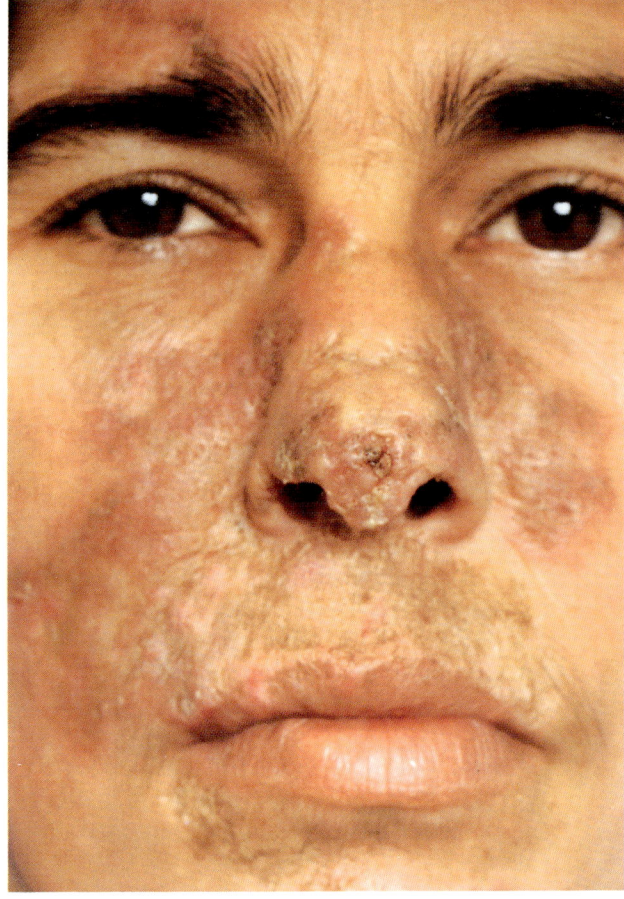

FIG. 4.40-B. A close-up shows the extensive scar tissue, as well as the active areas of disease.

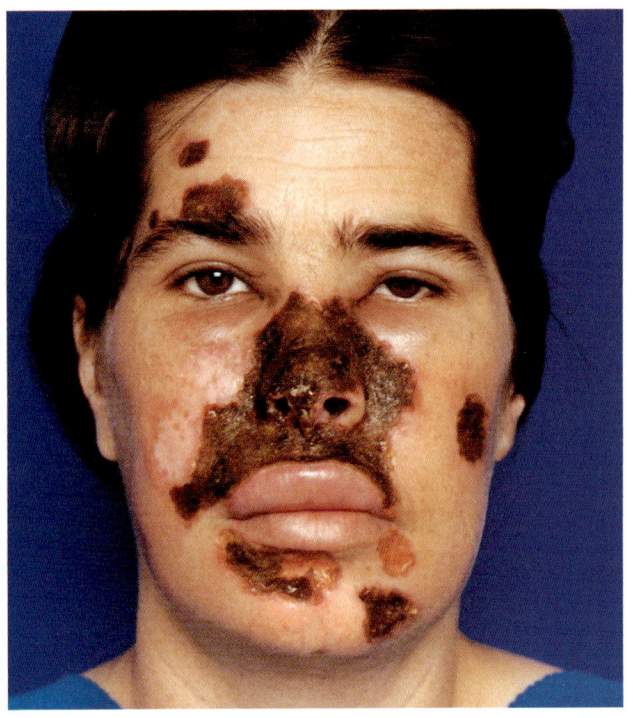

FIG. 4.40-C. Approximately one week after the dermabrasion, a thick eschar is present. Note the laser dermabraded test spots on the right cheek.

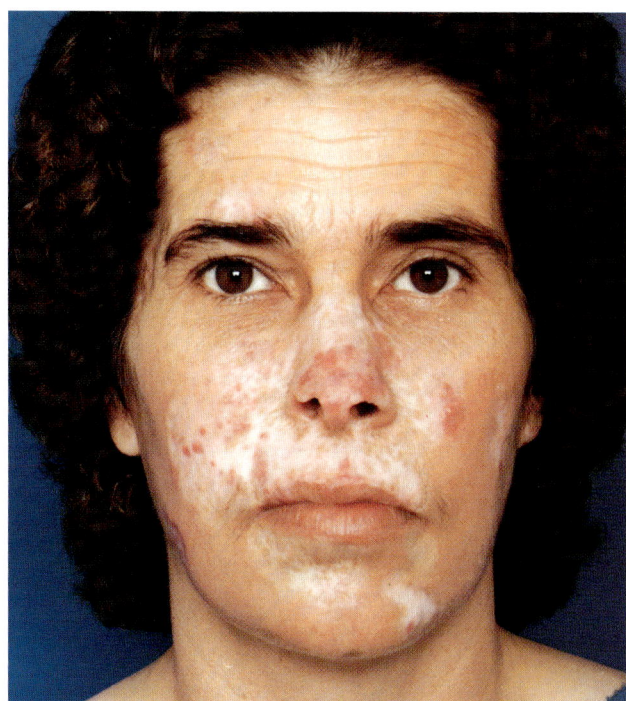

FIG. 4.40-D. Two years post-operation, some areas of residual lupus are showing up in the area that was treated.

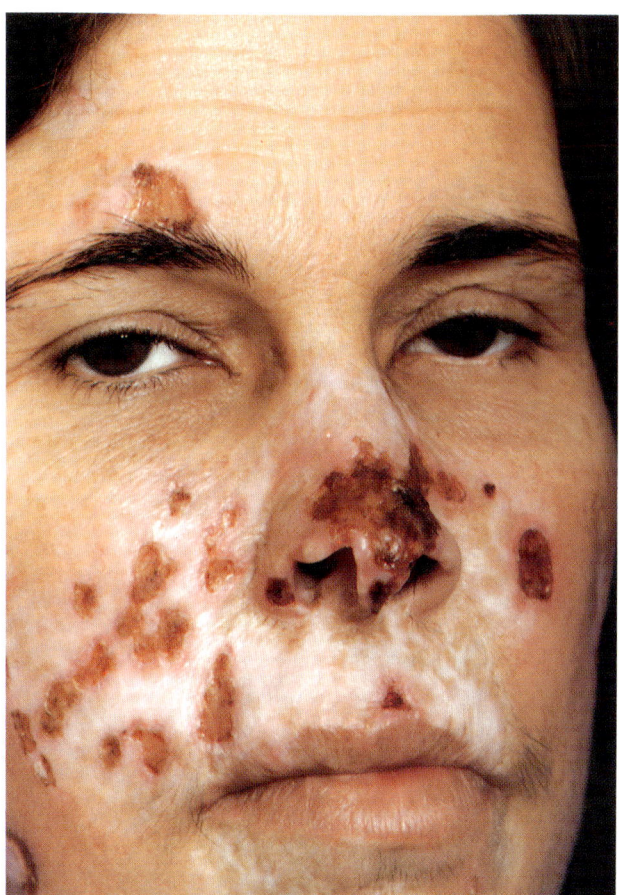

FIG. 4.40-E. Repeat laser dermabrasion in the areas of recurrence.

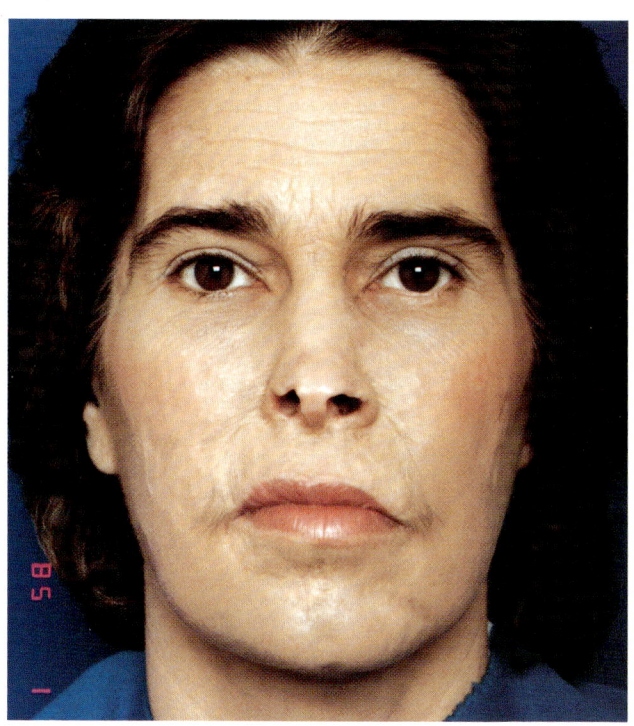

FIG. 4.40-F. Three years post-operation, marked improvement in the patient's condition is seen.

Case courtesy of *Darrell L. Henderson*, M.D.

CASE 4.41
Heterotopic Gastric Mucosa of the Tongue

REVIEW OF CASE. The patient is a 30-year-old woman with an anterior tongue mass which had been present for 9 months. The lesion was soft, grayish tan and polypoid. It measured 2 cm in diameter. The patient's main problem from the mass was difficulty with articulation. A biopsy performed in the office revealed gastric mucosa.

CHOICE OF LASER: CARBON DIOXIDE. The CO_2 laser was chosen because of its precise cutting ability and because of its hemostatic properties with associated decreased post-operative edema. This provides for a rapid, complication-free return of normal oropharyngeal physiology.

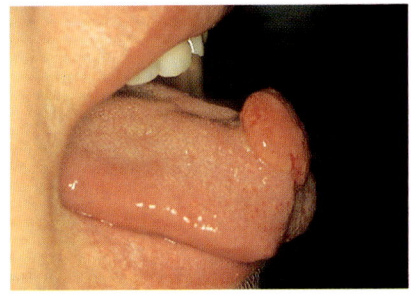

FIG. 4.41-A. The lesion can easily be seen on the anterior aspect of the tongue. As with any lesion, it is important to determine before definitive therapy is carried out whether the lesion is benign or malignant.

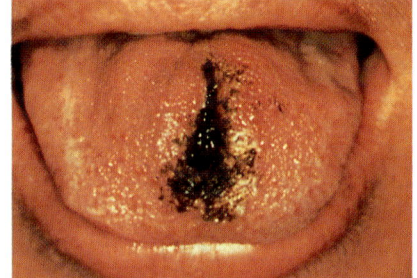

FIG. 4.41-B. This is the area of resection 6 hours after the procedure. As can be seen, there is minimal bleeding and minimal edema after the wedge resection. The resection was performed with the carbon dioxide laser using the hand piece with the laser set at 10 watts, continuous power. The resection was carried out under local anethesia in an outpatient setting. It must be emphasized that other tissues, as well as the eyes, of all persons in the room must be protected. This includes the patient's eyes. This also includes the teeth, since the laser impacts can cause crater-like defects in the enamel of the tooth.

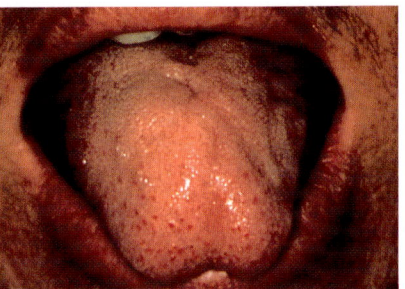

FIG. 4.41-C. This is the area of excision 14 days later. The excellent cosmetic and functional result this soon after surgery emphasizes the superiority of this method of treatment for lesions of the oral cavity.

Case courtesy of *Jack A. Coleman, Jr.,* M.D., *Robert H. Ossoff,* D.M.D., M.D., and *Wm. Russell Ries,* M.D.

CASE 4.42
Irritation Fibroma

REVIEW OF CASE. A 45-year-old white male presenting with a suspected irritation fibroma on the buccal mucosa. The patient had been aware of the lesion for about six months, and believed it had recently enlarged. The lesion was bothersome to the patient, prevented normal mastication, and was consistently bitten.

CHOICE OF LASER: CARBON DIOXIDE. A CO_2 laser was chosen to be used for the excisional biopsy of the lesion. The CO_2 laser has been shown and proven to be the laser of choice for intraoral soft tissue lesions and excisional biopsies of this nature. Advantages of the laser over conventional scalpel surgery are: (i) decreased to absent surgical and post-surgical bleeding, (ii) little chance for mechanical trauma to the tissues, (iii) sterilization of the wound site, (iv) minimal swelling and scarring, and (v) probably from the patient's point of view minimal to absent post-operative pain in the majority of cases. In addition no sutures are necessary as normally required with conventional scalpel surgery.

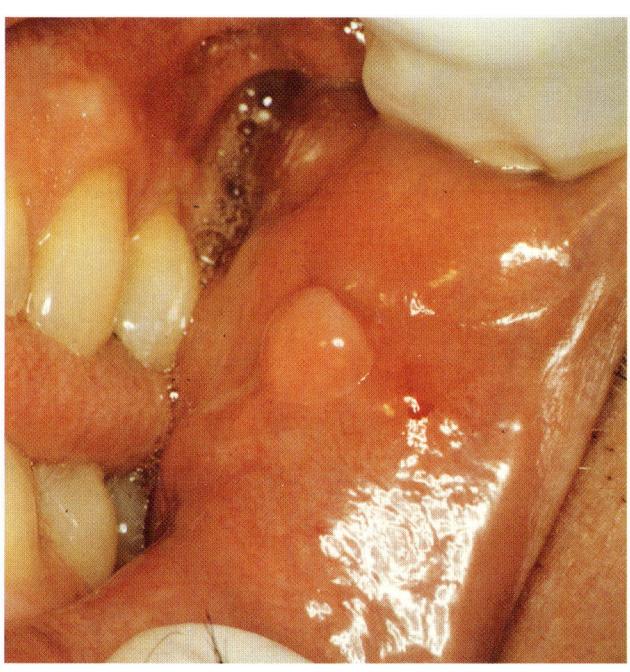

FIG. 4.42-A. A patient presenting with a suspected irritation fibroma on the buccal mucosa. The patient was unaware of how long the lesion had been present.

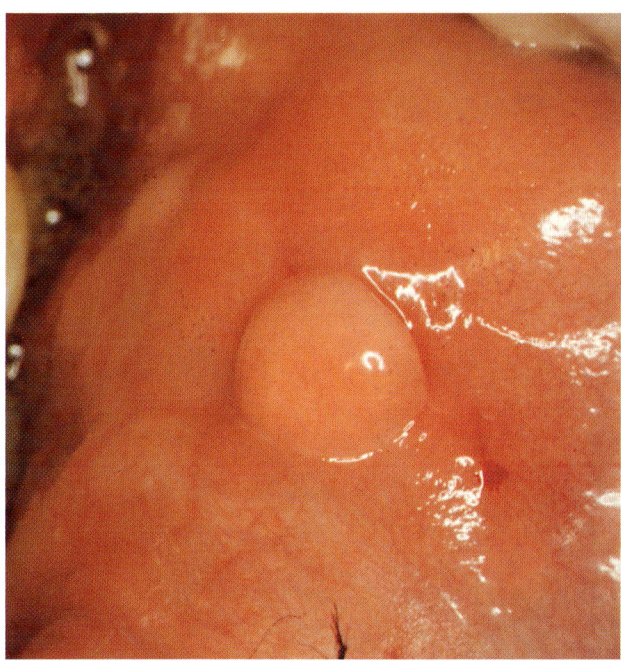

FIG. 4.42-B. Close-up view of Fig. A.

Case continues on following page.

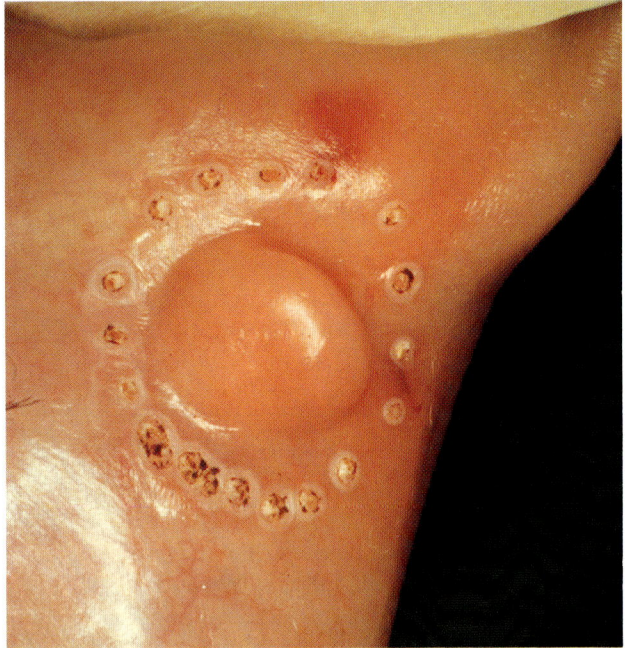

FIG. 4.42-C. Using a focused mode, pulsed, and 5 watts, the lesion can be outlined (although not necessary), and once outlined using 10 watts and a focused beam the area is circumscribed to create a cut into the tissue.

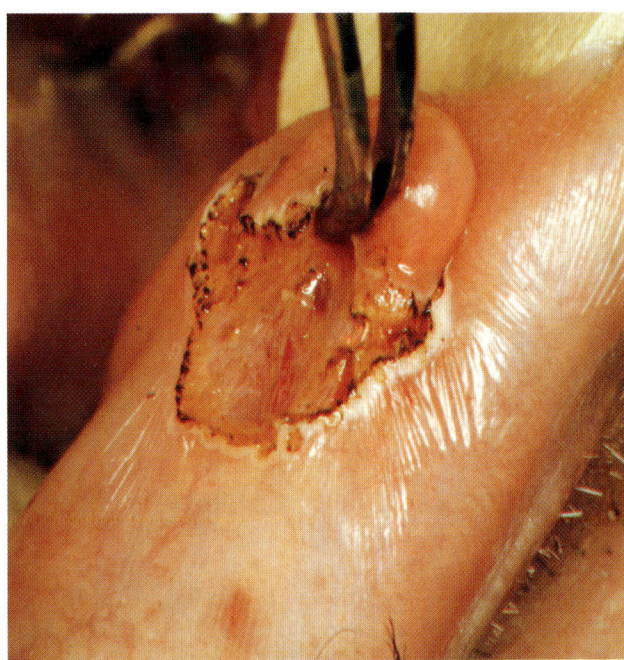

FIG. 4.42-D. Using a tissue pick-up an edge of the lesion is grabbed and lifted. Then using traction the lesion can be undermined using 10 watts, and a slightly defocused beam. Note the hemorrhage free nature of the biopsy in an area that normally bleeds easily.

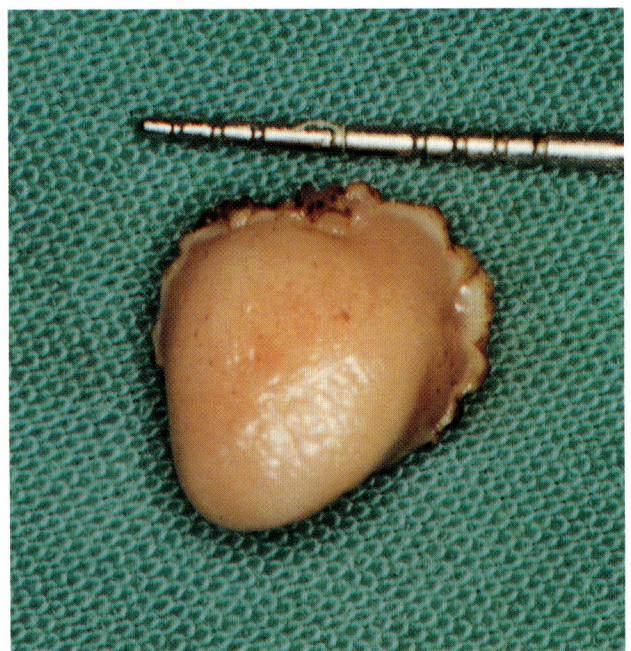

FIG. 4.42-E. The lesion is then removed, placed in formalin, and sent for biopsy.

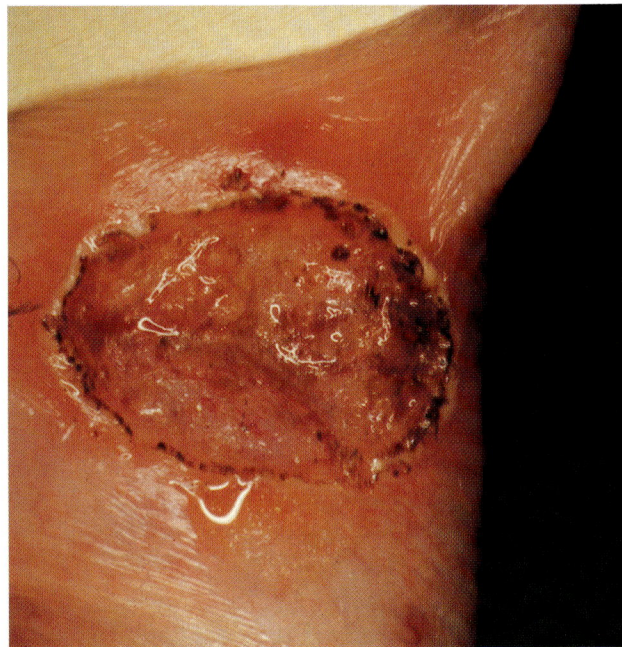

FIG. 4.42-F. The wound as it appears after lasing.

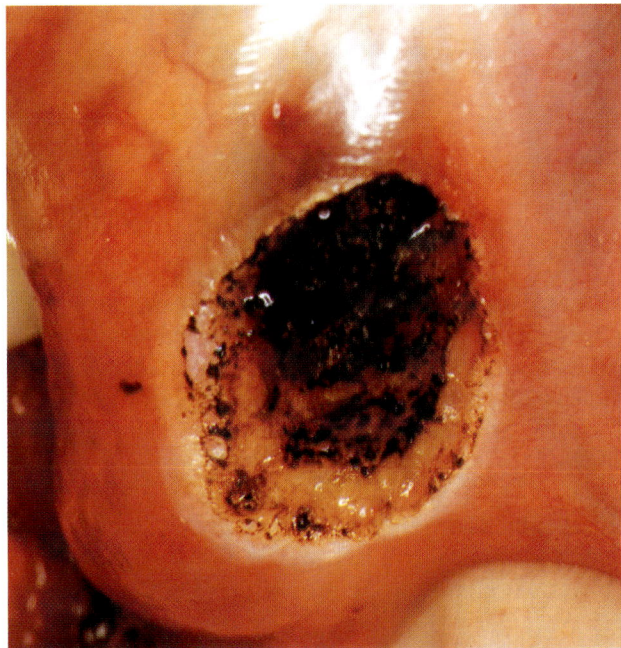

FIG. 4.42-G. To ensure a proper hemorrhage-free post-operative course, using 7 to 10 watts and a defocused beam, a "char layer" is then placed to ensure sealing of the vessels, and hence a hemorrhage-free area.

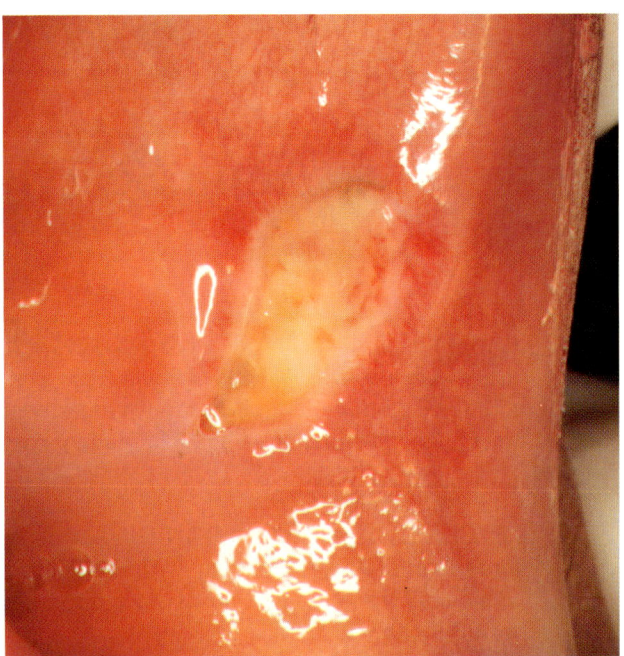

FIG. 4.42-H. The area as it appears one week post-operation. Laser wounds at the one week period have an "aphthous" appearance to them. The patient is in no discomfort.

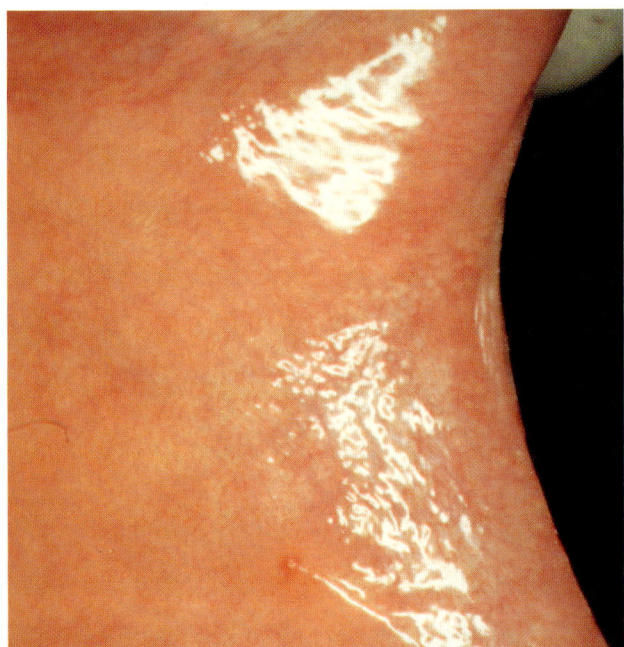

FIG. 4.42-I. The area as it appears two months post-laser surgery. Note that there is no scarring. Biopsy showed the lesion to be an irritation fibroma.

Case courtesy of *Robert M. Pick*, D.D.S.

CASE 4.43

Acne Scarring and Keloids

REVIEW OF CASE. The patient is a 25-year-old Hispanic male who has keloids as a result of acne, located between his eyebrows and mid face. Both lesions were vaporized with the CO_2 laser, with a 5 watt defocused beam, repeat mode, and exposure time of 0.2 second. Vaporization continued until excessive tissue was removed and the base of the treated area became the same level as the surrounding skin. The patient responded nicely with this treatment and stayed clear.

CHOICE OF LASER: CARBON DIOXIDE. The CO_2 laser was chosen because it is an excellent way to vaporize keloid tissue with the defocused beam. The rate of cure has been reported to be about 50%. In general, keloids are a difficult problem to treat and the CO_2 laser offers one more option for therapy.

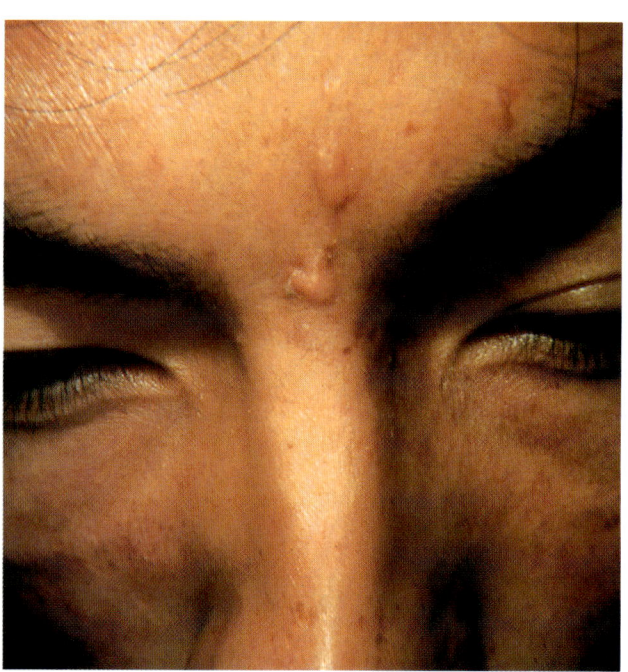

FIG. 4.43-A. Keloid between the eyebrows.

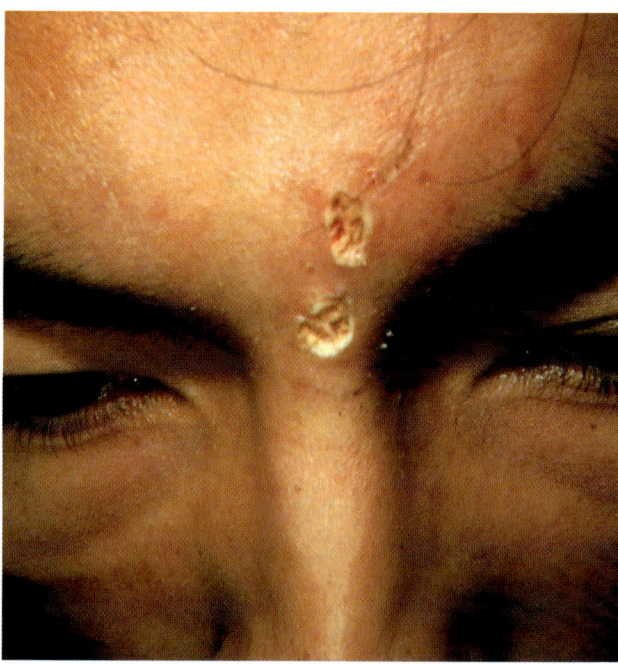

FIG. 4-43.B. The lesion was vaporized using the CO_2 laser with a 5 watt defocused beam in repeat mode and an exposure time of 0.2 second. The char was cleaned with hydrogen peroxide.

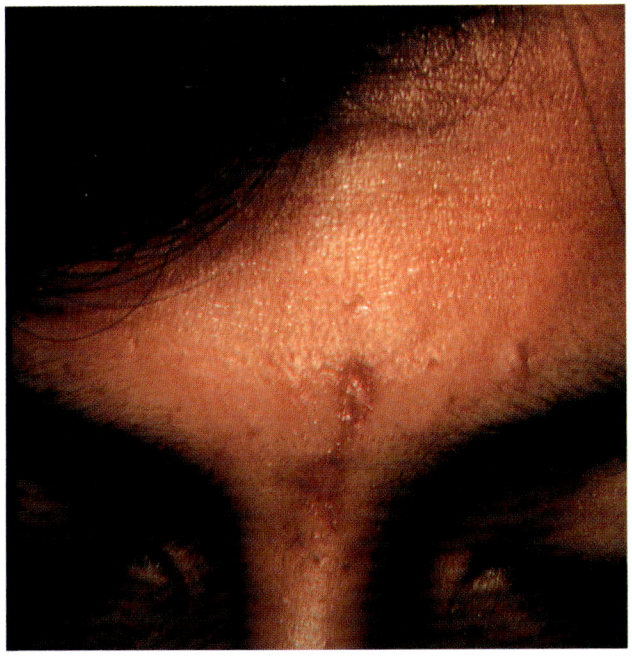

FIG. 4.43-C. One week post-treatment during the healing process.

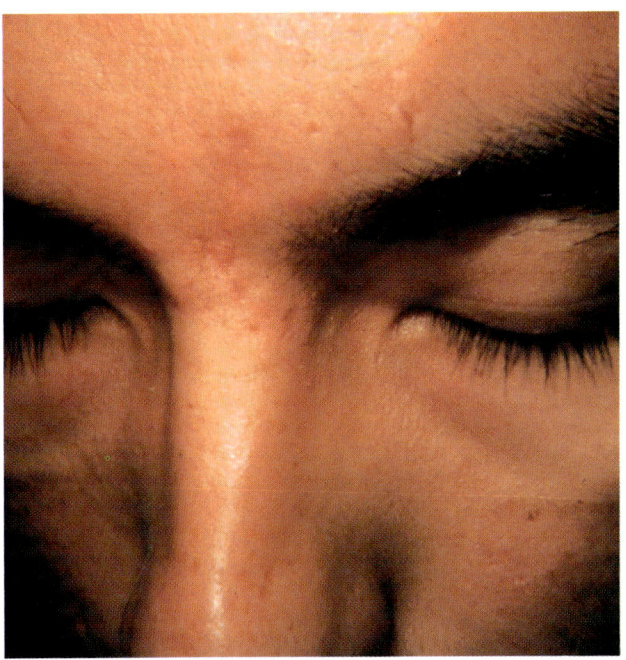

FIG. 4.43-D. Seven weeks post-treatment, the wound is healed with no keloid formation.

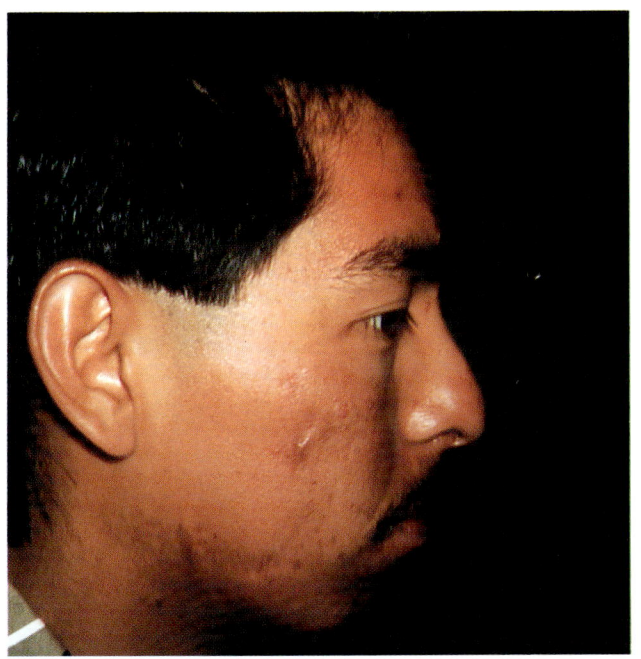

FIG. 4.43-E. Keloid mid face.

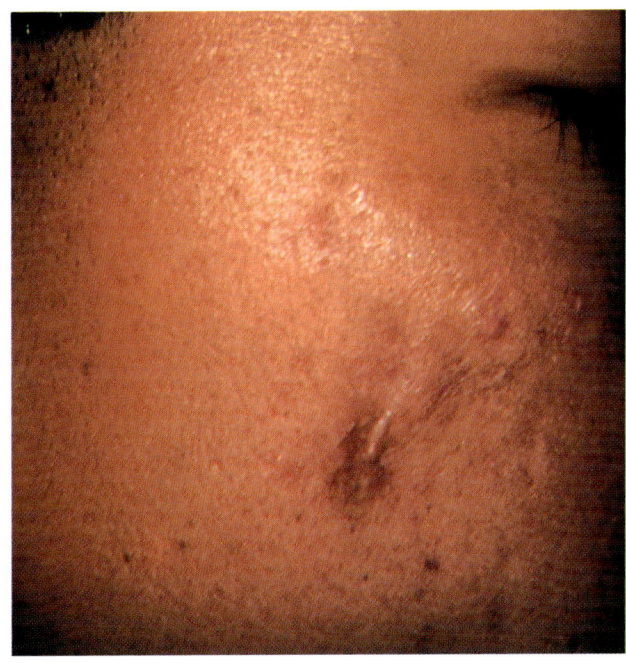

FIG. 4.43-F. Close up of Fig. E.

Case continues on following page.

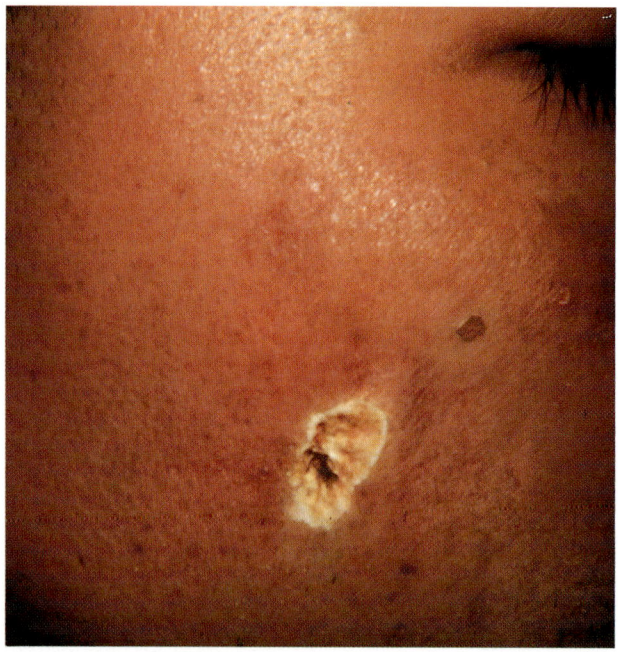

FIG. 4.43-G. After vaporization with the CO_2 laser. The same technique was applied as in Fig. B.

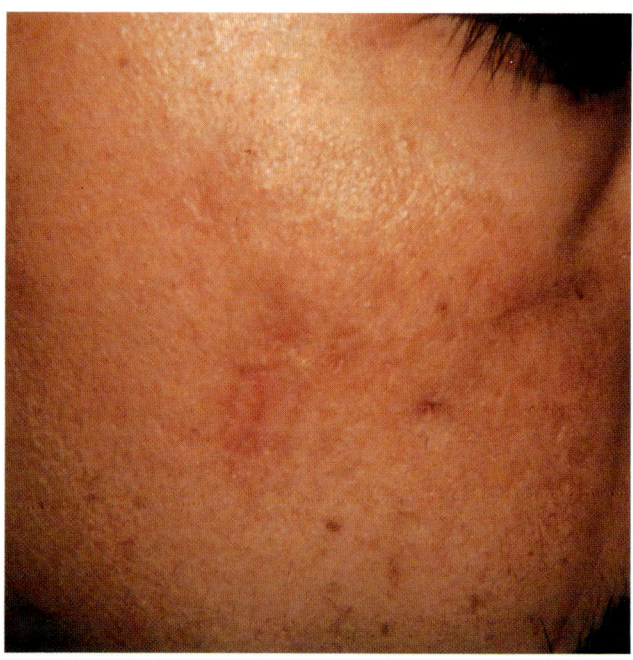

FIG. 4.43-H. Wound healed without keloid formation.

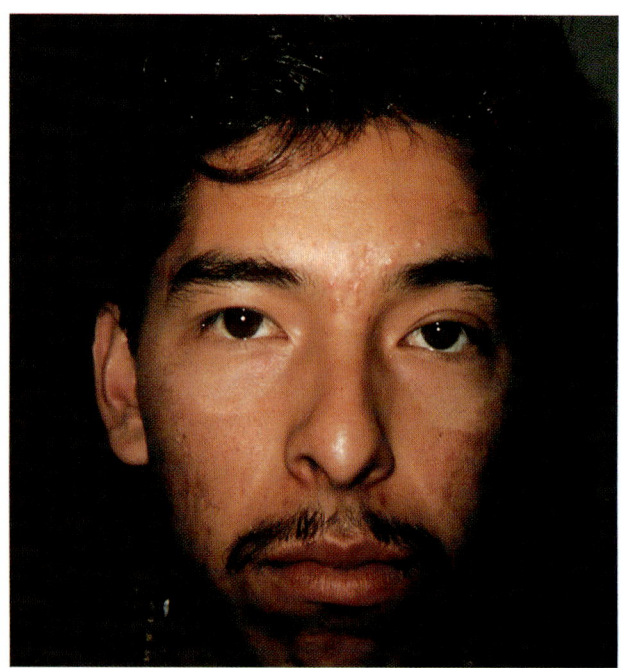

FIG. 4.43-I. Entire face three months post-treatment.

Case courtesy of **Syrus Rayhan,** M.D.

CASE 4.44
Keloid Scars

REVIEW OF CASE. This is a 17-year-old Mexican-American female with a 6 year history of recurrent bilateral ear lobe keloids, after ear piercing. The keloid scars have been treated 4 times previously, twice with surgical excisions and twice with steroid injections. The lesions recurred and continued to grow. The patient was disabled cosmetically with significant psychological impact.

CHOICE OF LASER: SUPER-PULSE CARBON DIOXIDE. The superpulse CO_2 laser emits at 10,600 nm mid-infrared range of the electromagnetic spectrum in a series of peak power bursts occurring very rapidly (ranging from 100–5000 cycles/sec with power outputs of 4–10 watts). Several studies suggest that the superpulse CO_2 laser has the ability to flash vaporize tissue, with less heat conduction into the surrounding tissue. The result is a clean surgical vaporization to a controlled depth, without charring, contraction of surrounding tissue, or significant protein coagulation in tissue adjacent to the target volume. Because there is less necrotic tissue to slough and less thermal damage to be repaired, the inflammatory response is lessened and scar formation is reduced.

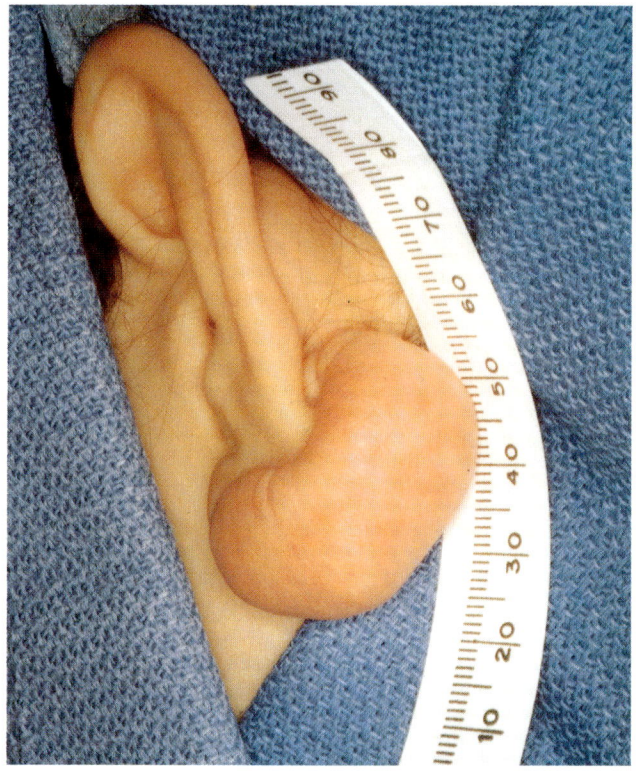

FIG. 4.44-A. Large recurrent right ear lobe keloid which has been treated four times previously, twice with complete surgical excision and twice with local steroid injections.

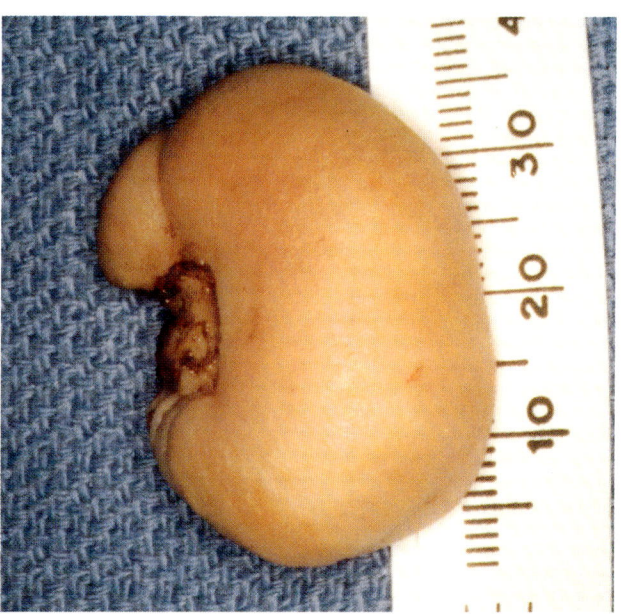

FIG. 4.44-B. Using an 8 watt superpulse CO_2 laser with a 500 watt peak power, 150 microsecond pulse-width, 250 Hz repetition rate and a focused spot size of 0.5 mm the keloid scar was excised using a hand-held piece. Care was taken to remain within the borders of the keloid, not violating normal surrounding tissue. Note the minimal amount of tissue charring. No bleeding occurred. The residual bed was paint-brushed using the superpulse CO_2 laser in defocused mode, at a power output of 4 watts.

Case continues on following page.

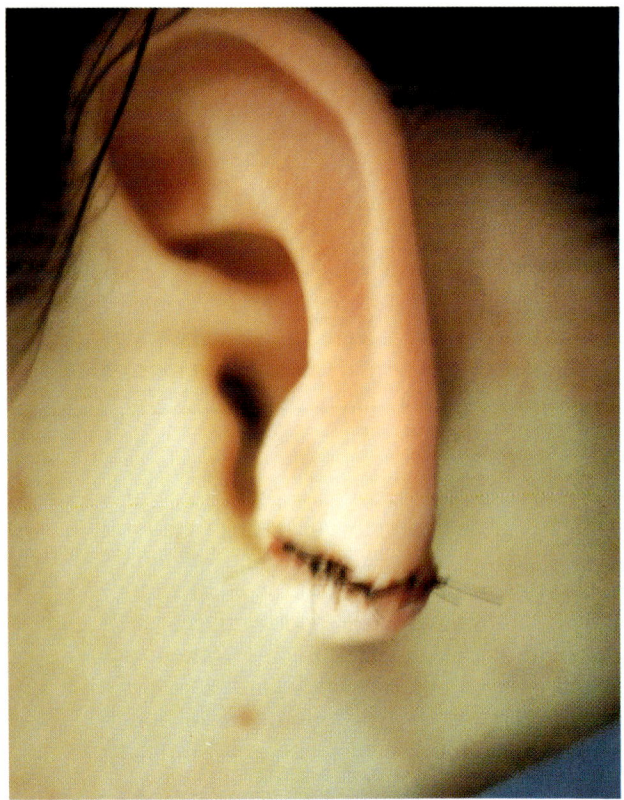

FIG. 4.44-C. The wound is closed with 6-0 nonabsorbable sutures. Sutures are left in place for 7–8 days post-laser treatment. After removal of the sutures, sterile-strips are applied for another 5 days.

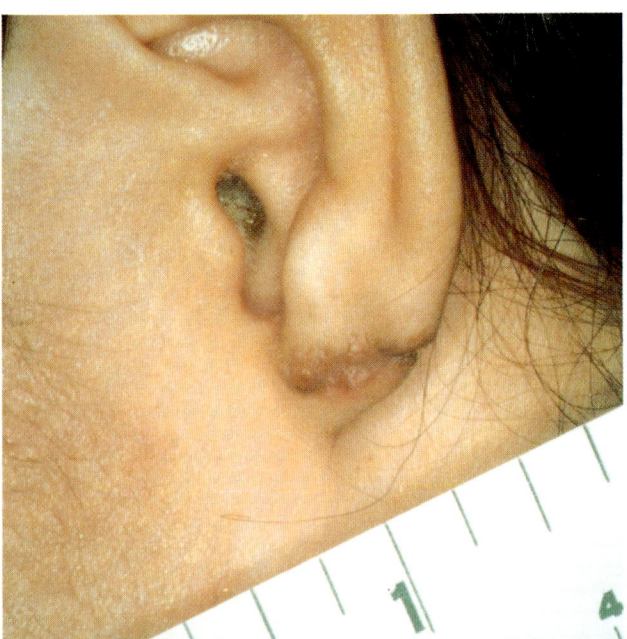

FIG. 4.44-D. Well-healed wound, two months after CO_2 laser excision, without any evidence of recurrences. The edges of the scar were not violated and are clearly seen. However, no regrowth is observed.

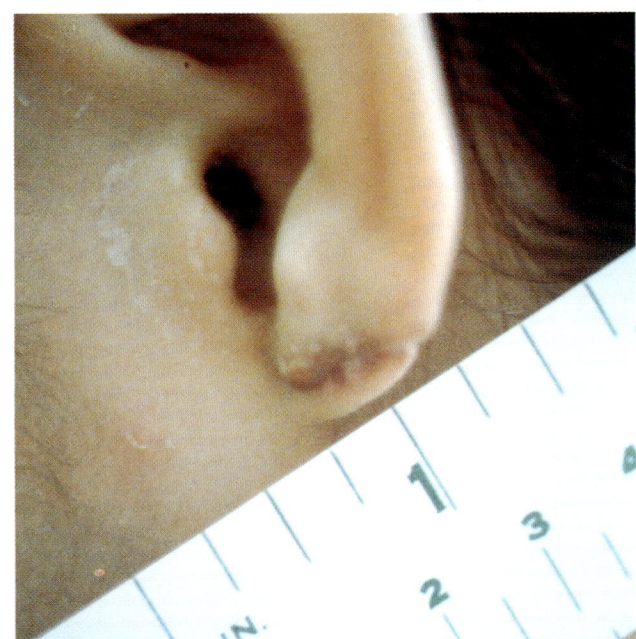

Fig. 4.44-E. No recurrences are seen even after one year post-treatment.

Case courtesy of *Dan J. Castro*, M.D.

CASE 4.45
Earlobe Keloid

REVIEW OF CASE. This healthy 22-year-old white female developed a tender, firm keloid on her right earlobe one year following ear piercing. This progressively enlarged over the next six years until it interfered with function due to increased sensitivity and pain. Previous treatment with potent topical and intralesional steroids produced no change in symptoms or size of this keloid.

CHOICE OF LASER: CARBON DIOXIDE. Energy from the mid-infrared CO_2 laser is selectively absorbed by the intracellular and extracellular water of soft tissues, including keloids, without significant thermal damage to the adjacent structures. Using a precisely focused beam of 0.1–0.2 mm in diameter and moderate power of 15–20 watts in a continuous discharge mode produces a sufficiently high irradiance of 50,000–150,000 watts/cm^2 to permit use of the laser as an incisional instrument that seals blood vessels up to 0.5 mm in diameter as the incision is made.

Previous laboratory research with another infrared laser, the Nd:YAG, has demonstrated that infrared energy can inhibit fibroblast activity and reduce collagen synthesis in cell cultures through a non-thermal mechanism that is, as yet, poorly understood. The concept of laser bioinhibition developed from this basic research data and has been applied to use of the CO_2 laser in a clinical setting to treat keloids. The theoretical possibility exists that CO_2 laser energy might be used to excise refractory keloids in a bloodless and atraumatic technique while simultaneously reducing the risk of recurrence through the possible inhibitory effect of this wavelength of light on fibroblasts.

ADDITIONAL INFORMATION. The usual safety precautions must be carefully followed to adequately protect the patient's eyes and guard against inadvertent ignition of dry surgical drapes or flammable antiseptic solutions during keloid excision.

If excision of an earlobe keloid results in a through-and-through perforation of the lobe, the defect is typically managed by immediately repairing only the anterior surface of the lobe and allowing the posterior aspect of the lobe to heal by second intention. This is done to reduce the time required for healing, but also to minimize the total amount of tension across the wound that would result from closure of both wound surfaces after surgery. Tension is one of the known causes of keloid formation and should be avoided if possible. If a non-perforating defect on either the anterior or posterior aspect of the earlobe is created following laser excision of a keloid, most wounds are generally allowed to heal exclusively by second intention without use of sutures. Postoperative use of flat, clip-on, compression earring devices are sometimes used to further reduce the risk of keloid recurrence.

It is most important to recognize that delayed keloid recurrences are possible even up to eighteen months post-operation. For this reason, cure rates with any surgical technique for the treatment of keloids must be established by careful and diligent long-term follow-up examinations.

POST-TREATMENT CARE. For those defects that will be allowed to heal by second intention, topical wound care consists of twice daily application of 3% hydrogen peroxide solution followed by application of a thin film of antibacterial ointment, and use of a nonstick dressing. For most patients, this will result in complete healing in two to three weeks.

For through-an-through defects that have been partially closed by suturing the anterior surface of the earlobe, the same wound care described above is utilized until the sutures are removed at seven days post-operation but continued to the posterior aspect of the lobe until this portion of the wound has healed by granulation and re-epithelialization, typically in two to three weeks.

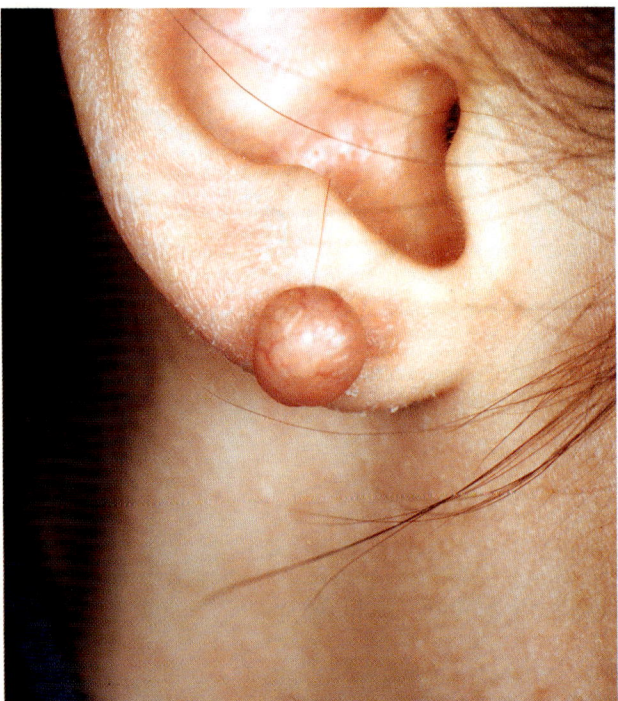

FIG. 4.45-A. Pre-operative appearance of a pedunculated, 1 cm, firm, skin-colored keloid on the anterior surface of the right earlobe.

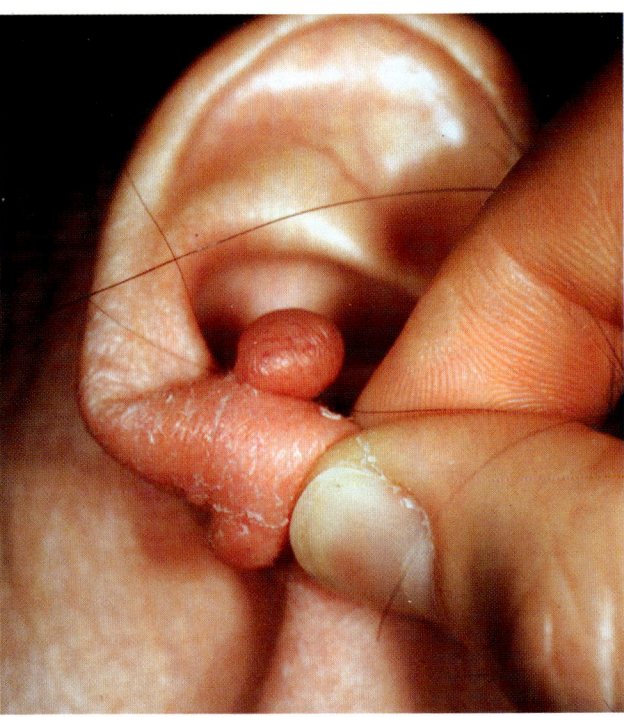

FIG. 4.45-B. With the earlobe held horizontally, the true extent of the keloid becomes apparent with the obvious large mass on the anterior surface (seen in Fig. A) and a smaller mass on the posterior surface of the lobe. Note the firm translobular component can also be readily identified on palpation.

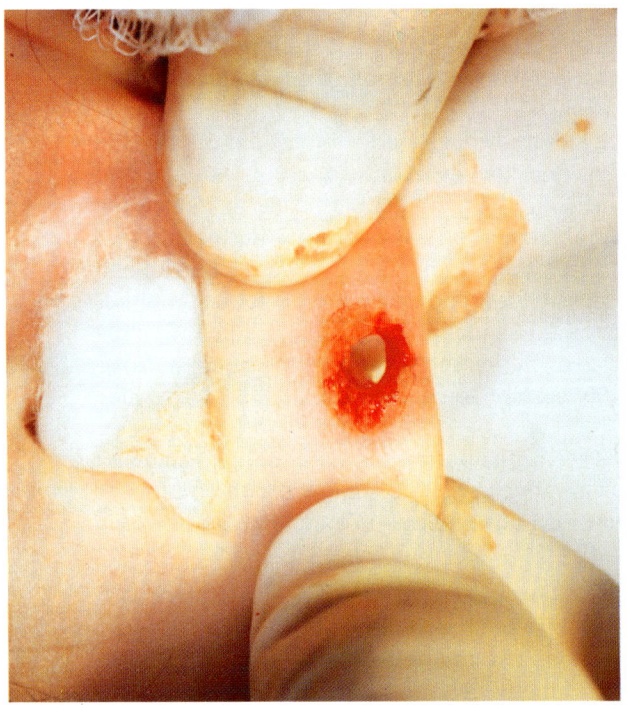

FIG. 4.45-C. After CO_2 laser excision with the focused beam, a through-and-through defect has been created.

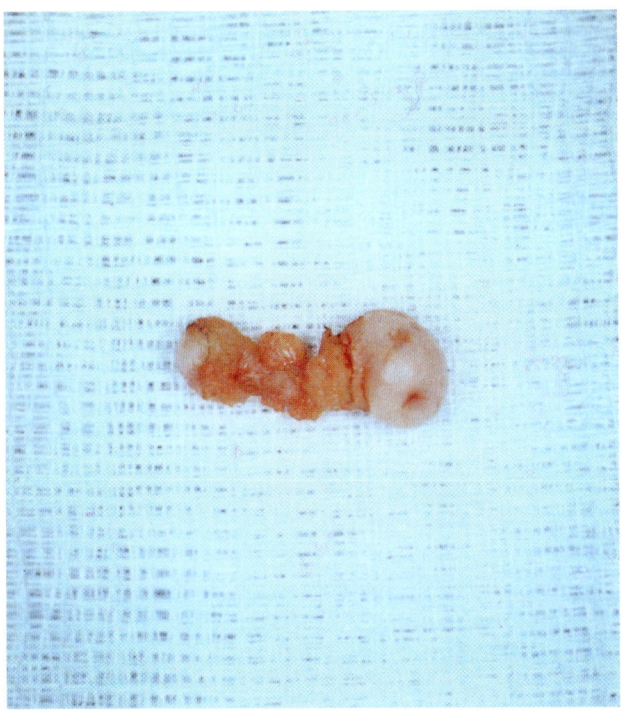

FIG. 4.45-D. Following laser excision, the dumb-bell shaped keloid with central translobular component can be seen on the gross specimen.

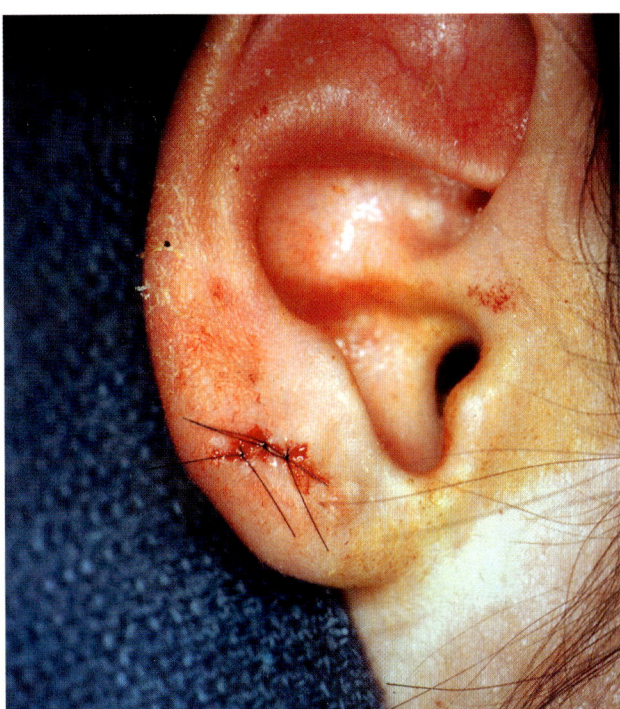

FIG. 4.45-E. Immediately after completion of the laser excision, the anterior surface of the defect has been repaired primarily with simple interrupted sutures. Note the posterior aspect of the defect will be allowed to heal by second intention.

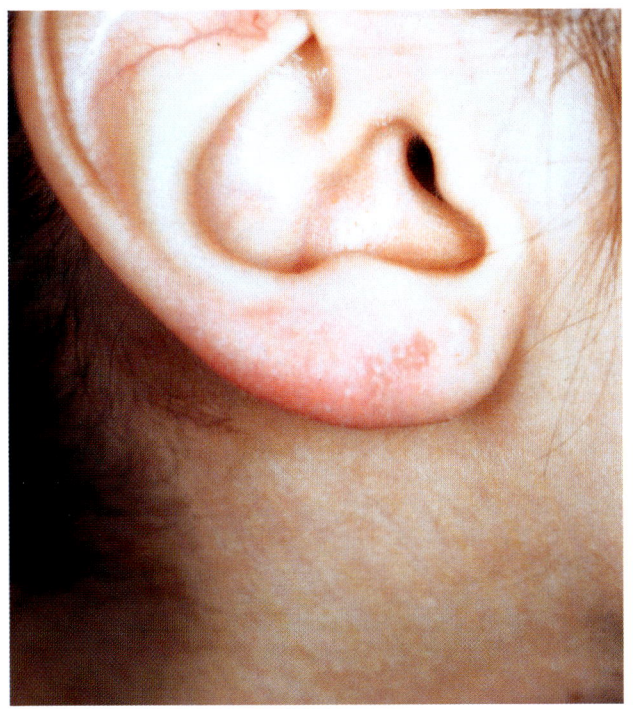

FIG. 4.45-F. The early cosmetic result is seen two months post-operation with a soft, flat, barely visible scar on the anterior surface of the earlobe and no evidence of recurrent keloid.

For literature pertaining to this case see References section.

Case courtesy of **Ronald G. Wheeland**, M.D.

CASE 4.46

Keloid

REVIEW OF CASE. A 32-year-old white male who underwent surgery some three years ago for removal of a sebaceous cyst on his neck. He developed a keloid, which was then treated unsuccessfully with another surgery and steroid injection.

CHOICE OF LASER: CARBON DIOXIDE. The CO_2 laser is the best laser for vaporization procedure.

ADDITIONAL INFORMATION. The treatment was performed with the CO_2 laser at 20 watts, continuous out of focus mode, in order to obtain a flat uniform vaporization of the lesion at its base. Immediately after the laser procedure, 60 mg of Depo-Medrol was injected underneath the lesion and repeated at monthly intervals thereafter for a total of 3 months. The success rate is not clear yet, and the patient should be informed that the procedure is still experimental.

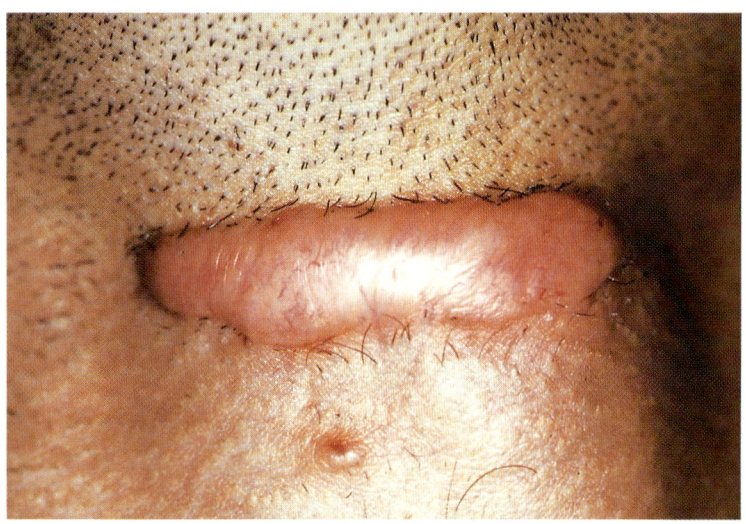

FIG. 4.46-A. Keloid of neck, front view.

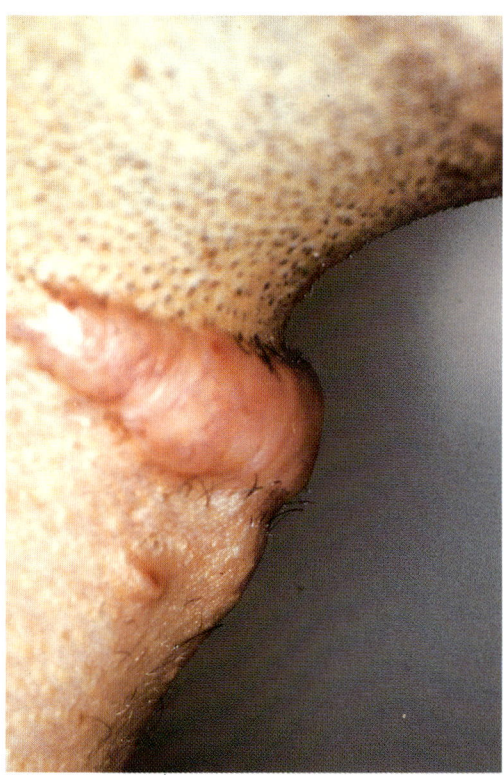

FIG. 4.46-B. Keloid of neck, side view.

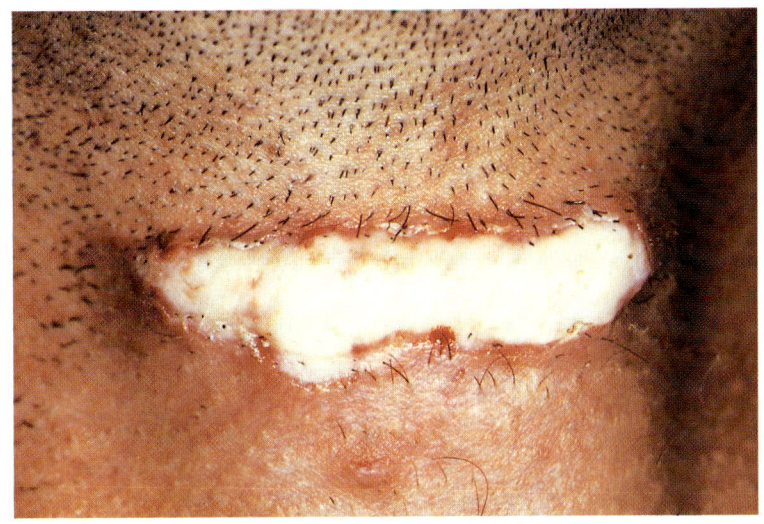

FIG. 4.46-C. Immediately post-treatment.

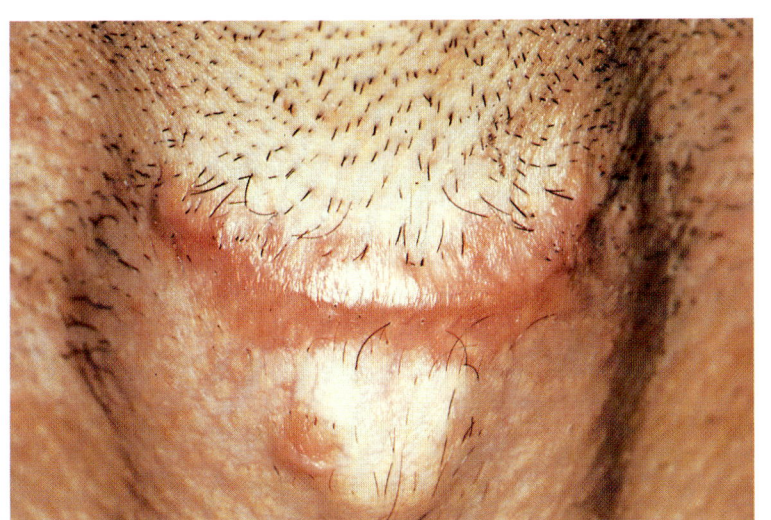

FIG. 4.46-D. One year post-treatment, front view.

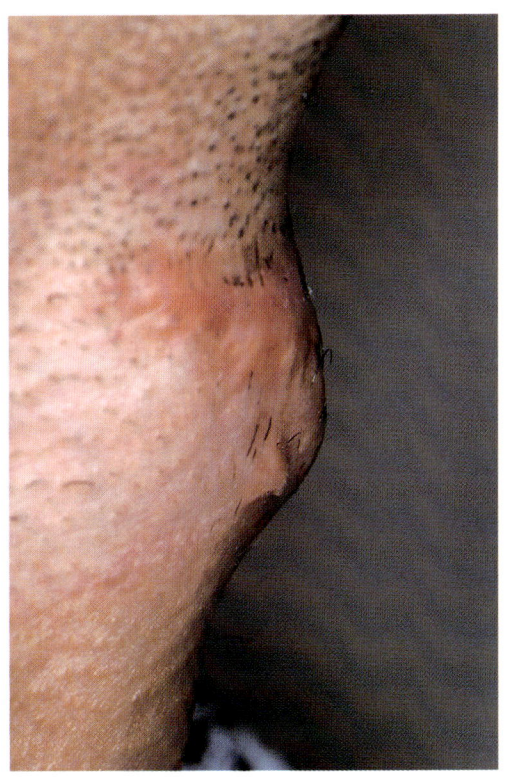

FIG. 4.46-E. One year post-treatment, side view.

Case courtesy of *Arie Orenstein,* M.D.

CARBON DIOXIDE LASER

CASE 4.47
Keloids

REVIEW OF CASE. This 30-year-old black male developed pseudofolliculitis barbae that resulted in localized follicular infection. When the infection resolved, scar tissue and keloid formation developed. Histology confirmed that the keloid resulted from follicular infection based on foci of ingrown hairs and pus within the keloid.

CHOICE OF LASER: CARBON DIOXIDE. The CO_2 laser was chosen to excise the keloid because of the minimal peripheral damage that results from its use. There is usually no need to use electrosurgery for hemostasis. The power setting used is 20 watts with a continuous beam that is focused to 0.1 mm. The lesion was excised down to the subcutaneous fat leaving behind no palpable keloid. The wound was allowed to heal by second intention, and preferably *no* sutures were necessary. Granulation and re-epithelialization occurred in approximately six weeks. The resulting scar was wide but flat and asymptomatic. The cosmetic end point was considered acceptable for someone with a tendency for keloids. Follow-up six months post-operation revealed slight thickening of the scar, and was treated with intralesional steroids.

ADDITIONAL INFORMATION. Some surgeons make the mistake of simply shaving the keloid flat with the skin surface using the laser. When keloid is left behind either after shave excision or vaporization with the laser, recurrence would be more likely. In addition, it is important to pre-select which keloids are more likely to respond based on anatomic location. Lesions on the face and earlobe respond best, while lesions on the chest, shoulders, and back respond poorly. Primary closure causes excessive pressure or stretch on the wound edges and may result in hypertrophic scarring. Often, intralesional steroids are used immediately post-operation and during follow-up. Pressure garments may also be required. Use of the CO_2 laser alone is clearly not the only important part of treating keloids. Recurrence of keloids may develop as much as two years post-operation. Cure rates are unclear at this time but, given the difficult nature of treating keloids, CO_2 laser excision is at least comparable to standard surgical excision, intralesional steroids, or radiation therapy.

POST-TREATMENT CARE. Antibiotic ointment (2% erythromycin in petrolatum) and nonadherent gauze normally are used for six weeks. Periodic intralesional steroid injections and pressure garments as needed.

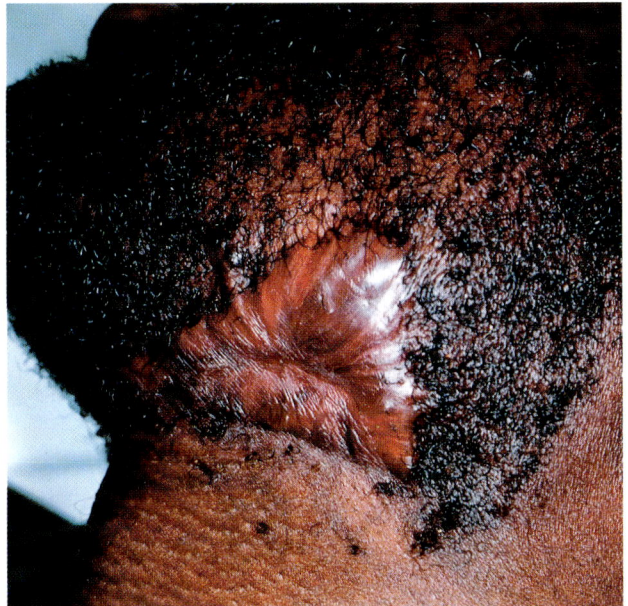

FIG. 4.47-A. Keloid pre-operation, left cheek. Patient has another keloid on the right side.

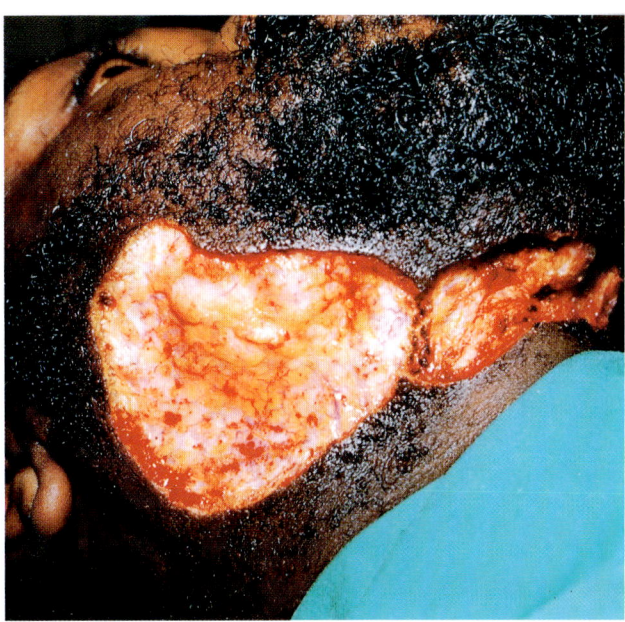

FIG. 4.47-B. Immediate post-operative result of keloid on the right jaw and neck. Note the bloodless field and excision taken down to the subcutaneous fat.

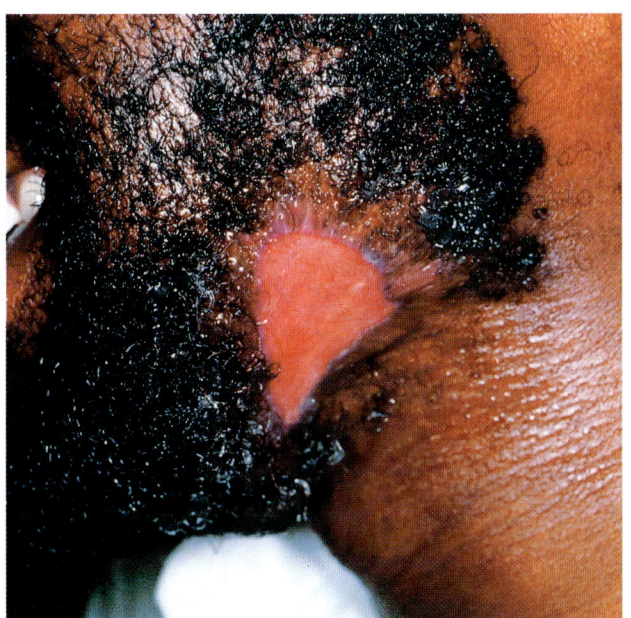

FIG. 4.47-C. Five weeks post-operation; granulation is complete but re-epithelialization will take another two weeks.

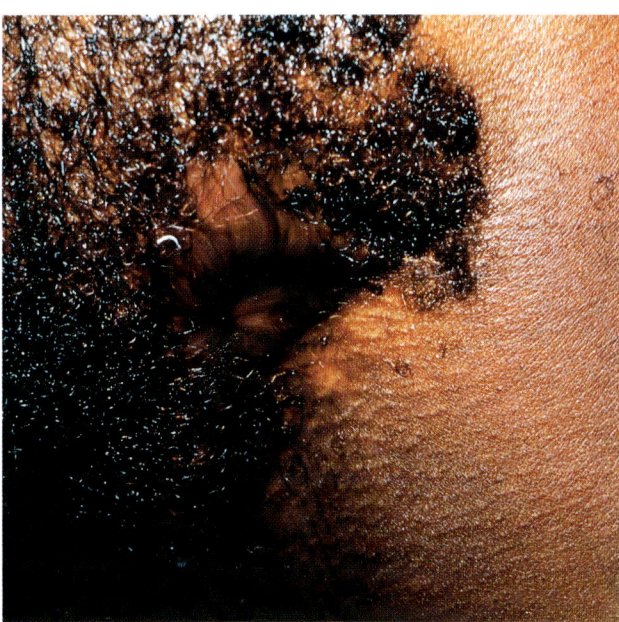

FIG. 4.47-D. Six months post-operation; flatter, asymptomatic, smaller scar. Slight thickening has developed which can be treated with repeated intralesional injections of glucocorticoid.

Case continues on following page.

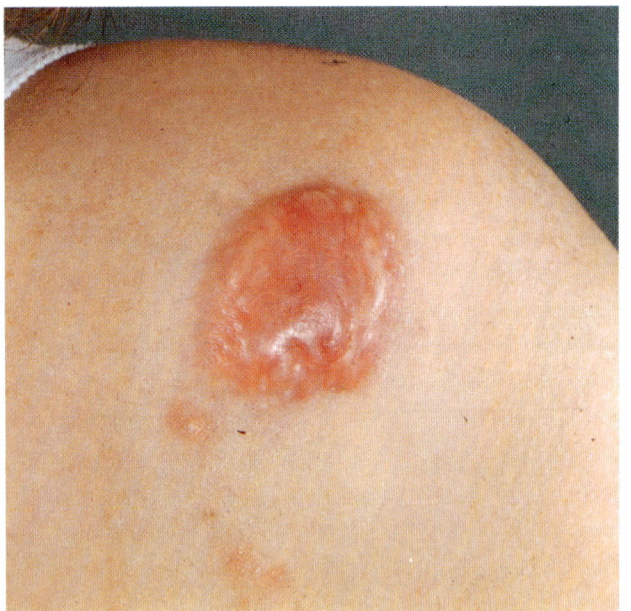

FIG. 4.47-E. A different patient with a keloid on the shoulder as a result of acne. This is a difficult location to treat as recurrences are common.

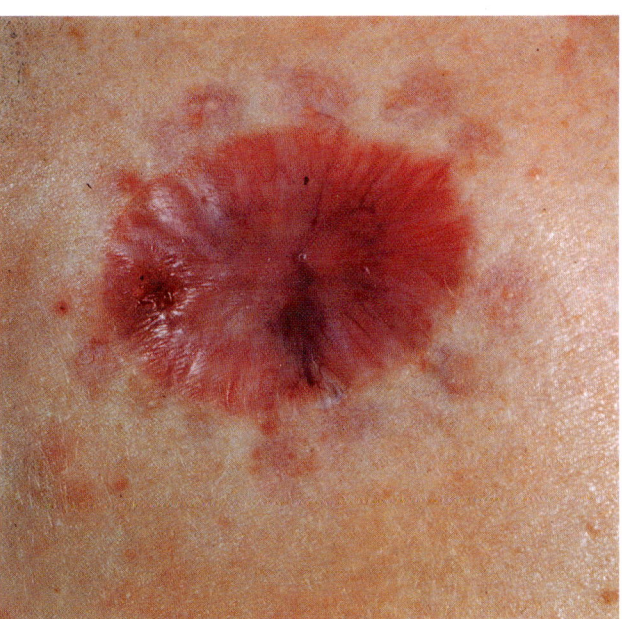

FIG. 4.47-F. Same patient as in Fig. E. Six weeks post-operation; while still wide, the scar is flatter. Sometimes recurrences can be treated with intralesional steroids, but in this case the keloid returned but only half as thick.

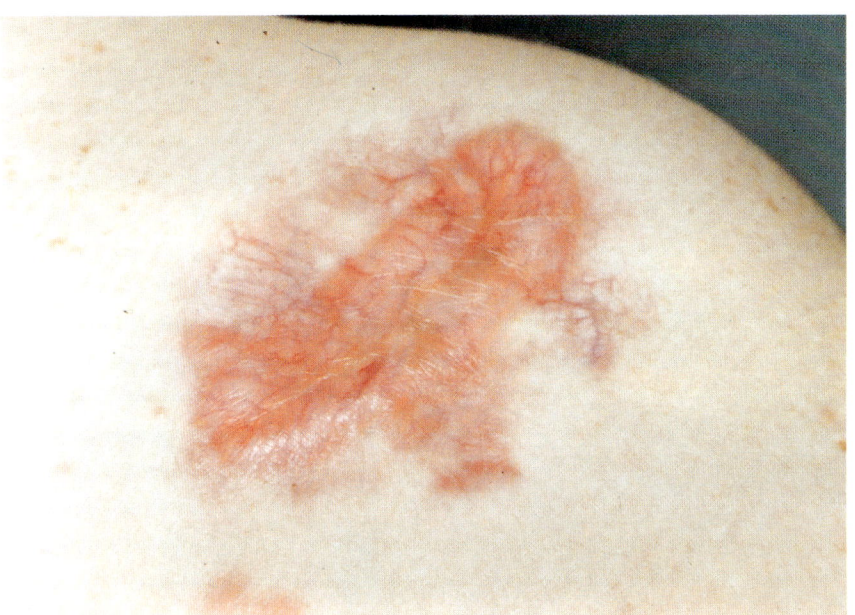

FIG. 4.47-G. Same patient as in Fig. E. Six and one-half months post-operatively. Partial recurrence has been treated by intralesional glucocorticoid injections.

Case courtesy of *Randall K. Roenigk,* M.D. and *Philip L. Bailin,* M.D.

CASE 4.48
Multiple Keloids

REVIEW OF CASE. This 45-year-old black female began to develop keloids spontaneously in 1987 in the beard area of the neck and chin. They did not respond to either topical or intralesional steroids and had become very painful, developing multiple abscesses.

CHOICE OF LASER: CARBON DIOXIDE. The CO_2 laser was chosen to treat these keloids because of the author's previous success in treating such lesions. In addition, the patient was further motivated to pursue this type of therapy because of the successful treatment of similar keloids in her sister by CO_2 laser excision. Although the use of this laser is not universally accepted for the treatment of keloids, many treatment failures may be due to differences in technique, or speed with which the excision is carried out. When used properly, the CO_2 laser will cause minimal thermal damage, and because it lies in the infrared area of the electromagnetic spectrum, it may have additional inhibitory effects of fibroblast activity.

ADDITIONAL INFORMATION. Although CO_2 laser excision has been extremely rewarding for most of this author's keloid patients, there are those who continue with proliferative growth of their scars. These patients may require intralesional steroid treatment indefinitely. Two important points to be made for successful keloid removal are: (i) The excision must be carried out rapidly and effectively so as to minimize thermal damage to the surrounding tissue, and (ii) all of the fibrosed tissue must be removed totally in order to maximize the potential for success.

POST-TREATMENT CARE. The wounds are coated with a nonsensitizing antibacterial ointment such as Polysporin or Batroban. This is covered with Vigilon and then with a bulk dressing. The dressing is left in place for 24 hours. The dressing is then removed, and the wound is cleansed with hydrogen peroxide and a similar dressing is reapplied. This process is repeated for 5–7 days. Following this, the Vigilon may be replaced by a nonstick telfa dressing and the wound may be cleansed with either peroxide or a mild Hibiclens solution.

Case continues on following page.

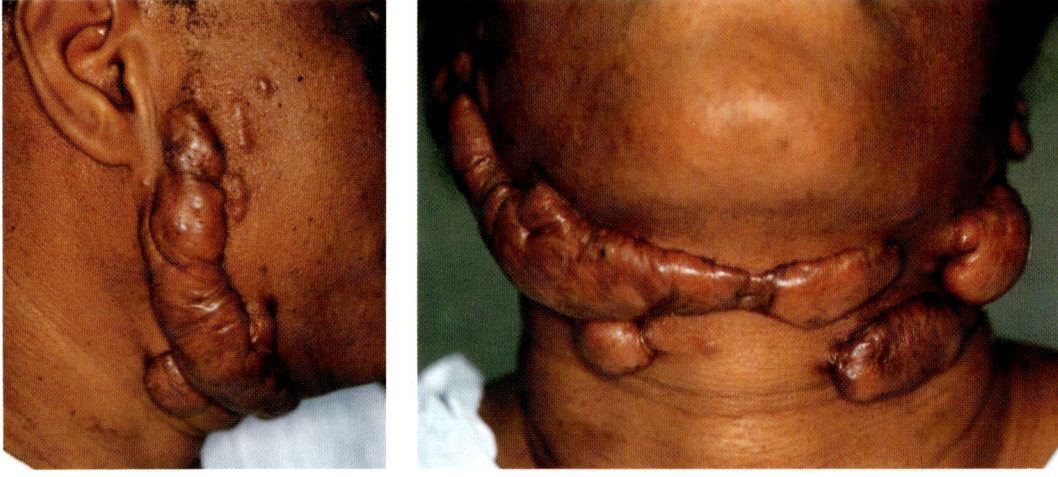

FIG. 4.48-A. Panoramic view of the extent of involvement by keloids in this patient.

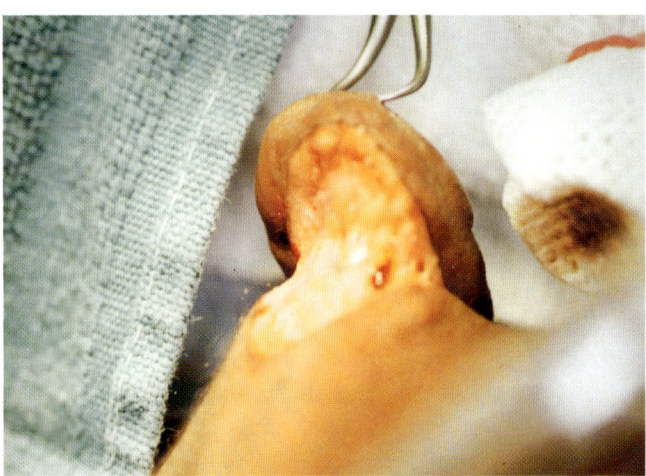

FIG. 4.48-B. Operating at 10 watts of power, with a 0.1 mm spot in the continuous mode, the initial cutaneous incisions are made, which are followed by the actual excision process which is carried out at 20 watts of power.

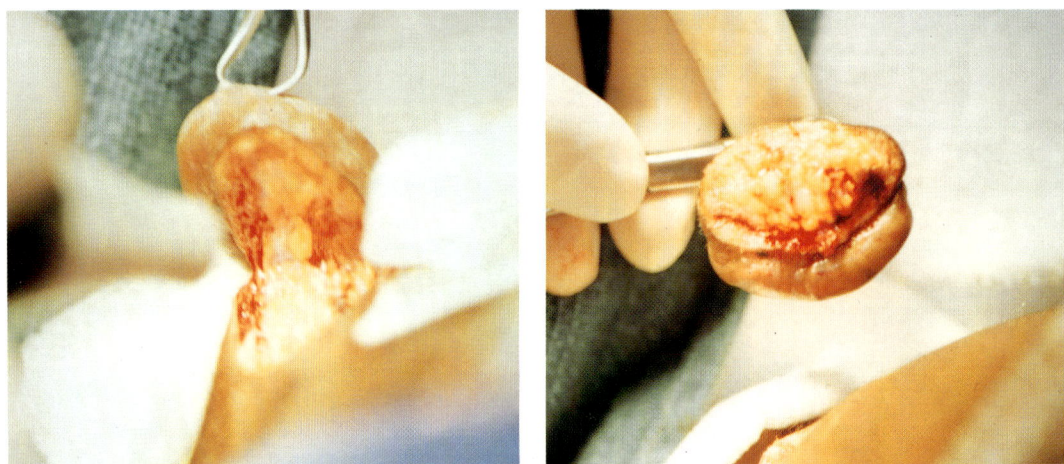

FIG. 4.48-C. Once each individual keloid is removed, the wound is carefully palpated for any evidence of residual keloid. Any such residual tumor is then further excised. Should additional hemostasis be necessary, the laser can simply be defocused for sealing of larger vessels. For small arterioles, electrocautery may be necessary.

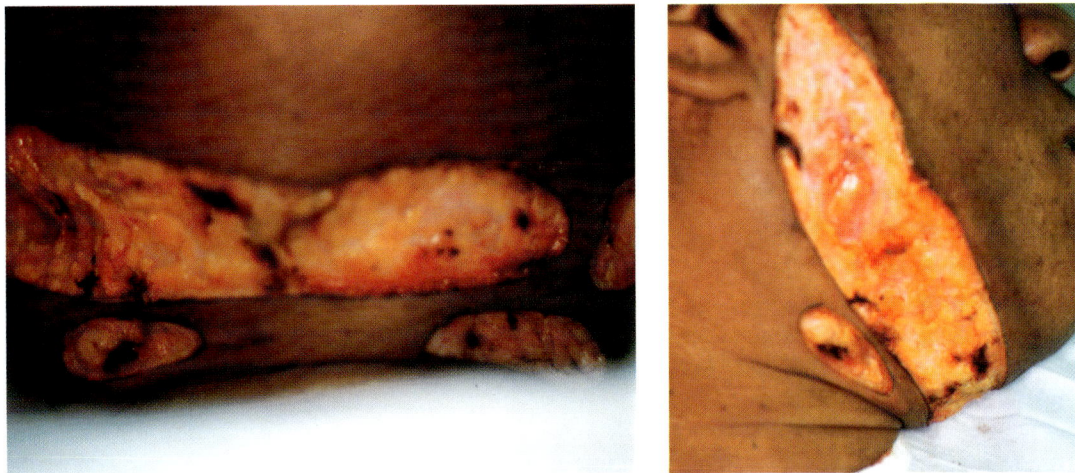

FIG. 4.48-D. Appearance of the open wound once keloid removal has been completed.

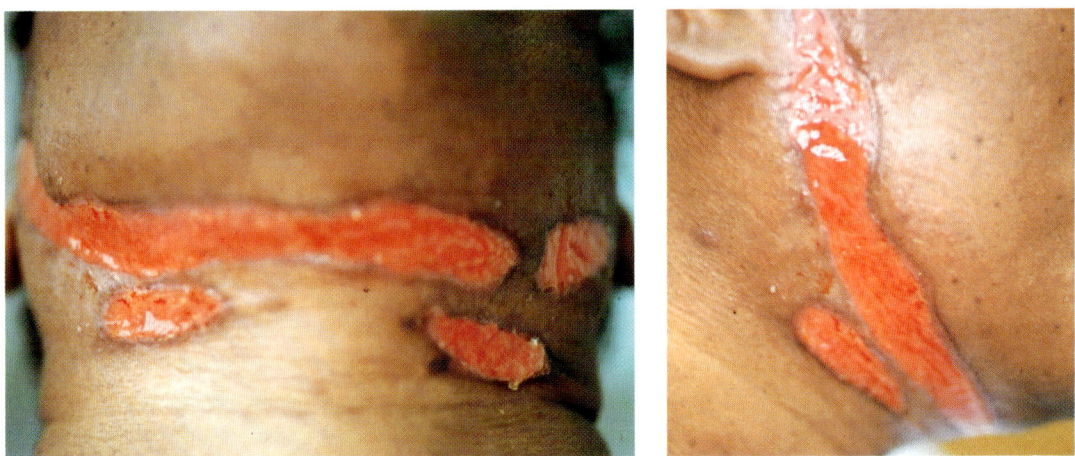

FIG. 4.48-E. Appearance of the patient one month after keloid removal showing excellent granulation and contraction and flattening of the wounds.

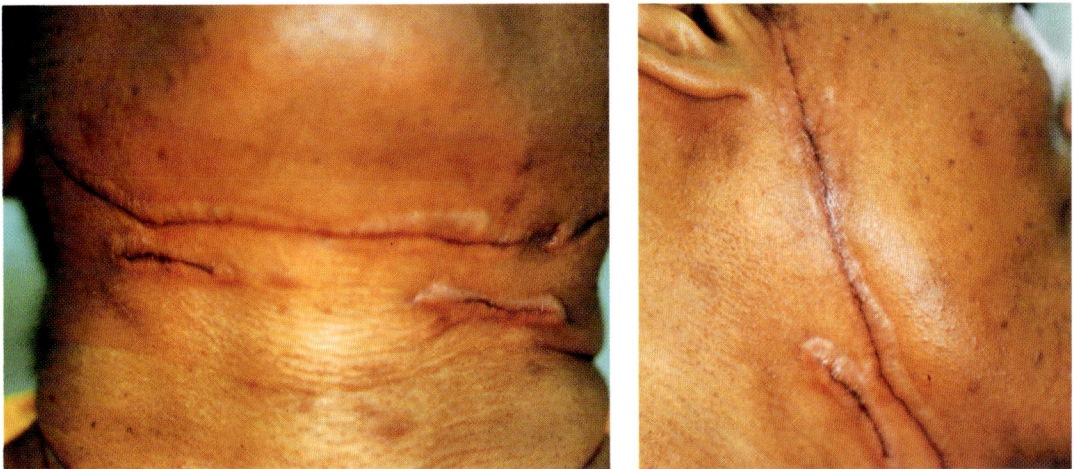

FIG. 4.48-F. Appearance of the wounds three months after the surgery revealing the excellent result. Such wounds must be carefully monitored for the development of any thickening of the scar. Any such hypertrophic cicatrix should then be injected intralesionally with triamcinolone acetonide at a concentration of no less than 40 mg per cc. Such injections may be necessary at four week intervals and should be carried out until the thickening has ceased.

Case courtesy of *John Louis Ratz, M.D.*

CASE 4.49

Lichen Planus

REVIEW OF CASE. A 52-year-old white female who was unaware of how long her lesions had been present. However, recently she complained of an itching and burning sensation in this area.

CHOICE OF LASER: CARBON DIOXIDE. A CO_2 laser was chosen to be used for the biopsy of the lesion, and for the "peel" and ablation of the rest of the lesion. A "peel" is accomplished using the laser highly out of focus at a low wattage and causing the tissue to blister, and therefore able to be peeled away. The CO_2 laser has been proven to be the laser of choice for intraoral soft tissue lesions and lesions of this nature. Advantages of the laser over conventional scalpel surgery are: (i) Decreased to absent surgical and post-surgical bleeding, (ii) little chance for mechanical trauma to the tissues, (iii) sterilization of the wound site, (iv) minimal swelling and scarring, and (v) probably from the patient's point of view minimal to absent post-operative pain in the majority of cases. Because of the systemic nature of these lesions they can often recur with frequency. Due to the lasers benign ability of removing these types of lesions, when they do recur patient's are less apprehensive to have the procedure re-performed.

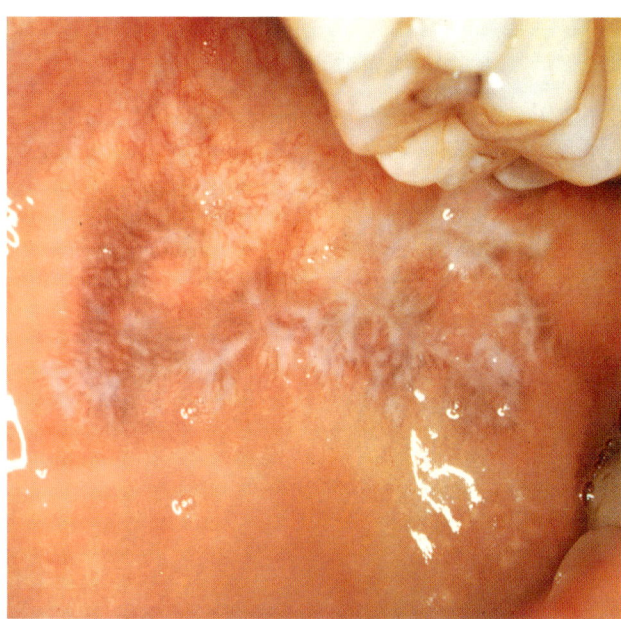

FIG. 4.49-A. The area on the patient's buccal mucosa showing a suspected lichen planus. Note the classic Wickham's striae. The patient's chief complaint was that the lesion itched.

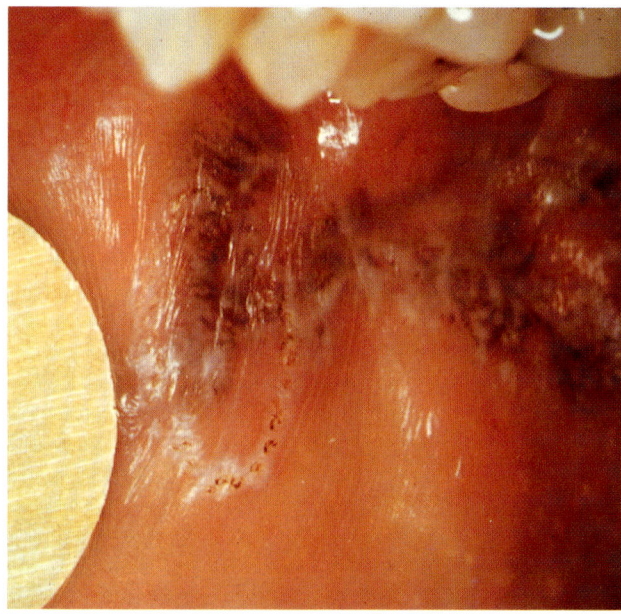

FIG. 4.49-B. The area to be biopsied is outlined using a pulsed mode, slightly defocused, and 5 watts of power. Note that normal margins will be taken as well as pathologic tissue.

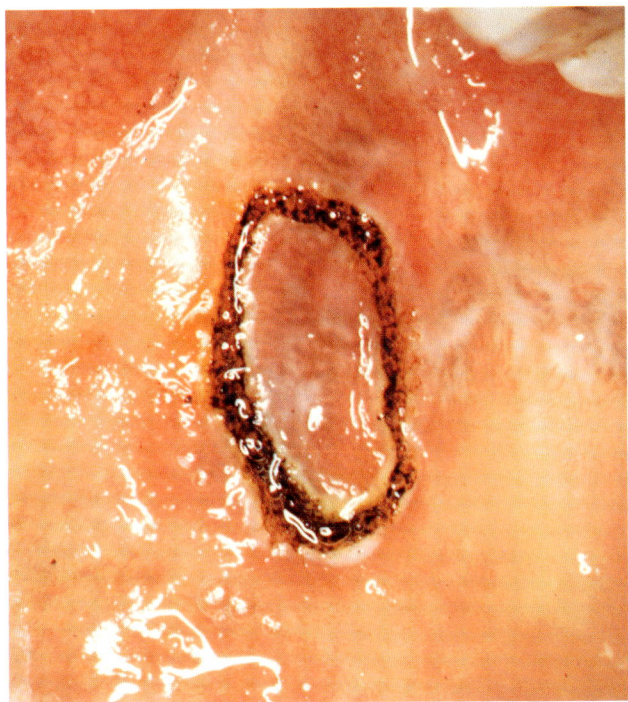

FIG. 4.49-C. Using 7 watts, and a focused beam the area to be biopsied is definitely outlined. Again, note that the bottom one-third of the biopsy contains normal tissue.

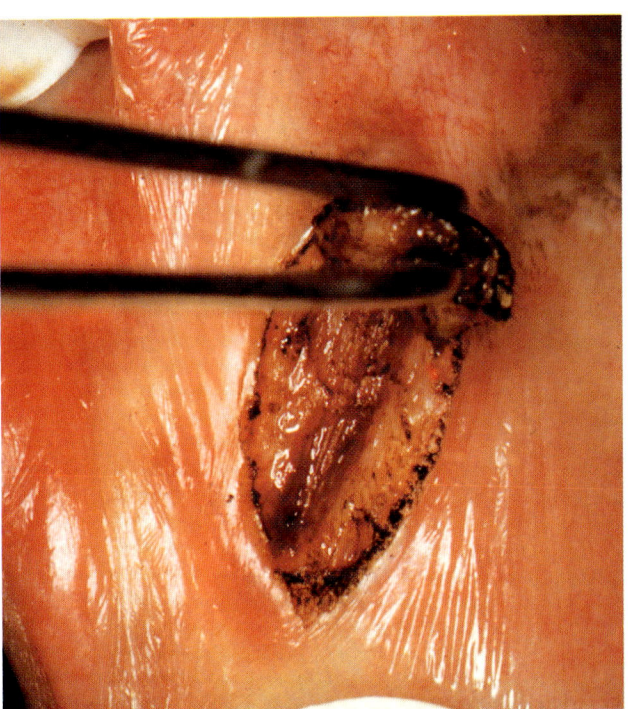

FIG. 4.49-D. Using a tissue pick-up an edge of the lesion is grabbed and lifted. Then using traction/counter-traction the lesion can be undermined using 10 watts, and a slightly defocused beam. Note the hemorrhage-free nature of the biopsy in an area that normally bleeds easily.

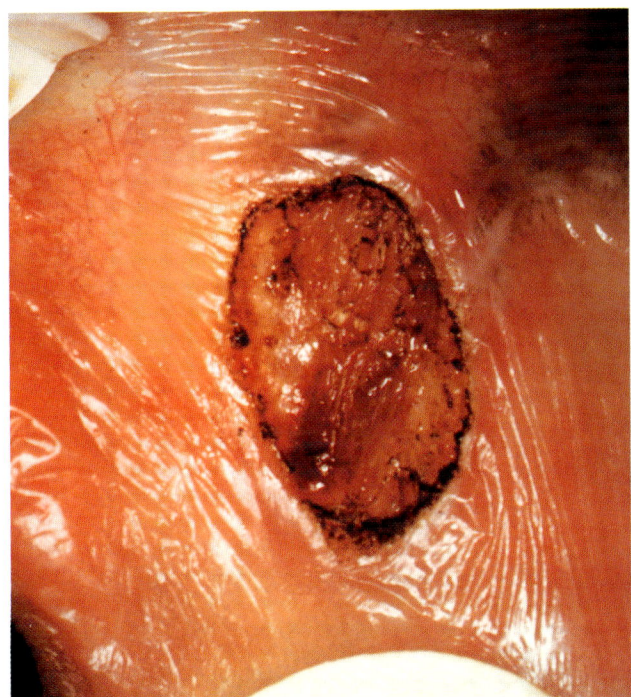

FIG. 4.49-E. The area of the incisional biopsy immediately after lasing. Note the hemorrhage-free nature of the wound in an area that normally bleeds easily.

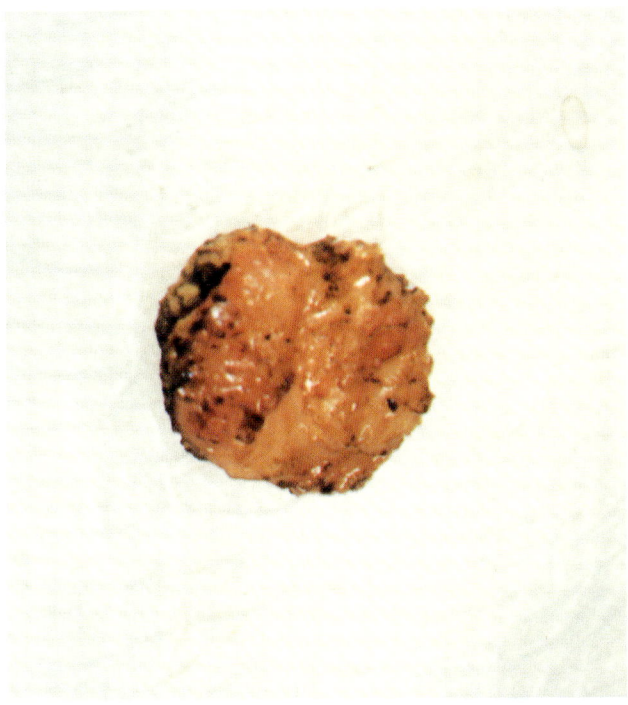

FIG. 4.49-F. A connective tissue view of the lesion before being sent for biopsy.

Case continues on following page.

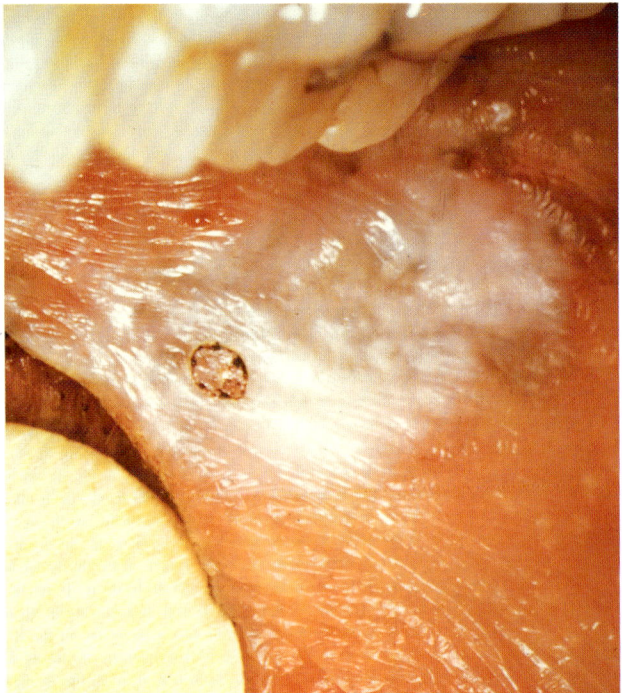

FIG. 4.49-G. To further remove the rest of the suspected lesion, using a highly *defocused* beam, 7 watts, the area is lased until the tissue blisters.

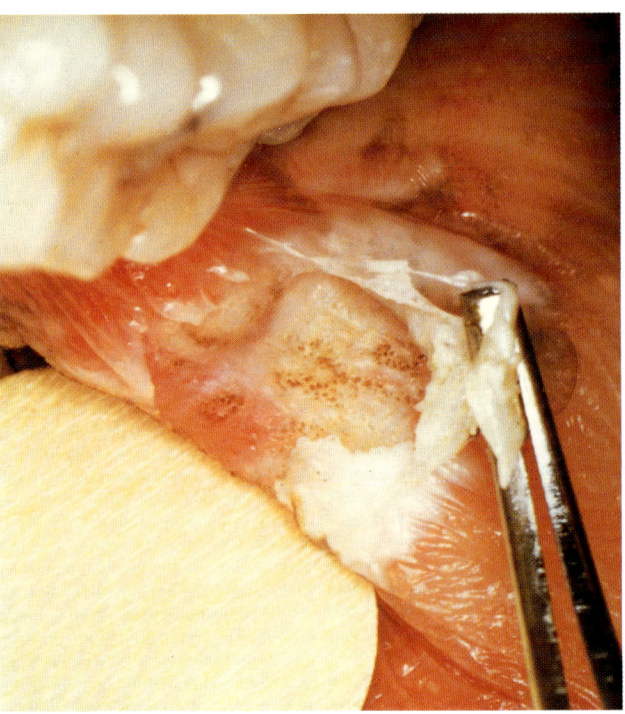

FIG. 4.49-H. Using a tissue pick-up or a curved hemostat the blistered area can be "peeled" away exposing underlying tissue. If the tissue appearance is not healthy, additional lasing may be necessary.

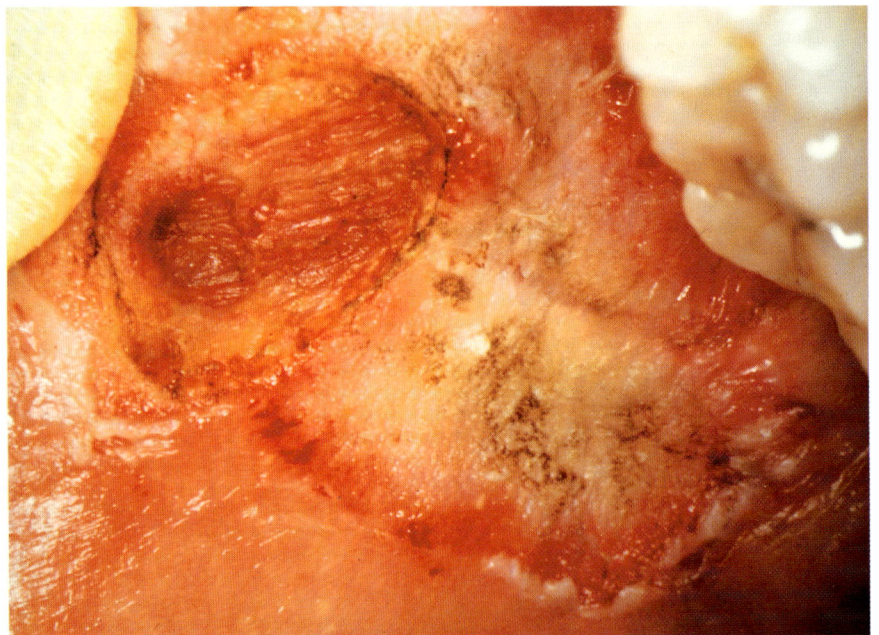

FIG. 4.49-I. The area of the biopsy and laser peeling. As with most intraoral lesion removal, at this point using a 7 to 10 watt defocused beam, the "char layer" will be placed to ensure effective coagulation and a hemorrhage-free post-operative course. Biopsy proved the lesion to be lichen planus.

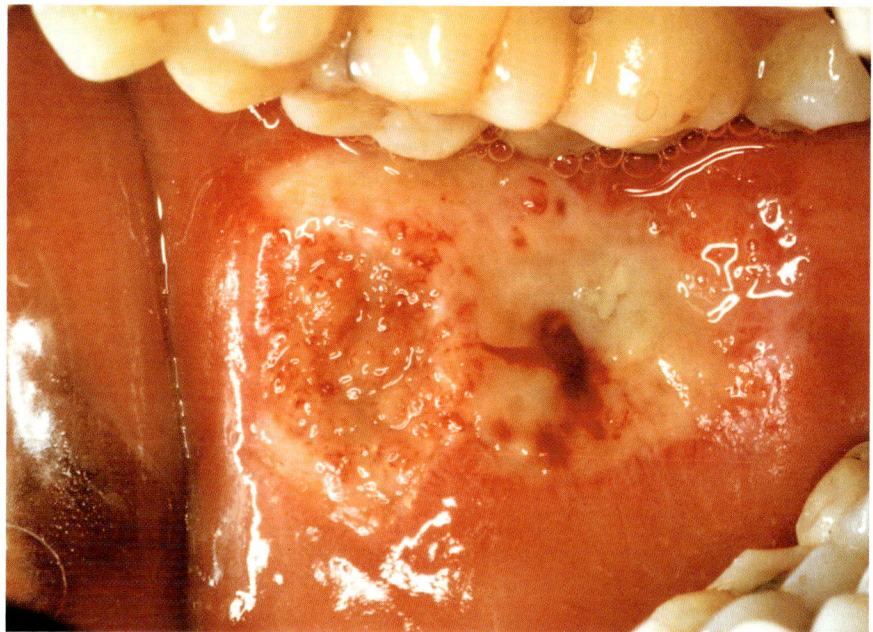

FIG. 4.49-J. The appearance of the lesion at one week. As with most intraoral laser wounds they have a whitish "aphthous-like" appearance. However, the patient is in no discomfort.

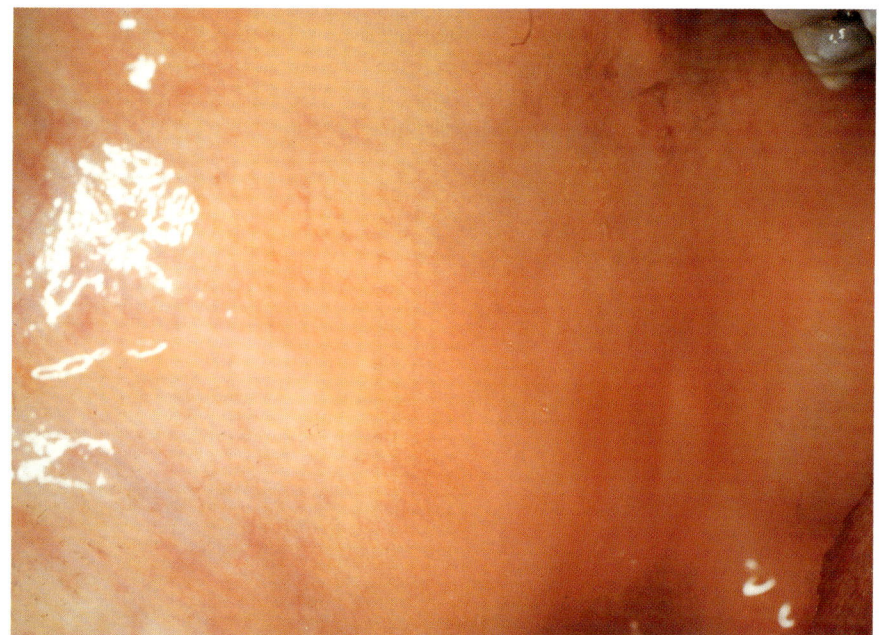

FIG. 4.49-K. The same patient three months after laser surgery. Because of the systemic nature of lichen planus, patients need to be informed of its recurrence rate.

Case courtesy of **Robert M. Pick**, D.D.S.

CASE. 4.50
Partial Radical Nail Excision

REVIEW OF CASE. This is a 67-year-old female who suffered a traumatic injury to the lateral aspect of the right index finger a number of years previously. At that time, the nail plate was injured and was sutured. The resulting nail growth was erratic with a separated piece along the lateral aspect of the nail. The lesion was refractory to local measures and was constantly being caught in the patient's clothing. Therefore partial radical nail excision was planned.

CHOICE OF LASER: CARBON DIOXIDE. The CO_2 laser permits a variety of procedures to be performed on the nails and nail bed with little bleeding and morbidity. The procedure is greatlly facilitated by the fact that it is possible to destroy the nail matrix and diseased portions of the nail bed without the need of counter incisions proximal to the subungual fold. Post-operatively, the wounds are easily cared for and the patients may resume their normal activities immediately.

ADDITIONAL INFORMATION. Digital block anesthesia was accomplished with 1.5% Carbocaine and a Penrose drain tourniquet was put in place. The area was prepared and draped in sterile fashion. The pre-operative view is demonstrated in Fig. A. A CO_2 laser was used with a 125 mm handpiece (0.2 mm spot size) at 25 watts continuous power. The nail is first scored along the proposed line of resection by placing the laser beam parallel to the long axis of the nail (Fig. B). The portion of the nail to be removed is grasped (Fig. C) and the laser is used to facilitate the avulsion of the nail. A Senn retractor is then used to raise the subungual fold (Fig. D) and the laser is used in a pulsed fashion to destroy the underlying nail matrix. Figure E demonstrates the completed result after the removal of the tourniquet. The patient is advised to keep the area clean and to use an antiseptic ointment until complete healing occurs.

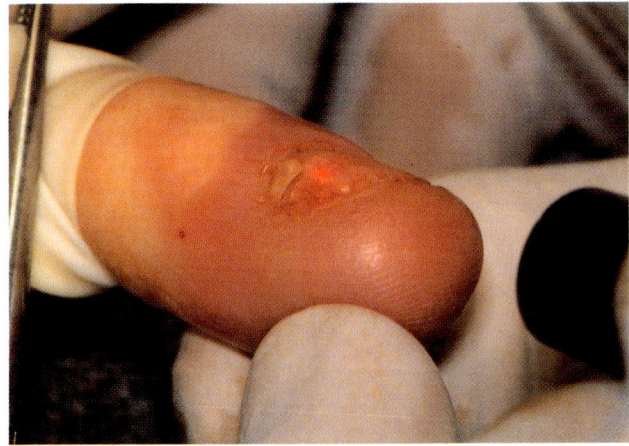

FIG. 4.50-A. Pre-operative appearance of the nail. Note abnormal pattern of nail growth.

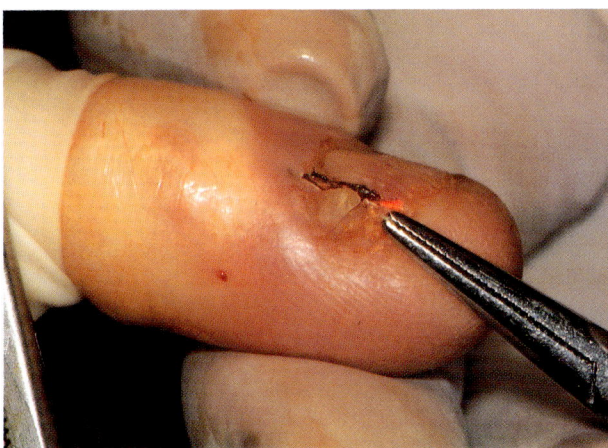

FIG. 4.50-B. The nail is scored with the CO_2 laser by holding the laser beam parallel to the long axis of the nail and thereby separating the diseased portion of nail from the nail portion which will remain in situ.

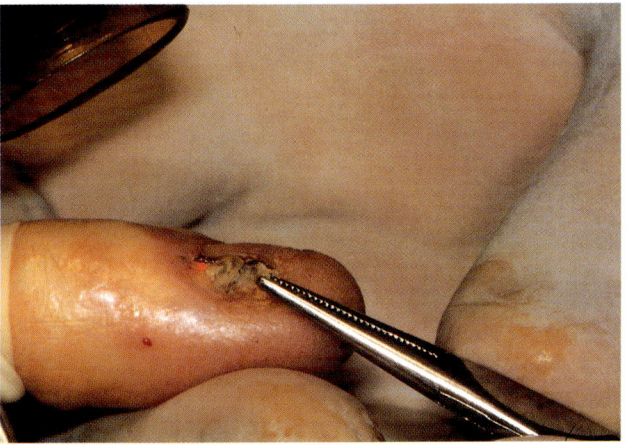

FIG. 4.50-C. The diseased portion of the nail is grasped with a clamp and will be dissected by using the laser to separate it from the underlying tissues.

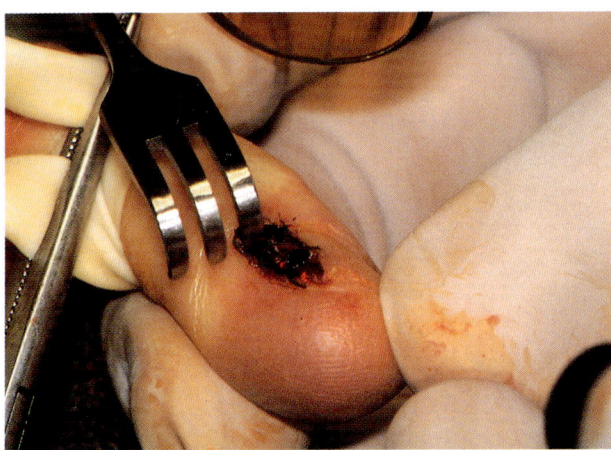

FIG. 4.50-D. A Senn retractor is used to retract the subungual fold and to permit destruction of the underlying nail matrix.

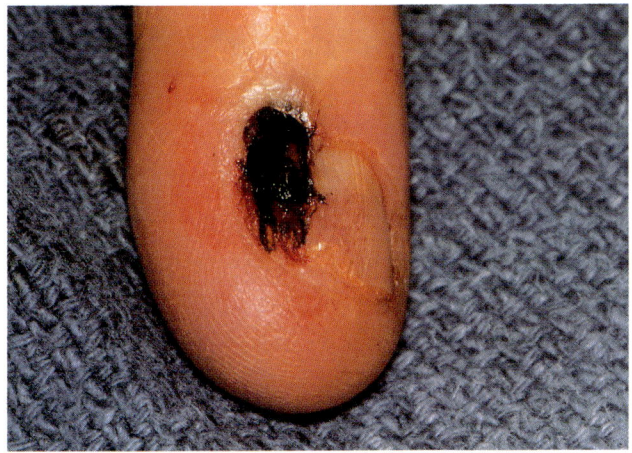

FIG. 4.50-E. The immediate post-surgical result is shown following the removal of the tourniquet.

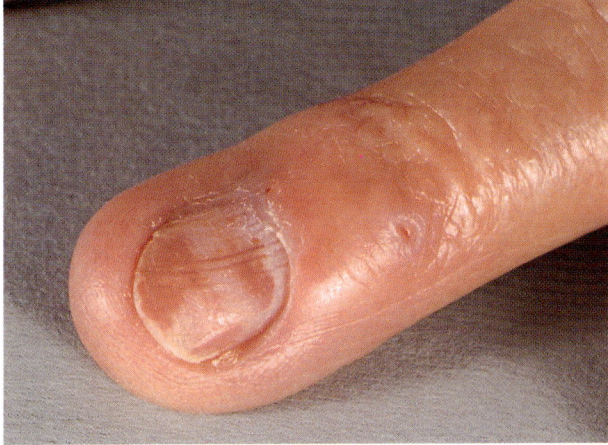

FIG. 4.50-F. The late post-operative view is shown at one year.

Case courtesy of *Raymond J. Lanzafame, M.D.*

CASE 4.51
Nevocellular Nevus

REVIEW OF CASE. This patient is a 30-year-old female presenting with a nevocellular nevus about 12 mm in size on the left nasolabial fold. The lesion first appeared at infancy and gradually grew larger.

CHOICE OF LASER: CARBON DIOXIDE. With the CO_2 laser, successive transpiration therapy is possible, and compared with electrocoagulation, microscopic removal of the lesion can be performed. In case of large bosselated lesions, treatment can be done in a short period of time with the CO_2 laser after excising a part of the lesion. Post-operative pain, swelling, and bleeding are almost nonexistent, and the results are extremely good.

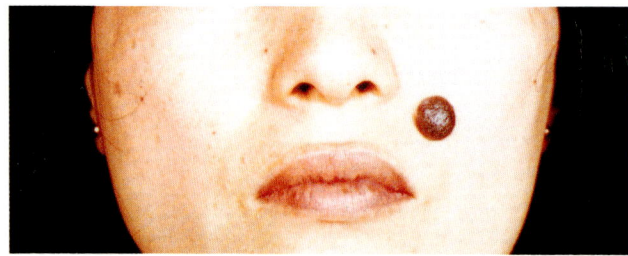

FIG. 4.51-A. Pre-operative view.

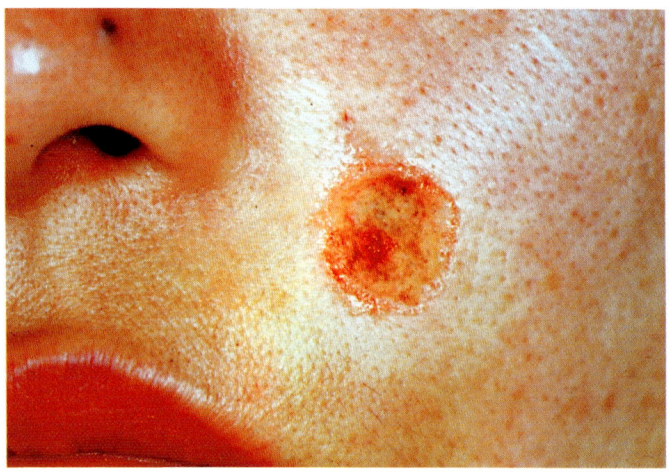

FIG. 4.51-B. Immediately after being treated with the CO_2 laser.

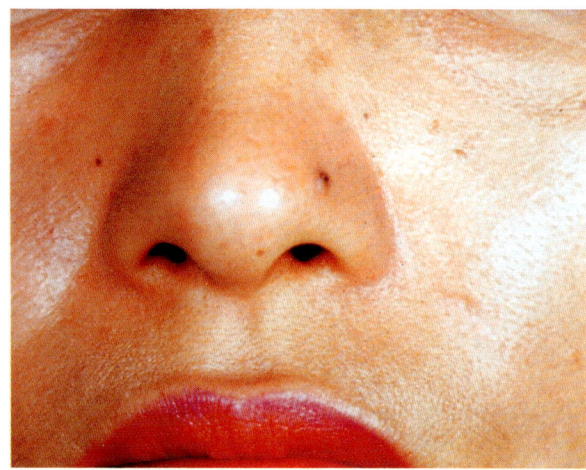

FIG. 4.51-C. One year after operation. Although a slight scar remains, the results are satisfactory.

Case courtesy of **Taichin Morita,** M.D., **Hiroto Yamada,** M.D., **Muneo Miyasaka,** M.D., **Ryuzaburo Tanino,** M.D., and **Mitsuhiro Osada,** M.D.

CASE 4.52

Neurofibromatosis

REVIEW OF CASE. This is a 44-year-old white female who developed lesions of neurofibromatosis at the age of 16. There is no family history of the disease. The patient's major complaint was that because the lesions were increasing in size and some of the lesions were growing between her toes, causing pain, it was hard for her to dress. She was not able to find employment because of the lesions on her face. Pathology on a large lesion revealed no change toward malignancy.

CHOICE OF LASER: CARBON DIOXIDE. The CO_2 laser was chosen because several hundred lesions could be vaporized or excised in one session. Because the CO_2 laser seals lymphatic and blood vessels, there is less chance of swelling and bleeding.

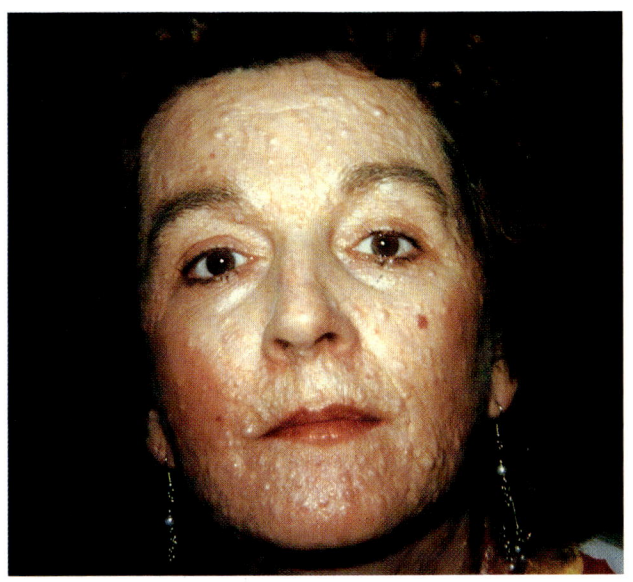

FIG. 4.52-A. Neurofibromatosis on face.

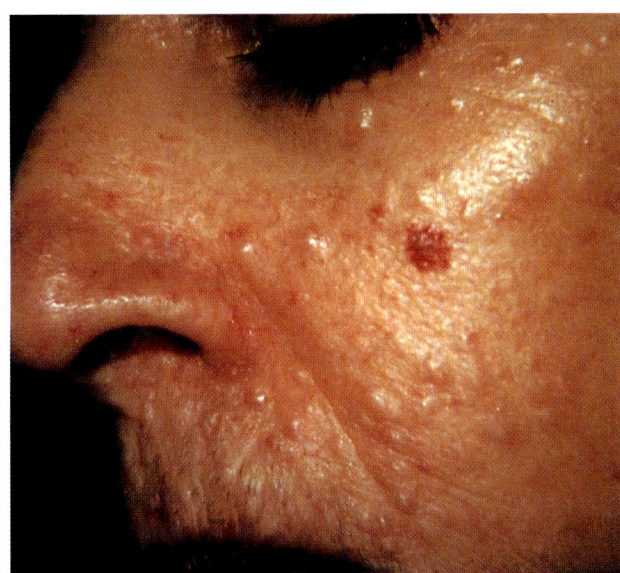

FIG. 4.52-B. Close-up of Fig. A.

Case continues on following page.

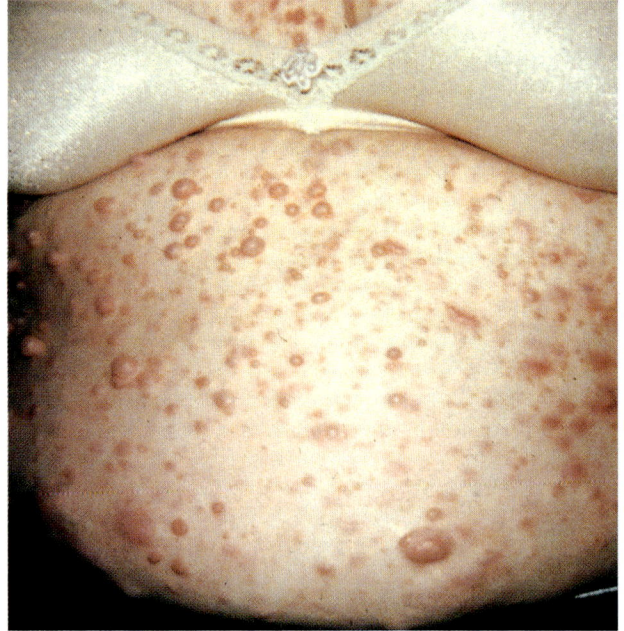

FIG. 4.52-C. Widespread lesions including involvement on the abdominal area.

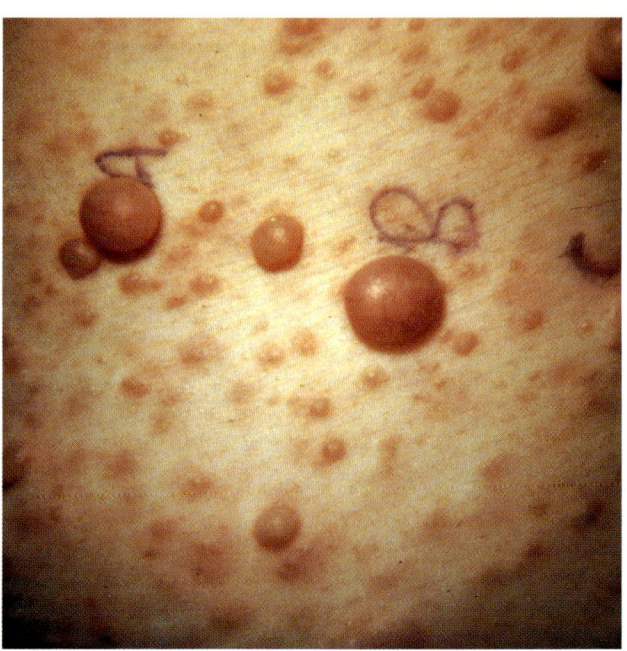

FIG. 4.52-D. Close-up of Fig. C.

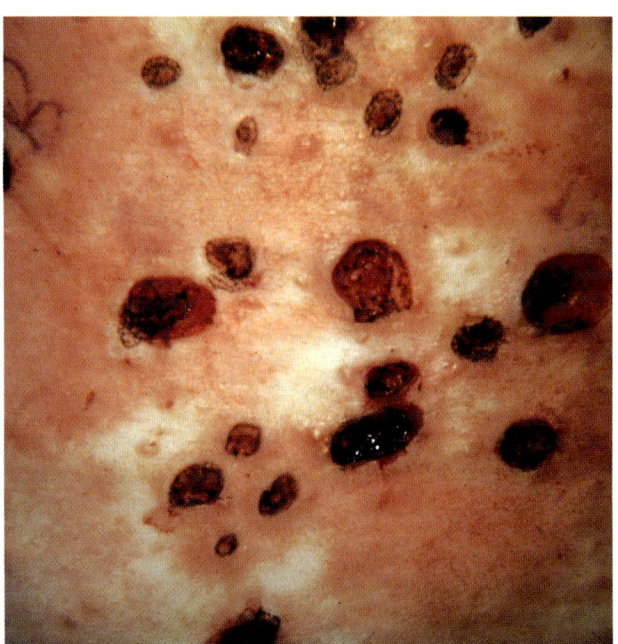

FIG. 4.52-E. Under general anesthesia, the lesions were vaporized using a CO_2 laser with a 10 watt defocused beam.

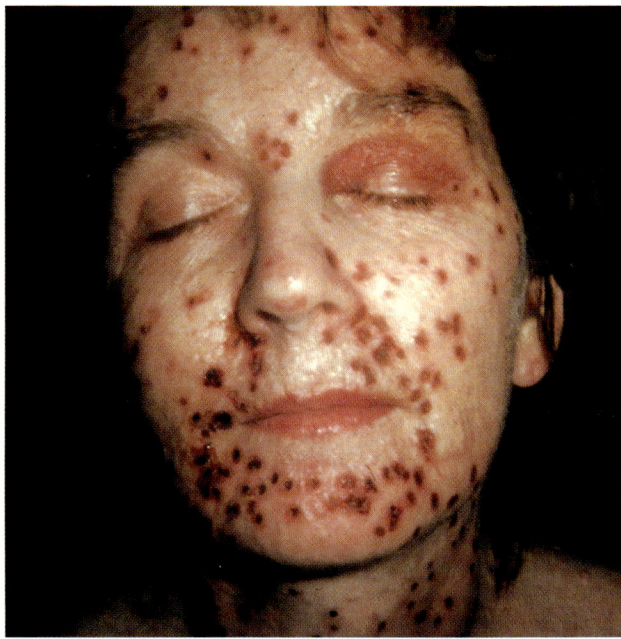

FIG. 4.52-F. The same technique was used in Fig. E to vaporize lesions on the face and neck.

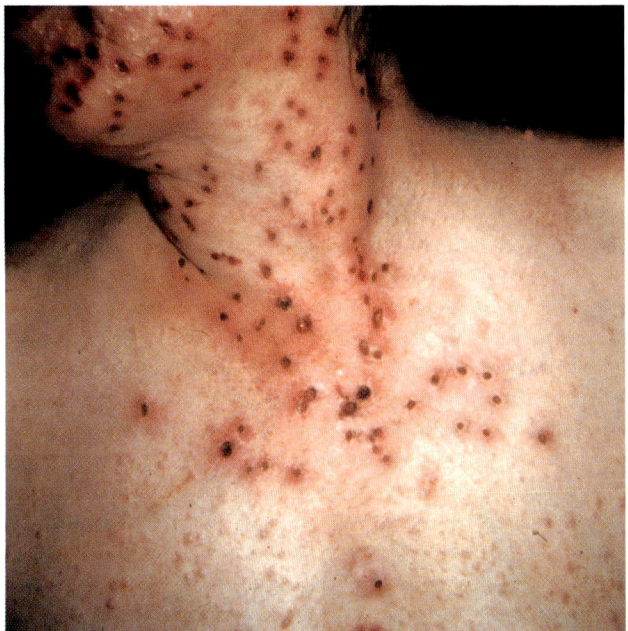

FIG. 4.52-G. Neck region after vaporization of lesions using the CO_2 laser with a 10 watt defocused beam.

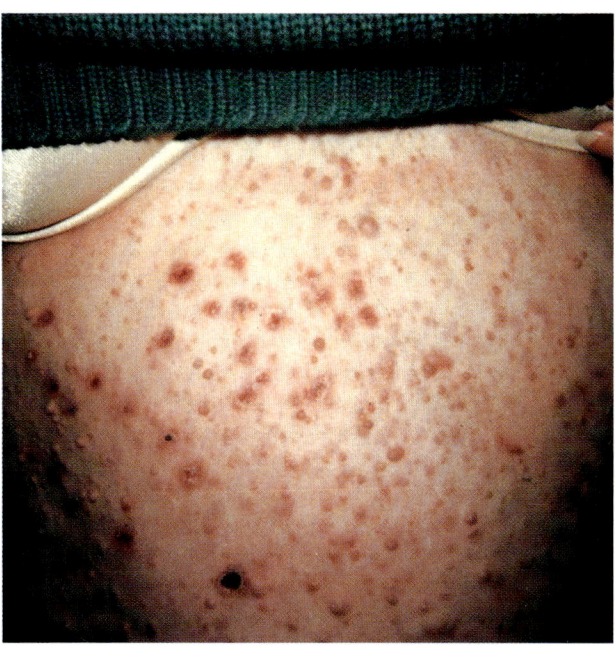

FIG. 4.52-H. Abdomen, one week post-laser treatment in healing stage.

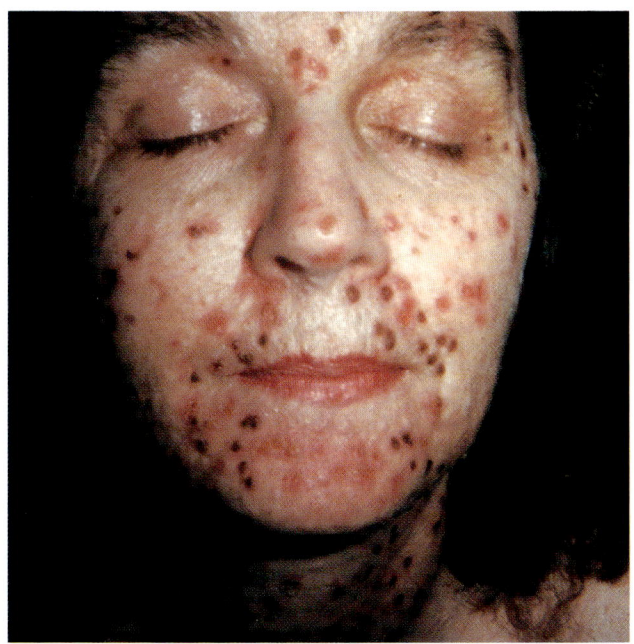

FIG. 4.52-I. Face, one week post-laser treatment in healing stage.

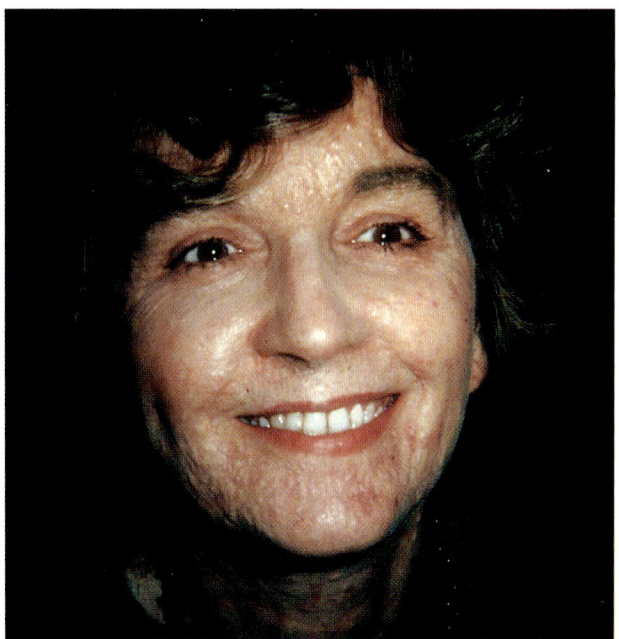

FIG. 4.52-J. Face, nicely healed with a much better cosmetic result.

Case courtesy of *Syrus Rayhan,* M.D.

CASE 4.53
Multiple Cutaneous Neurofibromata

REVIEW OF CASE. This is a 43-year-old female nurse with von Recklinghausen's disease (peripheral neurofibromatosis, NF-1), an autosomal dominant disorder whose gene is located on the long arm of chromosome 17. She desired removal of two large eyelid neurofibromata and wished to consider the treatment of thousands of growths present on all areas of the body. Some of the growths were symptomatic because of their location (eyelids, bottoms of the feet, scalp, and neck); others were bothersome because of their appearance and the inability to camouflage them with cosmetics.

CHOICE OF LASER: CARBON DIOXIDE. The CO_2 laser was chosen because of its versatile properties of cutting, vaporizing, and coagulating. Each of these properties has a use in treating the three types of neurofibromata seen:

(i) The pedunculated form is attached by a stalk. The retracted lesion is cut across at the attachment to the skin with 10 to 15 watts of focused beam. The coagulating properties stop any bleeding.
(ii) The common sessile form is partly above and partly below the skin surface. The slightly defocused beam vaporizes the portion above the skin (35 to 60 watts can be used depending on the operator's level of comfort). Squeezing on either side of the mass causes the subcutaneous portion to protrude into view, allowing it to be vaporized. The bleeding again is negligible due to the coagulating properties.
(iii) The subcutaneous form has the bulk of the tumor under the skin surface. A focused beam at 10 to 15 watts incises the skin over the mass. Pinching or squeezing the mass causes it to protrude through the incision, allowing it to be vaporized under direct vision, bleeding being controlled by the coagulating properties of the laser.

POST-TREATMENT CARE. Only large sessile lesions require suturing. Pain is minimal. Itching can be troublesome, requiring antihistamines (Hismanal) and topical antibiotic ointments.

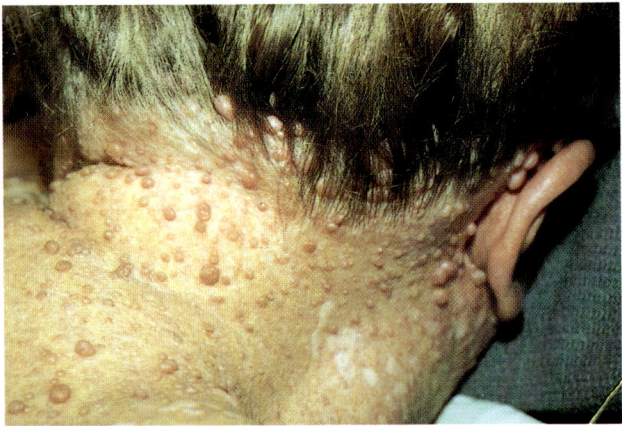

FIG. 4.53-A. Neurofibromata representative of the sessile, pedunculated, and subcutaneous forms. We advise picking a relatively inconspicuous area for a "test treatment" to insure that the patient's expectations are in line with the surgical result. The test treatment can be performed under local anesthesia if desired. Definitive treatment, with the removal of 1,000 to 1,500 lesions, is best accomplished under general anesthesia as an outpatient. This requires about 1½ hours of operating time, and is always associated with a "smoke" smell which is objectionable to the awake patient.

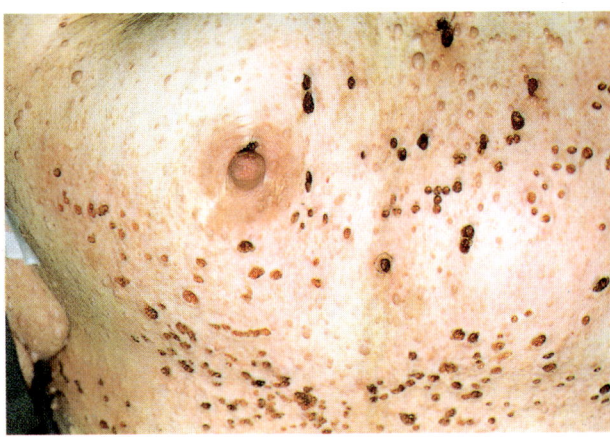

FIG. 4.53-B. Immediate appearance of treatment area showing residual ash and absence of bleeding.

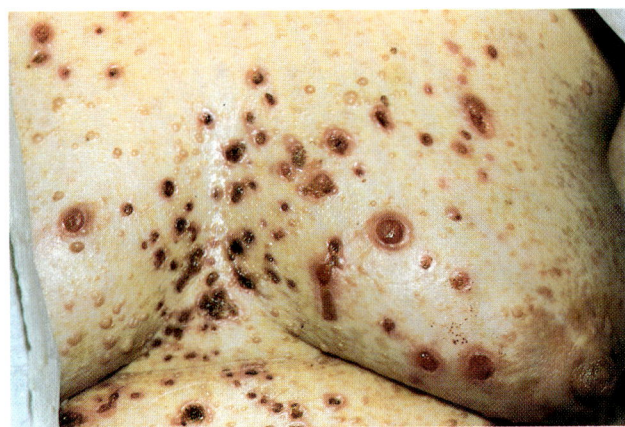

FIG. 4.53-C. Eight days after treatment. Erythema and ash are apparent. Approximately six weeks is required for healing. The flat pink scars mature and fade over the next year.

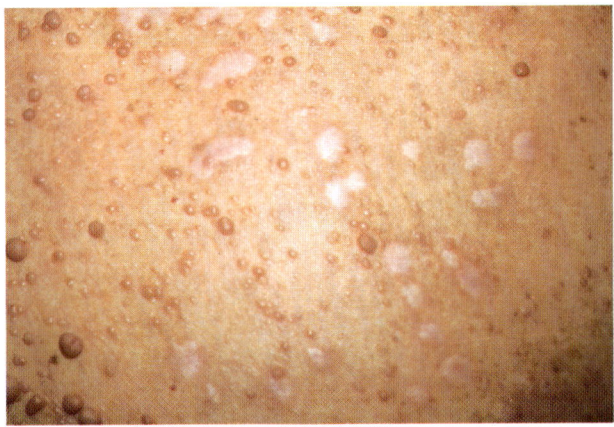

FIG. 4.53-D. Test area one year after treatment showing mature flat, depigmented scars adjacent to untreated neurofibromata. This mediocre speckled appearance is a trade-off for the multiple growths which are so detestable to the patient.

Case courtesy of *David W. Becker, Jr.*, M.D.

CASE 4.54

Onychocryptosis

REVIEW OF CASE. This is a 50-year-old male with chronic ingrown nails. The nail plate has been removed twice in the past 3 years. The nail plate regrew and was still incurvated producing periodic pain and drainage.

CHOICE OF LASER: CARBON DIOXIDE. The CO_2 laser was chosen to photovaporize the nail matrix cells. It has been shown that the laser is able to destroy these cells so the nail plate remains permanently narrower. The fact that the laser seals lymphatics and nerve endings also provides more comfortable wound healing with less pain and edema. This produces faster healing time.

POST-TREATMENT CARE. Apply a mild compression dressing with antibacterial cream to the area for the first 24 hours. The area can be bathed in 24 hours, and the patient is instructed to reapply an antibacterial cream with a bandaid daily until the area is healed.

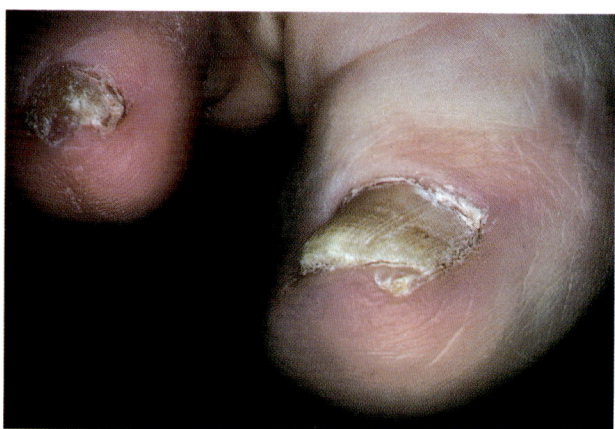

FIG. 4.54-A. Chronic onychocryptic medial nail border of the hallux.

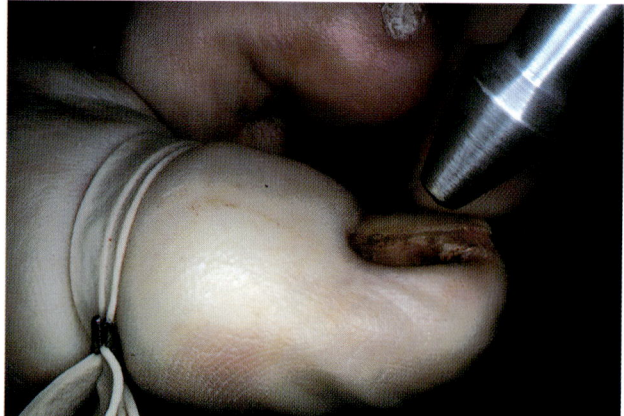

FIG. 4.54-B. The cryptic portion of the nail plate is split back through the root of the nail and avulsed. This leaves the normal portion of the nail plate intact. This allows for adequate exposure of the involved matrix area. Using a 10 watt focused CO_2 laser beam the matrix area and the exposed nail bed is photovaporized. Be sure to treat the underlying portion of the posterior skin fold as matrix cells are located in this area. A skin hook may be used to lift the posterior skin. Do not allow the laser beam to hit the skin hook and burn the normal tissue of the posterior skin fold. Curet the charred tissue down to the healthy nail bed.

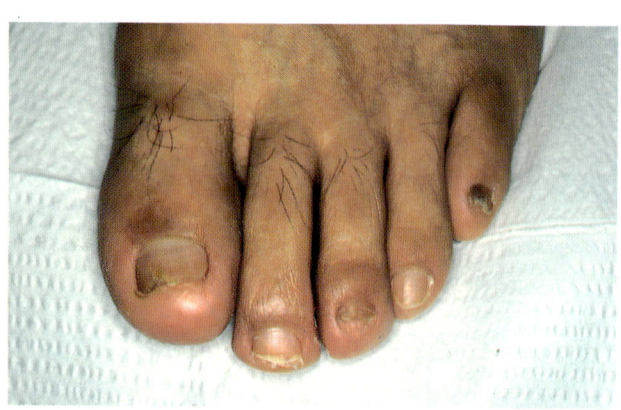

FIG. 4.54-C. Normal nail plate regrown with a narrower width.

Case courtesy of *Elston Rothermel,* D.P.M.

CASE 4.55

Painful Red Nose

REVIEW OF CASE. This is a 60-year-old female with a many year history of frequent, painful, vascular discoloration of the nose. Previous treatment was attempted with tetracycline and argon laser tracing of individual telangiectasia with no noted improvement. The patient complained of episodic stinging and violaceous color changes which could last minutes or hours and occur multiple times daily. No clear association with physiologic or environmental stimuli could be discovered.

CHOICE OF LASER: CARBON DIOXIDE. The CO_2 laser was chosen to uniformly ablate the epidermis and the superficial nasal vessels within the upper dermis that were suspected of giving rise to pain and vascular discoloration. Reports have been published of red nose syndrome patients improving after superficial nasal tissue vaporization with the CO_2 laser.

POWER SETTING. 15 watts, continuous wave, spot size 3–4 mm.

ADDITIONAL INFORMATION. The procedure is performed using a 15 watt continuous wave and a spot size of 3–4 mm. One or two passes maximum is sufficient over the central nose and tip. Pause to wipe away the epidermis after the first pass. A single pass should only be performed at the junctions of other cosmetic units to achieve unnoticeable blending.

Patients selected for this treatment must be fair complected. Otherwise the reduction of melanocytes will result in a strikingly hypopigmented nose. See the patient at least every three weeks during the first two months. Any sign of scar tissue formation may be treated immediately with intralesional steroids.

POST-TREATMENT CARE. Antibiotic ointment and nonadherent dressings for moist healing are used until re-epithelization is complete.

Case continues on following page.

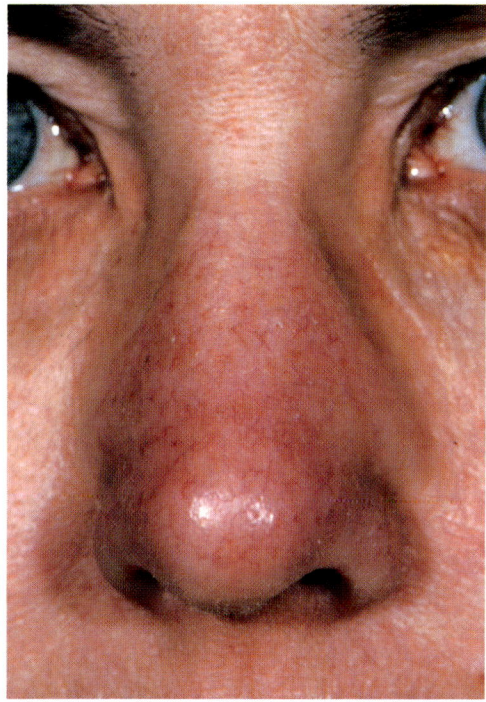

FIG. 4.55-A. Painful red nose, noninflamed state.

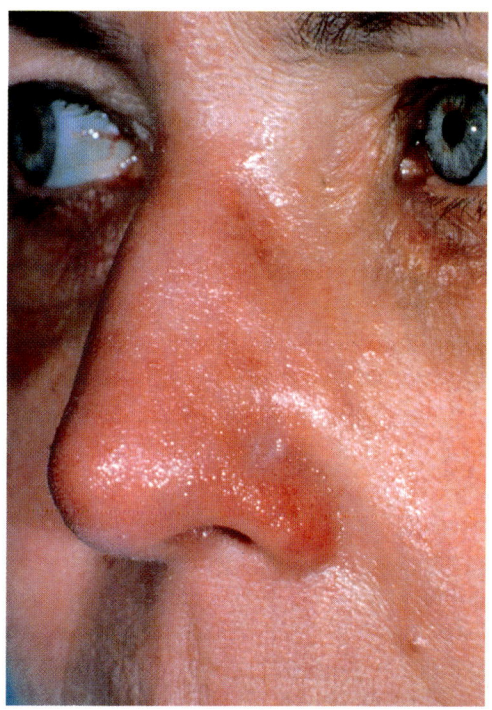

FIG. 4.55-B. After two passes over the body of the nose and one pass at junctions of cosmetic units.

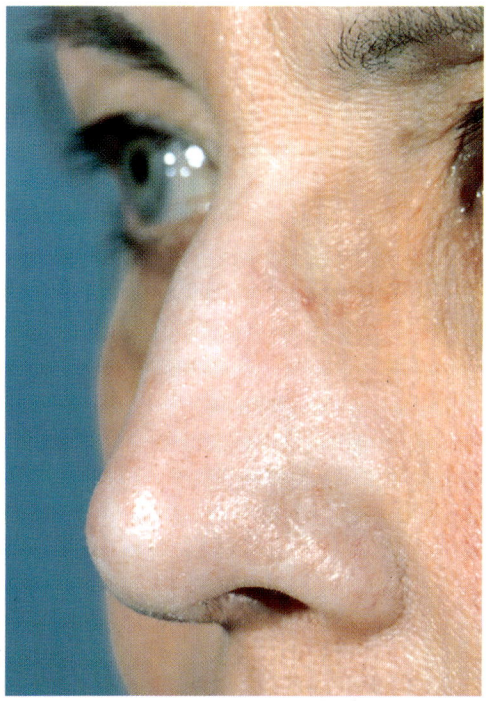

FIG. 4.55-C. Smooth transition into adjacent cosmetic unit.

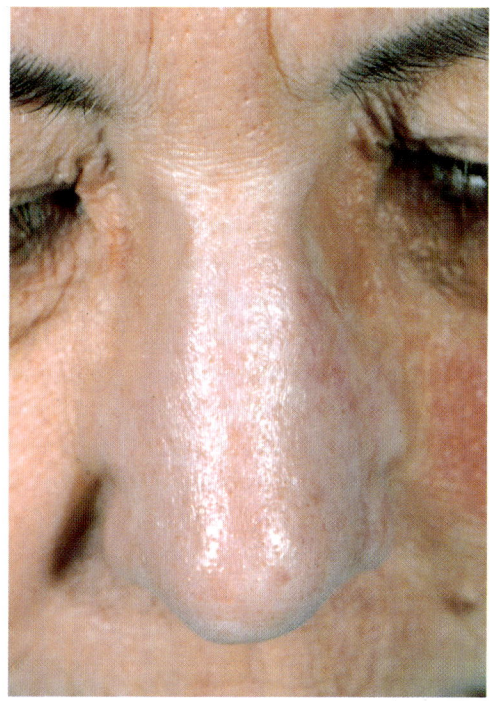

FIG. 4.55-D. Mild hypopigmentation nonevident in fair-complected patients.

Case courtesy of *Timothy J. Rosio,* M.D.

CASE 4.56
Periapical Granuloma (Oral)

REVIEW OF CASE. A 72-year-old female was referred for evaluation and treatment of an acute exacerbation of a periapical lesion associated with the left maxillary canine tooth. Clinical examination revealed a fluctuant swelling of the buccal vestibular mucosa consistent with an acute periapical abscess. An antibiotic regimen was initiated and the patient was rescheduled for surgical treatment.

CHOICE OF LASER: CARBON DIOXIDE. The rationale for CO_2 laser application in endodontic periapical surgery includes the following: improved hemostasis and visualization of the operative field, potential sterilization of the contaminated root apex, and potential reduction of post-operative pain.

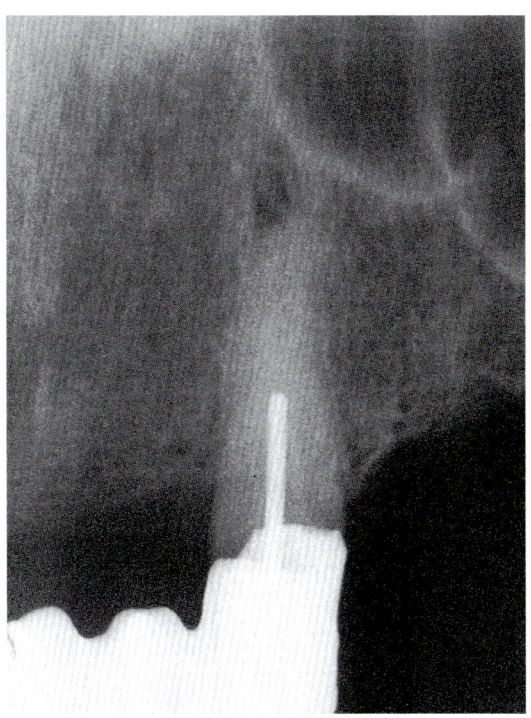

FIG. 4.56-A. Pre-operative radiograph of tooth displaying radiolucent area at root apex. The tooth has been endodontically treated previously (1979) and supports a maxillary anterior bridge prosthesis.

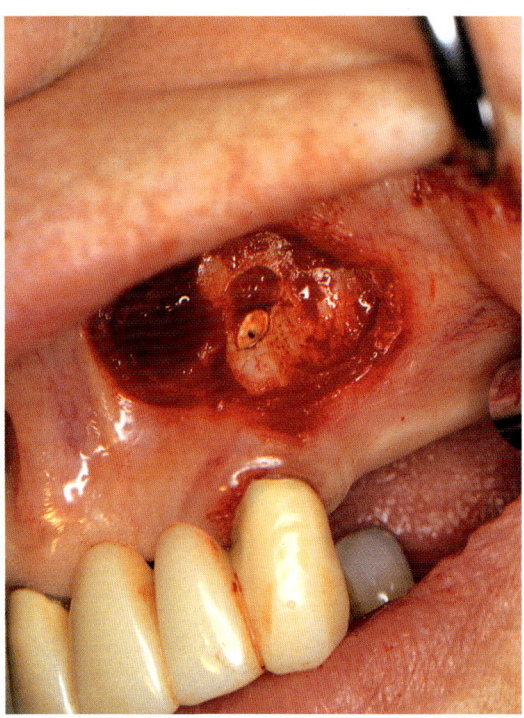

FIG. 4.56-B. Incision of the oral mucosa with reflection of tissue flap. Maxillary cortical bone exposed revealing intra-osseous lesion. Incision made with a 0.25 mm focal spot, 4 watts, continous mode.

Case continues on following page.

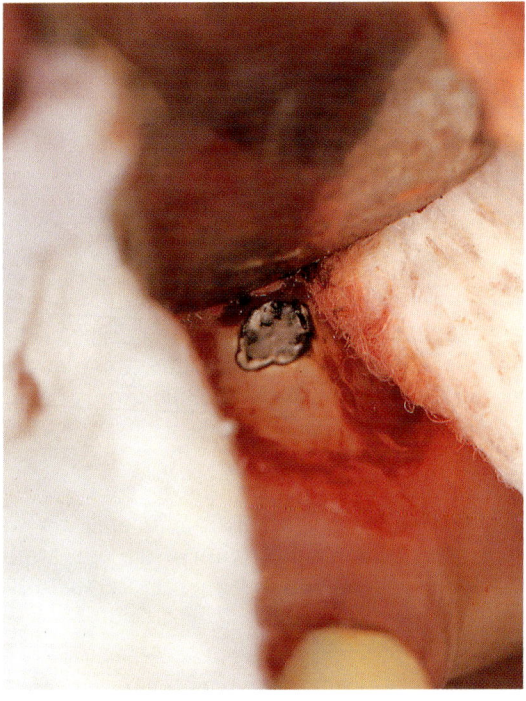

FIG. 4.56-C. Root apex lased at 10 watts in focus, 0.25 mm focal spot. Lesion vaporized at 5 watts unfocused in continous mode. Note carbonized root apex.

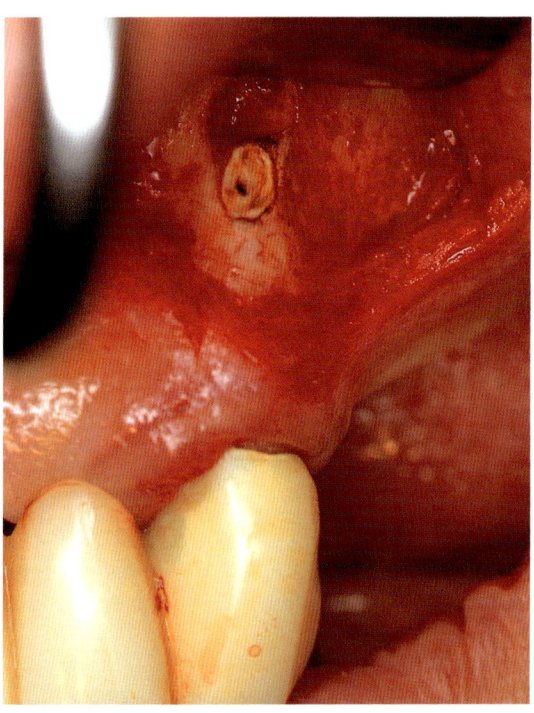

FIG. 4.56-D. Carbonized material removed and root prepared for retrograde filling.

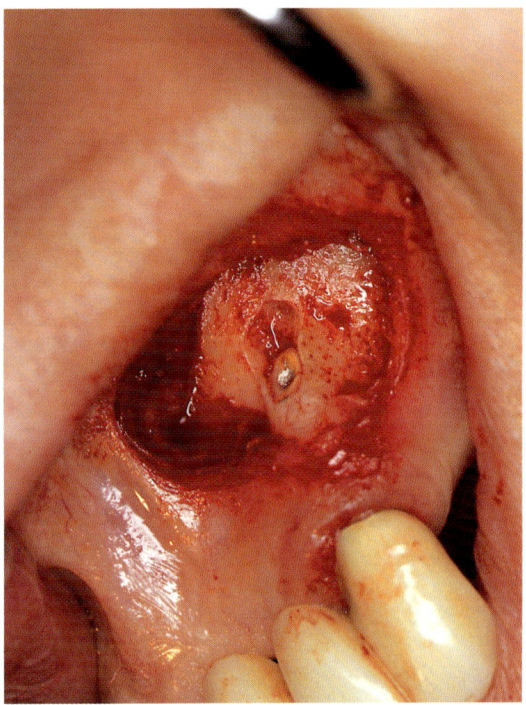

FIG. 4.56-E. A retrograde amalgam filling was placed to seal the root apex.

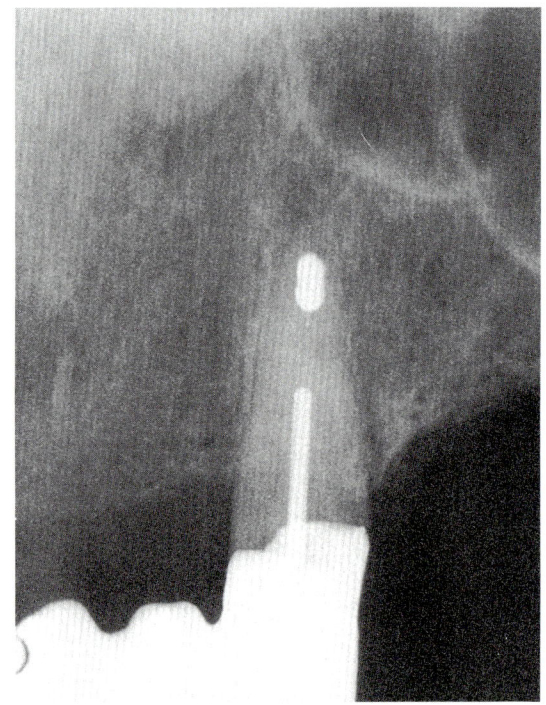

FIG. 4.56-F. Six months post-treatment radiograph reveals osseous regeneration.

Case courtesy of *Leo J. Miserendino*, D.D.S.

CASE 4.57

Pincer Nail Deformity with Onychocryptosis

REVIEW OF CASE. An elderly gentleman presented with a long history of pain around his right great toenail, and a history of intermittent ingrown toenail. Physical examination revealed a pincer nail deformity with extreme curvature of the nail plate, and impingement into both lateral nail folds. The patient desired permanent removal of the offending nail (matricectomy).

CHOICE OF LASER: CARBON DIOXIDE. The CO_2 laser affords many advantages over other techniques of nail matricectomy:

(i) The germinative epithelium (matrix) for the nail can be vaporized, with limited damage to non-matrix tissue. This is in distinct contrast to chemical matricectomy in which there is substantial tissue necrosis involving the lateral and posterior nail folds.
(ii) The CO_2 carbon laser ablation of the matrix can be achieved by directing the beam deep into the matrix horns without incising and reflecting the posterior nail folds, as is required with cold steel (surgical) matricectomy.

ADDITIONAL INFORMATION. Insertion of cotton-tipped (dry) applicators between lateral-posterior nail folds and matrix for several minutes prior to treatment permits better visualization of the matrix. Overtreatment of the matrix area can result in destruction of underlying phalangeal periosteum.

POST-TREATMENT CARE. Remove pressure dressing in 24 hours. Soak treated digit in a dilute solution of chlorhexidine (or povidone-iodine) and water two to three times per day. Follow soaks with hydrogen peroxide swab of treatment area, then application of an antibiotic ointment. Follow-up visits are weekly until site is completely healed.

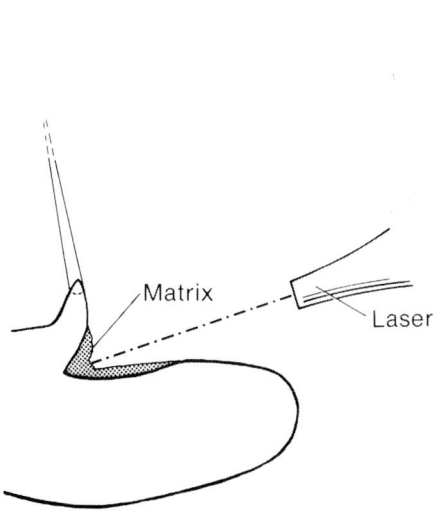

FIG. 4.57-A. Diagram depicts retraction of the posterior nail fold and reflection of matrix onto the undersurface of the posterior nail fold.

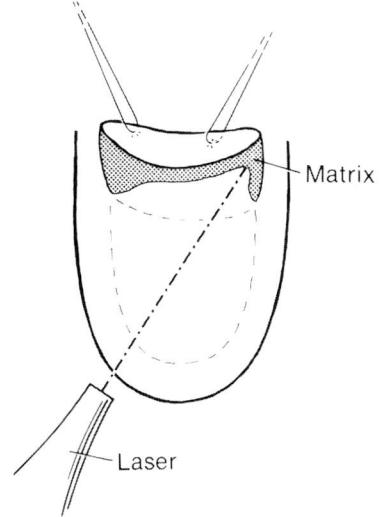

FIG. 4.57-B. Diagram depicts extension of matrix into lateral horns, which must be ablated for successful permanent nail removal.

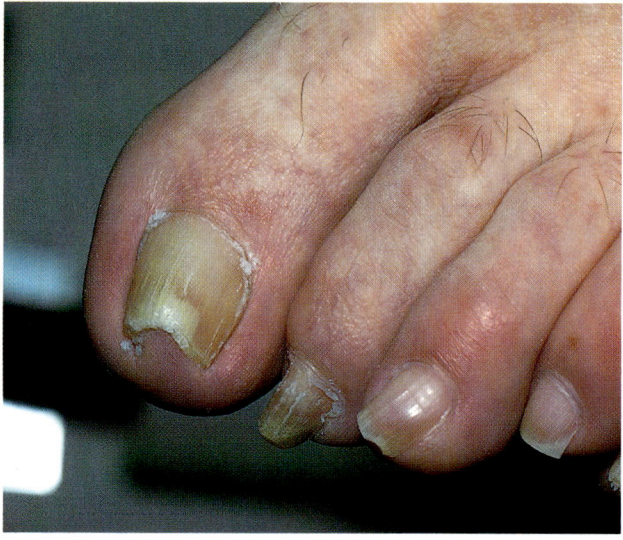

FIG. 4.57-C. Patient with pincer nail deformity of left great toenail.

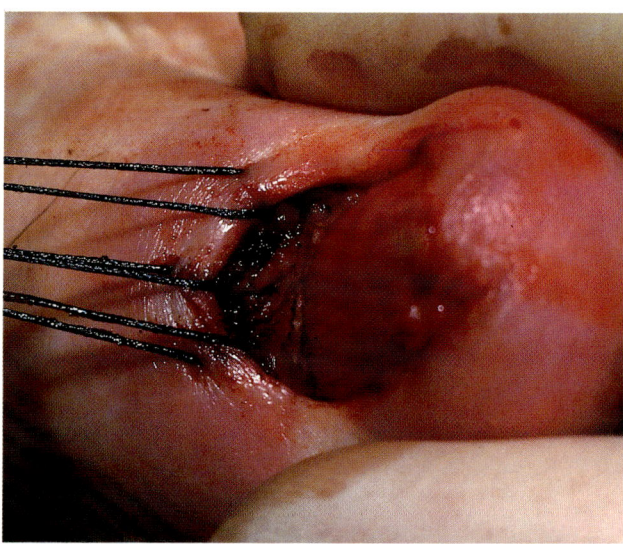

FIG. 4.57-D. After digital block anesthesia, the nail has been avulsed. 4-0 Silk sutures are placed in the posterior nail fold to permit retraction and better visualization for treatment of the matrix. The matrix has a white, shiny surface.

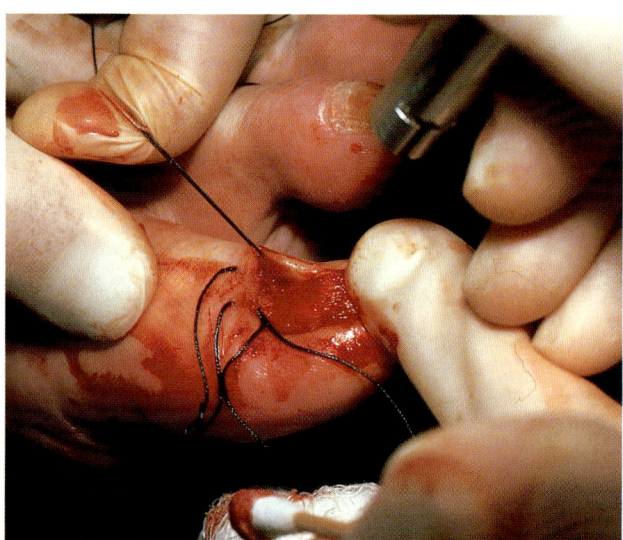

FIG. 4.57-E. Matrix immediately following CO_2 vaporization in a continuous mode at 5 watts of power with a 2 mm spot size.

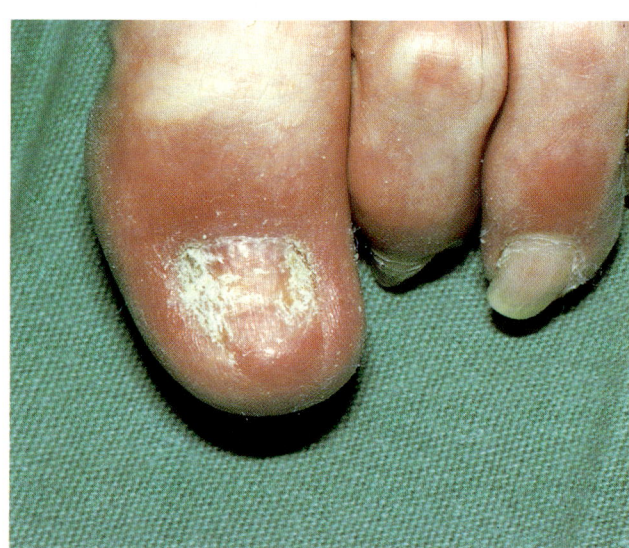

FIG. 4.57-F. Six months post-operation. Hyperkeratosis represents pseudonail arising from nail bed.

Case courtesy of *Barry Leshin*, M.D.

Reprinted with permission of Elsevier Science Publishing Company, Inc., © 1988.
For literature pertaining to this case see References section.

CASE 4.58

Pilar Cyst of the Scalp

REVIEW OF CASE. This patient complained about an enlarging non-painful mass present in the scalp. This mass was constantly being traumatized by a comb or brush.

CHOICE OF LASER: CARBON DIOXIDE. While removal of pilar cysts is simple through traditional methods, the CO_2 laser provides a relatively bloodless and quick method to remove these hereditary, multiple, cystic lesions of the scalp.

ADDITIONAL INFORMATION. After local anesthetic, an incision is made through the skin and cyst sac using a CO_2 laser at 10 watts of pulsed or continuous power focused to a 0.3 mm spot. Using a blunt instrument (hemostat or small blunt undermining scissors) the cyst sac is separated from the adjacent and underlying tissues and extracted through the incision. A few nylon sutures are used for closure. This procedure can be done quickly requiring 2–3 minutes per cyst.

POST-TREATMENT CARE. Standard post-operative wound care after minor skin incisional surgery is provided and sutures are removed in 8–10 days.

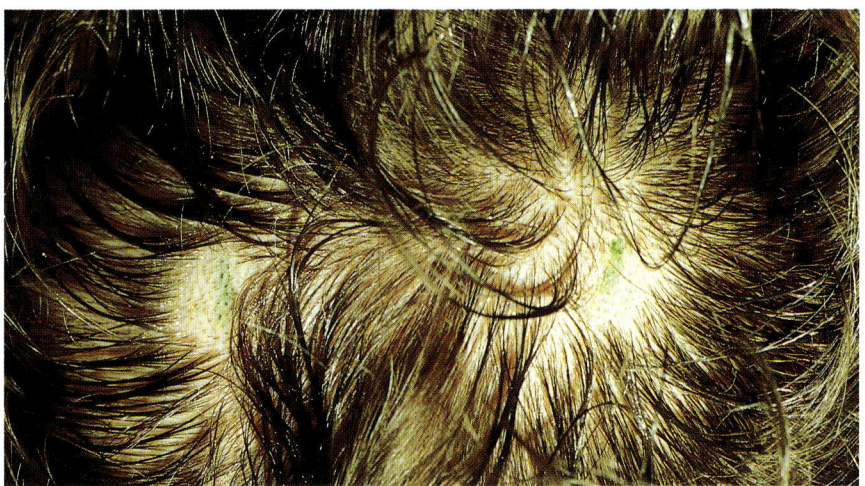

FIG. 4.58-A. Pre-operative pilar cyst of the scalp.

Case continues on following page.

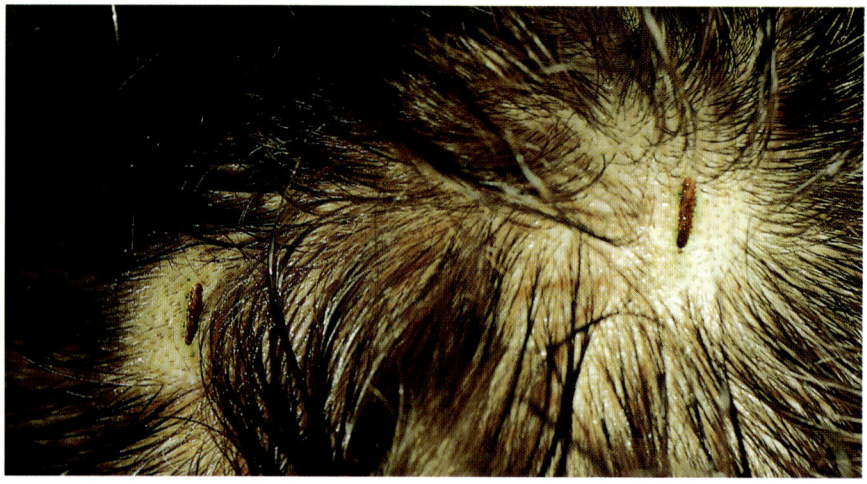

FIG. 4.58-B. Laser incision intraoperatively. Note the lack of bleeding in normally vascular area.

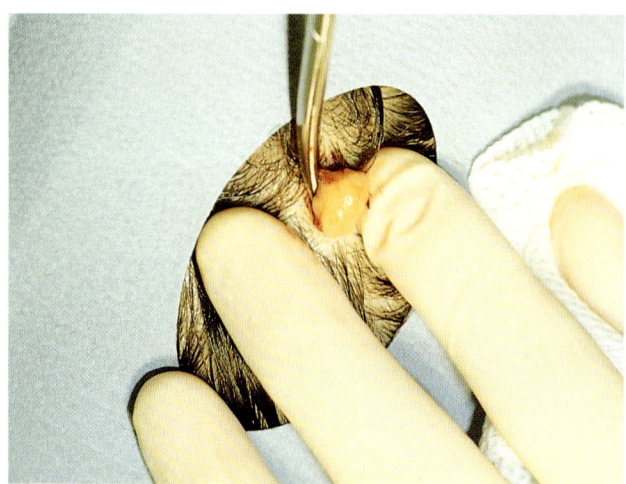

FIG. 4.58-C. Cyst sac extraction accomplished with small curved scissors.

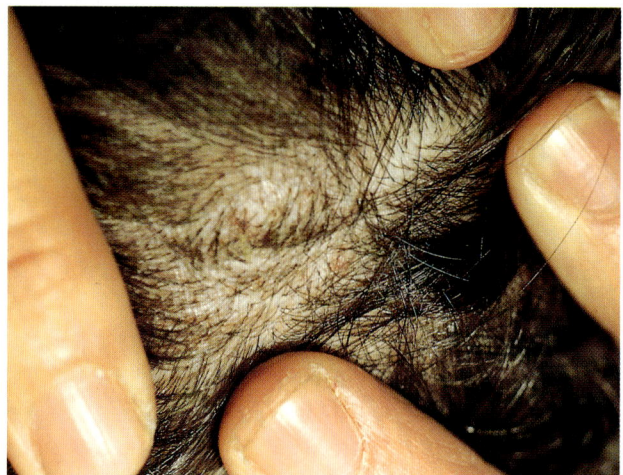

FIG. 4.58-D. One month post-operation.

Case courtesy of *Mark B. Taylor*, M.D.

CASE 4.59

Post-Thermal Hypertrophic Scar

REVIEW OF CASE.   This is a 45-year-old male who had sustained thermal burns over multiple areas of his body from hot tar in September 1979. He was in intensive care for thirty days. After he eventually healed, he had extensive hypertrophic scars over many areas of his body. He was treated with triamcinolone injections, Z-plasties, pressure wraps, and other conservative measures.

The burns were 2½ years old. There was a considerable amount of burning, stinging, and itching, as well as pain and contracture in many of the scars of his body.

CHOICE OF LASER: CARBON DIOXIDE.   Post-thermal hypertrophic scars have been treated extensively with both the argon and the CO_2 laser. The CO_2 laser was chosen because of it's greater predictability, higher power output, and the ease of obtaining a small spot size. The argon laser can be used with equal success, as long as a 0.2 mm spot size handpiece is available and the laser is putting out a minimum of 4.5 watts. The CO_2 laser, because of its higher power output is capable of being used at a 0.05 second interval to a 0.1 second interval but the argon laser must be used at 0.5 to 1.0 second intervals in order to obtain high enough power densities. This gives less precision in its treatment.

ADDITIONAL INFORMATION.   After general anesthesia is achieved, all of the areas of the body are chilled with ice. The CO_2 is used in a hand held manner and tiny holes are drilled into the scar spaced apart by 3 mm to 4 mm. The smallest possible hole of vaporization is desired with the smallest possible zone of white thermal damage surrounding this. It is absolutely imperative that normal, uninjured tissue be present between the thermal white halo zone around a lasered spot and the next adjacent thermal damaged zone. It is in this area that the physiology of the fibroplast is changed so as to retard collagen synthesis. If the areas of thermal damage coalesce together, too much damage will have occurred and instead of improving the scar, one is actually cooking it and will make the scar worse. In treating it, the laser should be moved around on the scar at random so as to allow cooling between spots and the area should be iced periodically. If superpulse mode is available on the laser, it should be used, as this lessens thermal damage. In general, the higher the power and the shorter the time interval, the less thermal damage there will be and the better the result will be.

Post-operatively, the area is iced for another hour and then gentamicin ointment is used in the post-operative period.

Under general anesthesia, as high as 30% to 50% of the body has been treated by this technique. Triamcinolone injections have been used on some patients but normally in thermal burns, the area is much too large to be able to effectively utilize triamcinolone. Unlike keloid scars, these hypertrophic scars are not dependent upon periodic reinjections of triamcinolone.

Unlike the drilling of the holes with the argon laser, the CO_2 laser will occasionally perforate a small vessel with resultant bleeding. Compression and ice will usually control this problem.

Laser treatment of these lesions usually is followed by very prompt relief of paresthesias, such as stinging, itching, burning, and tightness within a two to four week period of time. Usually, in eight weeks, a marked flattening of the lesion is recognized. It may be necessary to repeat the treatment on two to three subsequent occasions. Once the hypertrophic scar process is reversed, it will *not* recur, as do keloid scars.

Case continues on following page.

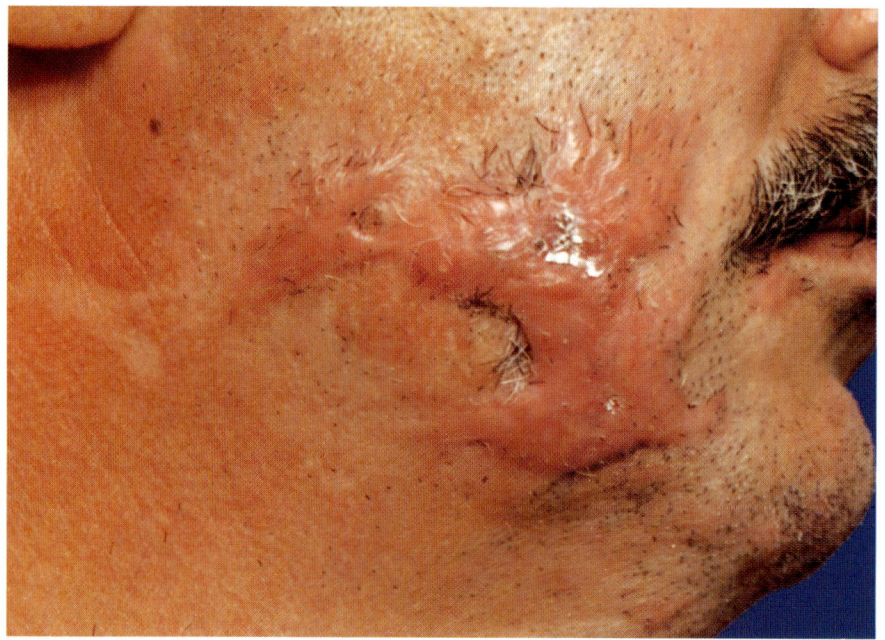

FIG. 4.59-A. A thick hypertrophic post-thermal scar on the patient's right cheek 2½ years after injury.

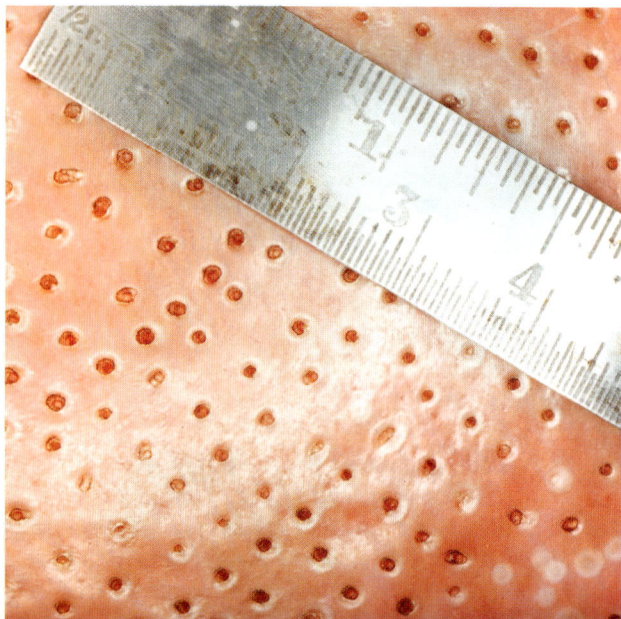

FIG. 4.59-B. A magnified view of one area of a typical hypertrophic scar. Notice the central area of vaporization surrounded by the small thermal area of damage. There should be normal uninjured tissue between the spots. Note also areas in the picture where the thermal damage coalesces without a normal zone. This area will not be improved and laser treatment will probably have to be repeated at a later time.

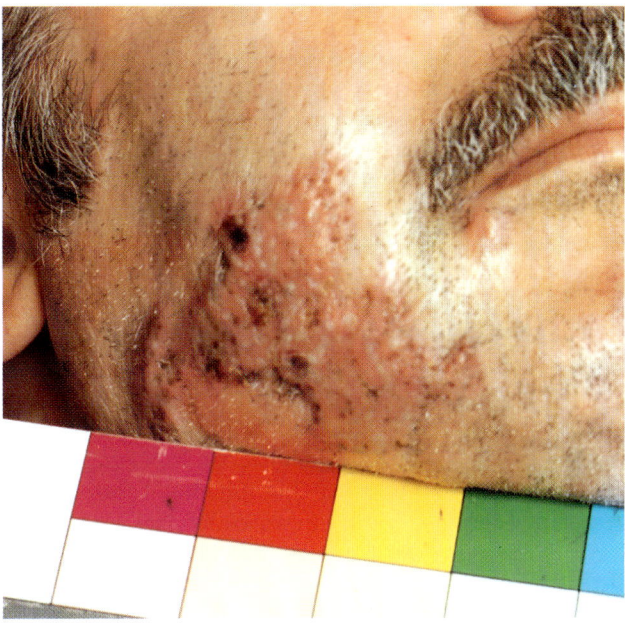

FIG. 4.59-C. Note the marked flattening of this scar at a period of only two months following laser impaction. The small areas of vaporization have broken up the long bands of collagen in the fashion of minute "Z-plasties" and collagen synthesis has been drastically reduced.

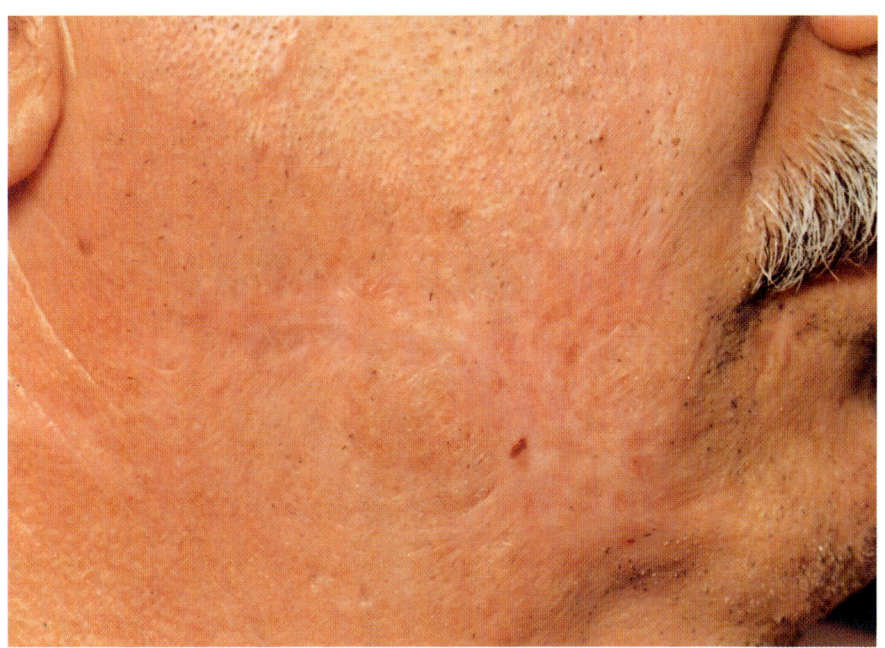

FIG. 4.59-D. The patient's scar eight years later has shown no tendency for recurrence and there has been no need to inject at intervals with triamcinolone, as is necessary with keloid scars.

Case courtesy of *Darrell L. Henderson*, M.D.

CASE 4.60

Rhinophyma, Large Size

REVIEW OF CASE. This 59-year-old white male presented with a large rhinophyma present for many years. Medical treatment caused improvement of the inflammatory portion of his acne rosacea, but extensive scar and sebaceous hyperplasia resulted.

CHOICE OF LASER: CARBON DIOXIDE. The reasons for using the CO_2 laser are the same for this case as for the case of moderate-sized rhinophyma. However, for patients with large-sized rhinophyma, the laser can be used as both an excisional tool as well as a vaporizational tool. It would take an excessive amount of time to vaporize the large nodules of sebaceous hyperplasia and scar tissue. Using a power setting of 15 to 20 watts with a continuous beam in a focused mode, incisions can be made with the CO_2 laser to debulk the nose. Once this is complete, more precise removal of tissue can be performed in the defocused mode to contour the nose to a cosmetically acceptable shape.

ADDITIONAL INFORMATION. Be careful not to be overzealous with the amount of tissue excised. It is generally prudent to perform a second procedure rather than be overly aggressive the first time.

POST-TREATMENT CARE. Antibiotic ointment (2% erythromycin in petrolatum) and nonadherent gauze. The wound is cleansed two to three times daily with peroxide. Extensive paranasal and periorbital edema may result which in some cases is treated prophylactically with intramuscular short-acting glucocorticoid or a short course of prednisone. Normally the pain, if any, is minimal and re-epithelialization is complete in four weeks.

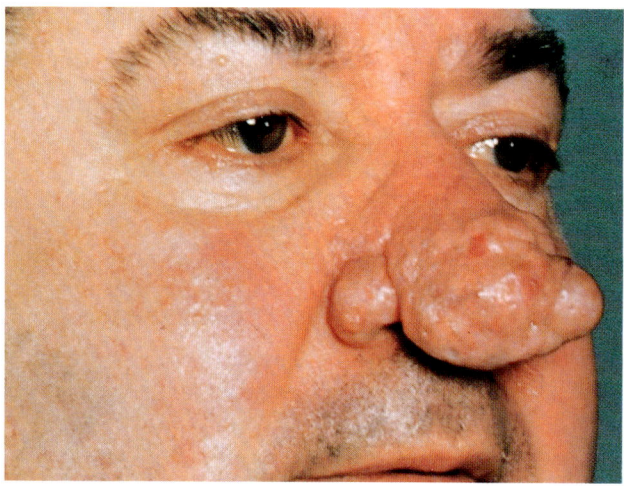

FIG. 4.60-A. Pre-operative rhinophyma.

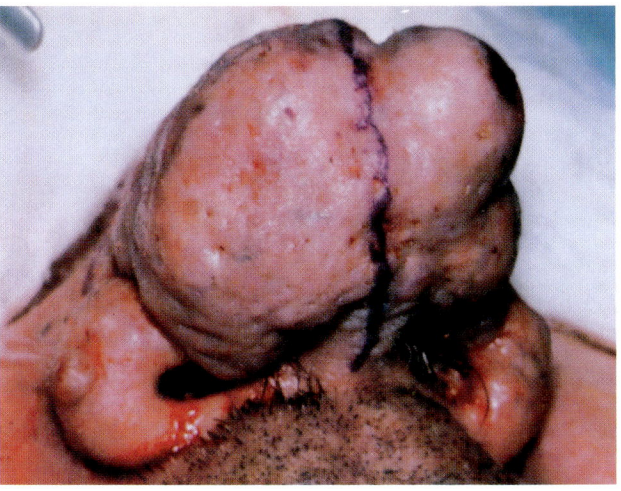
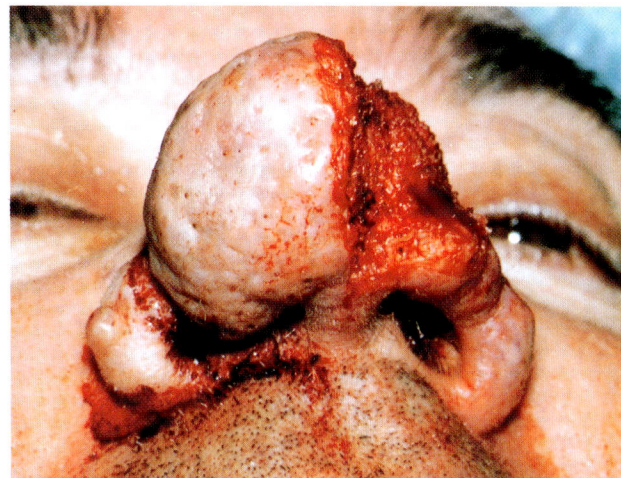
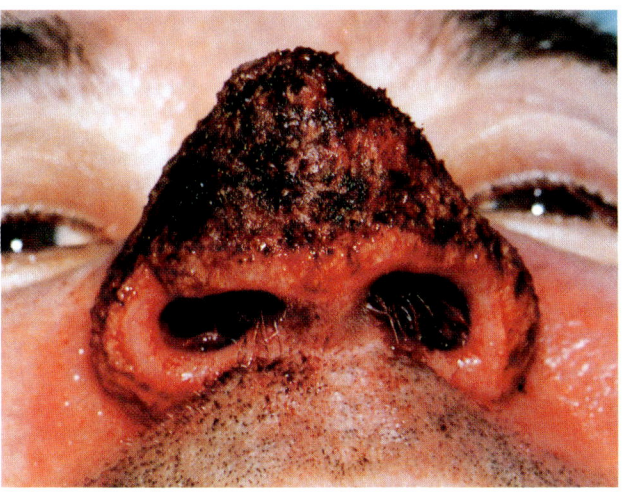

FIG. 4.60-B. Intraoperatively. **Top Left:** Incision planned. **Top Right:** Half of the rhinophyma removed by CO_2 laser excision with a focused beam. **Bottom:** Immediate postoperative result after vaporization with a defocused beam. Char has not been washed off yet.

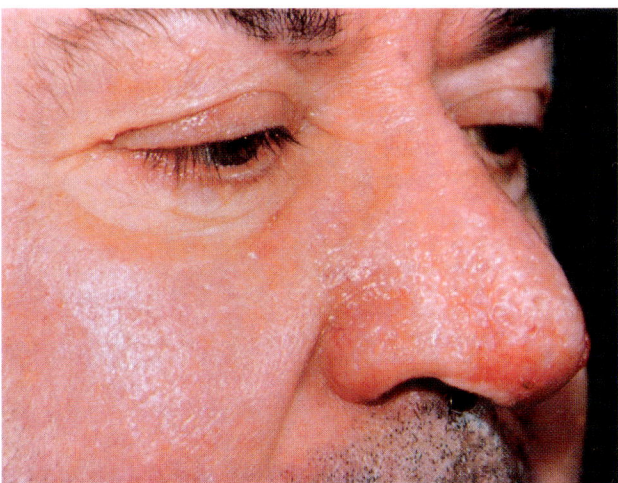
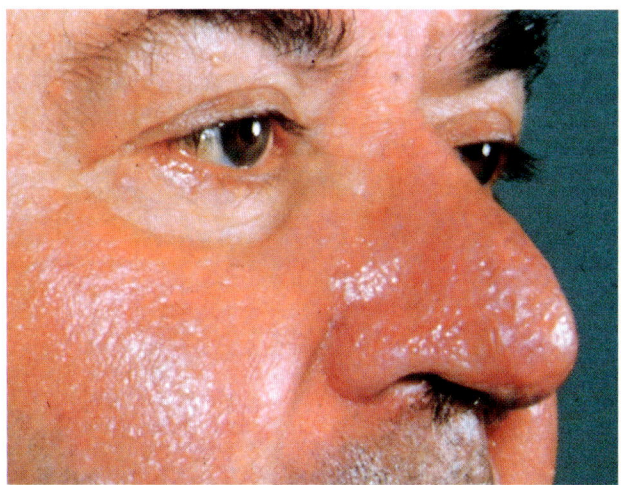

FIG. 4.60-C. Post-operatively at 5 weeks; some erythema and edema persists, but epithelialization is complete and the cosmetic appearance is much improved.

FIG. 4.60-D. Post-operatively at 10 weeks; good cosmetic result, erythema and edema resolving, color and skin texture match well.

Case courtesy of **Randall K. Roenigk,** M.D., and **Tom D. Wang,** M.D.

CASE 4.61

Rhinophyma, Moderate Size

REVIEW OF CASE. This 69-year-old white male has a moderate-sized rhinophyma. Medical therapy resulted in clearing of the inflammatory portion of his rhinophyma leaving him with classic sebaceous gland hypertrophy and scar tissue.

CHOICE OF LASER: CARBON DIOXIDE. Decortication of the nose is an old procedure for rhinophyma performed with a variety of instruments. A heated scalpel (Shaw scalpel), electro-sectioning, dermabrasion, and standard cold steel surgery have all been used with good success. I find the CO_2 laser to be best because of both the high degree of precision and the completely bloodless field. This allows treatment of rhinophyma with a local anesthetic (nasal block) in an office/outpatient setting. Attention need not be paid to small capillary oozing, and far more time can be spent removing precise small amounts of tissue as is cosmetically appropriate. The power settings will vary, normally at 15 watts with a continuous beam in a defocused mode.

ADDITIONAL INFORMATION. Do not vaporize deeper than the pilosebaceous unit, otherwise an abnormally smooth second-intention scar will result. While vaporizing with the laser, the skin is dehydrated and contracts. This causes the sebaceous glands to extrude sebum. This is a sign that the pilosebaceous unit is still present. If the surgeon is more aggressive and vaporizes beyond the point (deeper) where the sebum extrudes from the pores, a poor scar may result. In addition, the pilosebaceous pores on the nose often are dilated after this procedure. This is predominately due to the larger size of the sebaceous glands in rhinophyma. In most cases this is not a source of concern and patients are very pleased with the result. A smaller rhinophyma, especially in younger patients, should be treated cautiously as dilated pores in these cases may not be acceptable cosmetically.

POST-TREATMENT CARE. Antibiotic ointment (2% erythromycin in petrolatum) and non-adherent gauze. The wound is cleansed two to three times daily with peroxide, and re-epithelialization is complete in approximately three to four weeks. Reactive erythema and a small degree of swelling may last for several months after re-epithelialization is complete.

For literature pertaining to this case see References section.

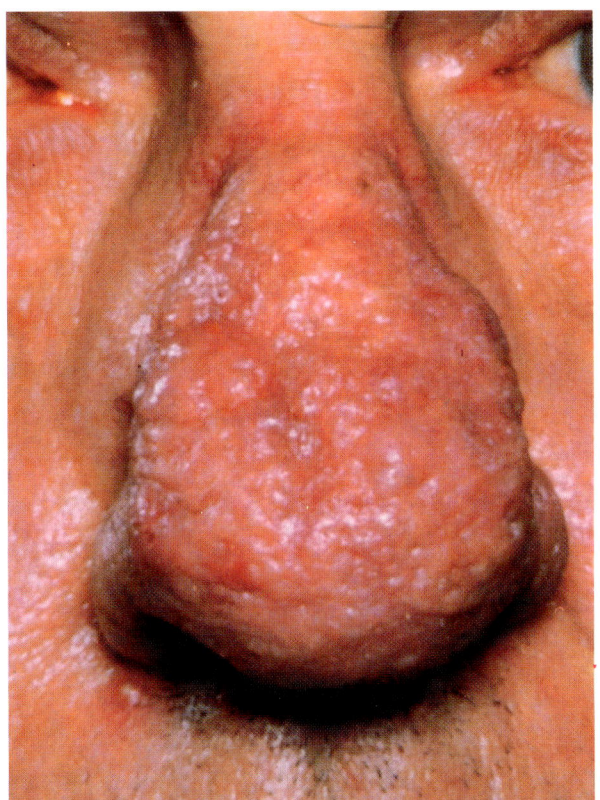

FIG. 4.61-A. Front view of rhinophyma pre-operation.

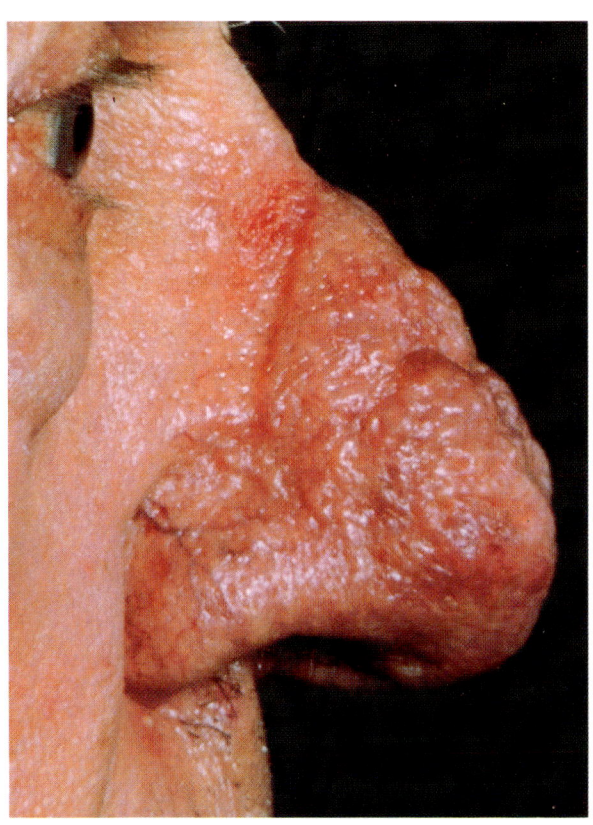

FIG. 4.61-B. Side view of rhinophyma pre-operation.

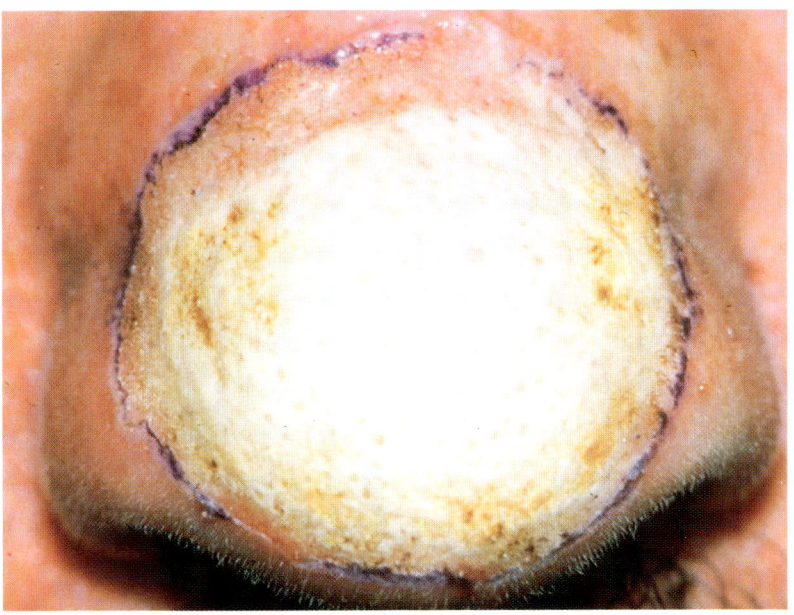

FIG. 4.61-C. A different patient, immediately post-operation; the char is wiped off leaving a completely bloodless field.

Case continues on following page.

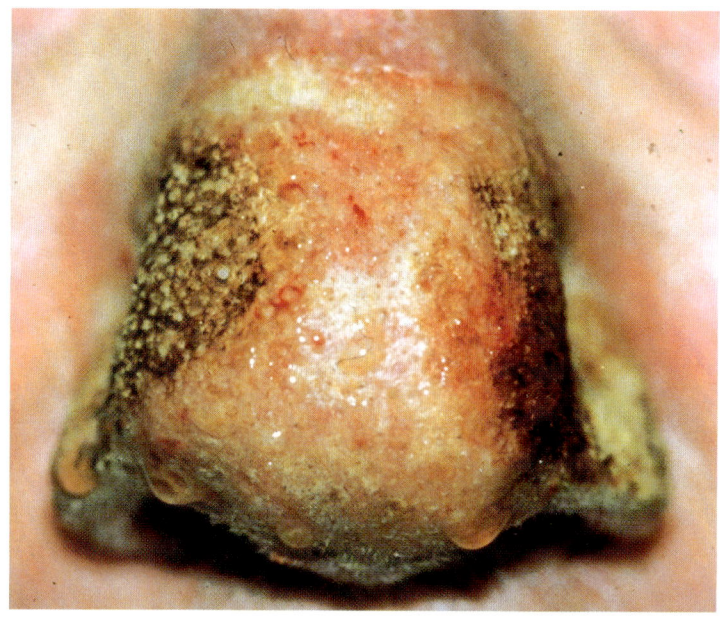

FIG. 4.61-D. Another patient several hours post-operation. Rhinophyma is usually asymmetric requiring that the surgeon have a good cosmetic sense when "sculpting" the nose. Lymphatic drainage begins and must be cleansed regularly to avoid crust formation.

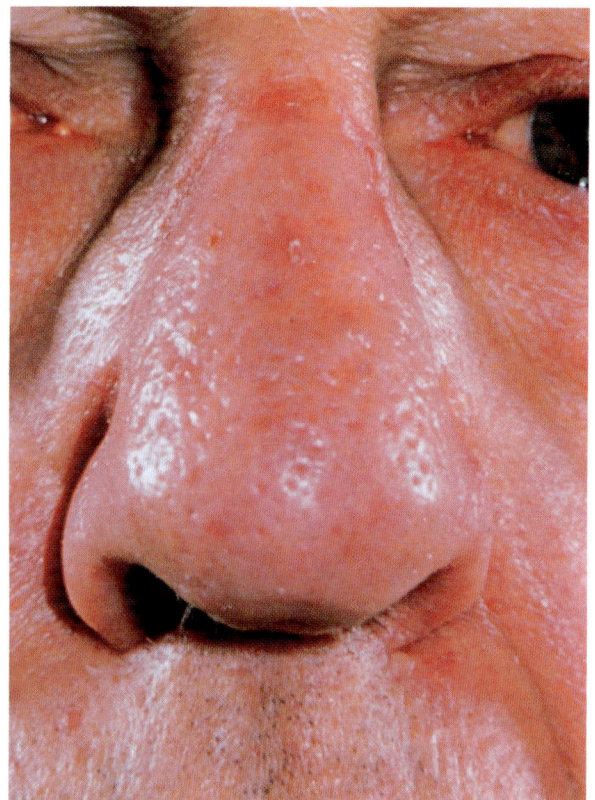

FIG. 4.61-E. Front view, patient in Fig. A, three months post-operation.

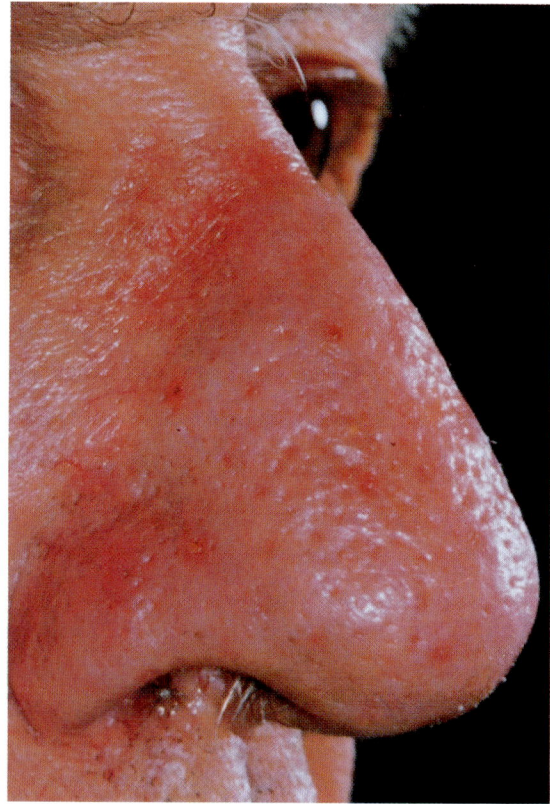

FIG. 4.61-F. Side view, patient in Fig. A, three months post-operation.

Case courtesy of **Randall K. Roenigk**, M.D.

CASE 4.62
Pigmented Seborrheic Keratosis

REVIEW OF CASE. The patient is a 44-year-old Hispanic female who had developed a pigmented macular lesion on the left lower eyelid one year ago. It is growing and becoming darker. A biopsy was done to rule out the possibility of malignancy. Pathology revealed pigmented seborrheic keratosis.

CHOICE OF LASER: CARBON DIOXIDE. The CO_2 laser was chosen to photovaporize the lesion because with low power and vaporization, the lesion can be removed with minimum or no scarring. Although this could have been treated with liquid nitrogen, there is a chance of hypopigmentation. It could have also been done with a curet but there is a higher chance of damaging the dermis and causing scarring than with the laser technique.

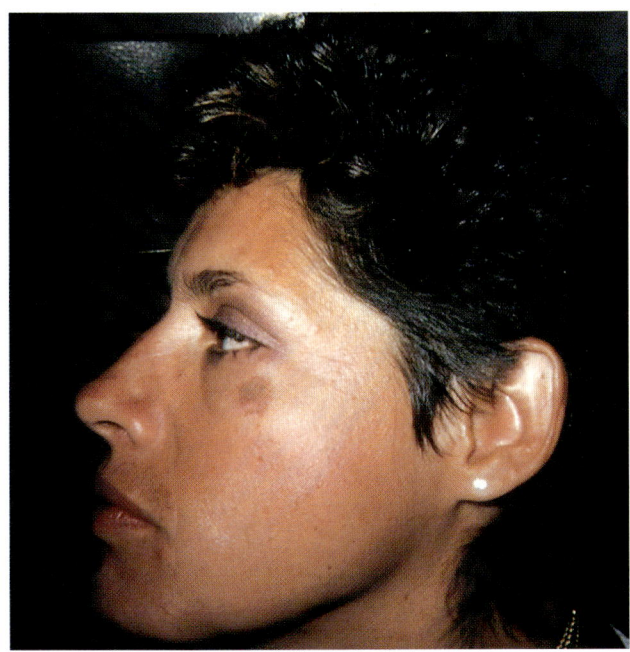

FIG. 4.62-A. Pigmented lesion on the left lower eyelid getting larger and darker. A shave biopsy was performed at the lower corner of the lesion to rule out malignancy.

Case continues on following page.

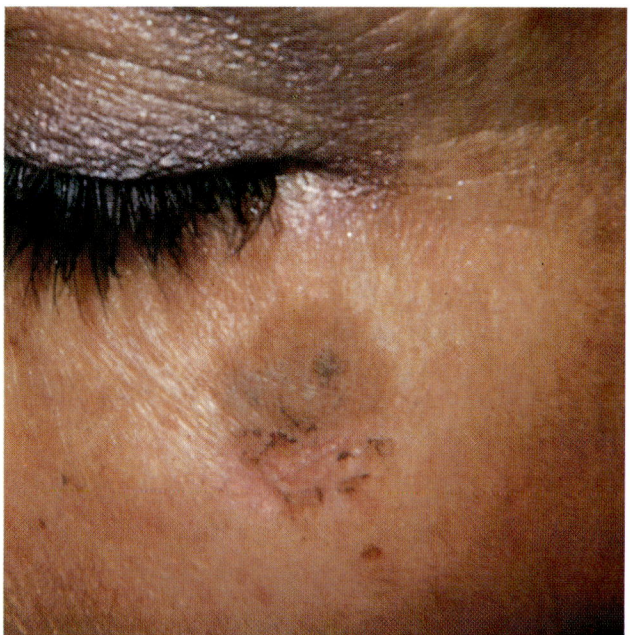

FIG. 4.62-B. Close-up of Fig. A.

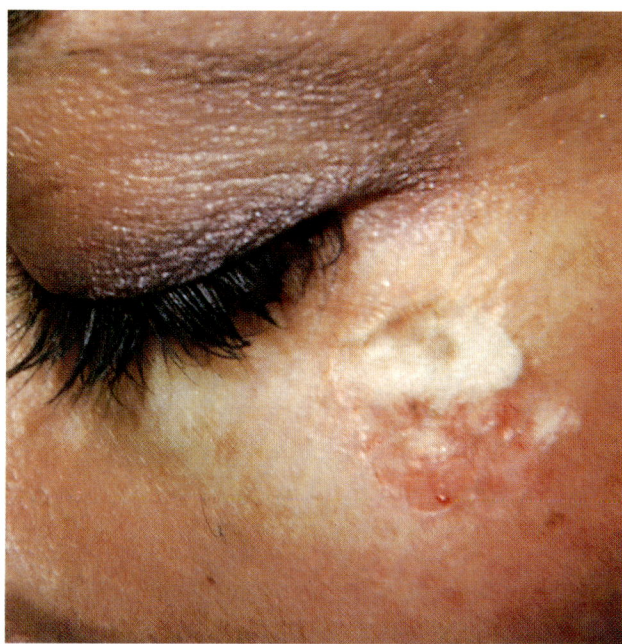

FIG. 4.62-C. The lesion was vaporized with the CO_2 laser defocus beam, power of 2.2 watts. Note with this power, epidermis warms up and sloughs easily with a cotton tip and normal saline.

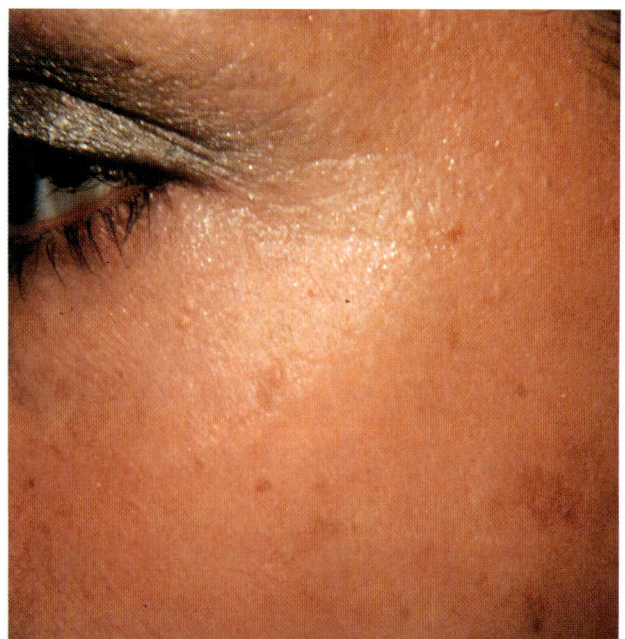

FIG. 4.62-D. Healed lesion without scarring, recurrence, or color change.

Case courtesy of **Syrus Rayhan,** M.D.

CASE 4.63
Facial Syringomas

REVIEW OF CASE. This is a 42-year-old white American female, working as a model, with a 30 year history of bilateral lower eyelid syringomas. These have been treated three times previously with sharp excision, electrodessication, and curettage without success. The syringomas recurred rapidly and the patient was cosmetically disabled.

CHOICE OF LASER: CARBON DIOXIDE. The superpulse CO_2 laser emits at 10,600 nm mid-infrared range of the electromagnetic spectrum in a series of peak power bursts occurring very rapidly (ranging from 100–5000 cycles/sec with power outputs of 4–10 watts). Several studies suggest that the superpulse CO_2 laser has the ability to flash vaporize tissue, with less heat conduction into the surrounding tissue. The result is a clean surgical vaporization to a controlled depth, without charring, contraction of surrounding tissue, or significant protein coagulation in tissue adjacent to the target volume. Because there is less necrotic tissue to slough and less thermal damage to be repaired, the inflammatory response is lessened and scar formation is reduced.

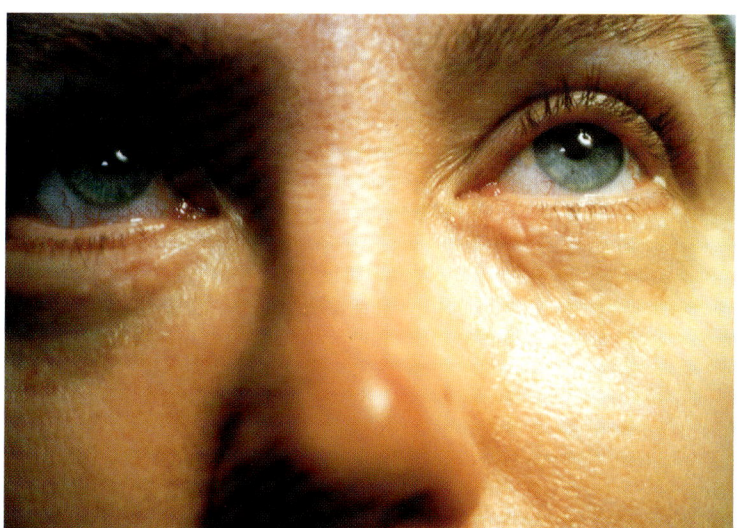

FIG. 4.63-A. Recurrent bilateral lower eyelid syringomas after failed attempts of sharp excision, electrodessication, and currettage. There are approximately 50 lesions, cream-colored, each 1–5 mm in size.

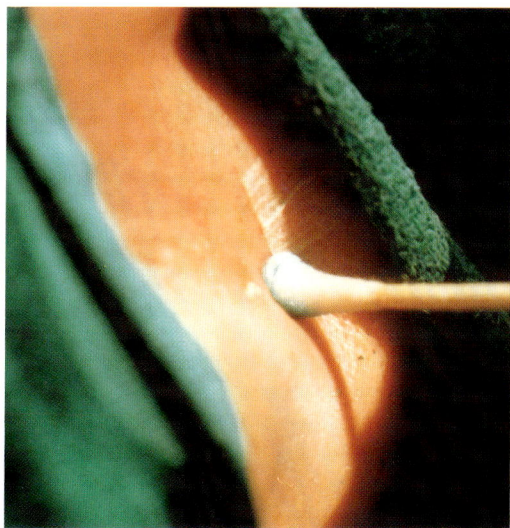

FIG. 4.63-B. The patient elected to have general anesthesia. A standard upper and lower eyelid blepharoplasty was performed prior to CO_2 laser treatment of the syringomas. Methylene blue is brush-painted over the lower eyelids, and then cleaned with normal saline.

Case continues on following page.

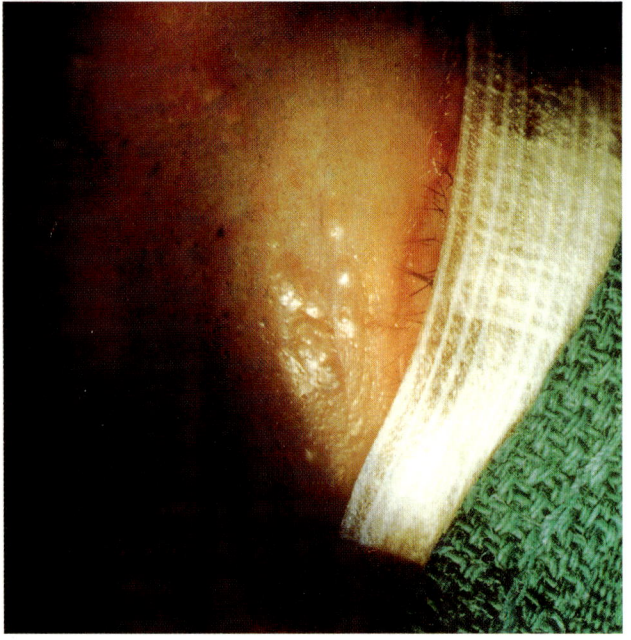

FIG. 4.63-C. After cleansing the excess of methylene blue not absorbed by the normal tissue, the syringomas are highlighted and their borders are clearly visible.

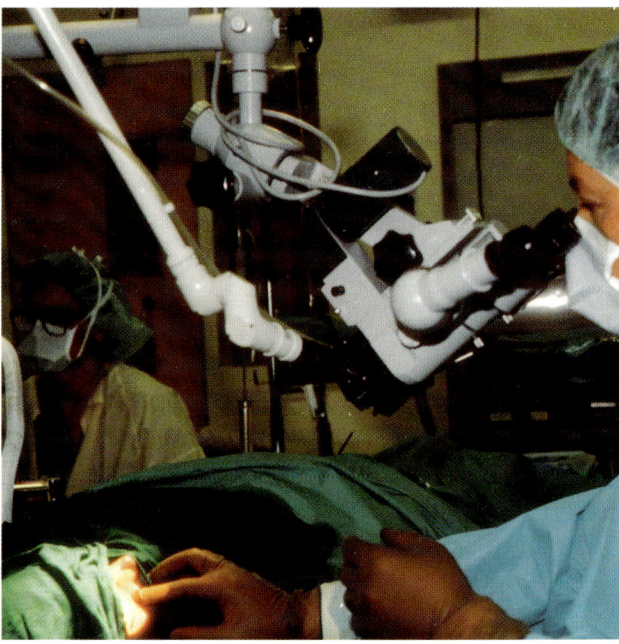

FIG. 4.63-D. The superpulse CO_2 laser is connected to a standard operating microscope. With a power output of 6 watts, 150 ms, and a spot size of 0.2 mm, each lesion was photoevaporated using two to four pulses.

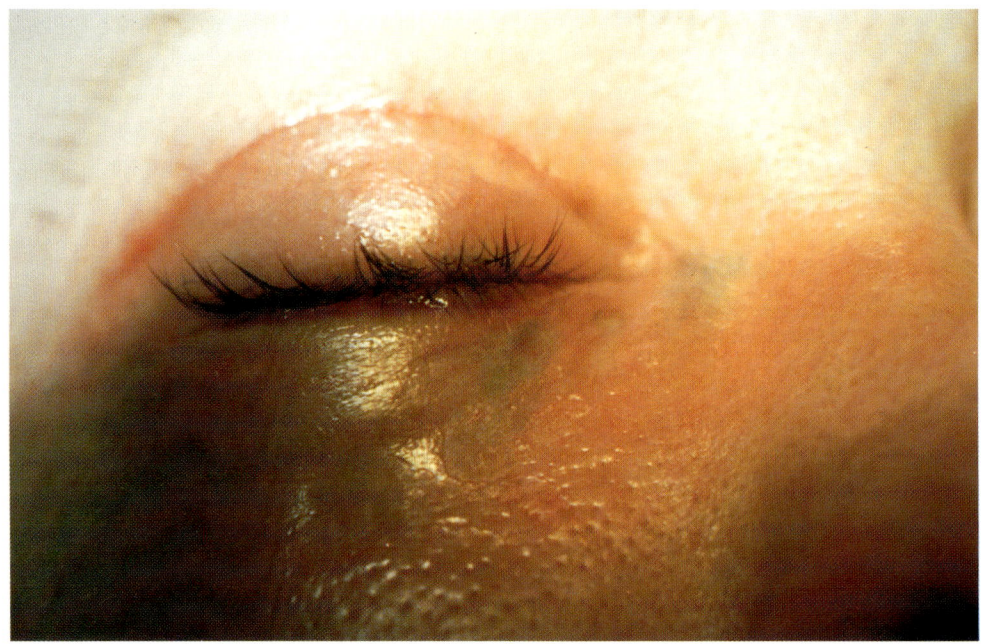

FIG. 4.63-E. Appearance of the lower eyelids immediately post-CO_2 laser treatment. Minimal swelling is observed. Polysporin ointment is applied locally.

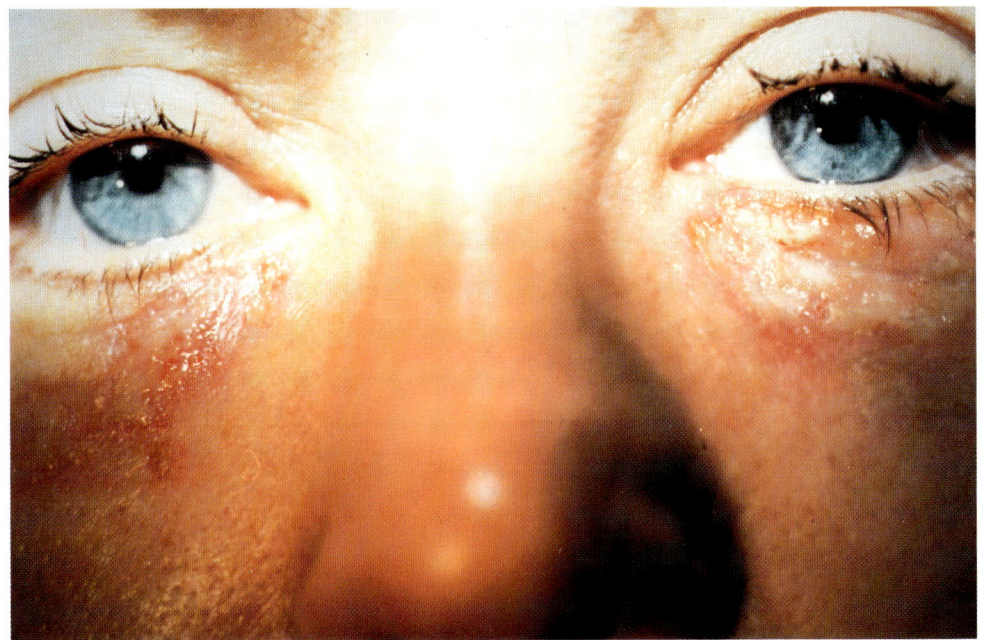

FIG. 4.63-F. One week post-CO_2 laser treatment of the lower eyelid's syringomas. Superficial scabs are formed. The patient denied any pain.

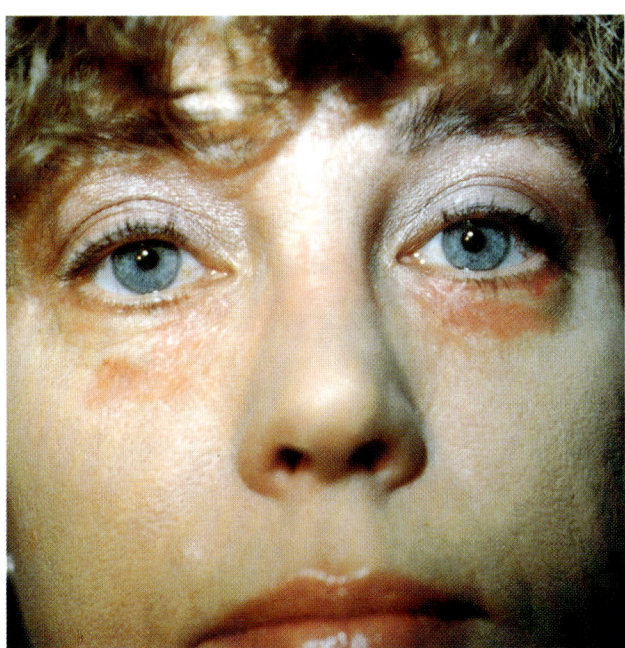

FIG. 4.63-G. Some of the scabs are still present at three weeks post-CO_2 laser treatment.

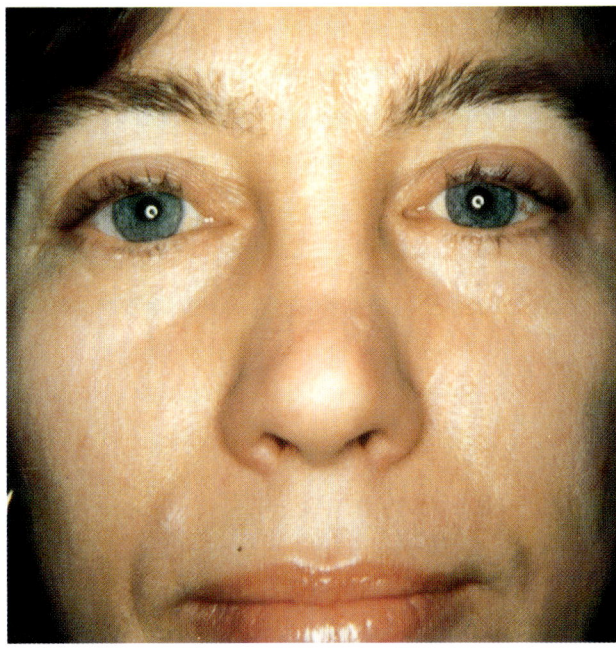

FIG. 4.63-H. Complete healing was observed at one month post-laser treatment with no recurrences even after a two year follow-up as seen in this picture. No scars were observed.

Case courtesy of *Dan J. Castro*, M.D.

CASE 4.64

Syringoma

REVIEW OF CASE. This is a 36-year-old white female with an increasing number of syringomas on both eyelids. She wanted to receive treatment.

CHOICE OF LASER: CARBON DIOXIDE. The CO_2 laser was chosen because with the defocused CO_2 laser beam and vaporization, the lesions can be vaporized. Therapy at this site usually heals nicely.

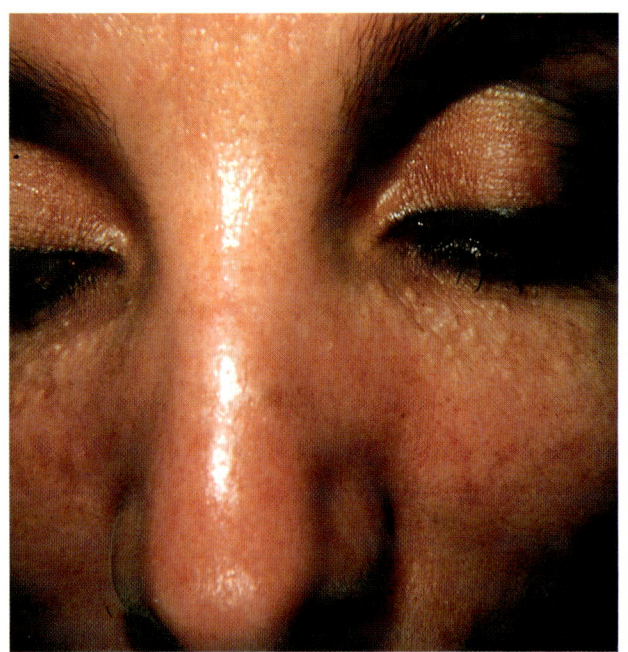

FIG. 4.64-A. Syringomas on both lower eyelids.

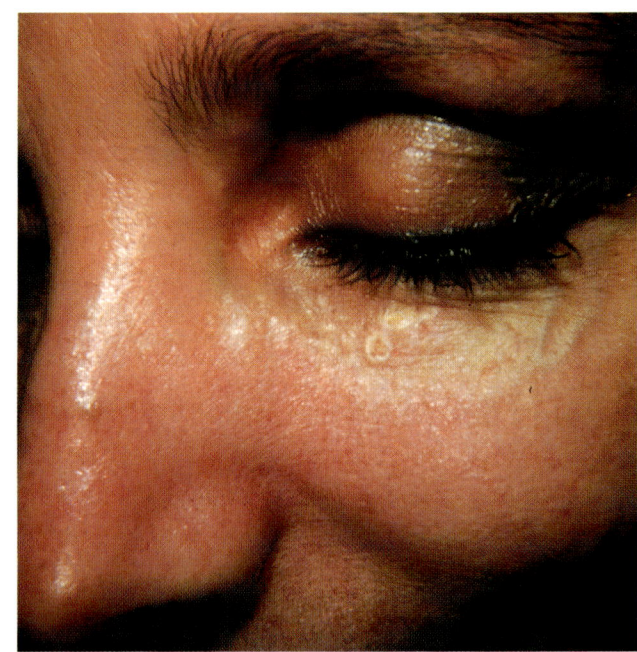

FIG. 4.64-B. Close-up of Fig. A.

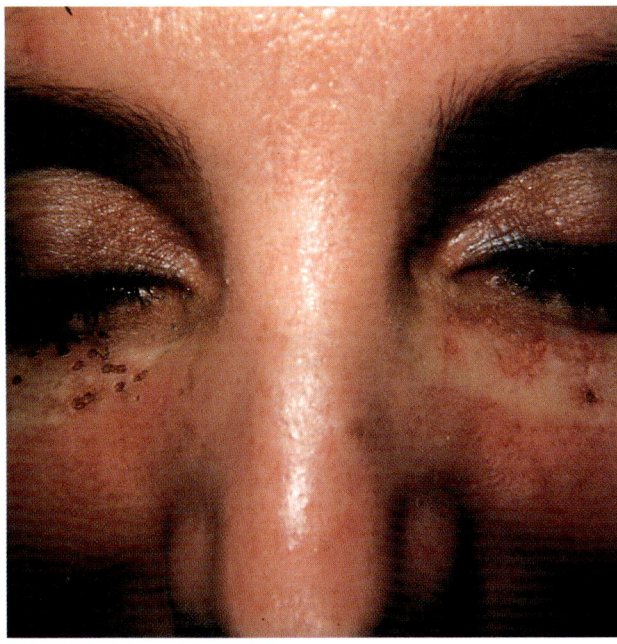

FIG. 4.64-C. Under local anesthesia, the lesions were vaporized using the CO_2 laser with a 5 watt defocused beam and an exposure time of 0.2 second.

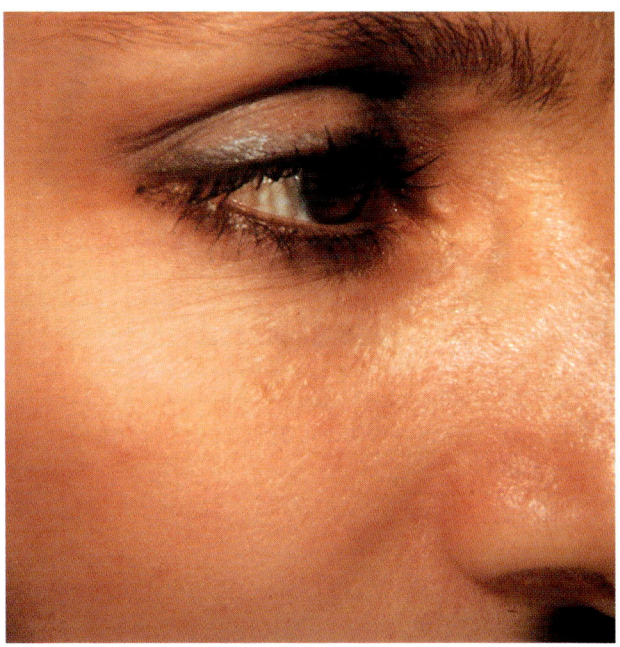

FIG. 4.64-D. Right lower eyelid four weeks after treatment.

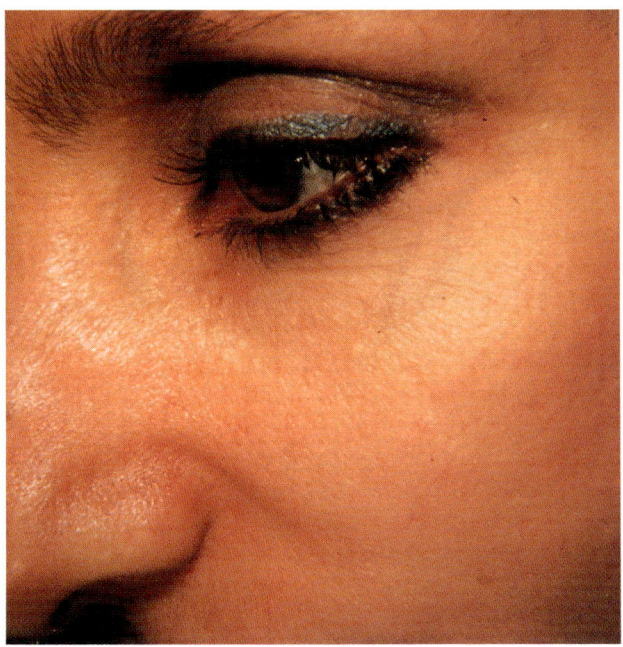

FIG. 4.64-E. Left lower eyelid four weeks after treatment.

Case courtesy of *Syrus Rayhan*, M.D.

CASE 4.65
Trichoepithelioma

REVIEW OF CASE. This healthy 34-year-old Hispanic female began to notice the development of many small asymptomatic skin colored papules around her nose at puberty. Since that time there has been a slow, but progressive, increase in both the size and number of lesions, restricted to the perinasal area. No other family members are similarly affected and she has had no prior medical or surgical treatment. A biopsy confirmed the clinical impression of multiple trichoepitheliomas.

CHOICE OF LASER: CARBON DIOXIDE. Treatment of localized or diffuse small cutaneous appendigeal tumors like trichoepitheliomas, syringomas, tricholemmomas, and sebaceous hyperplasia can be extremely difficult. Superficial dermabrasion may be effective for treating large areas of involvement, but the relatively large size of the diamond fraises and wire brushes makes treatment of small, localized areas far more difficult. In addition, bleeding that occurs during dermabrasion may interfere with the surgeon's ability to detect residual areas of involvement and reduce the effectiveness of the procedure while increasing the likelihood of recurrences due to incomplete removal of lesions.

The CO_2 laser can be used with a low power setting of 4–5 watts and a relatively large beam of 2 mm, to deliver short pulses of 0.1–0.2 second of low-irradiance energy (130–160 watts per cm^2). In this way, the invisible, mid-infrared laser energy precisely vaporizes soft tissue to a depth of 0.1 mm without bleeding. The selective absorption of this wavelength of light by intracellular and extracellular water minimizes thermal conduction to the surrounding normal tissue which speeds wound healing and minimizes the risk of developing adverse textural changes or scarring. This technique also provides the surgeon with the greatest opportunity to remove all abnormal tissue since there is, in most cases, no bleeding. Compared to the imprecise and non-selective injury resulting from electrosurgical techniques or cryosurgery, the laser technique provides excellent cosmetic results with minimal post-operative pain and rapid healing.

ADDITIONAL INFORMATION. Local anesthesia or regional nerve blocks must be utilized for this procedure since the discomfort of the exposure to CO_2 laser energy is intolerable, even by the most stoic patient. The volume of the injected local anesthetic agent elevates the skin surface and may obscure some of the smaller lesions. For this reason, it is appropriate to pre-operatively mark each individual lesion with a surgical marking device to reduce the risk of failing to treat any small areas of involvement inadvertently. After each lesion has been superficially vaporized, the debris and char is removed by lightly scrubbing with a cotton-tipped applicator soaked in 3% hydrogen peroxide. This further improves visibility and allows the surgeon to more easily identify residual islands of tumor cells due to the difference in color or texture.

In patients who have a dark complexion, post-inflammatory hyperpigmentation may result as a nonspecific reaction to this treatment. However, this color will fade spontaneously in most cases over a period of two to three months. Patients should limit unnecessary sunlight exposure following CO_2 laser vaporization so that additional irregularities in pigmentation will not develop.

For literature pertaining to this case see References section.

POST-TREATMENT CARE. Following laser vaporization, the open wounds are allowed to heal by second intention and are cleansed twice daily with 3% hydrogen peroxide solution and the base is then covered by applying a thin film of antibacterial ointment and a nonstick dressing. Wound healing, depending upon the size and location of the treatment site, as well as the depth of involvement, or number of treatment repetitions, typically requires two to three weeks. Use of oral medications for control of the minimal amount of pain is not usually necessary. The patient is instructed to avoid unnecessary sunlight exposure for six to eight weeks to reduce the risk of hyperpigmentation at the treatment site. Also, no makeup or other cosmetics should be used until the wound has completely re-epithelialized.

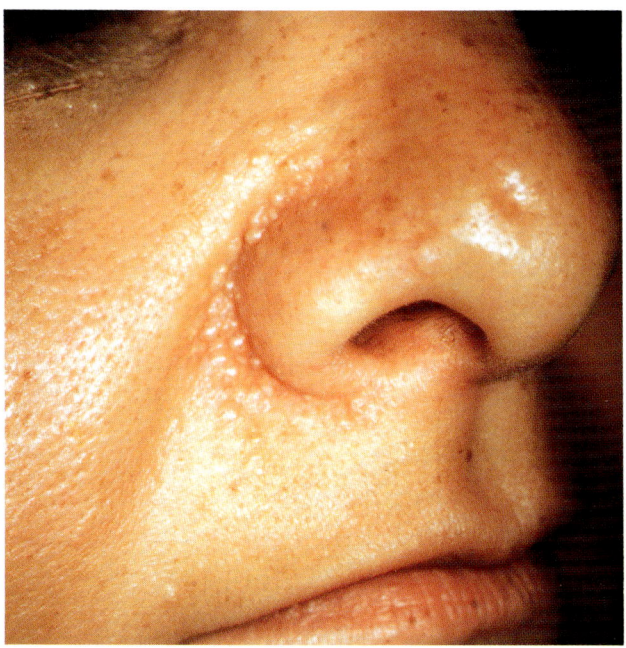

FIG. 4.65-A. Pre-operative appearance of the multiple skin-colored, 1–2 mm papules found grouped in the right nasolabial fold.

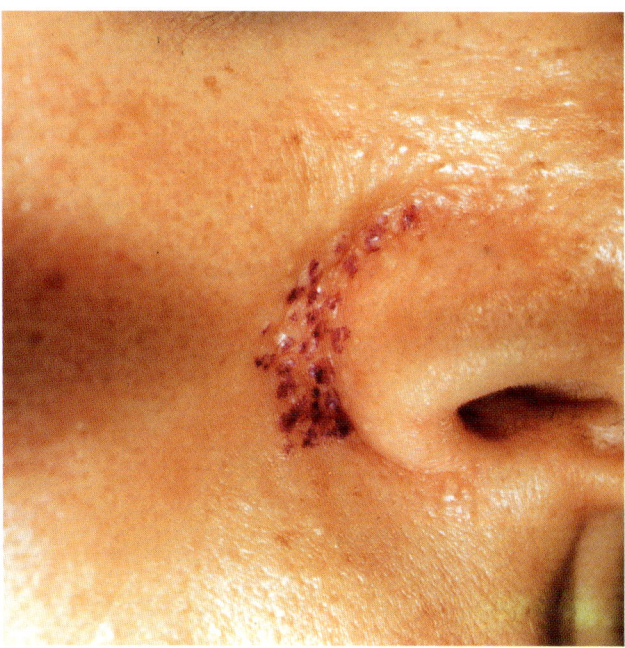

FIG. 4.65-B. Individual lesions have been marked with gentian violet prior to injection of the local anesthetic agent to assist in identification of all tumors at the time of laser surgery.

Case continues on following page.

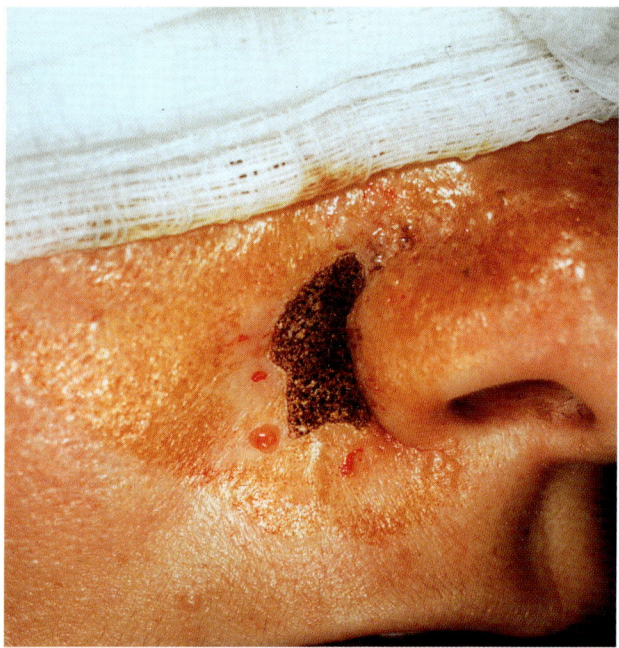

FIG. 4.65-C. After initial laser vaporization the surface of the treatment site shows a light char.

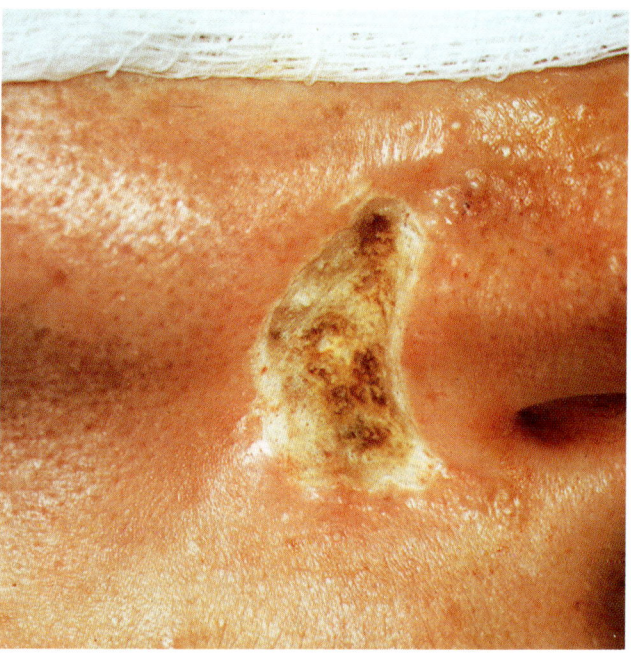

FIG. 4.65-D. After a second laser treatment repetition followed by cleansing of the wound with a solution of 3% hydrogen peroxide, complete removal of all tumors has been accomplished and the base is smooth in texture and white in color.

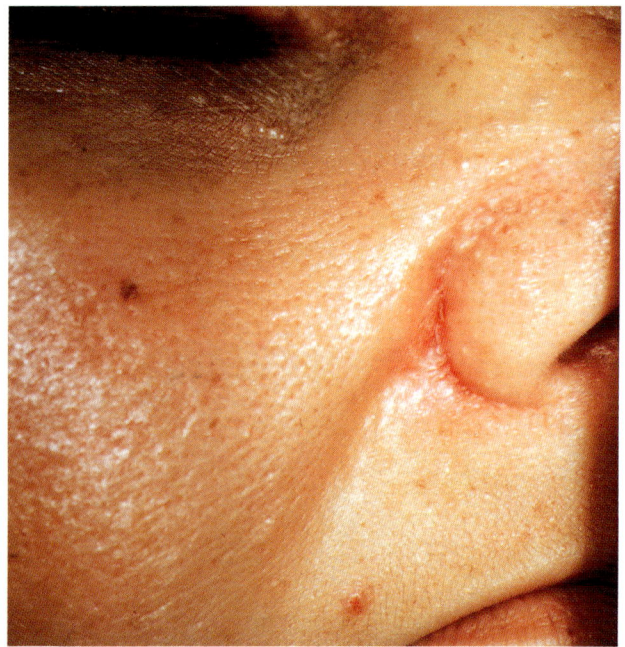

FIG. 4.65-E. The treatment site healed completely in two weeks and by six weeks post-operatively there is only slight residual erythema, with normal texture and no evidence of recurrent growth of trichoepithelioma.

Case courtesy of *Ronald G. Wheeland*, M.D., F.A.C.P.

CASE 4.66
Xanthelasma on Both Lower Eyelids

REVIEW OF CASE. This is a 56-year-old female presenting with xanthelasma on both eyelids. The patient desired removal of the xanthelasmas because of the cosmetic appearance.

CHOICE OF LASER: CARBON DIOXIDE. The CO_2 laser was chosen because with the defocused beam, the lesion could be vaporized. By using a magnifier, with a few passes of the defocused beam, the lesions can be removed. The wound, usually at this location heals nicely with secondary intention.

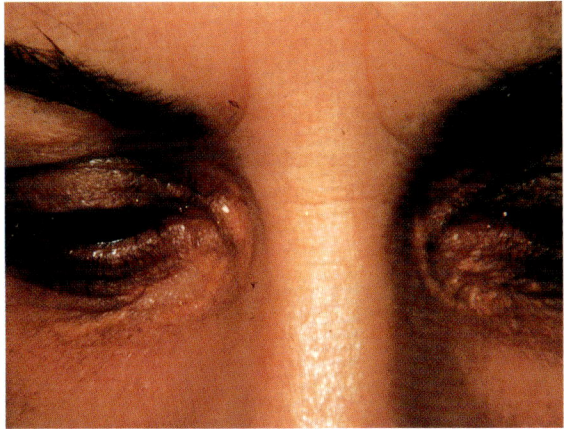

FIG. 4.66-A. Xanthelasma on both eyelids.

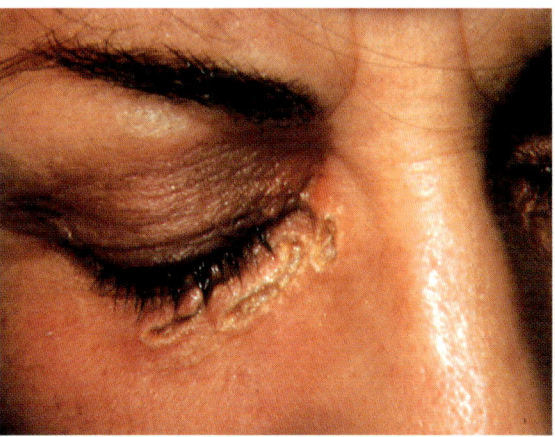

FIG. 4.66-B. One section of the lesion on the testing area was vaporized using the CO_2 laser with a 5 watt defocused beam.

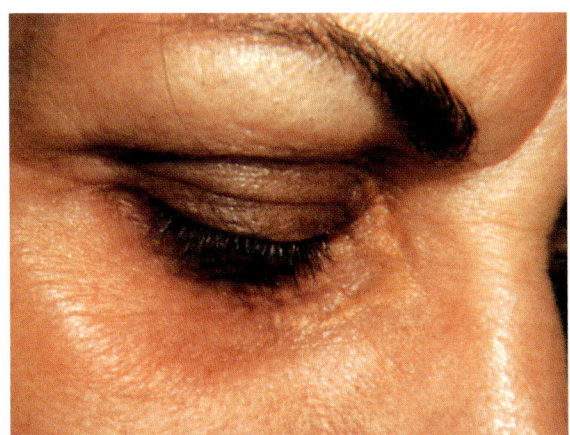

FIG. 4.66-C. The test area nicely healed.

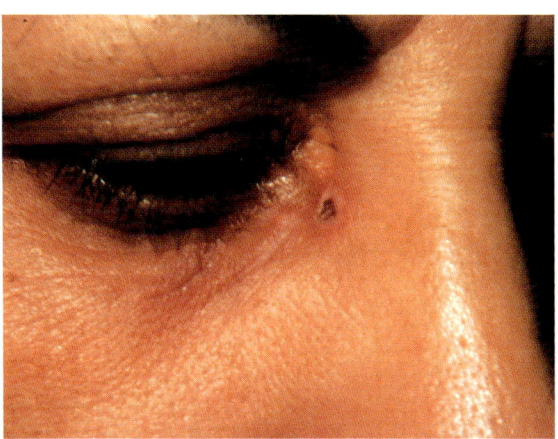

FIG. 4.66-D. Healing of test areas.

Case courtesy of *Syrus Rayhan*, M.D.

CASE 4.67
Basal Cell Carcinoma Left Parotid Area

REVIEW OF CASE. This 103-year-old female had a large infected fungoid mass of the left parotid area. She complained of pain and occasional bleeding.

CHOICE OF LASER: CARBON DIOXIDE. The CO_2 laser was used to excise the lesion precisely with a no-touch technique with free margins to avoid recurrence of the tumor. There is minimal bleeding and edema. The reduction of the bacterial count with flushing is helpful in the preparation of the area for reconstruction with a full-thickness skin graft.

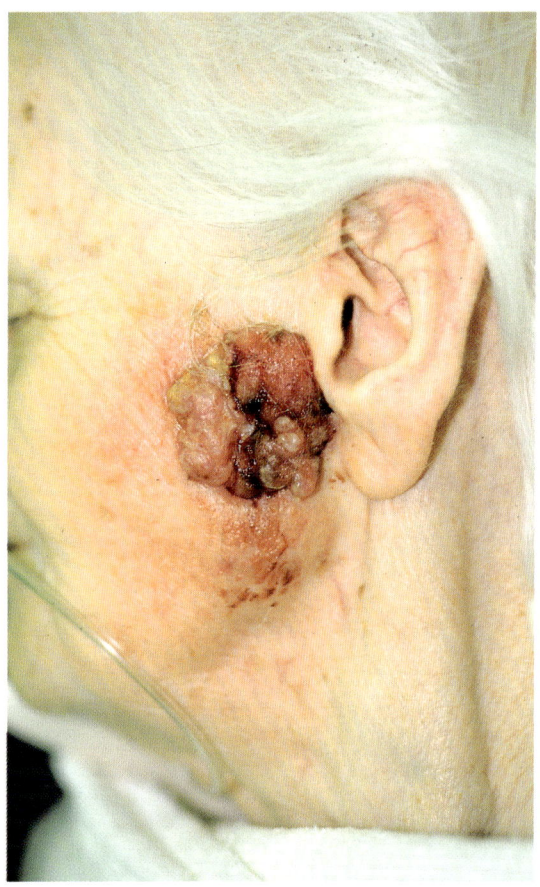

FIG. 4.67-A. Pre-operative view of the left parotid mass.

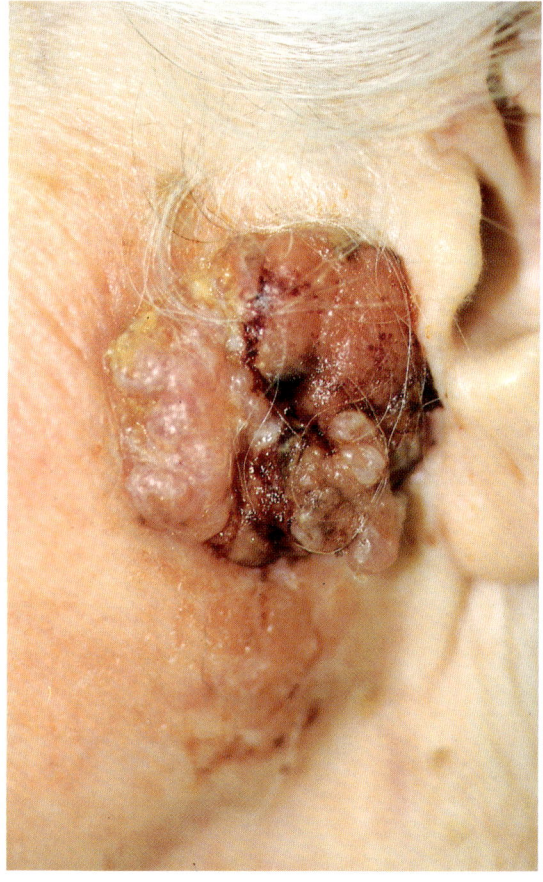

FIG. 4.67-B. Same as Fig. A.

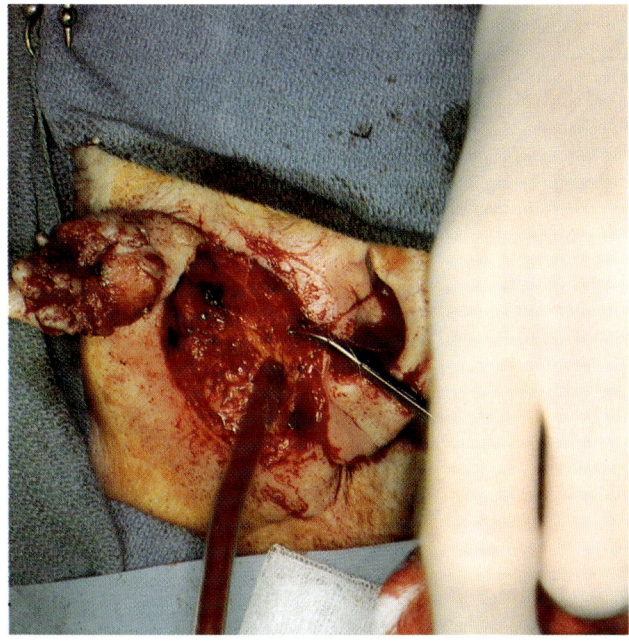

FIG. 4.67-C. The lesion was excised with the CO_2 laser using a 125 mm lens at 20 watts of power in a continuous mode.

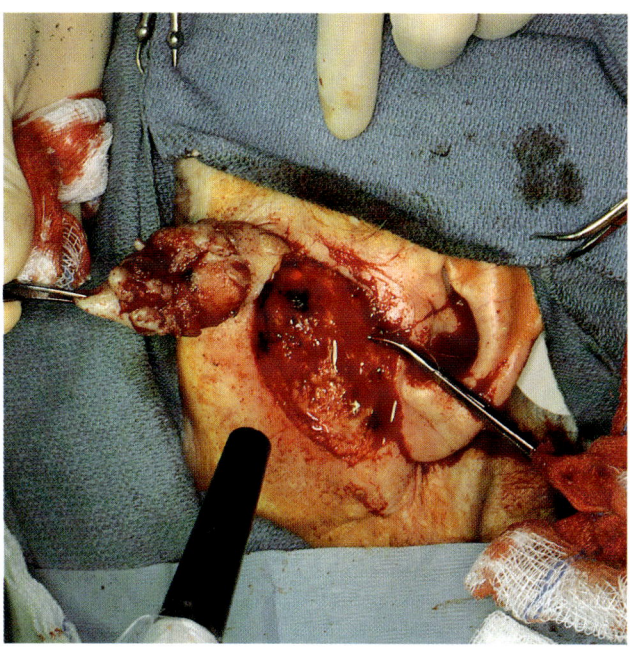

FIG. 4.67-D. Vaporization of the area using the CO_2 laser at 20 watts of power in a defocus mode to reduce the bacterial count.

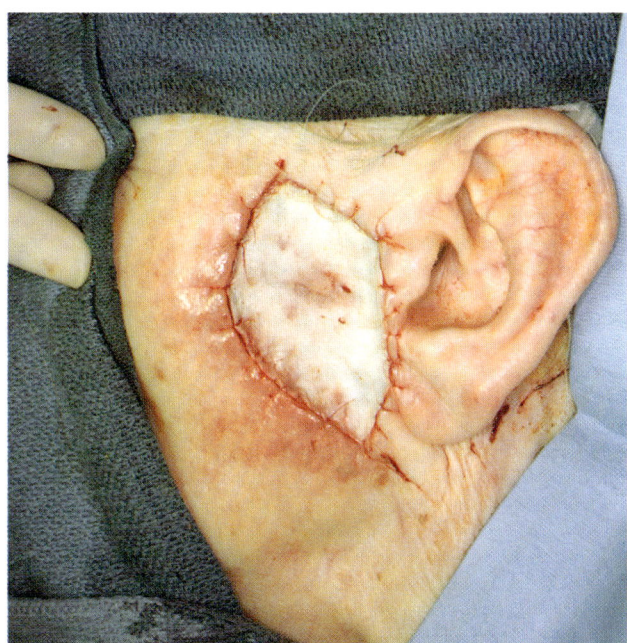

FIG. 4.67-E. The full-thickness skin graft in place over the defect.

FIG. 4.67-F. The graft is well established with no recurrence of the tumor.

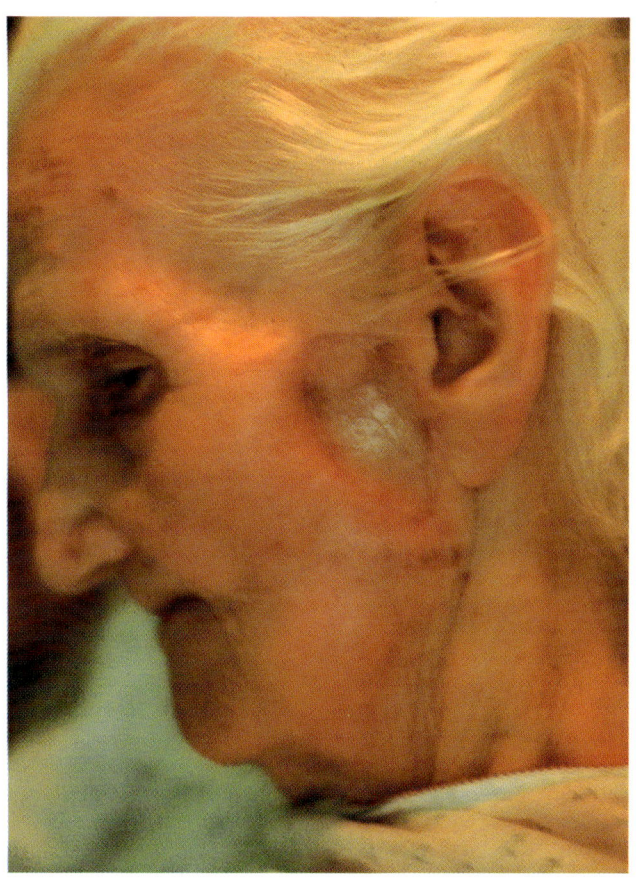

Case courtesy of *H. Raul Herrera*, M.D.

CASE 4.68

Blepharoplasty

REVIEW OF CASE. This 47-year-old female requested cosmetic blepharoplasty for moderate blepharochalasia. Examination demonstrated marked overhang of upper eyelid skin.

CHOICE OF LASER: CARBON DIOXIDE. The CO_2 laser when finely focused at the focal point produces a light beam which cuts and coagulates. Adjacent nerves and lymphatics are sealed, giving a more pain-free wound with less ecchymosis and edema compared to a standard scalpel incision.

ADDITIONAL INFORMATION. In this study, a comparison was made between CO_2 laser, blepharoplasty, and standard blepharoplasty. The CO_2 laser was used in the right upper eyelid and conventional scalpel technique was used in the left upper eyelid. In the right upper eyelid, skin only was incised with a scalpel and the remainder of the procedure including skin undermining and removal, muscle resection, and removal of fat pads was accomplished with the carbon dioxide laser. The patient was then observed immediately postoperatively, 1 day, 2 days, 4 days, 7 days, and weekly between 2 and 6 weeks. This study was done to assess whether carbon dioxide laser blepharoplasty produced superior results to standard blepharoplasty. No difference in patient comfort, pain, swelling, ecchymosis was noted.

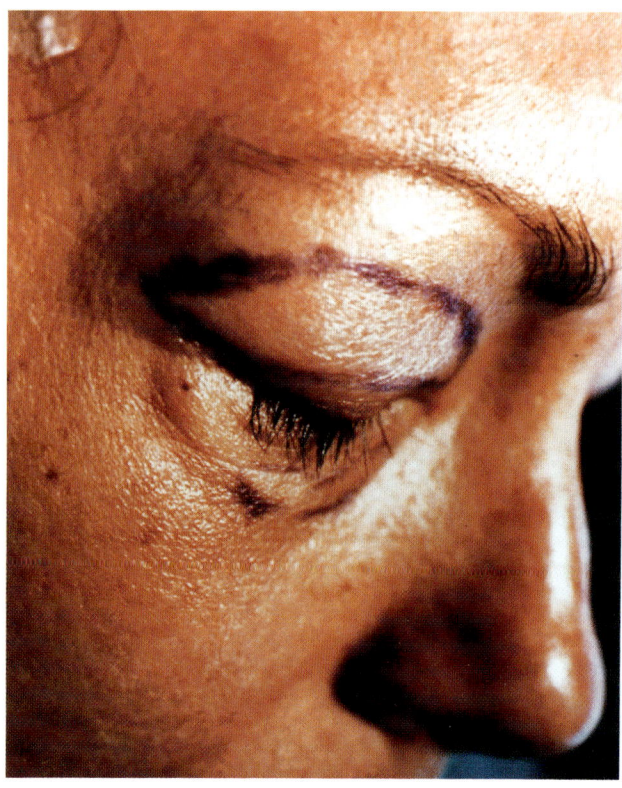

FIG. 4.68-A. Appearance of upper eyelid prior to surgery with amount of skin to be resected marked with gentian violet.

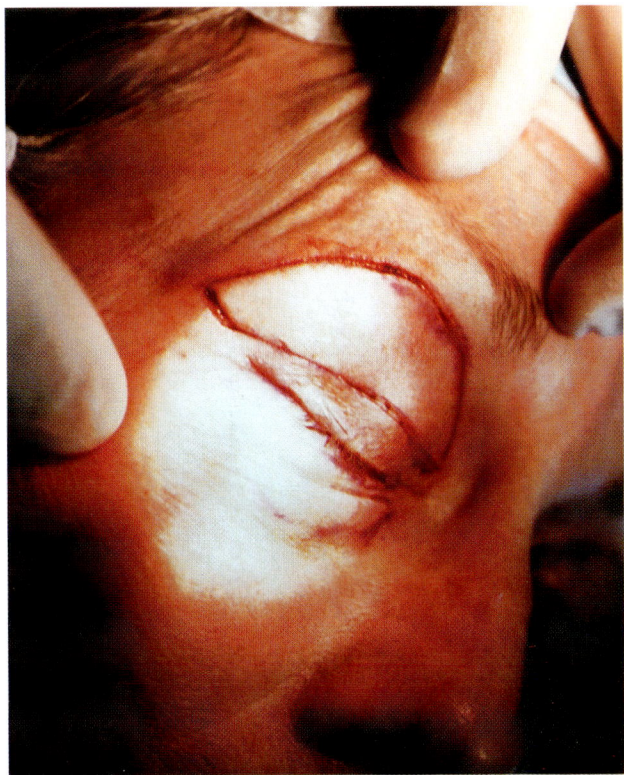

FIG. 4.68-B. Skin incised with scalpel.

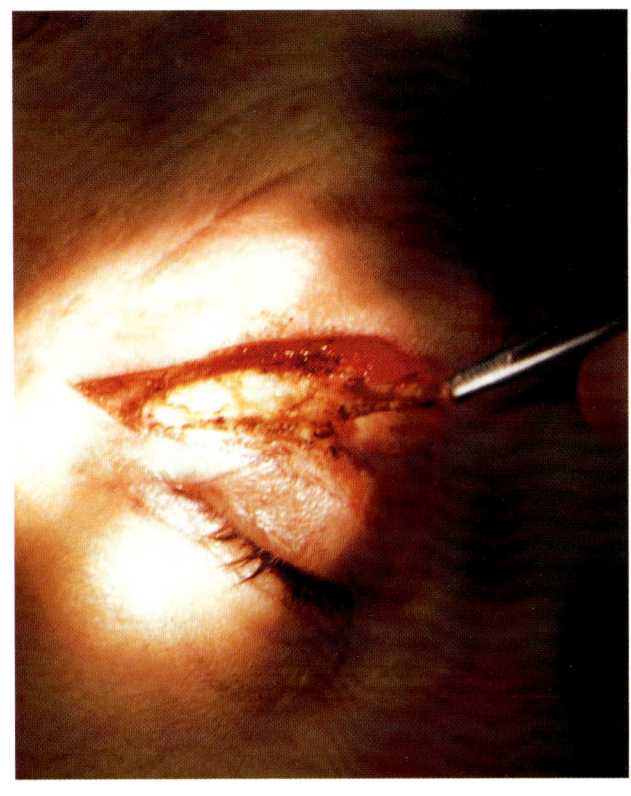

FIG. 4.68-C. Skin muscle flap dissected and removed with CO_2 laser.

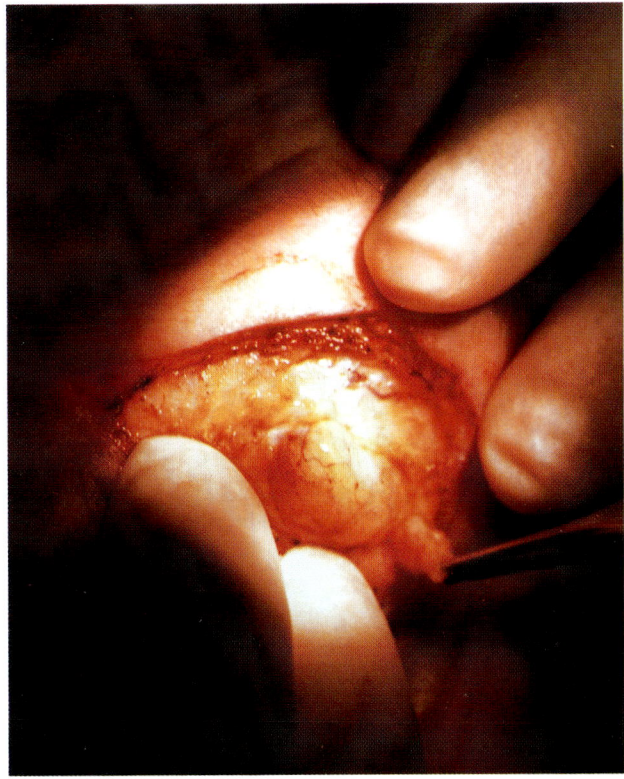

FIG. 4.68-D. Demonstration of fat herniation to be removed by laser.

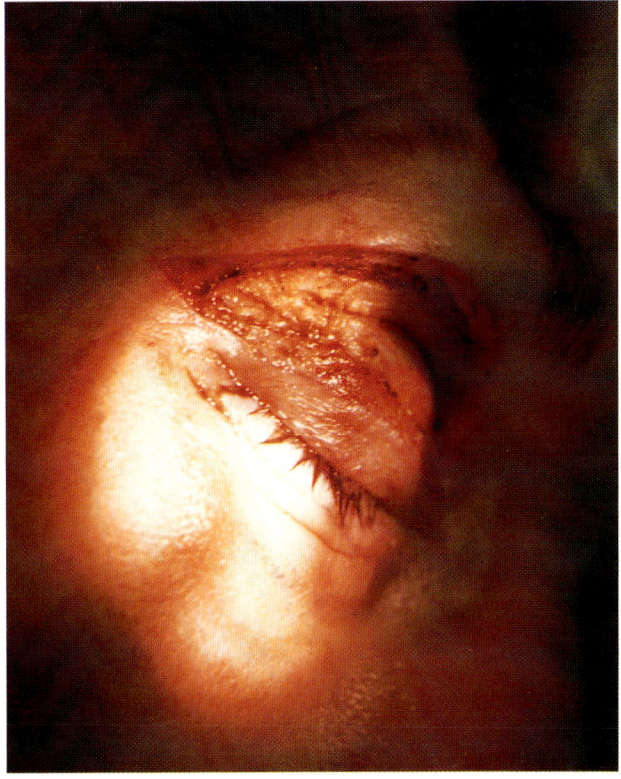

FIG. 4.68-E. Completed blepharoplasty prior to closure.

Case continues on following page.

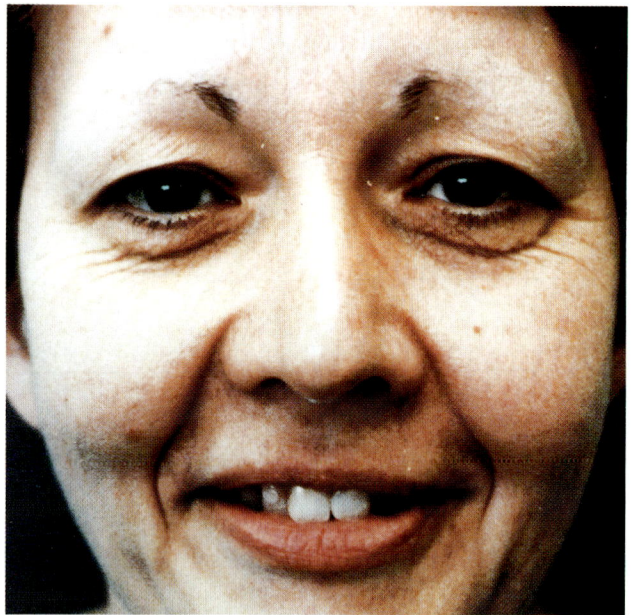

FIG. 4.68-F. Pre-operative appearance of patient.

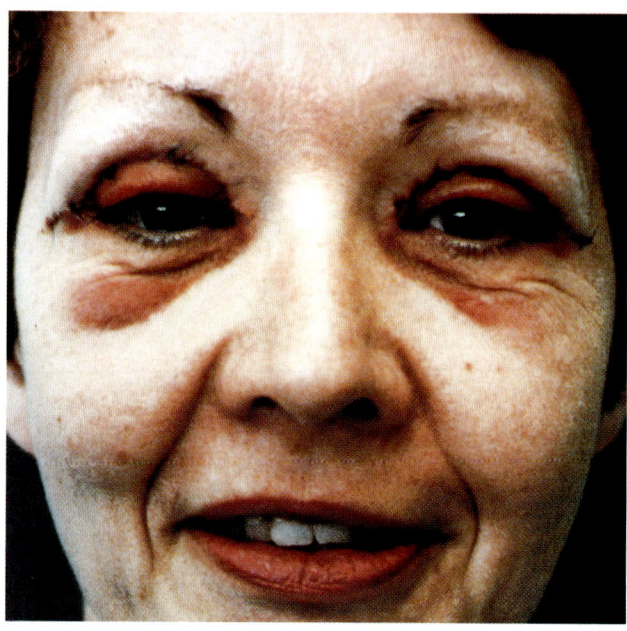

FIG. 4.68-G. Appearance one day following surgery—very little difference in upper lid edema, ecchymosis, or discomfort was noted.

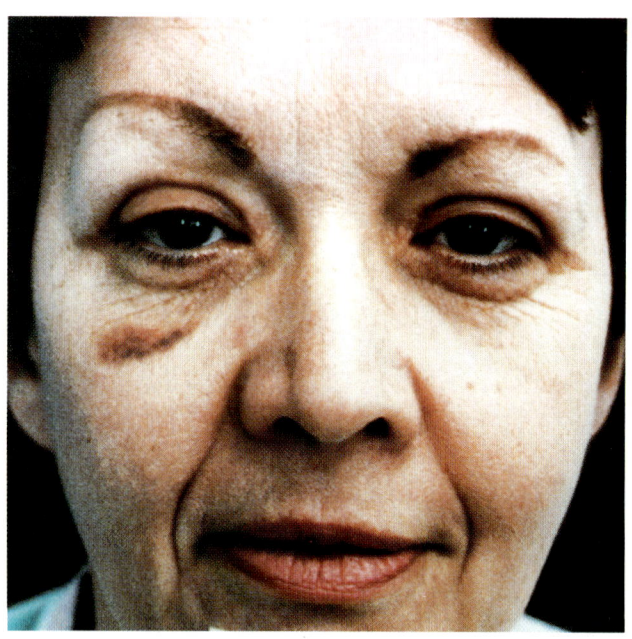

FIG. 4.68-H. Appearance after one week—minimal difference in upper lid swelling or discoloration is noted.

Case courtesy of *Harry Mittelman*, M.D., and *David B. Apfelberg*, M.D.

Reprinted with permission of Little, Brown and Company.
For literature pertaining to this case see References section.

CASE 4.69

Blepharopigmentation

Eyeliner Tattoo Removal

REVIEW OF CASE. Eyeliner tattoo was applied in a poor orientation to the lid margin and eyelashes resulting in an unwanted cosmetic result. The eyeliner tattoo was positioned above the base of the lashes by about 2–3 mm and was irregular in form. The patient desired removal of the tattoo because of the unnatural appearance.

CHOICE OF LASER: CARBON DIOXIDE. The CO_2 laser was chosen because of its proven effectiveness in vaporizing tissue-containing tattoo pigment. Because of the proximity to the lid margin and the eyelashes, extreme precision is necessary. The ability to focus the laser to correspond to the precise size of the tattoo line and to fire the laser in a series of 50 millisecond pulses allows removal of this tattoo with extreme precision. The superpulsed setting is chosen to minimize unwanted thermal damage to eyelid tissue underlying the tattoo. This is extremely important as well because of the very thin tissue of the eyelids.

ADDITIONAL INFORMATION. Because of the proximity to the lashes and the lid margin, extreme caution must be used to prevent damage to these structures and consequent loss of lashes or ectropion. Undertreatment is much preferable in this location rather than overtreatment. In fact, it probably is not necessary to completely remove the pigmentation as illustrated, as one case subsequent to this has been treated with only superficial vaporization of the tissue-containing pigment resulting in initial removal of only 50% of the pigment. It is preferable to re-treat remaining pigmentation six months later if necessary, rather than remove excess tissue. It should be mentioned that eye shields are necessary while performing this surgery.

POST-TREATMENT CARE. The patient was instructed to stand in the shower and allow water to run over the area gently for about five minutes twice per day. The wound was kept continuously coated with Polysporin ointment and bandaged.

Case continues on following page.

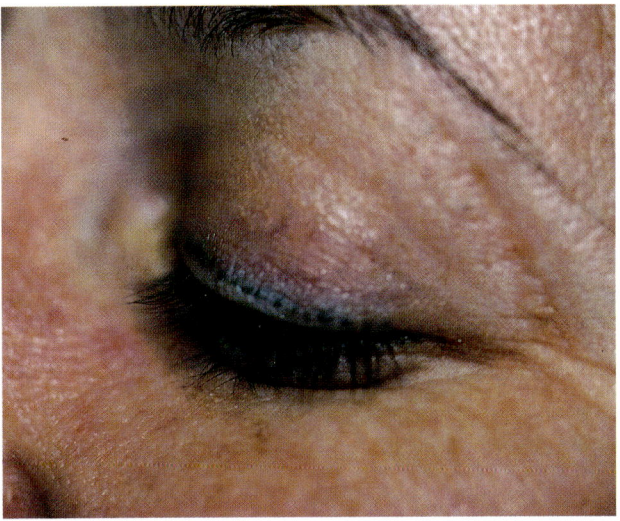

FIG. 4.69-A. Malpositioned eyeliner tattoo on the upper eyelid.

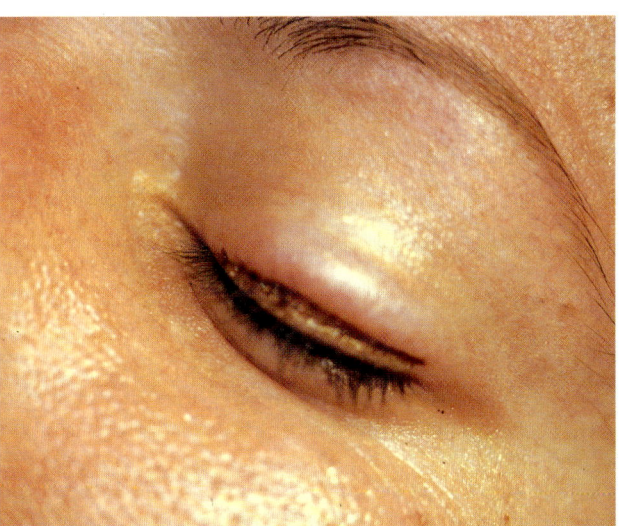

FIG. 4.69-B. Using a superpulsed CO_2 laser with settings of 80 watts pulse peaks, 300 microsecond pulses, and 500 Hz resulting in an average power of 12 watts and fired in repetitive 50 millisecond pulses, the tissue containing the tattoo pigment was vaporized after local anesthesia with 1% Xylocaine. This was accomplished by carefully tracing the tattoo line with the laser impacts, wiping the surface with cotton-tipped applicators soaked in normal saline, and repeating this process until the entire tattoo line was removed. This resulted in an open wound similar to an incision line, which was allowed to heal by secondary intention.

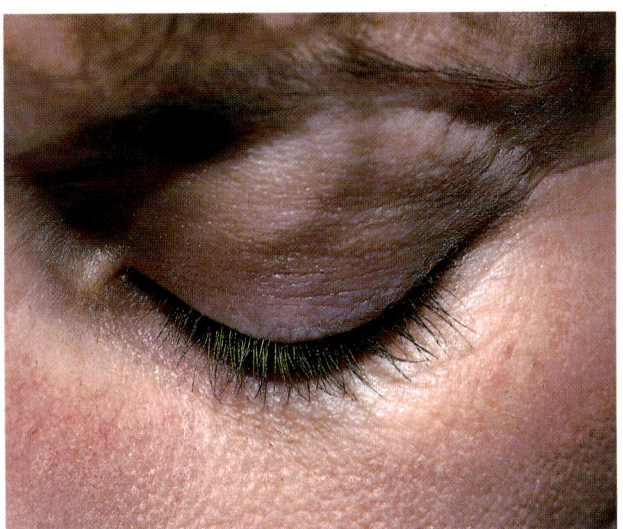

FIG. 4.69-C. The final result one year after the procedure.

Case courtesy of **Richard E. Fitzpatrick**, M.D., **Javier Ruiz-Esparza**, M.D., and **Mitchel P. Goldman**, M.D.

CASE 4.70

Tattoo Removal

REVIEW OF CASE. This 35-year-old white man had tattoo applied to the left deltoid area 18 years previously. He now finds the tattoo an embarrassment and wishes to have it removed.

CHOICE OF LASER: CARBON DIOXIDE. The CO_2 laser was chosen because of its proven effectiveness in vaporizing tissue containing tattoo pigment. Because the risk of unsightly scarring correlates with the depth of the wound, and deep pigmentation cannot be removed using the CO_2 laser without creating a deep wound, 50% urea ointment was added to leach out pigment from the laser wound.

ADDITIONAL INFORMATION. The urea ointment should be kept in the refrigerator with the cap tightly closed to prevent evaporation of moisture and further concentration or crystallization of the urea in order to avoid an irritating ointment.

POST-TREATMENT CARE. Bandages should be removed daily and the ointment washed off in the shower. The wound should then be patted dry and 50% urea ointment re-applied with the bandages.

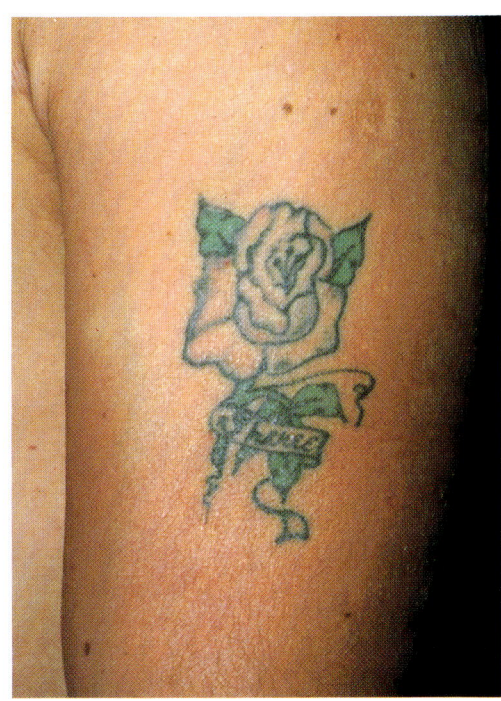

FIG. 4.70-A. Pre-operative tattoo on left deltoid area.

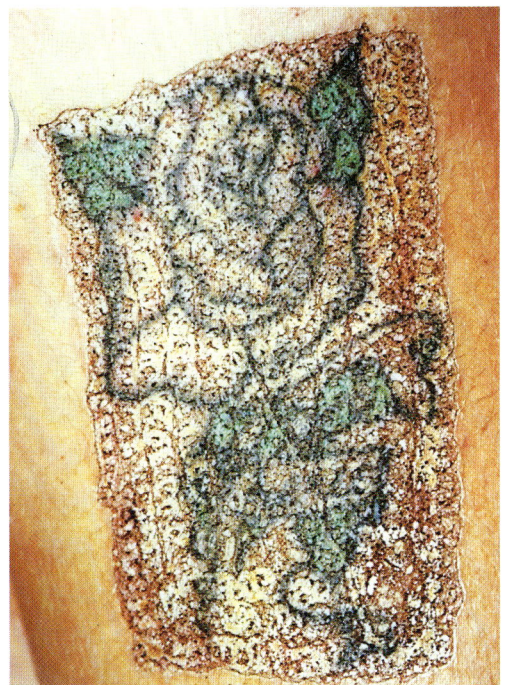

FIG. 4.70-B. Using a continuous CO_2 beam defocused to about 2.5 mm diameter and utilizing 12 watts of power the epidermal layer is vaporized over the entire area of the tattoo. This layer is easily removed by wiping with gauze sponges soaked in normal saline. It is important to note that the area vaporized is larger than the tattoo itself and with different borders, in order to avoid leaving a scar in the shape of the tattoo.

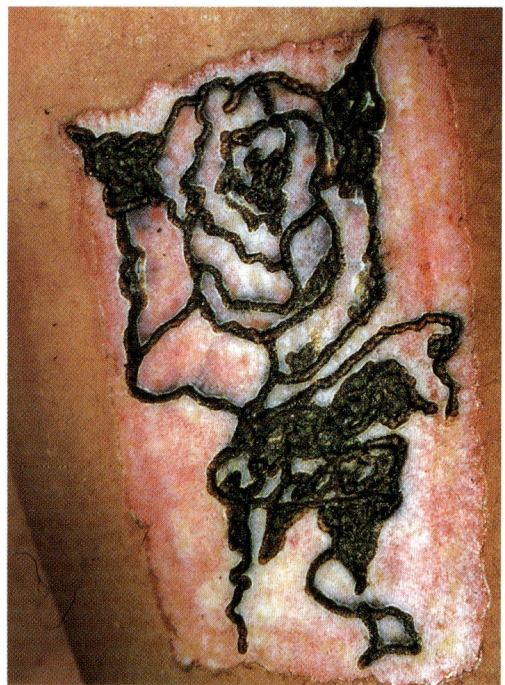

FIG. 4.70-C. The CO_2 laser is used again with the same power settings, but confined only to the areas of tattoo pigment. Once this area has been completely treated, the area is again wiped clean with normal saline on a gauze sponge to reveal the residual pigment. This process should be repeated until approximately 40% to 50% of the tattoo pigment is removed. Generally, this requires 2 or 3 passes over the pigment. Some darker and more deeply pigmented areas may require additional treatment to remove 50% of the pigment. It is important to note that no more than 50% of the pigment should be removed.

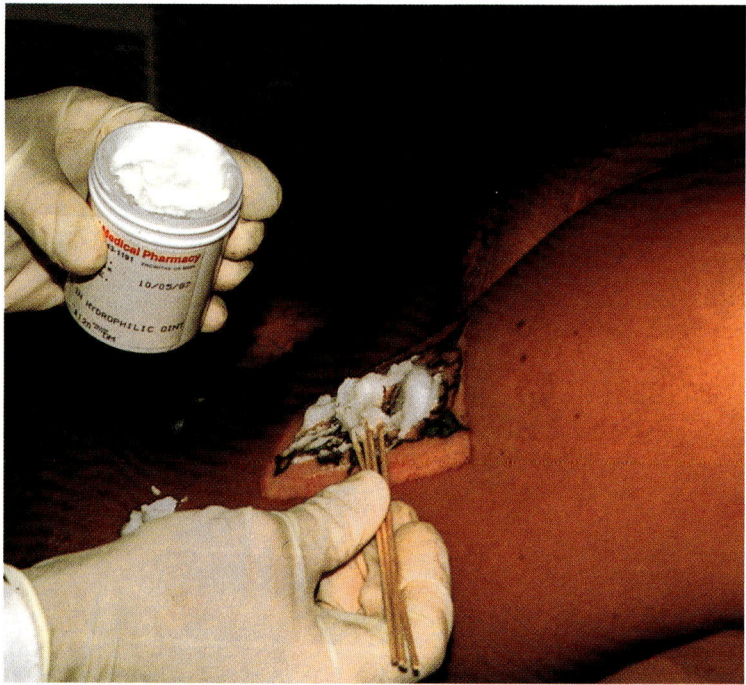

FIG. 4.70-D. Application of 50% urea in hydrophilic ointment is performed immediately post-operation and should completely cover the entire tattoo.

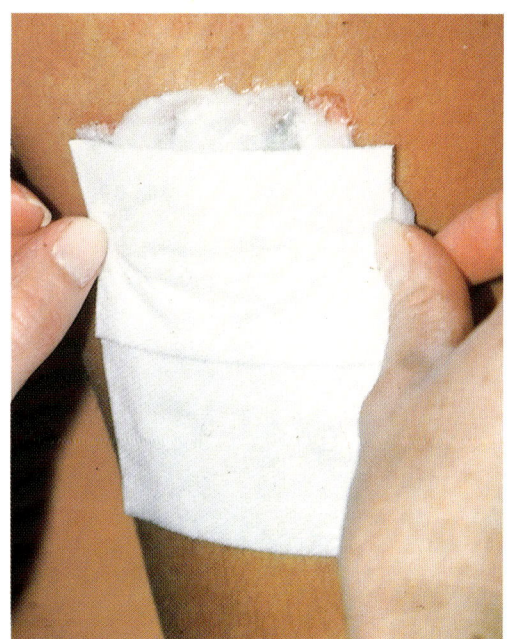

FIG. 4.70-E. Telfa is applied over the 50% urea ointment.

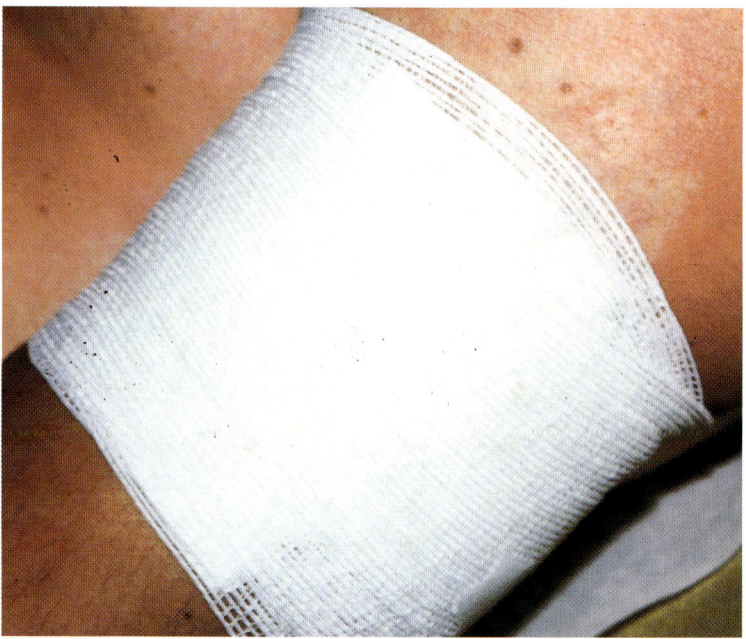

FIG. 4.70-F. Kling gauze is applied to hold the wound dressing in position.

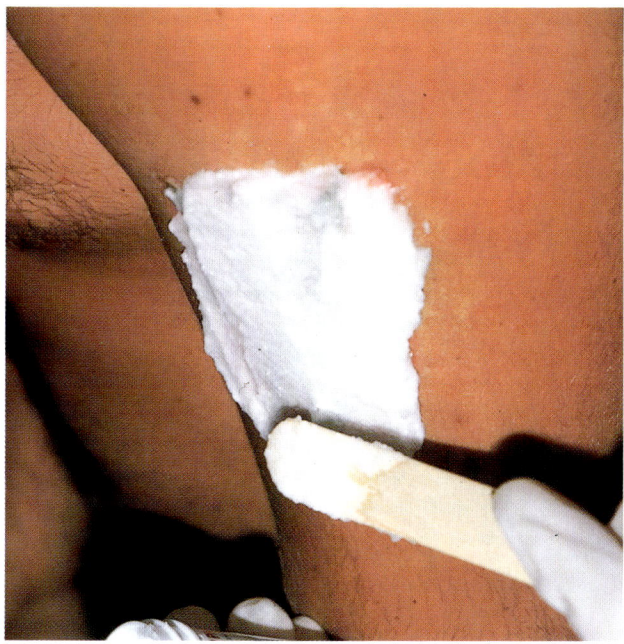

FIG. 4.70-G. The patient is instructed to change the bandage daily, washing off the ointment in the shower, patting the area dry, and then re-applying the 50% urea ointment and bandage.

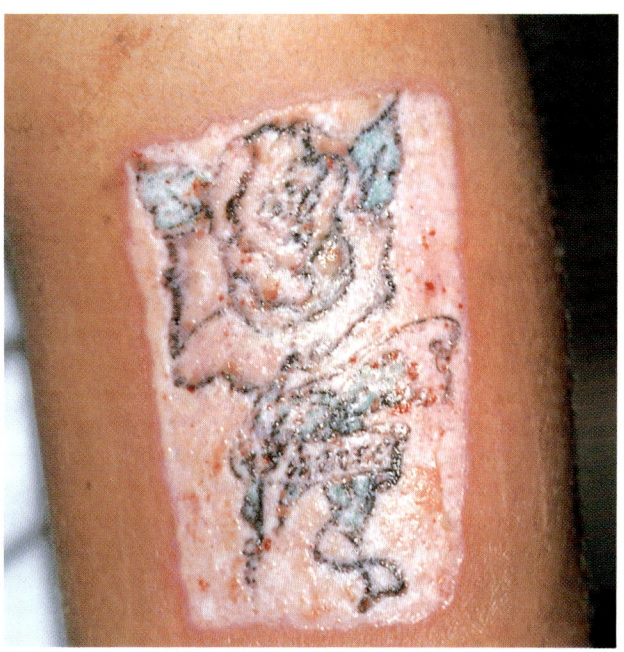

FIG. 4.70-H. The wound should be examined at the end of one week and each week thereafter until healed. The urea ointment should be continued to be applied to the tattoo pigment as long as there is a pigment extruded on the bandage daily.

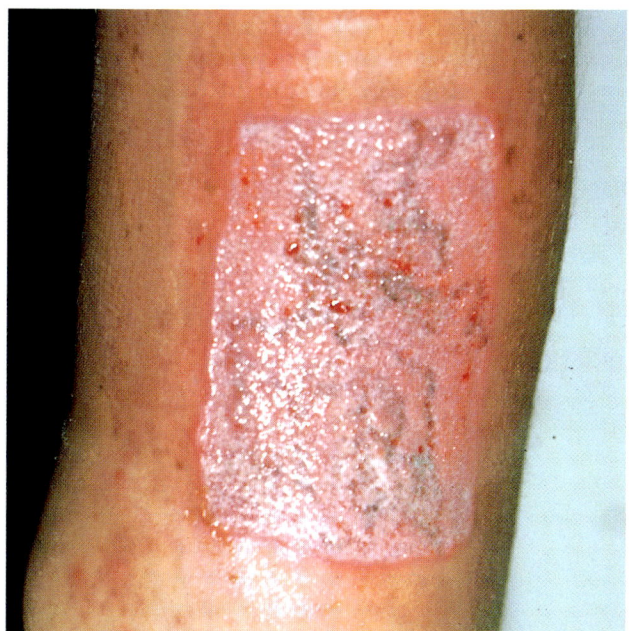

FIG. 4.70-I. At the end of one month over 90% of the pigment has been removed and the wound is healing well.

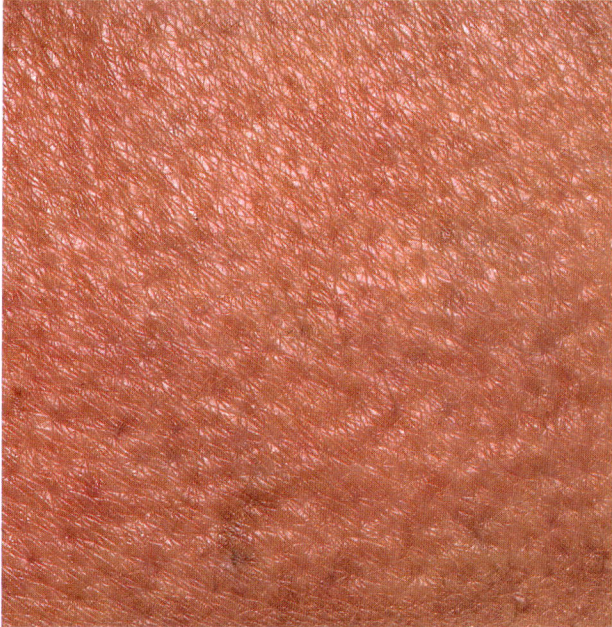

FIG. 4.70-J. Complete healing of the wound requires a period of 1 to 2 years and a decision to remove any residual tatto pigment is best deferred until that time.

Case courtesy of **Richard E. Fitzpatrick,** M.D., **Javier Ruiz-Esparza,** M.D., and **Mitchel P. Goldman,** M.D.

CASE 4.71
Decorative Tattoo

REVIEW OF CASE.   This is a 24-year-old female desiring removal of a decorative tattoo from the wrist for cosmetic reasons.

CHOICE OF LASER: CARBON DIOXIDE. CO_2 laser light is absorbed preferentially by water. The skin contains 70% to 90% water and will absorb CO_2 laser light and convert it to heat which has the ability to vaporize superficial skin layers. By defocusing the laser and rapidly passing it over the skin, external layers can be removed in a very selective fashion. Enclosed tattoo pigment in the upper dermis is progressively removed as each layer of skin is taken. Wound healing is usually prompt and pain and swelling are minimal. Laser power setting is 10 to 15 watts of continuous defocused power.

ADDITIONAL INFORMATION.   This laser is used with 10 to 15 watts of power. The defocused beam is passed back and forth across the area in a rapid "paint brush" manner producing a char. Each successive charred layer is then wiped with a saline/antibiotic solution revealing the deeper layers. Magnifying loupes of $\times 2.5$ are very helpful to assess tattoo pigment removal.

Removal of the most external or superficial skin layer often reveals the tattoo in even more brilliant detail and color since no overlying skin blocks its appearance. Each subsequent laser pass removes progressively more pigment. Often, 4–7 separate passes of the laser are required. One hundred percent of all pigment does not need to be removed. The inflammatory wound healing phase will subsequently cause residual particles to be shed. Extreme care must be taken not to completely penetrate the dermis and produce a full-thickness injury which will result in a hypertrophic scar.

POST-TREATMENT CARE.   A 50% urea solution is applied daily by the patient with a gauze bandage dressing. Daily showering with mild scrubbing of the area aids in removal of residual pigmentation. This daily washing and dressing change is discontinued in 7 to 10 days to allow re-epithelialization of the wound.

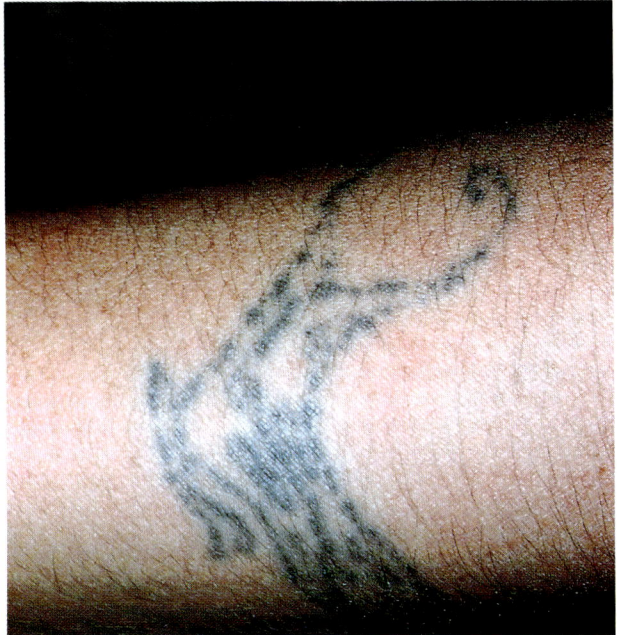

FIG. 4.71-A. Decorative tattoo of the wrist prior to treatment.

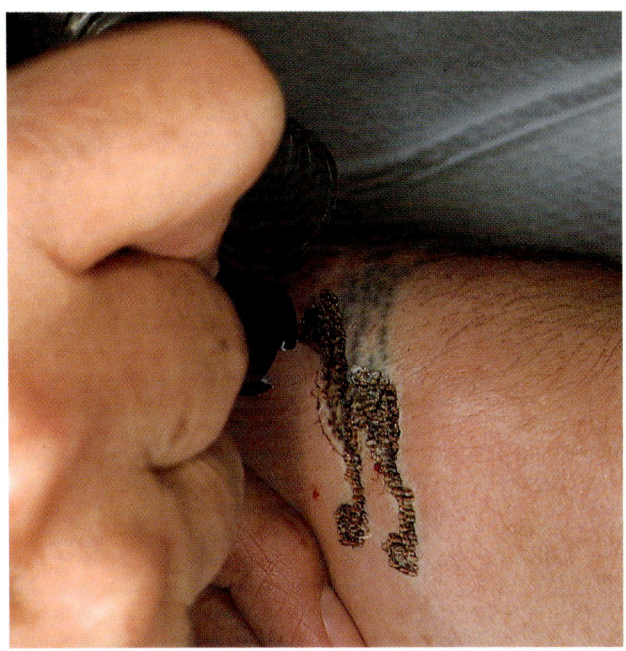

FIG. 4.71-B. The first or external layer of skin is removed.

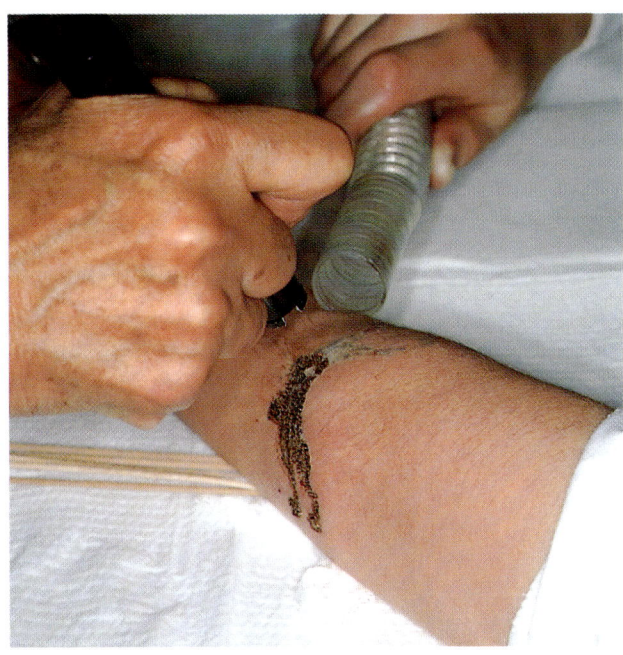

FIG. 4.71-C. The first or external layer of skin is removed. Note the smoke evacuator.

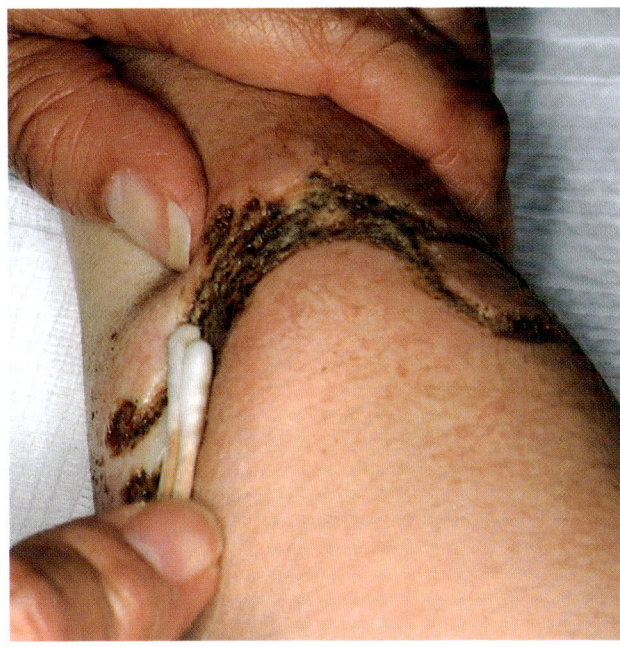

FIG. 4.71-D. The char is removed with a saline/antibiotic solution.

Case continues on following page.

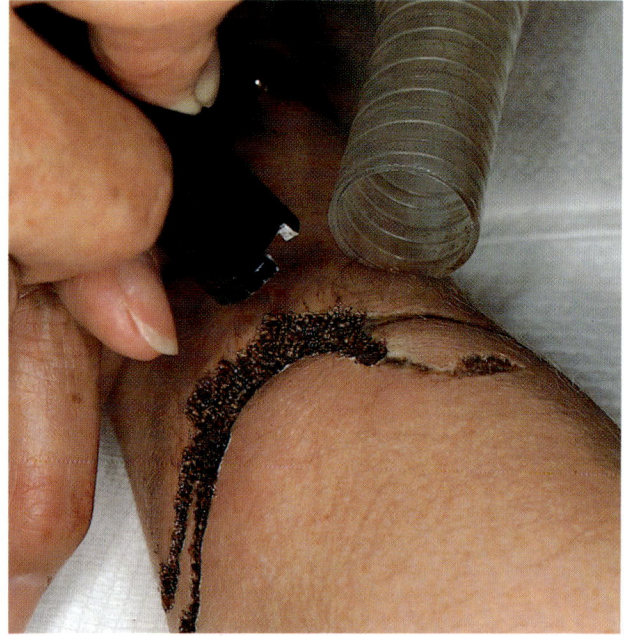

FIG. 4.71-E. The next layer of skin is removed.

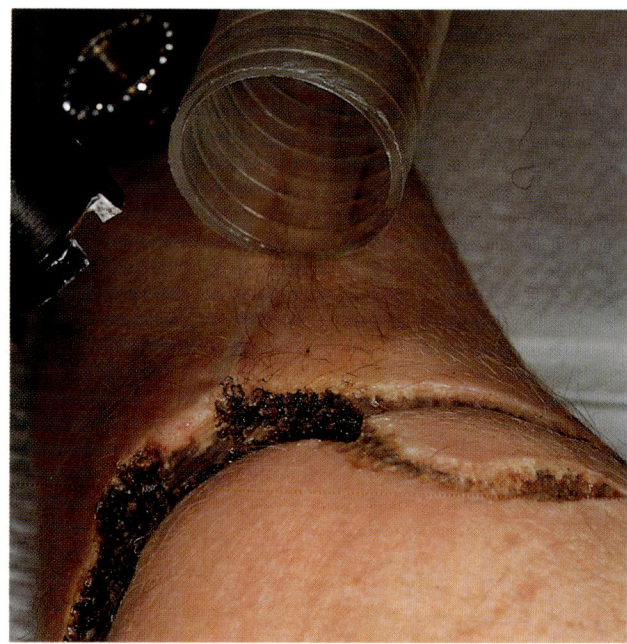

FIG. 4.71-F. Removal of another layer of skin.

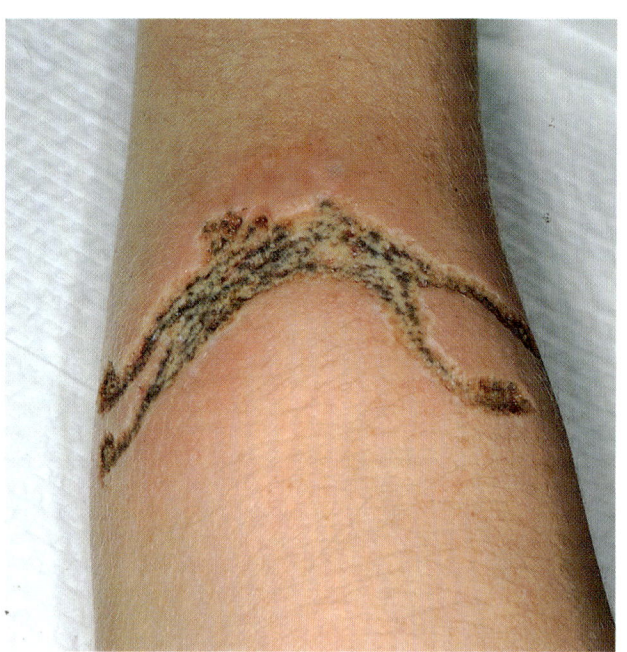

FIG. 4.71-G. Final removal of over 50% of the tattoo pigment but no full-thickness penetration of the dermis.

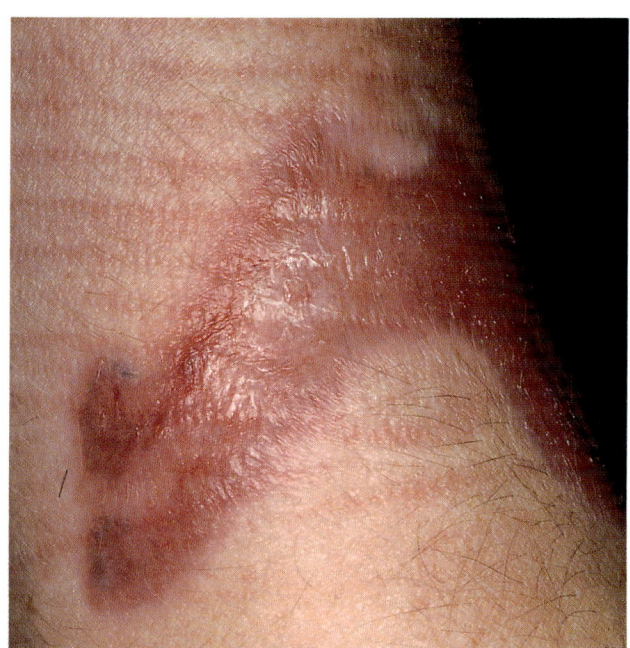

FIG. 4.71-H. Final clinical result demonstrating satisfactory clearing of the tattoo pigment with minor texture changes of the skin.

Case courtesy of *David B. Apfelberg*, M.D.

CASE 4.72
Chronic Chest Wall Ulcer

REVIEW OF CASE. This 57-year-old female had a history of an infected, painful ulcer of the right chest wall post-radiation of local recurrent breast carcinoma. There was necrotic tissue and exposure of the costal ribs.

CHOICE OF LASER: CARBON DIOXIDE. The CO_2 laser was selected to control the amount of bleeding, obtain adequate free margins, and to reduce the pain, edema, and bacterial contamination in preparation for the reconstruction with a latissimus dorsi myocutaneous flap.

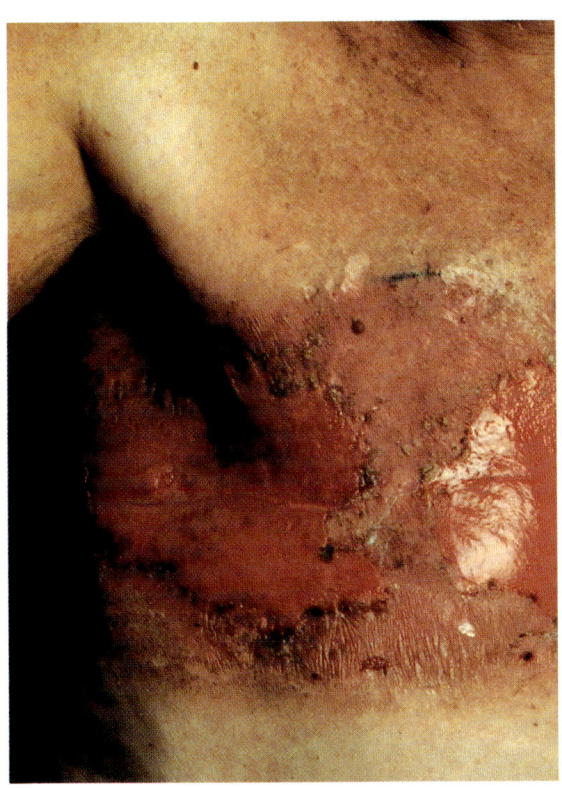

FIG. 4.72-A. Acute stage of ulcer post-radiation.

Case continues on following page.

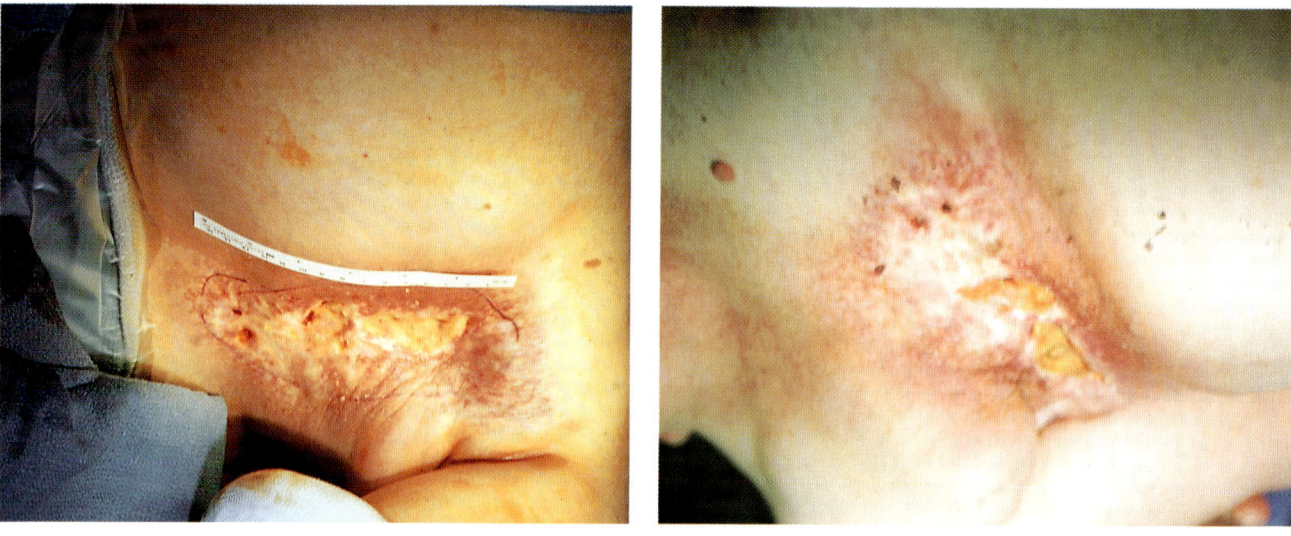

FIGS. 4.72-B, C. Chronic ulcers right chest wall.

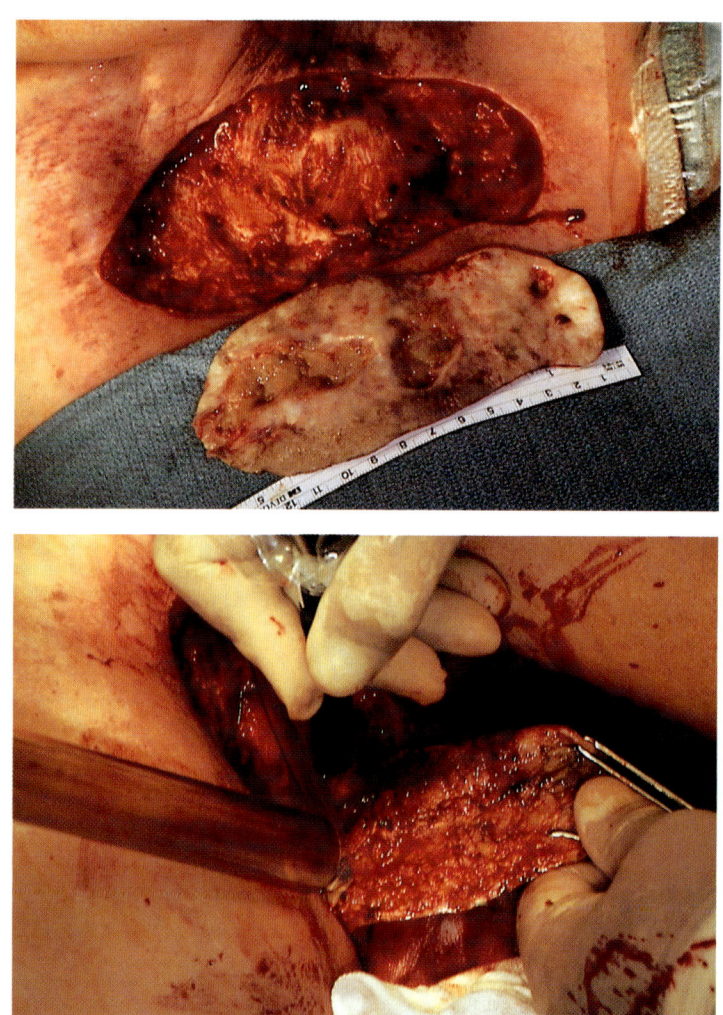

FIGS. 4.72-D, E. Precise excision using the CO_2 laser with a 125 mm lens at 30–40 watts of power in a continuous mode.

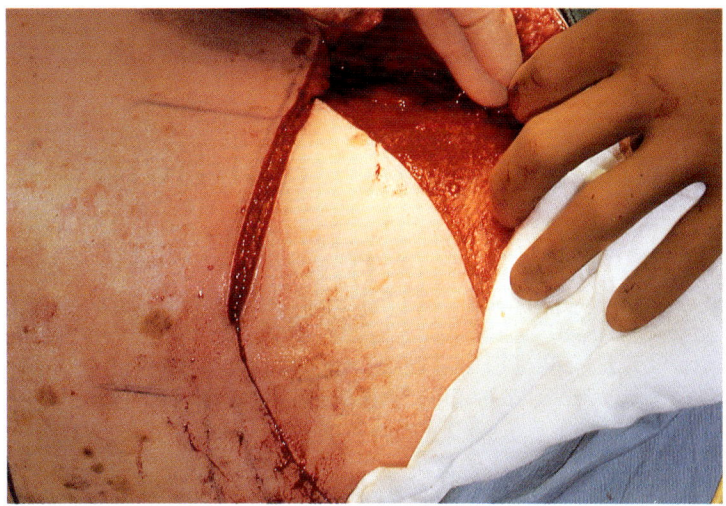

FIG. 4.72-F. Dissection of the latissimus dorsi myocutaneous flap using the CO_2 laser with a 125 mm lens at 30–40 watts of power in a continuous mode.

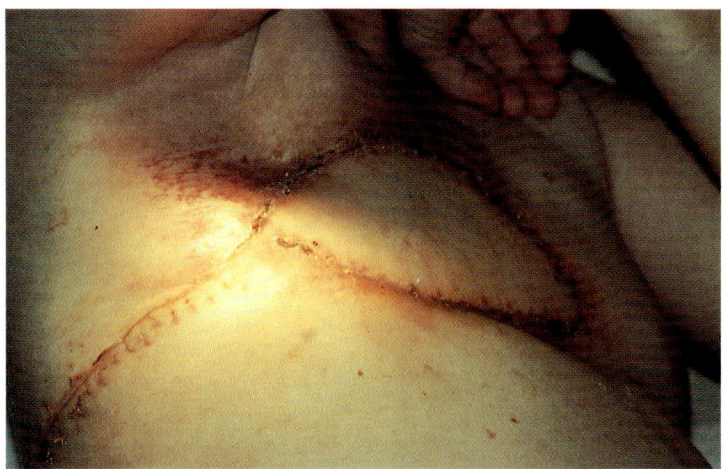

FIG. 4.72-G. Early post-operative wound.

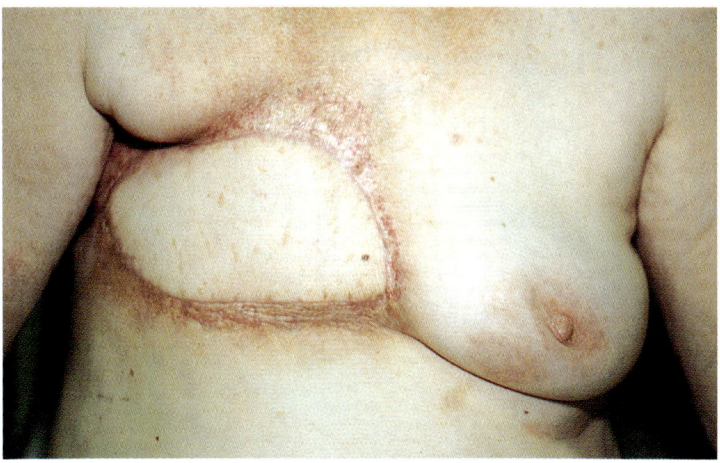

FIG. 4.72-H. Six months following surgery with wound completely healed.

Case courtesy of **H. Raul Herrera**, M.D.

CASE 4.73
De-epithelialization of Skin Flaps

REVIEW OF CASE. This young woman desired a reduction mammaplasty for symptomatic moderate macromastia. A standard inferior-based pedicle technique was chosen for preservation of nipple vascularization. De-epithelialization of the dermal pedicle prior to its being buried must first be performed to insure proper healing without risking development of epidermal retention cysts.

CHOICE OF LASER: CARBON DIOXIDE. Many techniques, usually using a sharp instrument, have been utilized for removing the epidermis prior to burying flaps in recontouring procedures or in breast reduction for formation of the dermal pedicle flap necessary for maintaining nipple viability. Frequently this is a tedious and time-consuming task. The CO_2 laser has an advantage not only in hastening this portion of such operations, but also preserves the circulation arising from the subdermal plexus.

Since the energy delivered by the CO_2 laser when used in a continuous defocused mode, is quickly dissipated in tissues of high water content such as the skin, surface vaporization of the epidermis results with a limited depth of penetration. Rapid skin de-epithelialization similar to a dermabrasion is then possible by serial paint brushing of the required region until the deeper dermis is delineated.

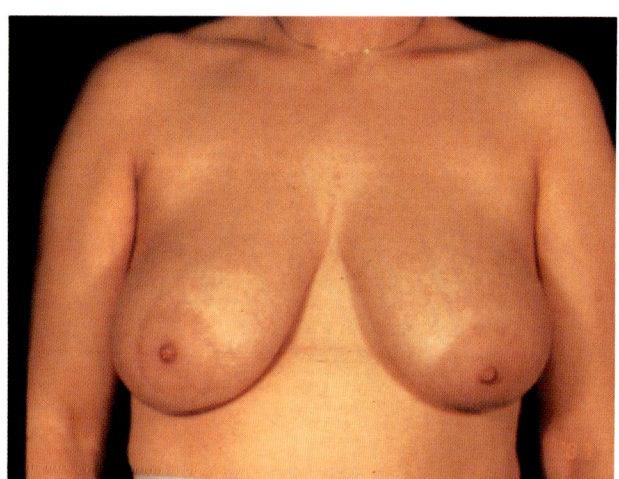

FIG. 4.73-A. Symptomatic bilateral moderate macromastia.

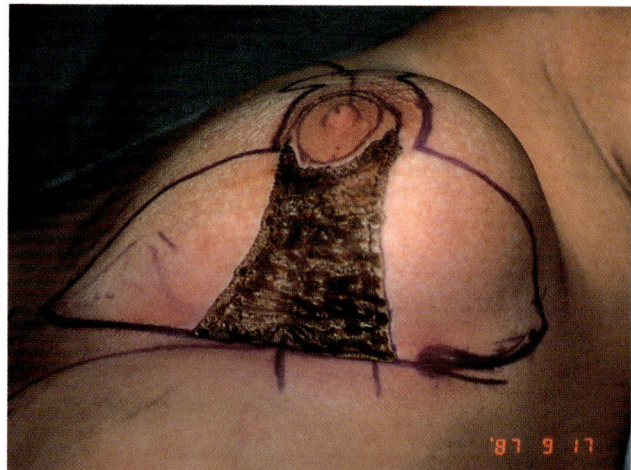

FIG. 4.73-B. After the desired markings for breast reduction have been drawn, the nipple-carrying dermal pedicle is de-epithelialized using the defocused beam of the CO_2 dioxide laser in continuous mode. The power setting is determined by the results of a spot test on adjacent skin that will be discarded, usually in the range of 20–40 watts. Remember that skin thickness varies from patient to patient.

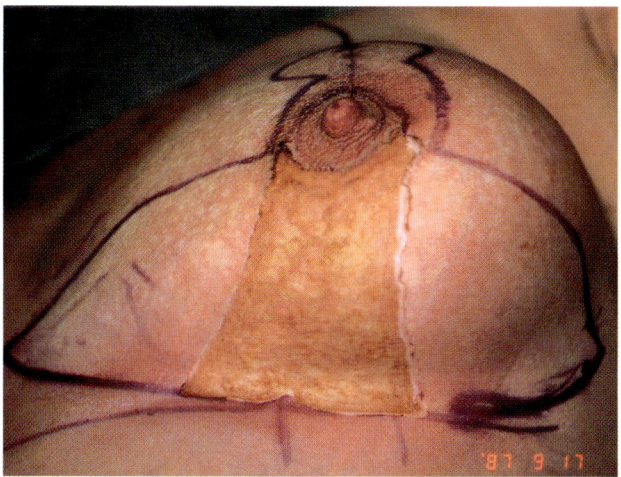

FIG. 4.73-C. The ash as seen in the previous figure has been wiped off exposing a yellow discolored dermis. This appearance assures adequate depth of de-epithelialization. The white color observed at the right hand vertical edge of the dermal pedicle implies that further vaporization must be performed to remove more epidermal elements, or the risk of retention cysts becomes increased.

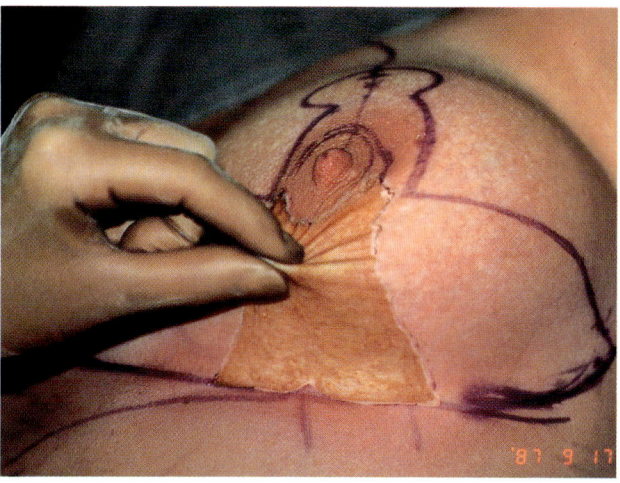

FIG. 4.73-D. The lasered area remains supple when pinched. Note that normal skin has been retained about the areola and the perimeter of the designed dermal pedicle. This is de-epithelialized with a cold steel scapel, although ultimate healing is no different with the laser early healing is delayed. This additional precaution permits early periareolar suture removal without risk of wound dehiscence.

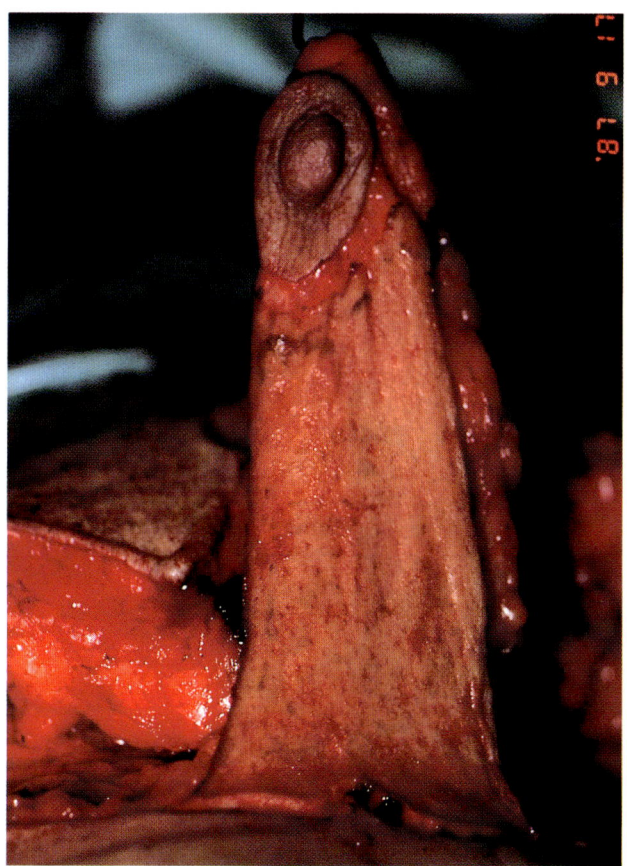

FIG. 4.73-E. The medial and lateral inferior breast quadrants have been excised in the reduction, baring the dermal pedicle that is now ready to be buried. The pink color of the nipple verifies adequacy of its vascularization.

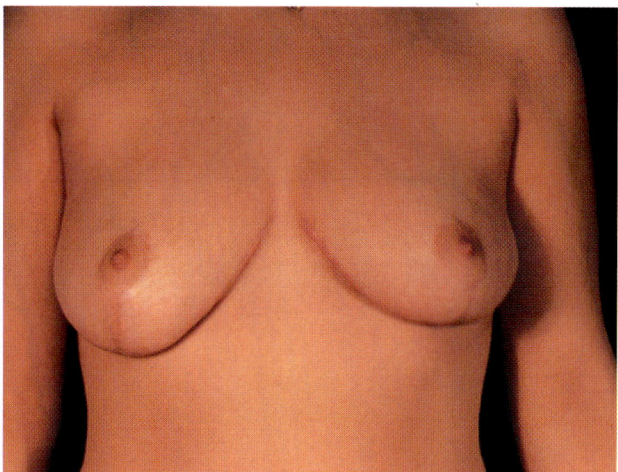

FIG. 4.73-F. Final result of breast reduction at seven months.

Case courtesy of *Geoffrey G. Hallock,* M.D.*,* and *David C. Rice.*

CASE 4.74

Dupuytren's Contracture of the Right Palm and Ring Finger

REVIEW OF CASE. This is a 68-year-old female with a Dupuytren's contracture compromising the right palm and ring finger. She was having limitation of the extension of her hand and pain on movement of the hand.

CHOICE OF LASER: CARBON DIOXIDE. The CO_2 laser was selected for precise excision of the fascial contracture with minimal trauma to the surrounding anatomical structures, particularly the nerves and vascular system. There is less post-operative pain and edema which enables the patient to begin early physiotherapy and obtain a more rapid recovery.

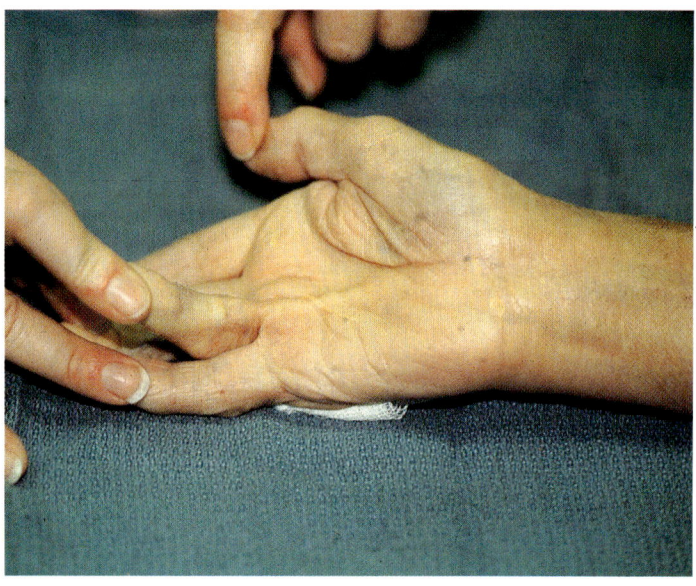
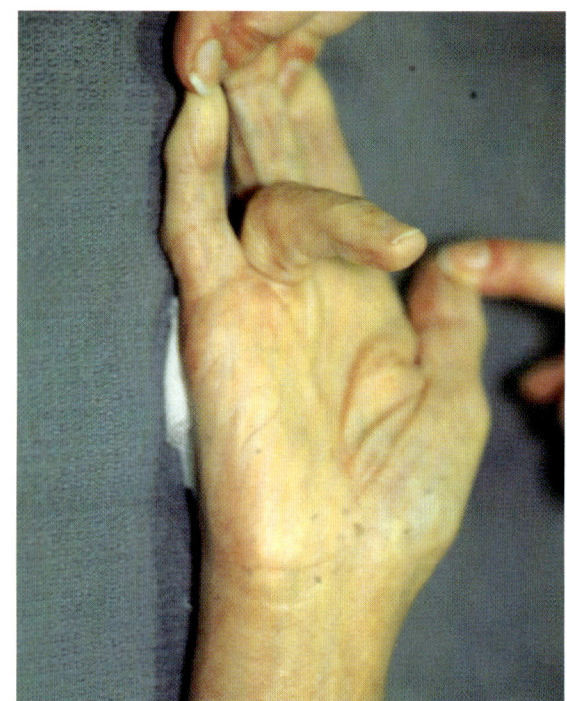

FIG. 4.74-A, B. The areas of the contracture compromising the right palm and ring finger.

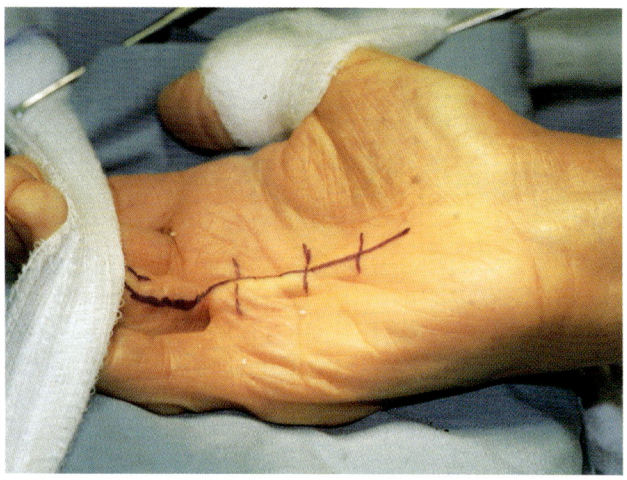

FIG. 4.74-C. Design of the skin flaps.

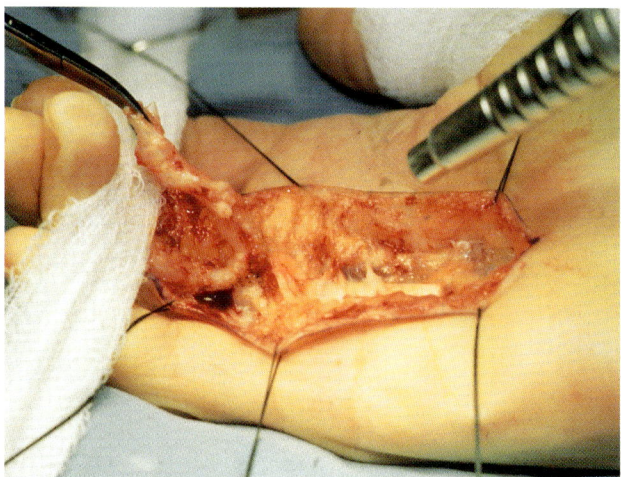

FIG. 4.74-D. The areas of the fascial contracture are excised with the CO_2 laser using a 125 mm lens at 10 watts of power in a continuous mode.

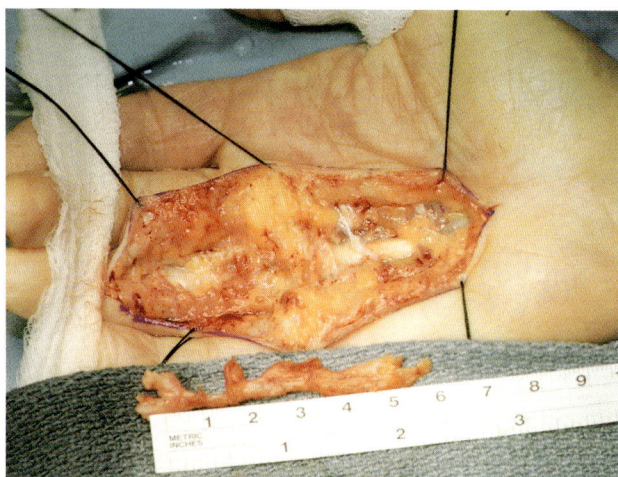

FIG. 4.74-E. Same as Fig. D.

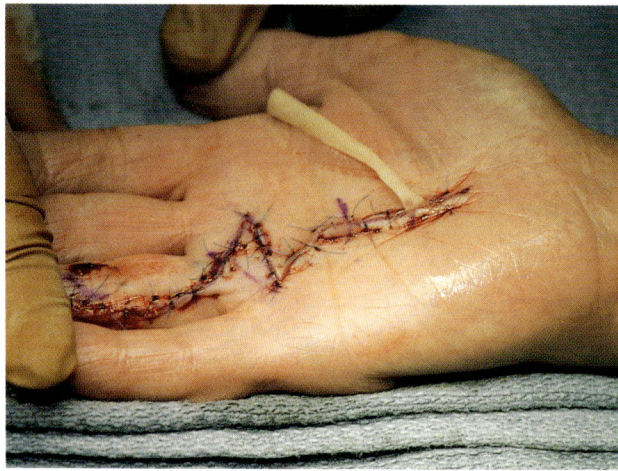

FIG. 4.74-F. Early post-operative result with minimal edema and tissue trauma.

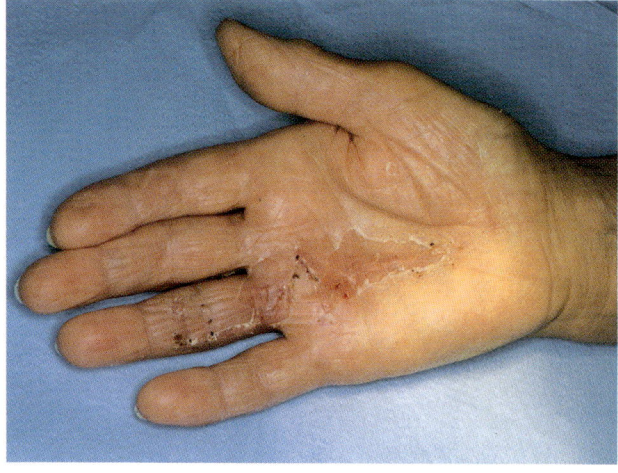

FIG. 4.74-G. Contracture fully released with complete extension present in the palm and fingers.

Case courtesy of *H. Raul Herrera*, M.D.

CASE 4.75
Fetal Surgery

REVIEW OF CASE. In utero surgery even for life-threatening developmental anomalies at this time must be classified as an experimental frontier. The role of the laser within this realm should be considered only as an investigational tool. Preliminary studies document some efficacy of the laser as a technique for incising and achieving hemostasis in these delicate tissues. Unfortunately, the minimum spot size presently available unavoidably produces a zone of tissue destruction extending into normal tissues.

CHOICE OF LASER: CARBON DIOXIDE. Modern microsurgical instruments currently utilized for gross surgery on these diminutive patients are often of equal size. Low energy CO_2 lasers may instead be used as a scalpel for precise cutting and hemostasis without requiring touching or distortion of the gelatinous fetus. Crude instrument handling on the other hand easily might result in tissue disintegration or crushing, or even expulsion of the fetus from the uterus, which invariably would result in its demise.

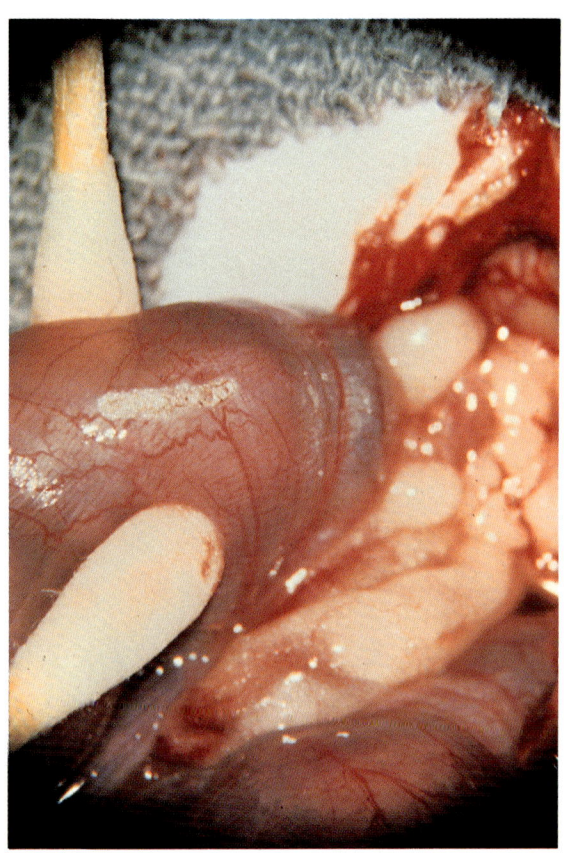

FIG. 4.75-A. Rat hysterotomy incision to permit access to the fetus is made on the antimesenteric border, midway between the applicators used here for stabilization of the uterus. The milliwatt CO_2 laser was utilized as a scalpel in continuous mode, 400 milliwatts of power, and the minimum spot size of 150 µm. (From ref. 1.)

Reprinted with permission of Alan R. Liss, Inc.
For literature pertaining to this case see Reference section.

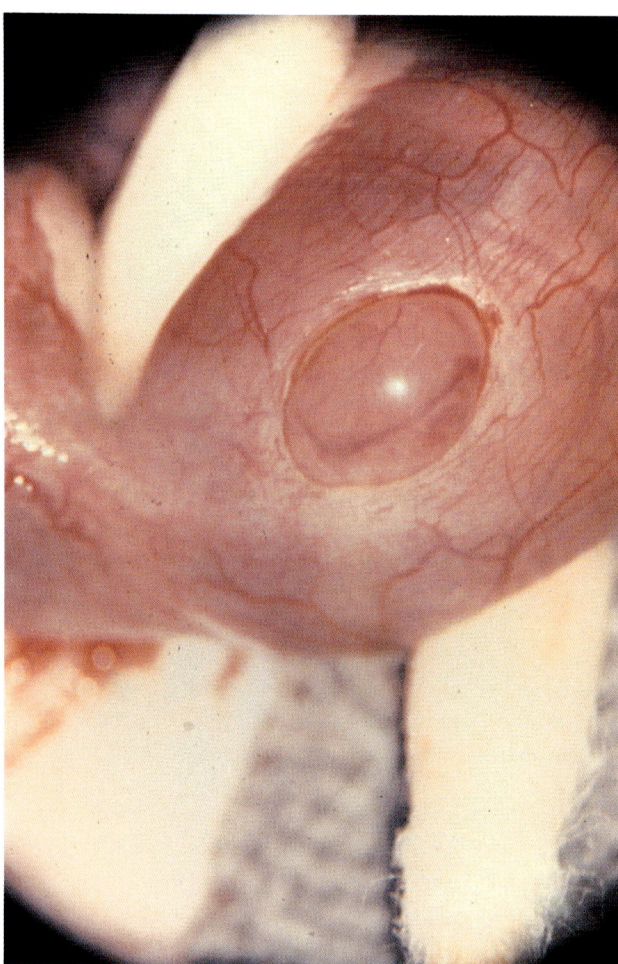

FIG. 4.75-B. The fetal head has been manipulated into the hysterotomy incision. In spite of numerous uterine wall vessels, no hemorrhage has occurred due to the hemostatic effect alone of the laser. (From ref. 1.)

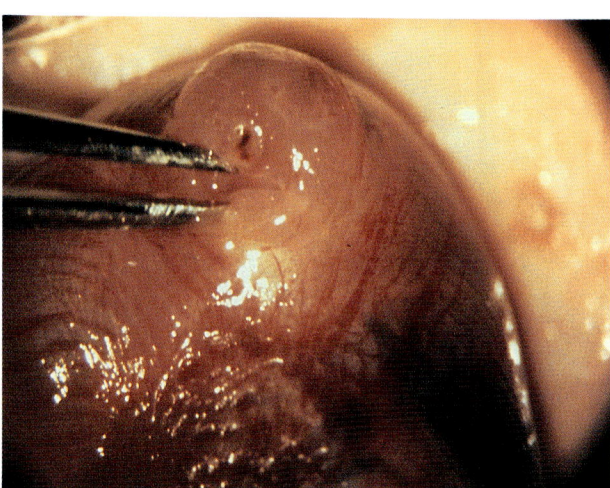

FIG. 4.75-C. The fetal snout now protrudes through the hysterotomy site, with forceps opening the mouth. A through-and-through laser incision of the upper lip has been created at the site of the char, prior to repair with microsutures. (From ref. 1.)

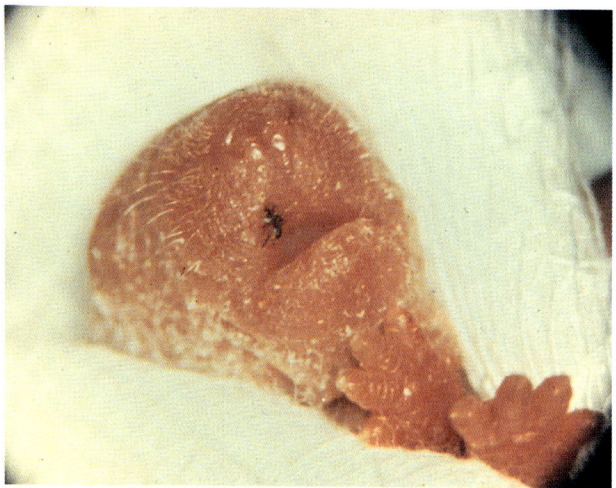

FIG. 4.75-D. Viable fetus six days after intrauterine laser lip division, three days postpartum. Sutures remain holding healed lip repair. (From ref. 1.)

Case courtesy of *Geoffrey G. Hallock,* M.D., and *David C. Rice.*

CASE 4.76

Excision of Ganglion of the Left Foot

REVIEW OF CASE. The patient is a 52-year-old female with a painful, slowly enlarging lesion of the lateral left foot. The lesion measured approximately 1.5 cm in diameter and was located over the navicular bone. The location of the lesion made it particularly difficult for the patient to wear shoes. Therefore surgical excision was warranted.

CHOICE OF LASER: CARBON DIOXIDE. The combination of the use of the CO_2 laser with regional anesthesia supplemented by local anesthesia permits the precise excision of the ganglion cyst and destruction of its point of origin. This technique not only provides for complete destruction of the lesion, but also reduces the likelihood of post-operative hematoma or late recurrence.

ADDITIONAL INFORMATION. The patient was placed in the supine position and sedated with midazolam 2 ml intravenously. Bier block anesthesia is utilized for the procedure. The operative site is prepared and draped in sterile fashion. Figure A demonstrates the location and pre-operative appearance of the lesion. The operative site is infiltrated with 0.25% bupivocaine so as to assist in the protection of the surrounding structures and to provide long-lasting post-operative analgesia. (Fig. B) A CO_2 laser is used with a 125 ml handpiece (0.2 mm spot) at 20–25 watts in continuous wave mode throughout the procedure. After the skin incision has been made, the lesion is carefully exposed (Fig. C) and dissected from the surrounding structures (Fig. D). The neck of the ganglion is exposed (Fig. E). The lesion is excised and the point of origination is then vaporized with the laser defocused to a 1 mm spot size (Fig. F) until any residual ganglion has been destroyed. The wound was closed with a continuous simple suture of 3–0 polypropylene suture material. The patient was placed in an ace bandage and instructed to keep the leg elevated for 12 to 24 hours.

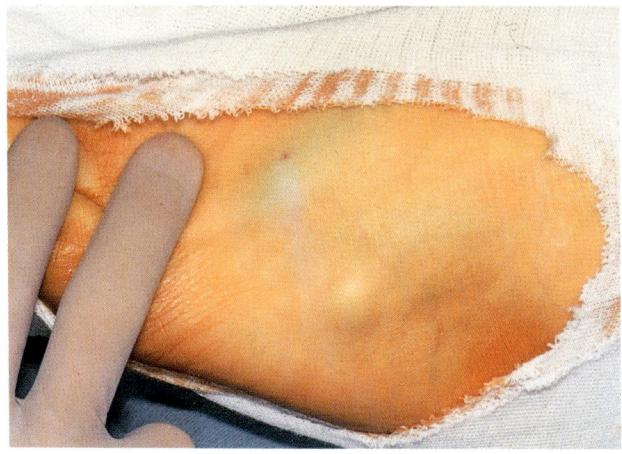

FIG. 4.76-A. Appearance of the lesion pre-operatively.

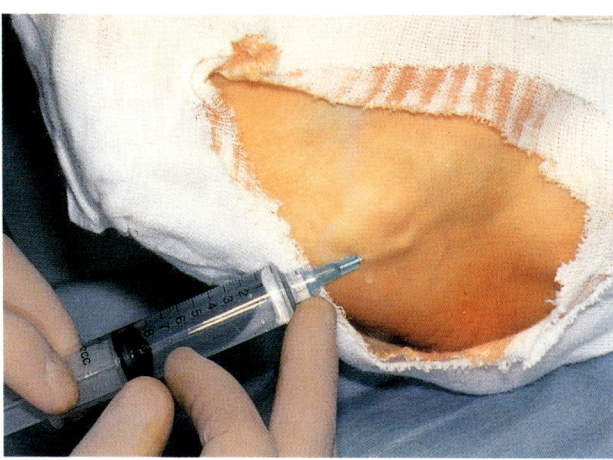

FIG. 4.76-B. The area surrounding the lesion is infiltrated with 0.25% bupivacaine following a Bier block.

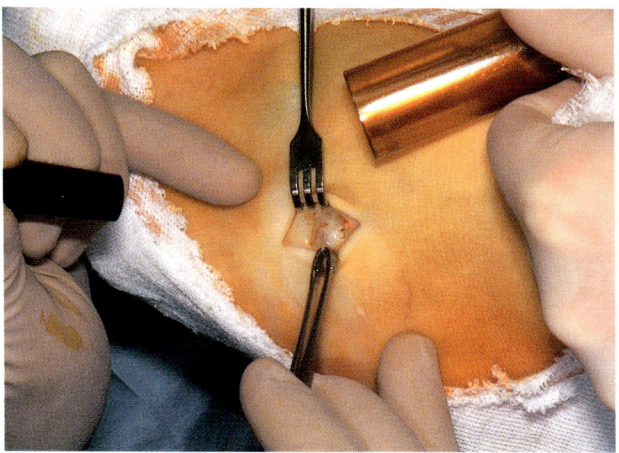

FIG. 4.76-C. The lesion is exposed and dissected from the surrounding tissues.

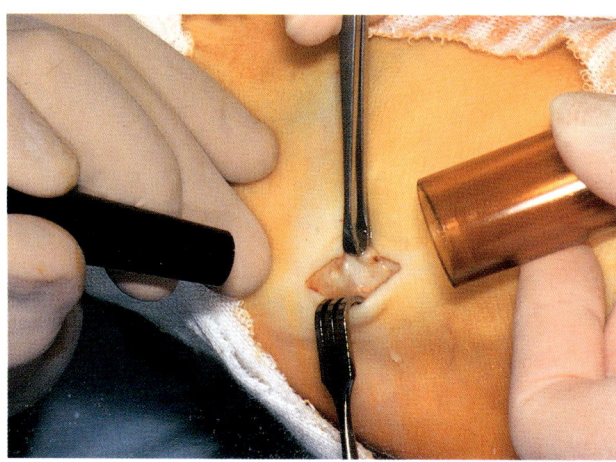

FIG. 4.76-D. The lesion is exposed and dissected from the surrounding tissues.

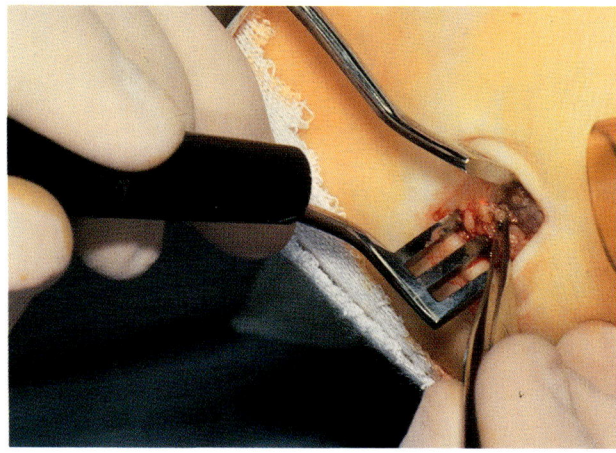

FIG. 4.76-E. The neck of the ganglion is traced to the area of the talonavicular joint.

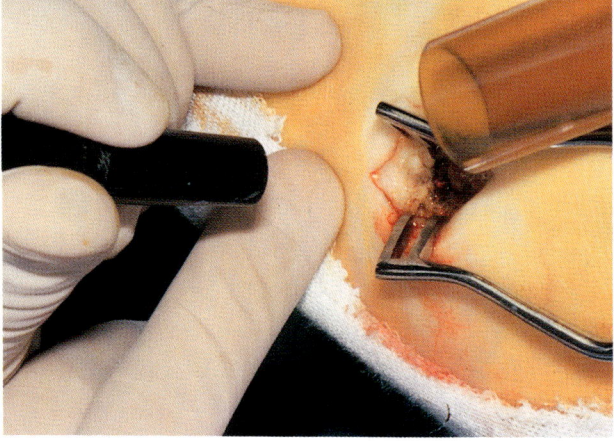

FIG. 4.76-F. The ganglion is excised and the base of the lesion (point of origin) is vaporized by defocusing the laser to a 1 mm spot size.

Case continues on following page.

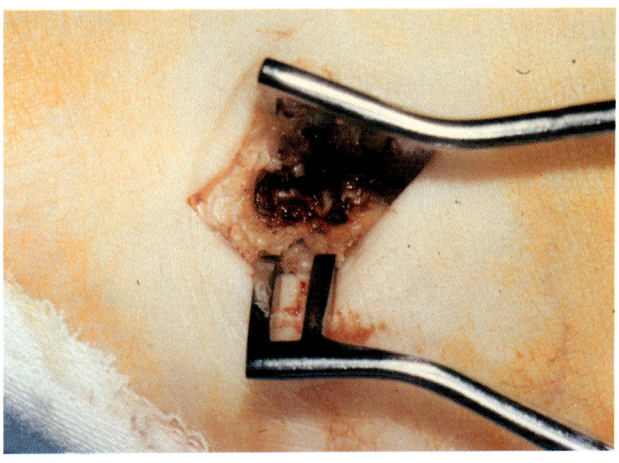

FIG. 4.76-G. The operative site following complete removal of the lesion and vaporization of the base.

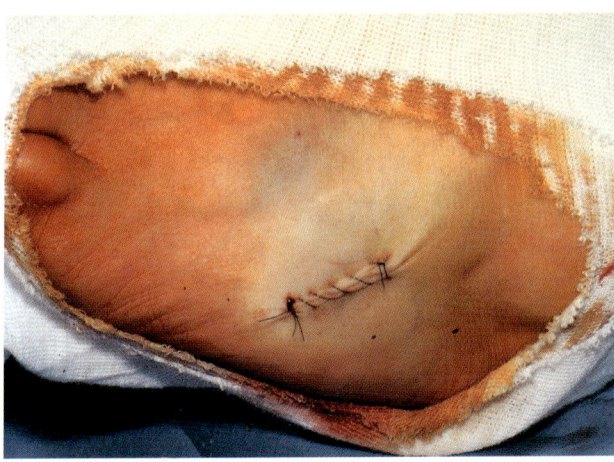

FIG. 4.76-H. The wound has been closed with continuous 3–0 polypropylene suture and the tourniquet has been released.

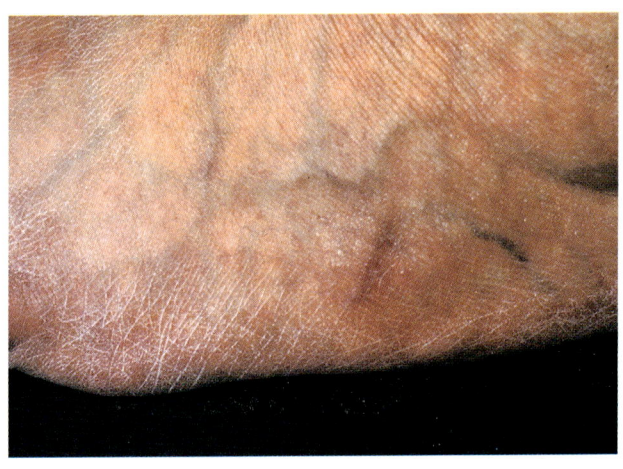

FIG. 4.76-I. The post-operative result one year.

Case courtesy of *Raymond J. Lanzafame*, M.D.

CASE 4.77
Bilateral Heel Ulcers

REVIEW OF CASE. This patient is a 72-year-old nursing home patient, nearly bedridden with bilateral heel ulcers. The patient was admitted to the hospital for debridement of ulcers and ulcer management.

CHOICE OF LASER: CARBON DIOXIDE. The CO_2 laser was chosen to allow surface debridement without damage to deeper layers and to sterilize the wound prior to application of dressings.

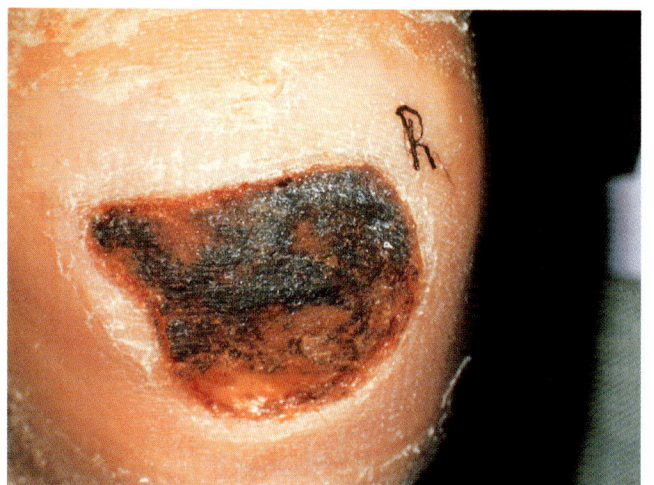 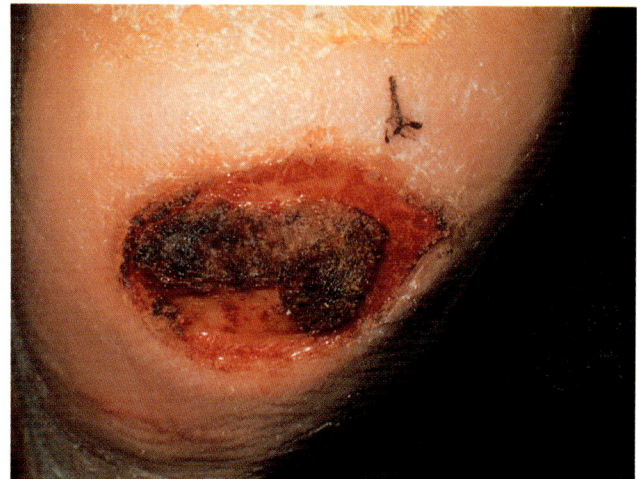

FIGS. 4.77-A, B. Heel ulcers after initial CO_2 laser debridement at 10 watts superpulse. Ulcers were then cureted of debrided tissue, rubbed with hydrogen peroxide, dried, and a hydrocolloid dressing applied.

Case continues on following page.

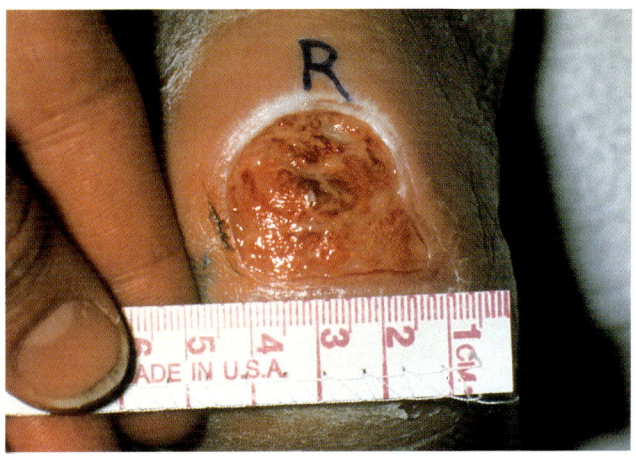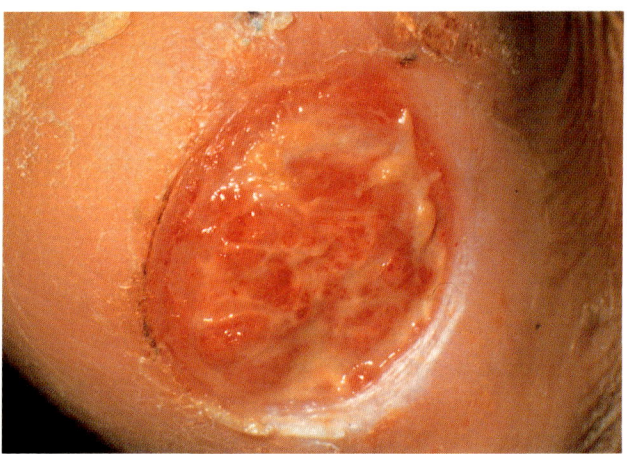

FIGS. 4.77-C, D. One week post-operation. Both ulcers appear clean, but the left ulcer is relased at biweekly intervals until a scab develops, while the right ulcer is not. Both ulcers continue to have hydrocolloid dressings applied.

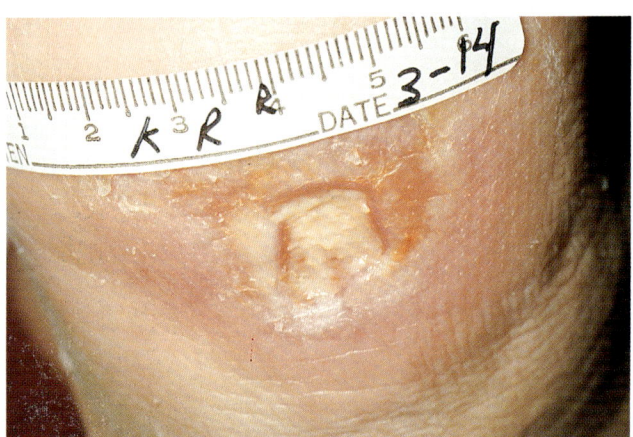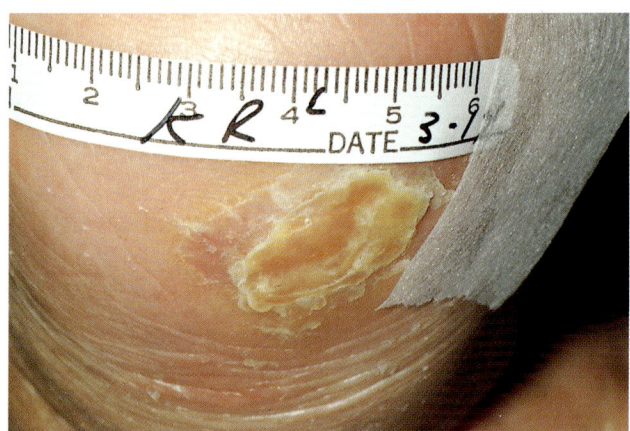

FIGS. 4.77-E, F. The same therapy is continued on the ulcers, which are now two months old. Lasing with the CO_2 laser at 5 watts superpulse was stopped on the left ulcer about one week previously.

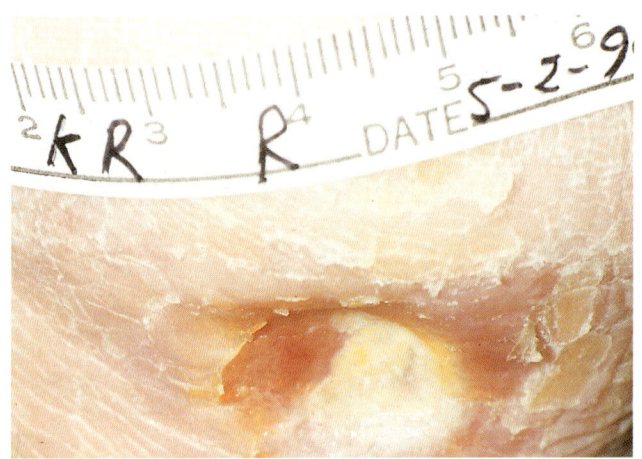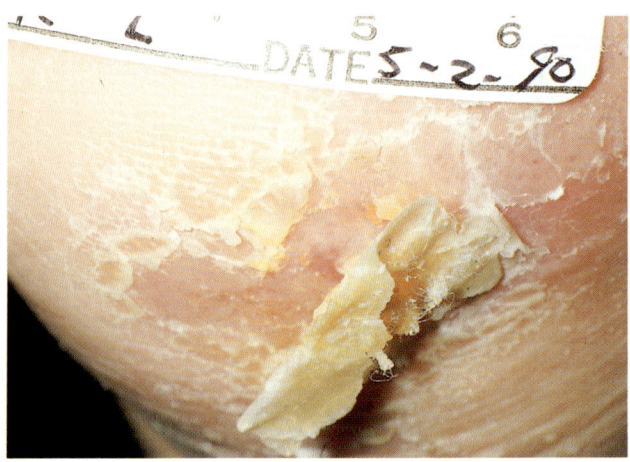

FIGS. 4.77-G, H. Both heel ulcers at four months post-operation, with patient treated as an outpatient except for initial three day admission. The right heel, which received only one early laser application is still not healed. The left heel ulcer is treated with the CO_2 laser until scab formation occurs.

Case courtesy of *Leonard S. Schultz, M.D.*

CASE 4.78

Right Foot Ischemic Ulcer

Secondary to Occlusive Peripheral Vascular Disease

REVIEW OF CASE. This 63-year-old white male presented with severe distal right leg ischemia without run-off amenable to bypass and a nonhealing lateral foot ulcer.

CHOICE OF LASER: CARBON DIOXIDE. For precise control of vaporization and superficial tissue and for sterilization of the ulcer bed.

ADDITIONAL INFORMATION. These lesions need to be dealt with aggressively, with complete debridement being the key to success. CO_2 lasing of the bone at 30 watts or less does not cause necrosis. Any carbonization on the bone will disappear within a few days as new tissue is formed.

POST-TREATMENT CARE. Specific wound care involves soap and water, half-strength hydrogen peroxide, antibiotic ointment, and roller gauze. An alternative would be soap and water, half-strength hydrogen peroxide, and a hydrocolloid dressing if no allergy is present.

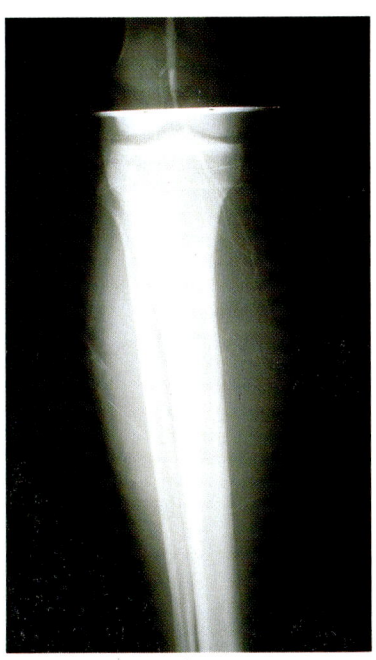

FIG. 4.78-A. Arteriogram showing only collateral vessel run-off distal to the knee.

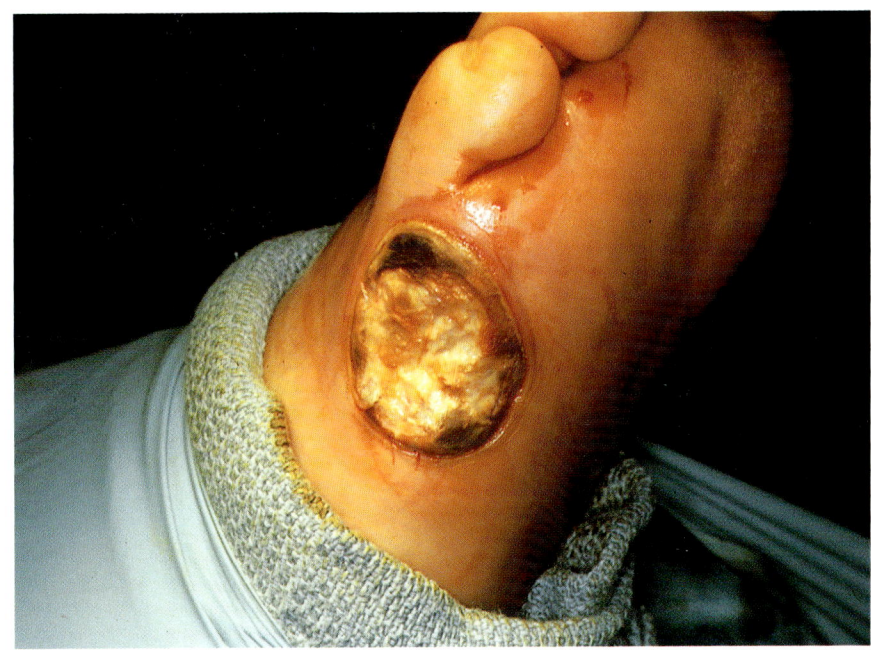

FIG. 4.78-B. Nonhealing right lateral foot ulcer.

Case continues on following page.

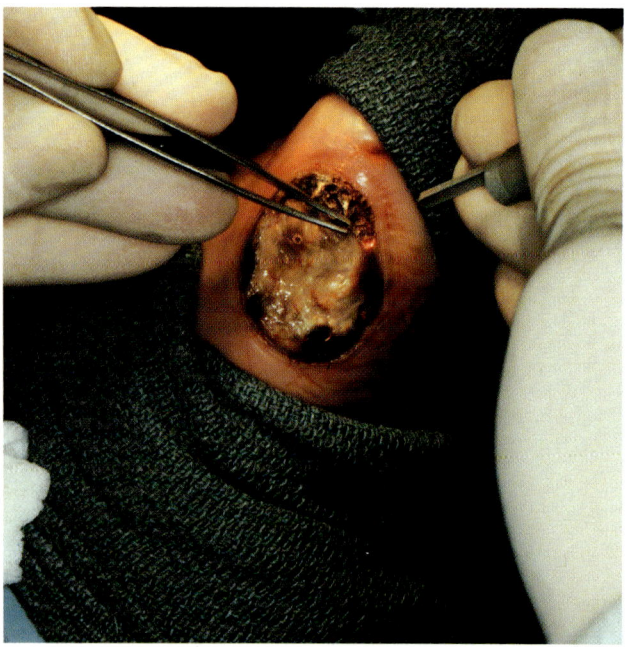

FIG. 4.78-C. Debridement with the CO_2 laser at 30 watts continuous mode after ankle block anesthesia.

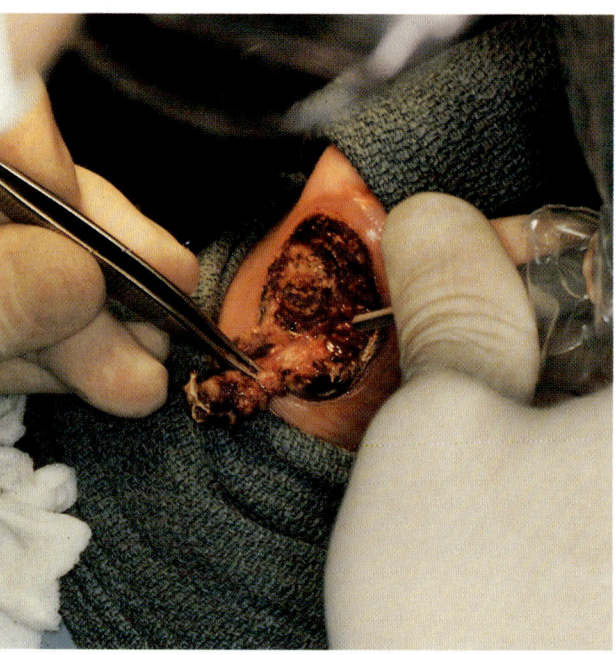

FIG. 4.78-D. Lasing continues down to the bone, including debridement of any tissue on the bone. Wattage is kept at 30 watts or less.

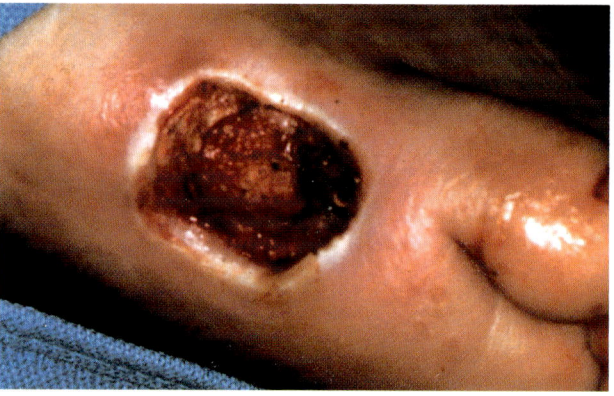

FIG. 4.78-E. Healing of the ulcer at two months.

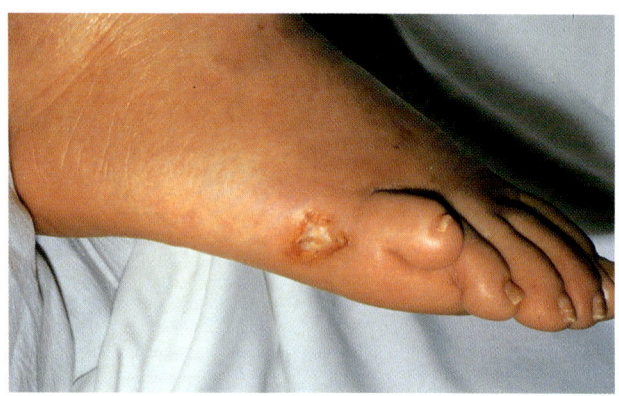

FIG. 4.78-F. Healing of the ulcer at four months.

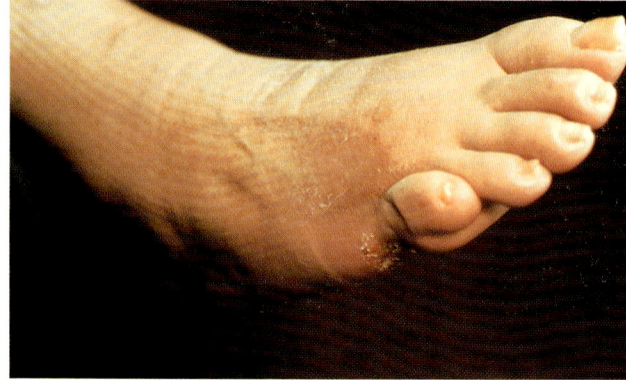

FIG. 4.78-G. Healing of the ulcer at five months.

Case courtesy of *Leonard S. Schultz*, M.D., and *John Graber*, M.D.

CASE 4.79
Laserbrasion of Acne Scars of the Face

REVIEW OF CASE. This 34-year-old female desired improvement of irregular facial skin contour resulting from acne scarring. She had relatively severe pustular acne as a teenager which left an irregular skin surface with numerous deeper areas. There had been no active acne or pustules for 5 years.

CHOICE OF LASER: CARBON DIOXIDE. The CO_2 laser light is absorbed preferentially by water. The skin contains 70% to 90% water and will absorb CO_2 laser light and convert it to heat, which has the ability to vaporize superficial skin layers. By defocusing the laser and rapidly passing it over the skin, external layers can be removed in a very selective fashion. Wound healing is usually prompt and pain and swelling are minimal. The power utilized is 10 to 15 watts of continuous power in a defocused mode.

ADDITIONAL INFORMATION. The laser is used with 10 to 15 watts of power. The defocused beam is passed back and forth across the area in a rapid "paint brush" manner producing a char. Each successive charred layer is then wiped with a saline/antibiotic solution revealing the deeper layers. Magnifying loupes of $\times 2.5$ allow for selective removal of "high points" while leaving deep areas untouched, thus achieving a uniform skin level.

POST-TREATMENT CARE. Copious irrigation with saline/antibiotic solution completes the procedure. Iced saline compresses and topical antibiotics or aloe vera gel are used for open treatment. Alternatively, artificial skin substitutes (Vigillon, Duoderm, Op-site, or pig skin) may be used.

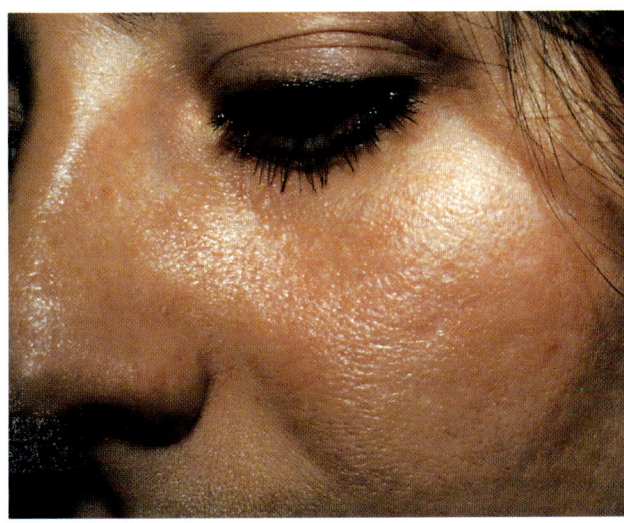

FIG. 4.79-A. Acne scars and irregular skin of the left cheek prior to the procedure.

Case continues on following page.

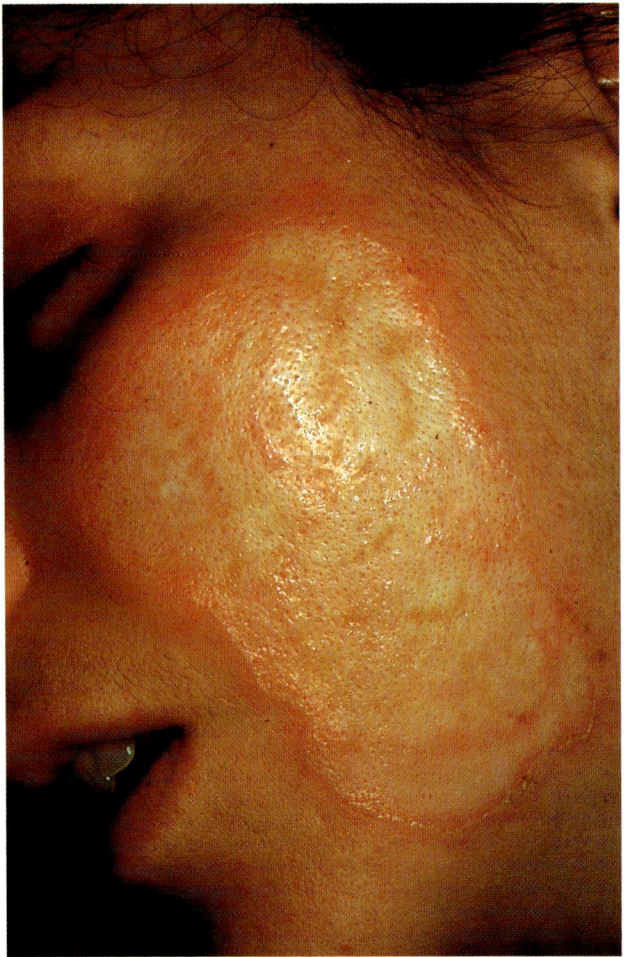

FIG. 4.79-B. Appearance immediately after laserbrasion demonstrating relatively bloodless removal of superficial skin layers.

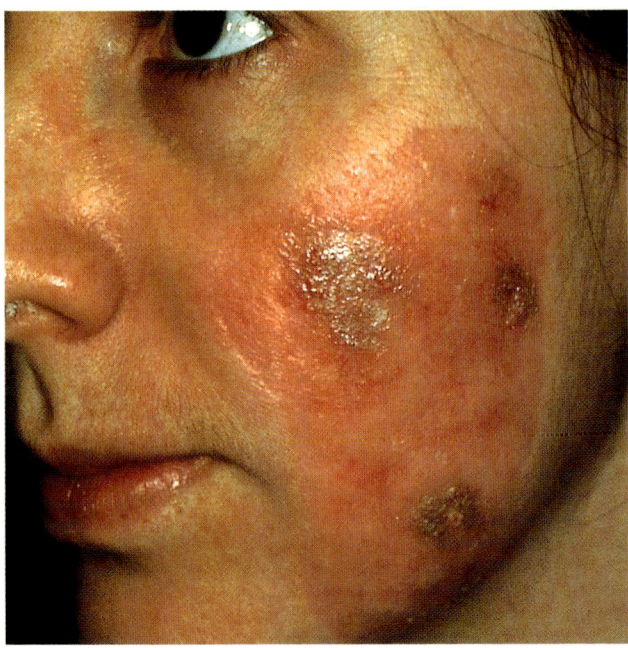

FIG. 4.79-C. Eschar of face separating at six days.

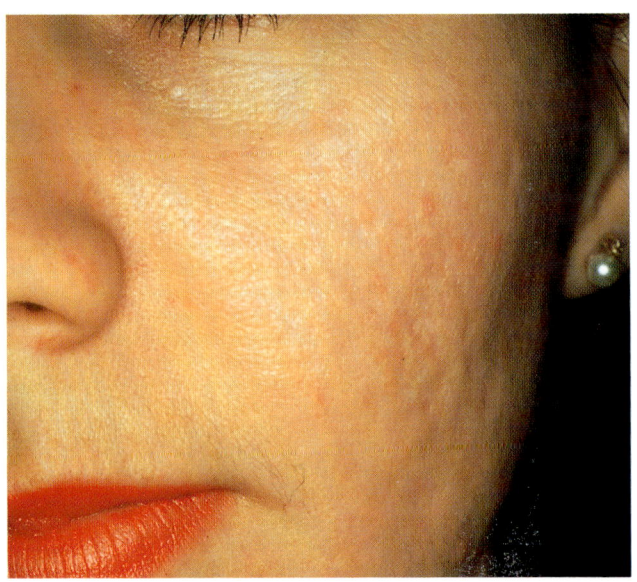

FIG. 4.79-D. Improvement eight weeks following treatment.

Case courtesy of *David B. Apfelberg*, M.D.

CASE 4.80

Lipoma Excision of the Anterior Chest

REVIEW OF CASE. This patient is a 43-year-old Hispanic female with a slowly, enlarging lesion of the right anterior chest in the area of the deltopectoral groove. The lesion was nontender and did not vary with the menstrual cycle. The lesion was not noted on mammography. The lesion was occasionally tender and was irritated by the patient's bra. Therefore the patient wished to have the lesion excised.

CHOICE OF LASER: CARBON DIOXIDE. The CO_2 laser is particularly useful in the excision of subcutaneous lesions such as lipomas. The laser enables the precise delineation of the extent of the lesion due to the excellent hemostasis and it's ability to dissect in the areolar plane. This is particularly useful in the excision of lipomatous lesions involving the back which may be poorly encapsulated and multilobulated.

ADDITIONAL INFORMATION. The skin incision was planned along the skin crease of the deltopectoral groove (Fig. A). The area was infiltrated with 0.25% Bupivacaine with epinephrine. The skin incision was made using a CO_2 laser with a 125 mm handpiece in focus (0.2 mm spot) (Fig. B). The skin incision was made at 25 watts using a continuous wave. The remainder of the dissection was completed at 25–40 watts continuously. The subcutaneous tissue was incised (Fig. C). The lobulated well-encapsulated lesion was dissected free from the surrounding tissue (Figs. D and E). Figure F shows the excised lesion and the surgical site immediately prior to closure. The wound was closed by approximating the subcutaneous tissue with interrupted undyed 3-0 polyglycolic acid suture and the skin was closed with a subcuticular suture of 4-0 polypropylene (Fig. G). The post-operative result is depicted in Fig. H.

Case continues on following page.

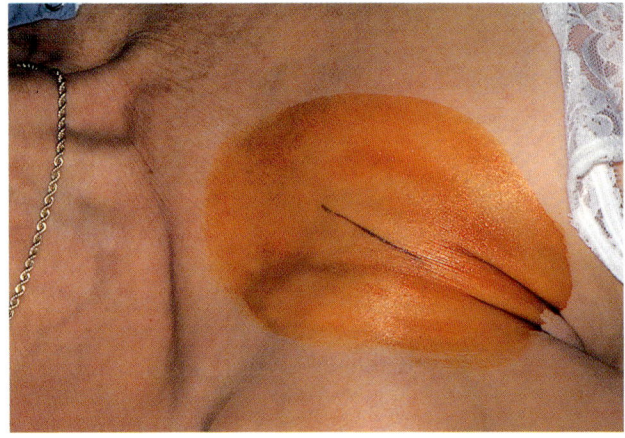

FIG. 4.80-A. Position of proposed skin incision for lesion of right deltopectoral groove.

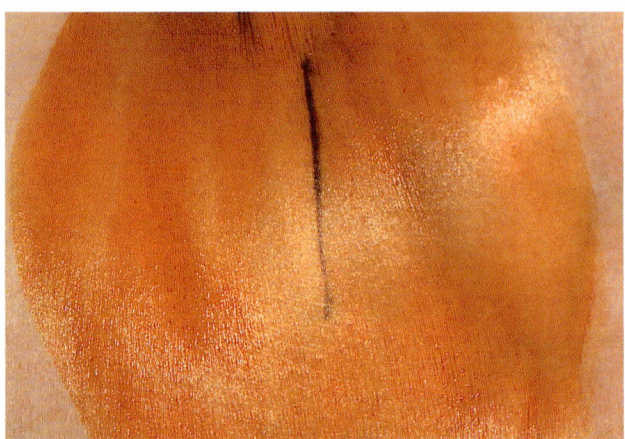

FIG. 4.80-B. Close-up view of operative site.

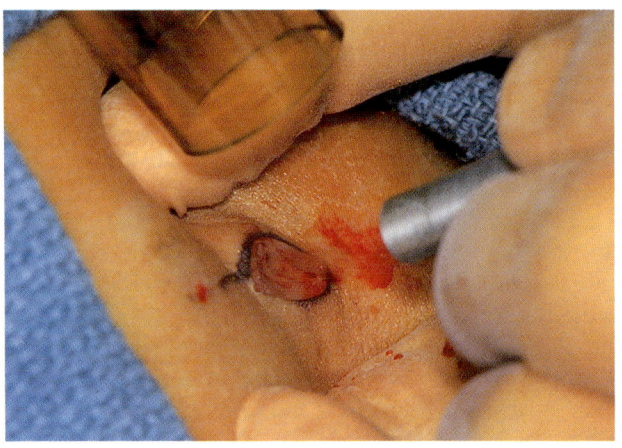

FIG. 4.80-C. Skin incision is made after infiltration with local anesthetic. The tissue is held under tension during the incision.

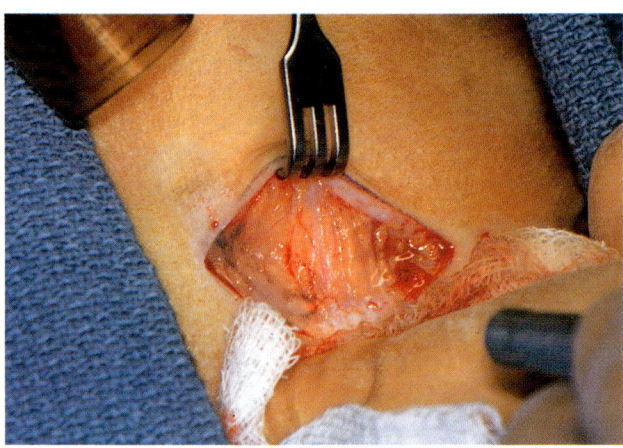

FIG. 4.80-D. The subcutaneous tissue is incised in order to expose the lesion.

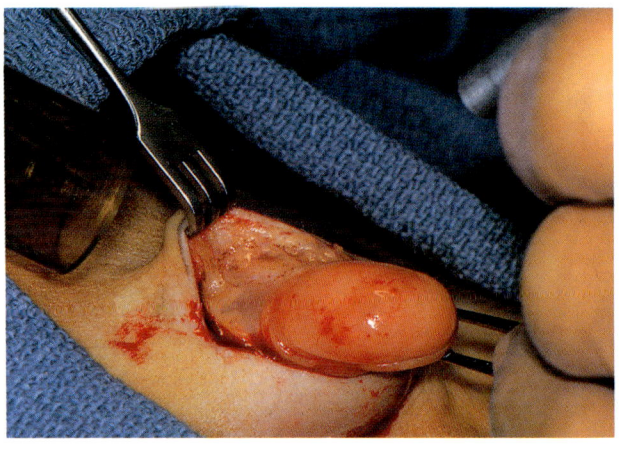

FIG. 4.80-E. The lesion is carefully dissected from the surrounding tissue.

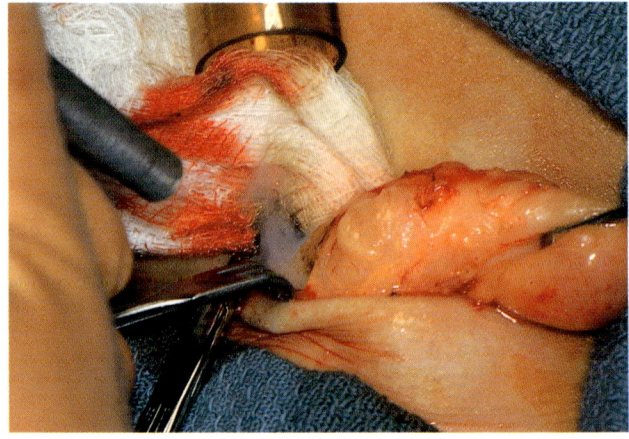

FIG. 4.80-F. Same as Fig. E.

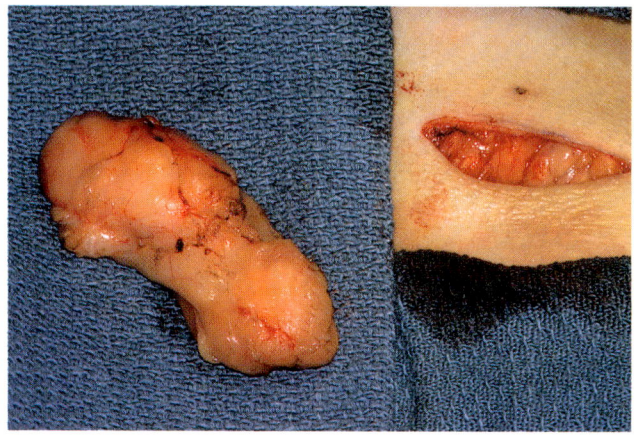

FIG. 4.80-G. Excised specimen and surgical wound.

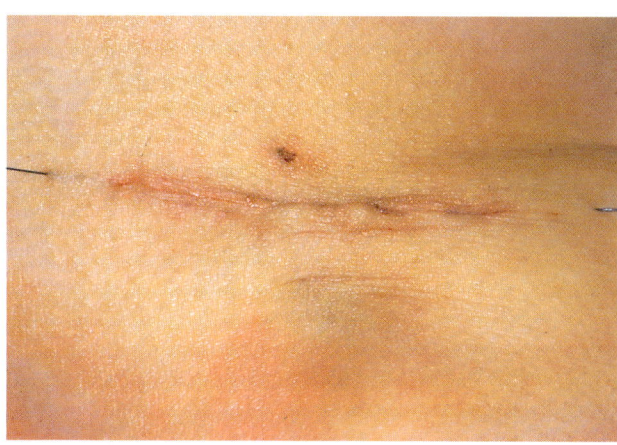

FIG. 4.80-H. The surgical wound after subcuticular closure.

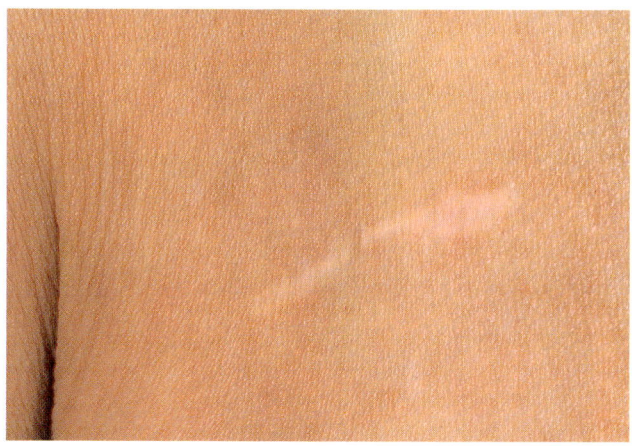

FIG. 4.80-I. Late post-operative result.

Case courtesy of *Raymond J. Lanzafame*, M.D.

CASE 4.81

Metastatic Squamous Cell Carcinoma of the Scalp

REVIEW OF CASE. This 69-year-old male presented with a history of a progressive growth of the mass of his scalp. He has a history of squamous cell carcinoma. He was complaining of pain and bleeding from the area.

CHOICE OF LASER: CARBON DIOXIDE. The CO_2 laser was chosen for the precise excision of the lesion with free margins. The lesion was excised deep through the bone to the dura. There was less bleeding and a lower incidence of recurrence. This provided adequate preparation of the area for a rotation flap closure and skin graft.

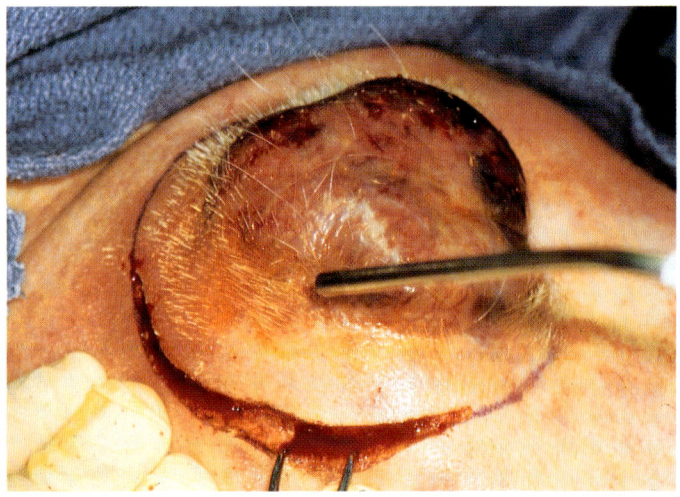

FIG. 4.81-A. Pre-operative scalp lesion.

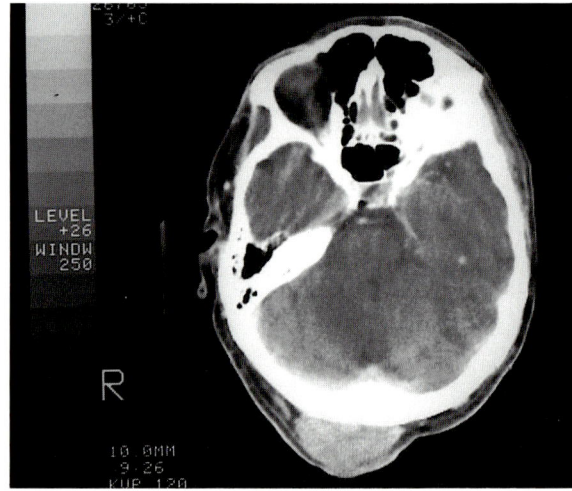

FIG. 4.81-B. CT Scan showing bony involvement of the mass.

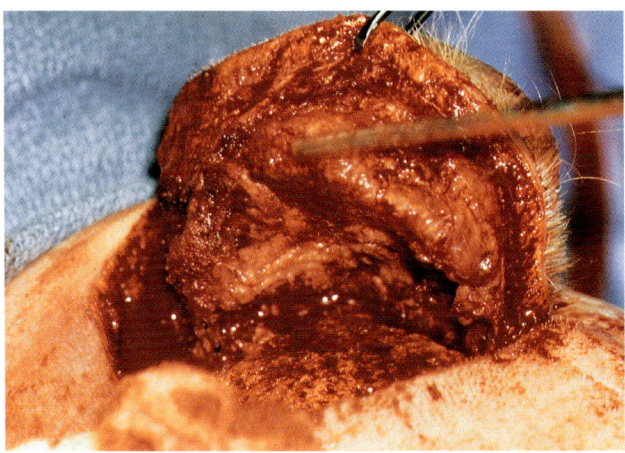 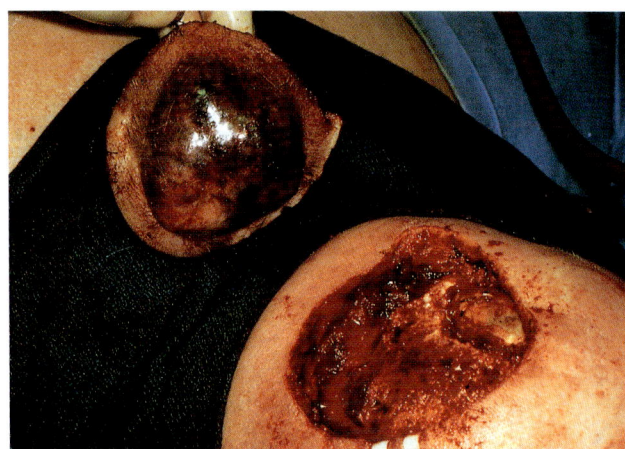

FIGS. 4.81-C, D. The tumor was precisely excised with the CO_2 laser with a 125 mm lens at 30 watts of continuous power. The excision was done through the bone to the dura. The margins were free of tumor.

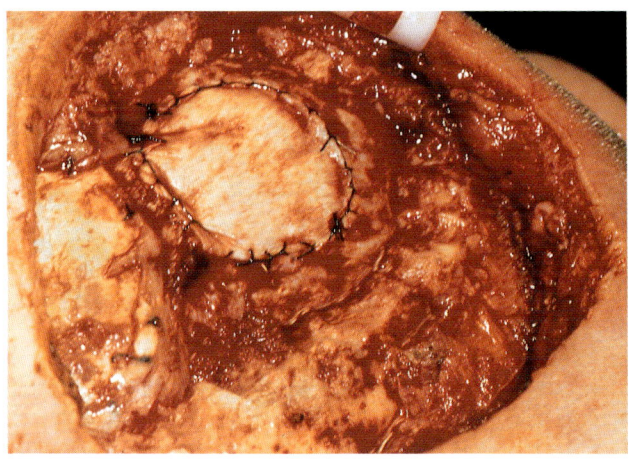

FIG. 4.81-E. The area was flushed with the CO_2 laser in a defocus position to reduce the bacterial count of the surgical bed in preparation of the reconstruction.

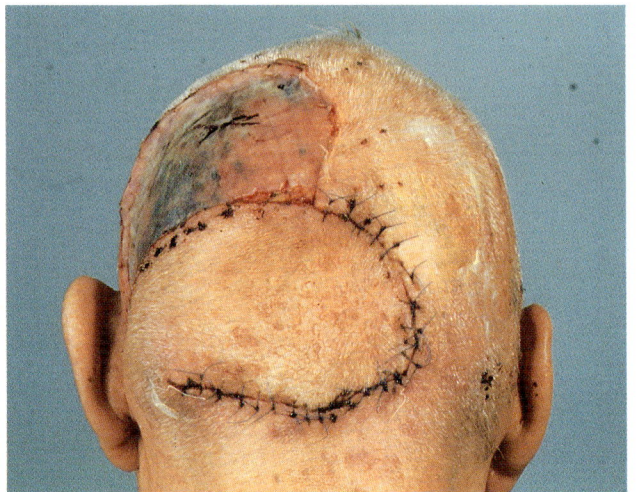 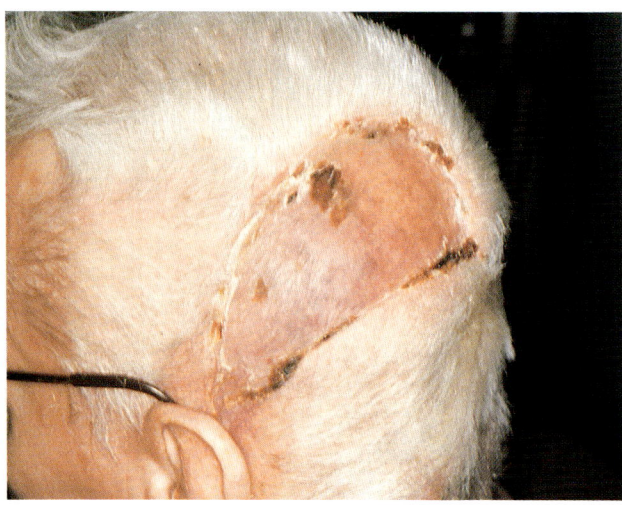

FIG. 4.81-F. Early post-operative wound.

FIG. 4.81-G. Late post-operative wound showing a well-established graft and flap with no recurrence.

Case courtesy of *H. Raul Herrera*, M.D.

CASE 4.82
Xanthelasma Palpebrarum

REVIEW OF CASE. This 45-year-old female presented with a long history of the development of yellowish flat plaques in the upper and lower eyelids. She had a positive family history of similar lesions. Serum cholesterol and lipid values were normal. Previous treatment had been unsuccessful.

CHOICE OF LASER: CARBON DIOXIDE. The CO_2 laser is hand-held perpendicular to the skin. Six to ten watts of defocused power is used to photovaporize the skin and underlying pigment. The laser is used in the superpulse capability which aids in the rapid vaporization and mechanical disruption of pigment but limits thermal injury thus diminishing chances for subsequent scarring. Multiple passes (4–6) of the laser in a "point brush" technique are required to remove all the pigment. Often exposed is the underlying dermis or occasionally the fascia overlying the orbicularis muscle. Gentle currettage with a small skin curette or cotton applicator removes charred pigment between laser passes.

ADDITIONAL INFORMATION. Adjacent areas must be draped with moist gauze for protection from stray beams. A protective scleral lens or corneal shield must be used to protect the eye. The operator and all personnel in the room must wear appropriate eye protection and masks, and adequate smoke evacuation is used to collect the laser plume.

POST-TREATMENT CARE. The laser wound is left exposed without bandages. Ice compresses, ophthalmic ointment, elevation, and rest for 2 to 4 days are recommended for proper healing. Full epithelization occurs in 7 to 10 days and red discoloration blends in 6 to 12 weeks. No ectropion at recurrence has been observed.

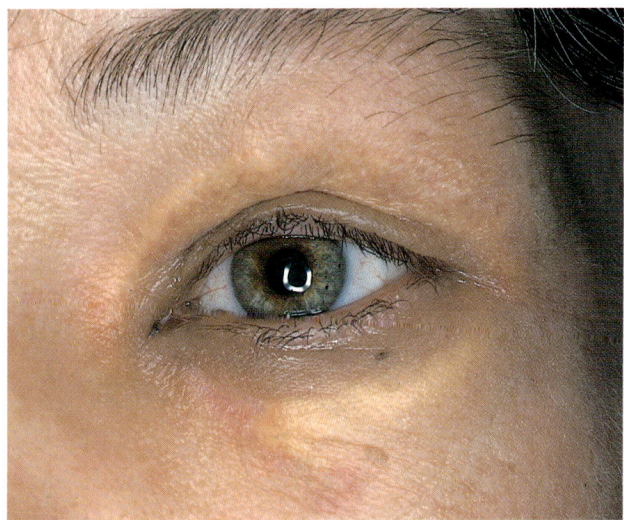

FIG. 4.82-A. Diffuse yellow xanthelasma pigment of entire left lower eyelid.

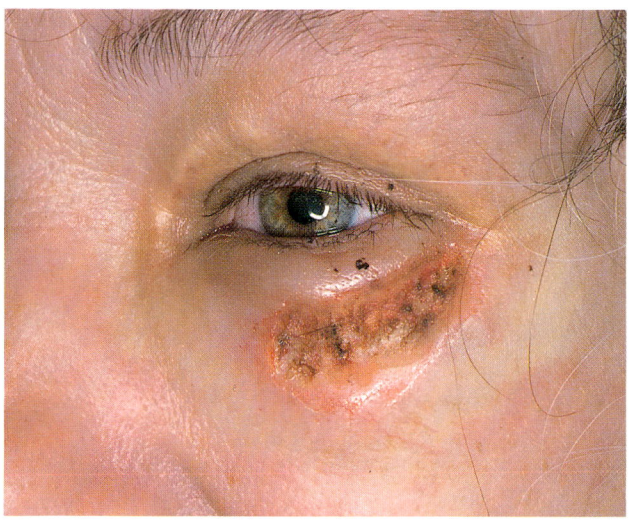

FIG. 4.82-B. Post-laser treatment appearance of wound 5 days following pigment vaporization.

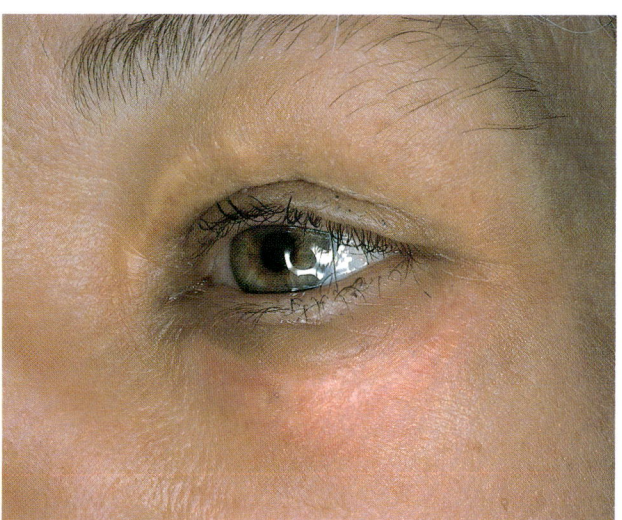

FIG. 4.82-C. Total re-epithelization and healing of eyelid without scar or ectropion 3 weeks after laser treatment.

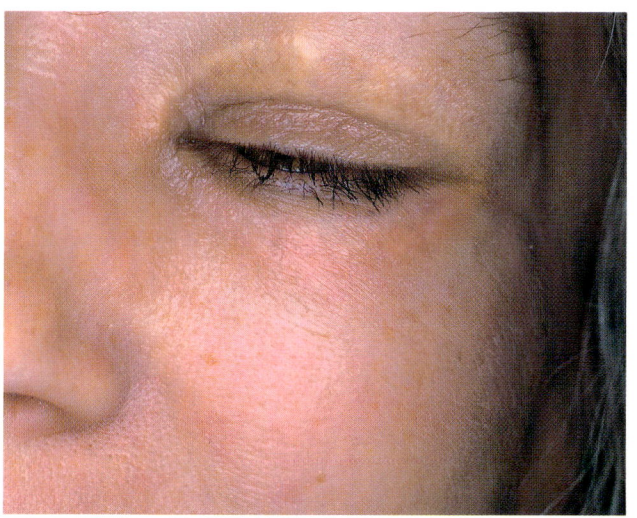

FIG. 4.82-D. Further blending and fading of treatment area 7 weeks after laser treatment.

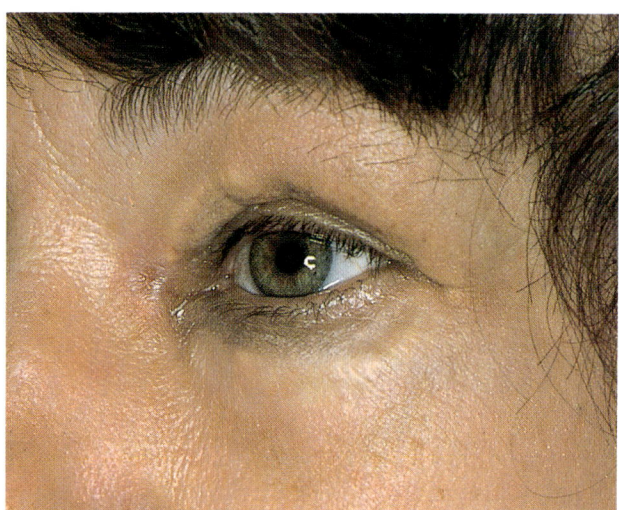

FIG. 4.82-E. Final appearance of eyelid 8 months following treatment. Skin has nearly normal color and texture without recurrence of xanthelasma.

For literature pertaining to this case see Reference section.

Case courtesy of *David B. Apfelberg*, M.D.

CASE 4.83
Mucous Cyst of the DIP Joint of the Right Middle Finger

REVIEW OF CASE. This is a 63-year-old male with a soft clear mass at the level of the DIP joint of the right middle finger. He was complaining of pain on motion of the joint.

CHOICE OF LASER: CARBON DIOXIDE. The CO_2 laser was selected to excise the cyst and vaporize the bony spur from the DIP joint with precision and minimal trauma. There is less postoperative pain and edema to facilitate more rapid use of the joint.

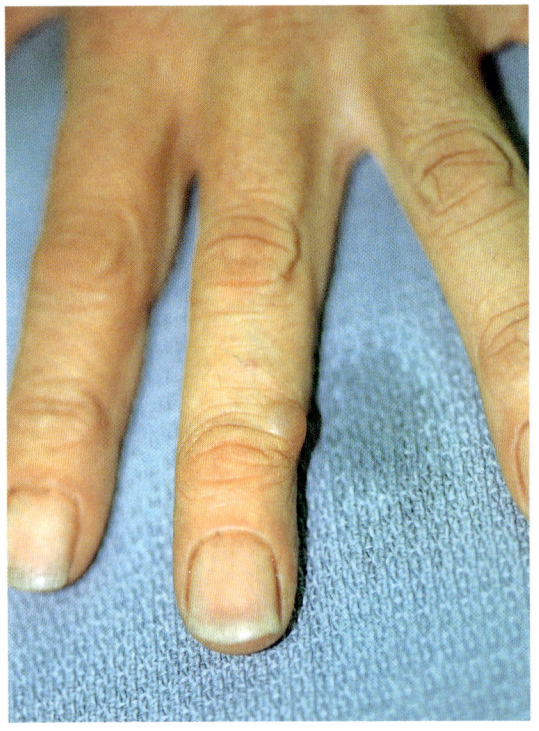

FIG. 4.83-A. Lesion of the DIP joint of the right middle finger.

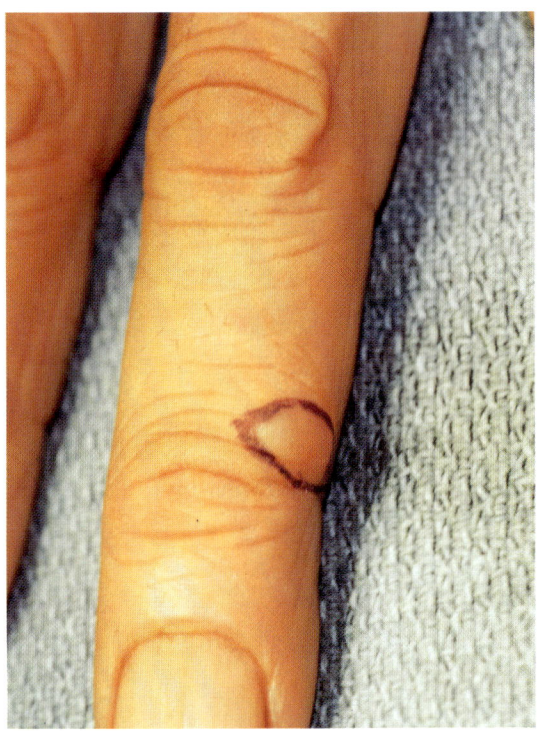

FIG. 4.83-B. Outline for the excision.

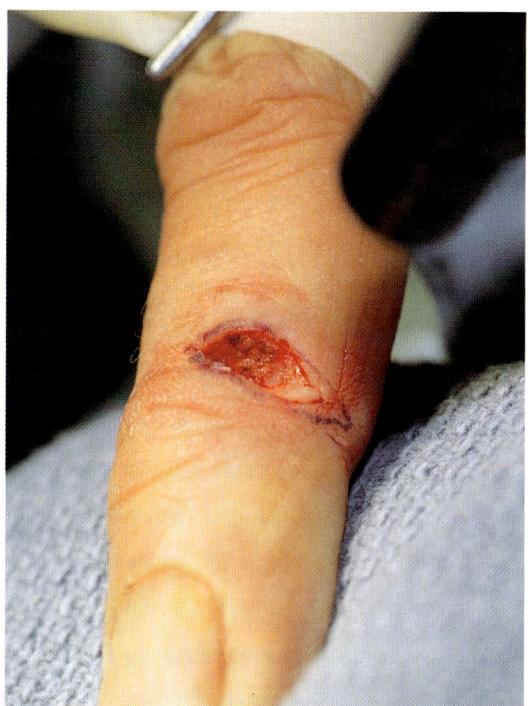

FIG. 4.83-C. Excision of the mucous cyst and vaporization of the osteophyte of the DIP joint with the CO_2 laser using a 125 mm lens at 10 watts of power in a continuous mode.

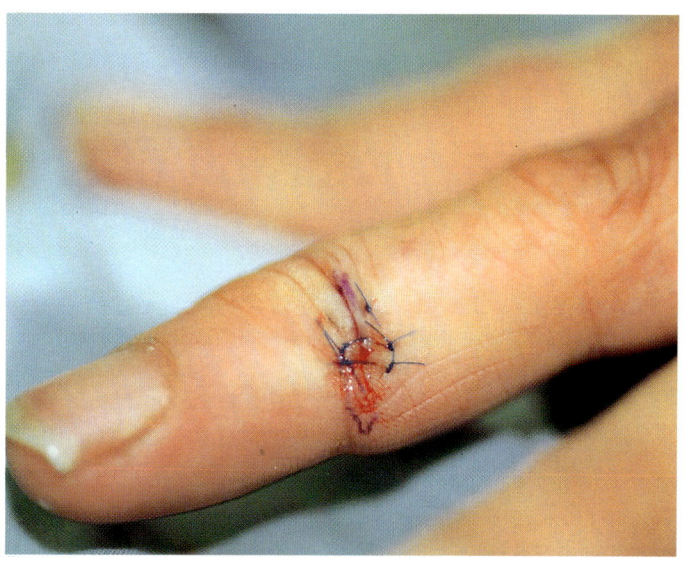

FIG. 4.83-D. Wound closure.

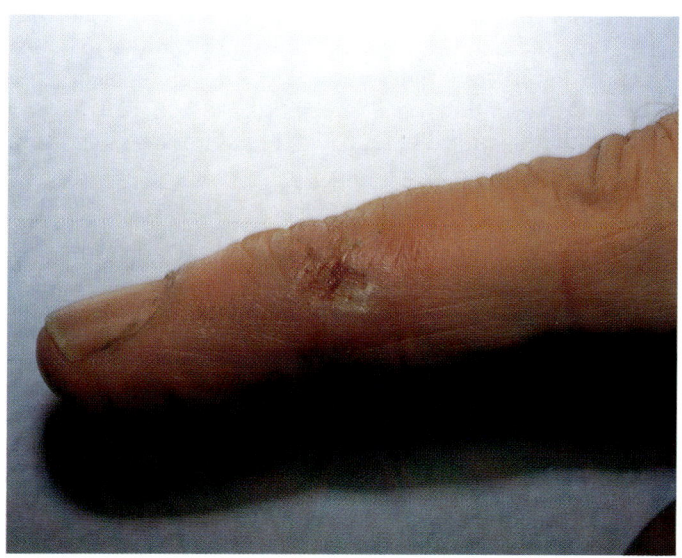

FIG. 4.83-E. Early post-operation with no evidence of recurrence and good motion without pain.

Case courtesy of *H. Raul Herrera*, M.D.

CASE 4.84
Excision of Sebaceous Cyst

REVIEW OF CASE. This is a 46-year-old male with multiple sebaceous cysts of the trunk. The lesion of greatest concern to the patient is located along the flank and is irritated by sitting and normal activity. In addition, the lesion has been inflamed three times previously requiring local therapy and antibiotic treatment. Examination demonstrates a 1.5 cm lesion of the right flank along the posterior axillary line at the level of T12. Chronic scarring from previous inflammation is obvious.

CHOICE OF LASER: CARBON DIOXIDE. The CO_2 laser facilitates excision of sebaceous cysts particularly in cases of prior inflammation and/or cyst rupture. The laser enables the cyst to be dissected with ease despite previous inflammation and scarification of the surgical site. The laser has the additional advantage of permitting the sterilization of the wound thereby reducing the possibility of post-operative complications.

ADDITIONAL INFORMATION. The area is prepared and draped in sterile fashion. The surgical site is infiltrated with a mixture of 1% Xylocaine with epinephrine and 0.5% Bupivacaine with epinephrine. The CO_2 laser is used with a 125 mm handpiece (0.2 mm spot size). The laser is set at 35 watts continuous mode. An ellipse of skin incorporating the obvious scar tissue is excised (Fig. A). The cyst is dissected free from the surrounding tissues (Figs. B and C). Hemostasis is secured and the base of the wound can be treated with defocused laser energy (5 mm spot size) to "sterilize" the wound site. Closure is accomplished with interrupted 3–0 polyglycolic acid sutures in the subcutaneous tissue (Fig. D). A subcuticular suture of 4-0 polypropylene is used as is shown in Fig. E and a Tegaderm dressing is applied (Fig. F). Post-operative result is shown in Fig. G.

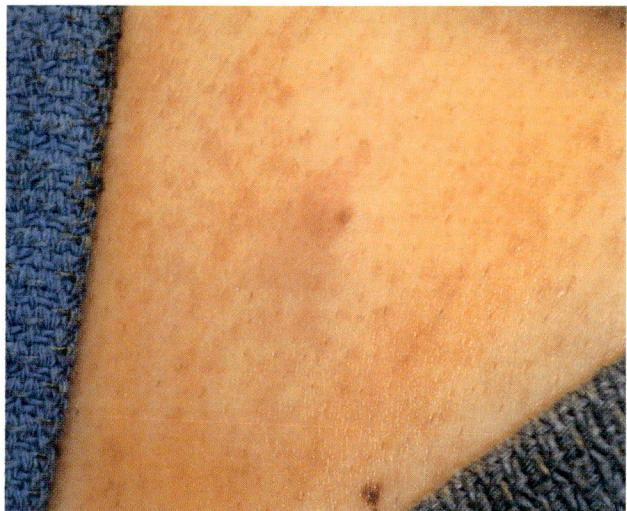

FIG. 4.84-A. Pre-operative appearance of the lesion.

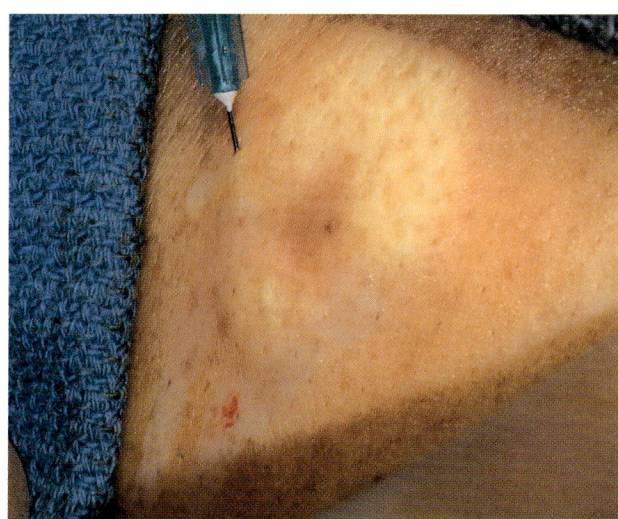

FIG. 4.84-B. The surgical site is infiltrated with local anesthetic.

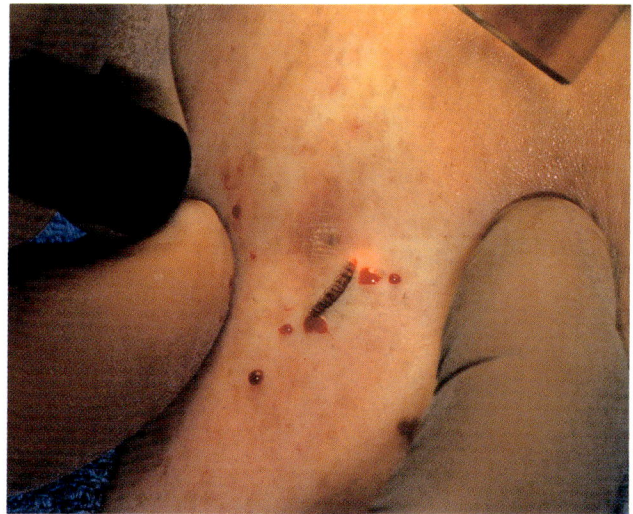

FIG. 4.84-C. The skin is incised with the CO_2 laser in focus.

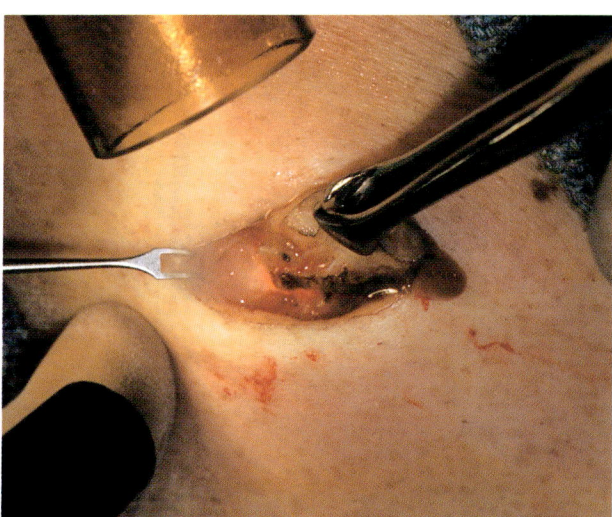

FIG. 4.84-D. The lesion is dissected from the surrounding tissues.

Case continues on following page.

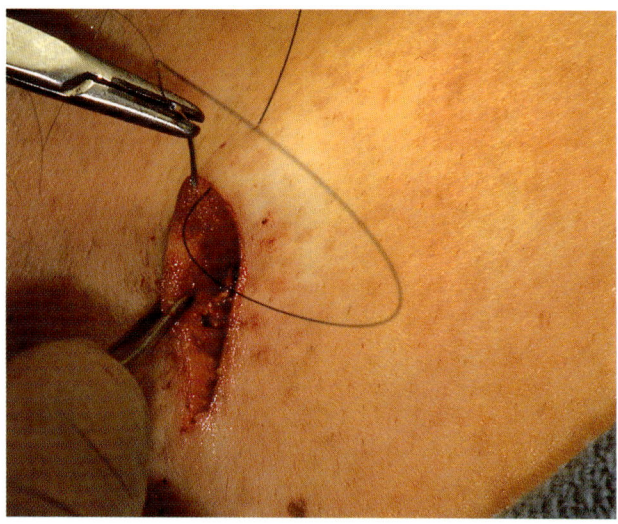

FIG. 4.84-E. The subcutaneous tissue is reapproximated with 3-0 polyglycolic acid suture.

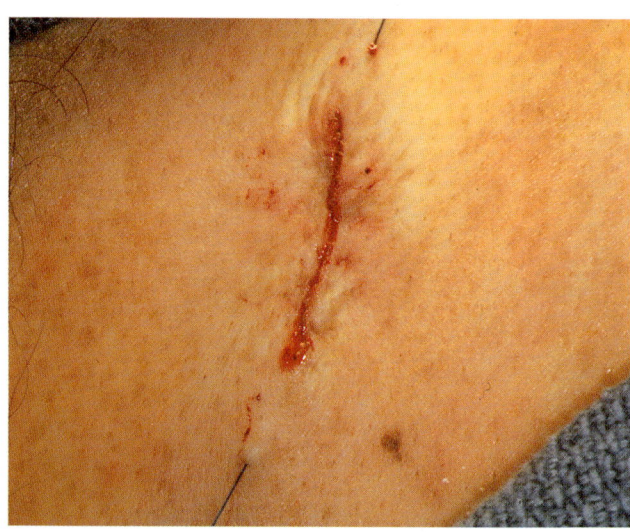

FIG. 4.84-F. A subcuticular closure is performed.

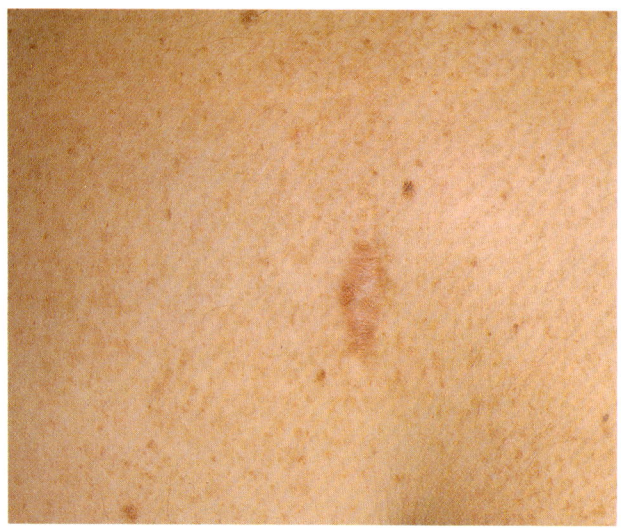

FIG. 4.84-G. Post-operative result.

Case courtesy of *Raymond J. Lanzafame*, M.D.

CASE 4.85
Left Preauricular Invasive Squamous Cell Carcinoma

REVIEW OF CASE. This 92-year-old nursing home patient presented with painful left preauricular invasive squamous cell carcinoma, previously irradiated with 5,000 rads to the area eight months before.

CHOICE OF LASER: CARBON DIOXIDE. The CO_2 laser is ideal for surface debridement and sterilization. General anesthesia is necessary. The key to success is aggressive lasing in a zone well beyond that of the original lesion. Tumor on bone can be lased at less than 30 watts without fear of bone necrosis.

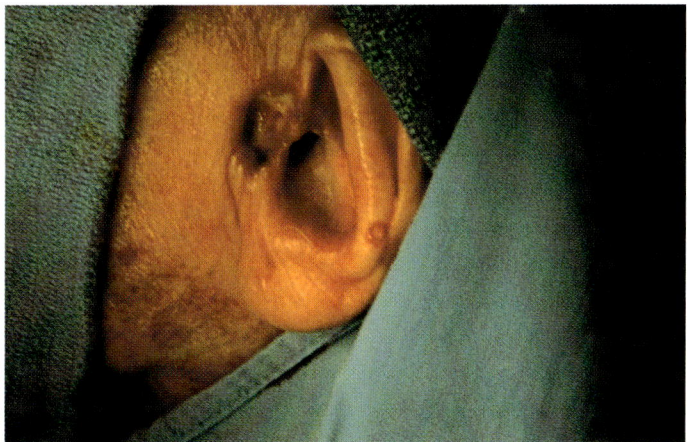

FIG. 4.85-A. 1.5 cm penetrating preauricular lesion.

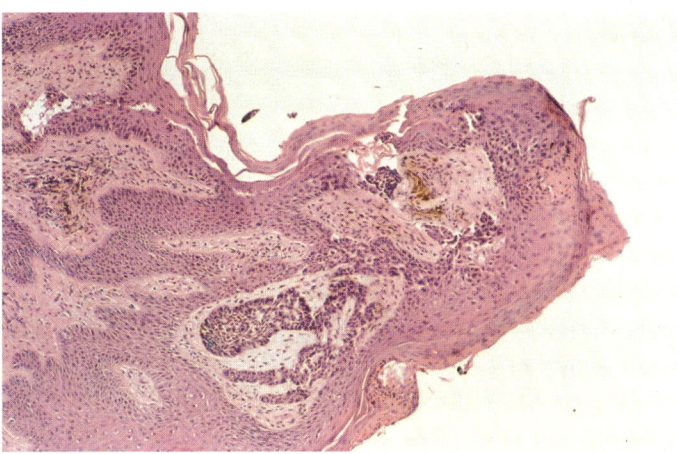

FIG. 4.85-B. Pathology slide of tissue taken at operation showing invasive nature of the lesion.

Case continues on following page.

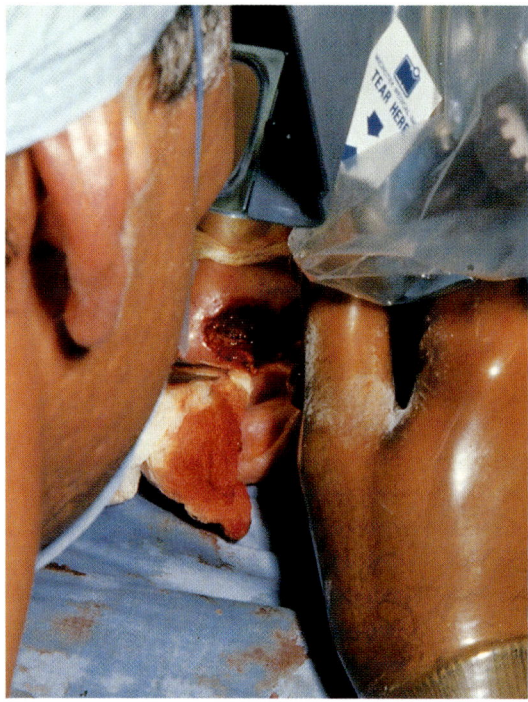

FIG. 4.85-C. Under high-power magnification, a hand-held CO_2 laser is set at 30 watts continuous power with the beam alternating between focused and defocused positions for incision and hemostasis, respectively.

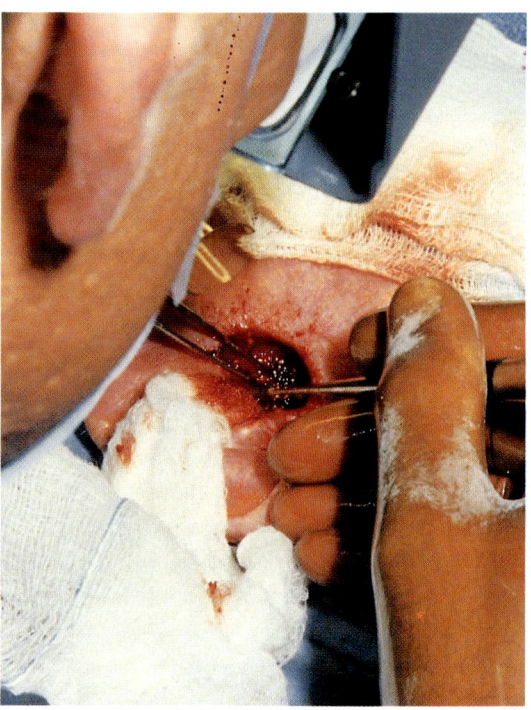

FIG. 4.85-D. After lasing, cureting of charred tissue is performed and the wound cleansed with hydrogen peroxide.

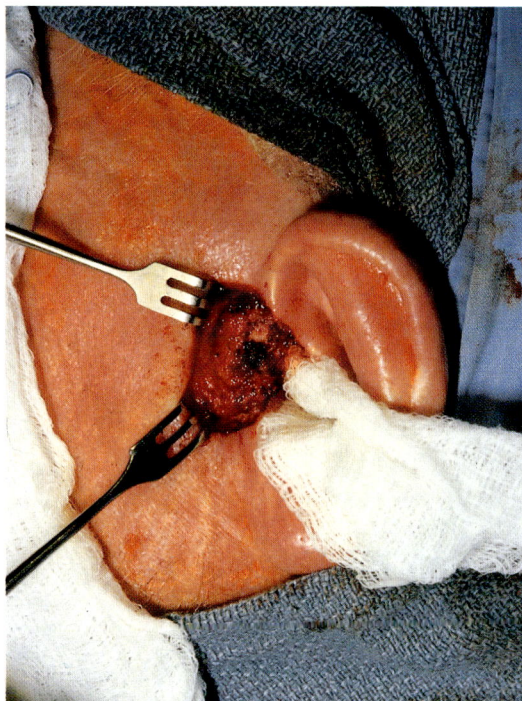

FIG. 4.85-E. Debridement is complete. One can see exposed bone at the base of the ulcer partially covered with char, indicating that the bone is readily lased to pursue necrotic tissue.

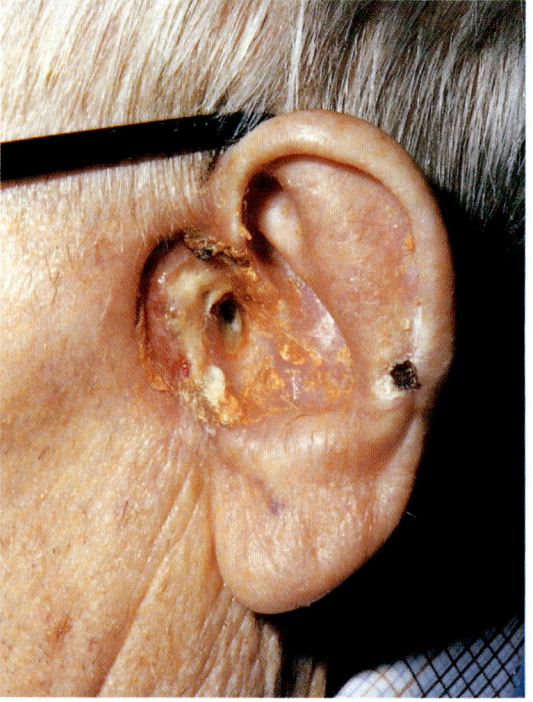

FIG. 4.85-F. The patient at two months post-operative, without pain and with new tissue formation in previously-irradiated field.

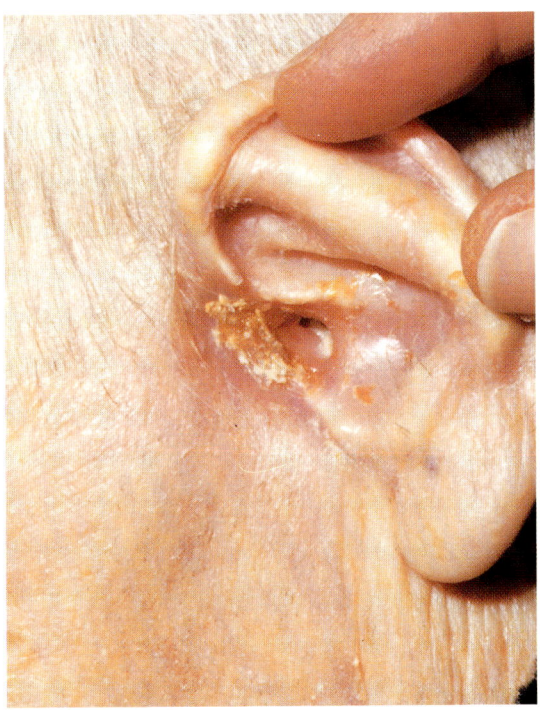

FIG. 4.85-G. Patient at four months post-operation.

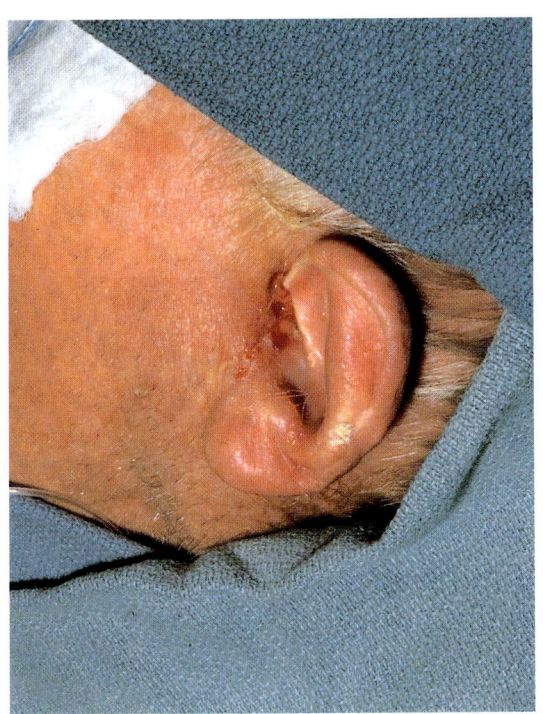

FIG. 4.85-H. Six months post-operation at time of repeat biopsy. Pathology report showed no regrowth of cancer.

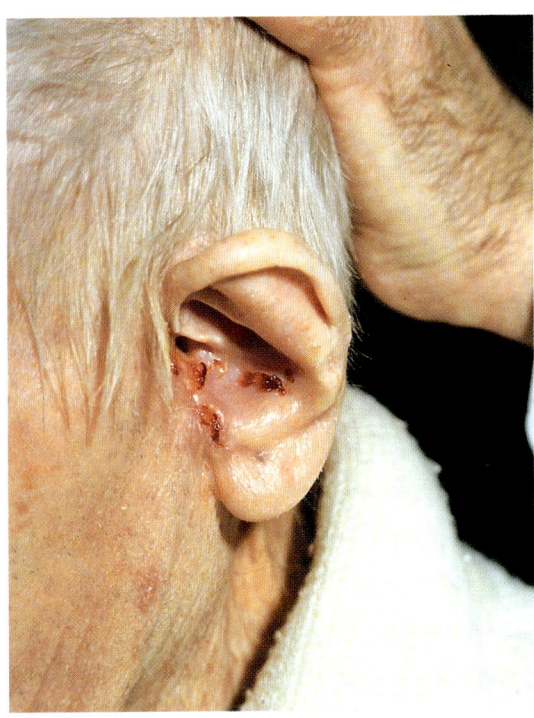

FIG. 4.85-I. Patient at nine months, still without evidence of recurrence. The patient died of unrelated causes three months later. The patient remained free of pain and tumor until his death.

Case courtesy of *Leonard S. Schultz, M.D.*

5

ARGON LASER

VASCULAR AND RELATED LESIONS
5.1 Acne rosacea
5.2 Angiofibroma
5.3 Angiokeratoma circumscriptum of the foot
5.4 Angiokeratoma circumscriptum of the thigh
5.5 Angiokeratoma of Fordyce
5.6 Anogenital/perineal strawberry hemangioma in infancy
5.7 Capillary hemangioma in infancy
5.8 Capillary and venous malformations
5.9 Hemangioma in growing phase: strawberry type
5.10 Periorbital/conjunctival strawberry hemangioma
5.11 Hemangioma of Vermilion
5.12 Lymphangioma of the Buccal Mucosa
5.13 Lymphangioma of the tongue
5.14 Post-rhinoplasty red nose
5.15 Port wine hemangioma of the face and neck
5.16 Port wine hemangioma of the chin and cheek
5.17 Port wine hemangioma of the right face
5.18 Port wine hemangioma with cavernous component of the lower lip
5.19 Port wine hemangioma of the face
5.20 Port wine hemangioma of the upper lip
5.21 Strawberry hemangioma in infancy: medial canthus and eyelid
5.22 Strawberry hemangioma in infancy: anogenital region
5.23 Strawberry hemangioma of the lip
5.24 Telangiectasia of the nose and face
5.25 Telangiectasia of the nose
5.26 Telangiectasia macularis erupta perstans: urticaria pigmentosa

5.27 Venous lake of the lower lip
5.28 Venous lake of the lip
5.29 Venous malformations

INFLAMMATORY/INFECTIOUS LESIONS
5.30 Verruca vulgaris of the finger

TATTOO
5.31 Decorative tattoo: comparison of argon and CO_2 lasers
5.32 Decorative tattoo (deltoid)
5.33 Decorative tattoo (upper arm)

MISCELLANEOUS
5.34 Adenoma sebaceum
5.35 Angiofibromas in a patient with tuberous sclerosis
5.36 Hypertrophic surgical scar
5.37 Keloid of the earlobe
5.38 Keloid of the pubic area
5.39 Linear hyperkeratotic nevus
5.40 Nevus of Ota
5.41 Nevus sebaceum
5.42 Nevus unilateralis
5.43 Papillomatosis of the lip in a patient with EEC syndrome
5.44 Seborrheic keratosis

SURGICAL PROCEDURES
5.45 Port wine hemangioma: Dot/pointillistic technique

CASE 5.1
Acne Rosacea

REVIEW OF CASE. This is a 62-year-old male with progressive development of red telangiectatic vessels on the dorsum of the nose and the cheeks. This was accompanied by an irregular and sebaceous character of the skin. There was progressive growth of the lesions and they became darker in color upon exertion or the consumption of alcohol. The patient requested treatment because of the cosmetic appearance of the lesions.

CHOICE OF LASER: ARGON. The argon laser produces visible blue-green light between 488–514 nm. Due to the absorption spectrum of hemoglobin and melanin which both absorb light at this wavelength, both vascular and pigmented lesions can be treated. The light is absorbed and converted to heat which has the ability to accomplish thermal photocoagulation to a depth of 1–2 mm of the upper dermis. Adjacent collagen and overlying dermis and epidermis may also be affected by the heat, producing a partial-thickness injury. Dermal appendages such as sweat glands and pilosebaceous glands are relatively resistant to argon laser energy and aid in the rapid healing of the laser wounds. The laser is most often used with a 1 mm spot size, 0.2 seconds exposure, and a power of 0.8–2 watts.

ADDITIONAL INFORMATION. The laser is hand held perpendicular to the skin at the focal length (2–4 cm from the skin surface) and slowly advanced according to the blanching of the lesion. Fine linear vessels are traced. Local anesthesia without epinephrine is most commonly used for adults, but children require sedation or general anesthesia.

POST-TREATMENT CARE. The wound is treated in an open wound fashion with the immediate use of ice compresses, followed by application of an antibiotic ointment. Alternatively, wounds in areas of trauma or in children may necessitate a sterile dressing.

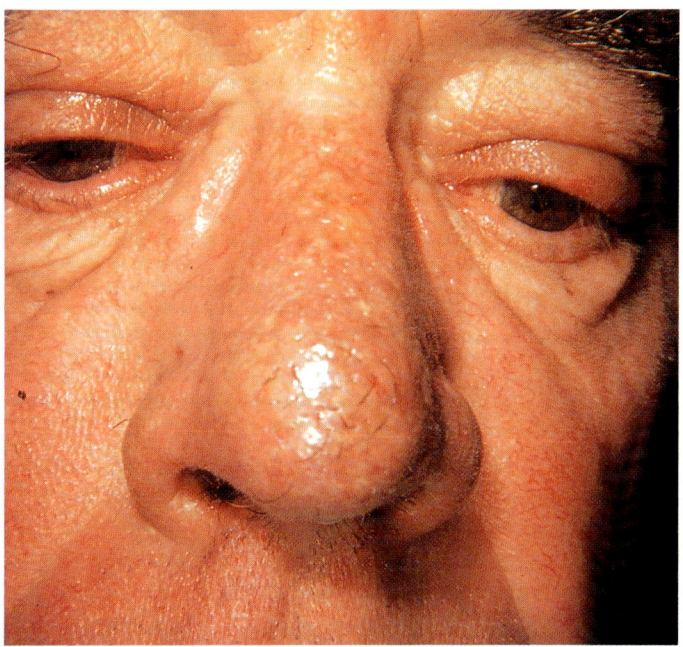

FIG. 5.1-A. Pre-treatment appearance of patient with acne rosacea of the nose and cheeks.

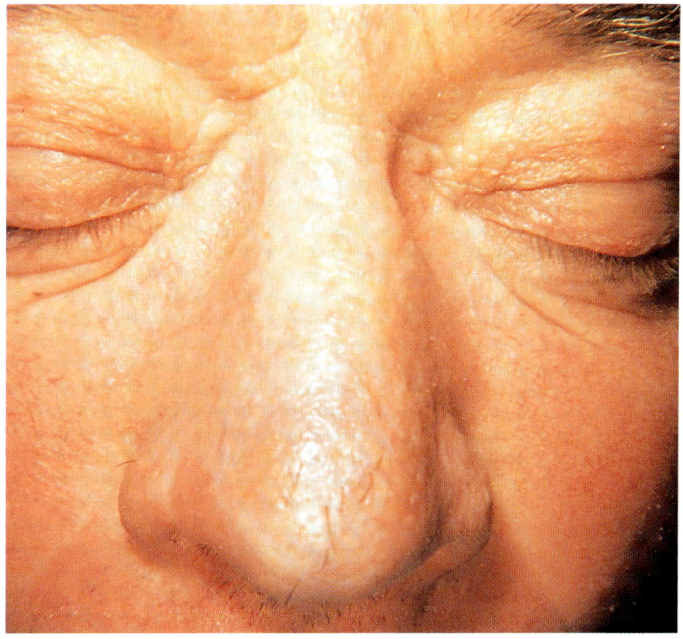

FIG. 5.1-B. One year following treatment, demonstrating the excellent blanching without recurrence of most of the vessels of the nose and cheek. The thickened acneiform sebaceous skin was not particularly affected by the argon laser treatment.

Case courtesy of *Lovic W. Hobby*, M.D.

CASE 5.2
Angiofibroma

REVIEW OF CASE. This is a 23-year-old female with a dark purple-red angiofibroma on the anterior tibial area of the leg. This area bled very easily following trauma.

CHOICE OF LASER: ARGON. The argon laser produces visible blue-green light between 488–514 nm. Due to the absorption spectrum of hemoglobin and melanin which both absorb light at this wavelength, both vascular and pigmented lesions can be treated. The light is absorbed and converted to heat which has the ability to accomplish thermal photocoagulation to a depth of 1–2 mm of the upper dermis. Adjacent collagen and overlying dermis and epidermis may also be affected by the heat, producing a partial-thickness injury. Dermal appendages such as sweat glands and pilosebaceous glands are relatively resistant to argon laser energy and aid in the rapid healing of the laser wounds. The laser is most often used with a 1 mm spot size, 0.2 seconds exposure, and a power of 0.8–2 watts.

ADDITIONAL INFORMATION. The laser is hand held perpendicular to the skin at the focal length (2–4 cm from the skin surface) and slowly advanced according to the blanching of the lesion. Fine linear vessels are traced. Local anesthesia without epinephrine is most commonly used for adults, but children require sedation or general anesthesia.

POST-TREATMENT CARE. The wound is treated in an open wound fashion with the immediate use of ice compresses, followed by application of an antibiotic ointment. Alternatively, wounds in areas of trauma or in children may necessitate a sterile dressing.

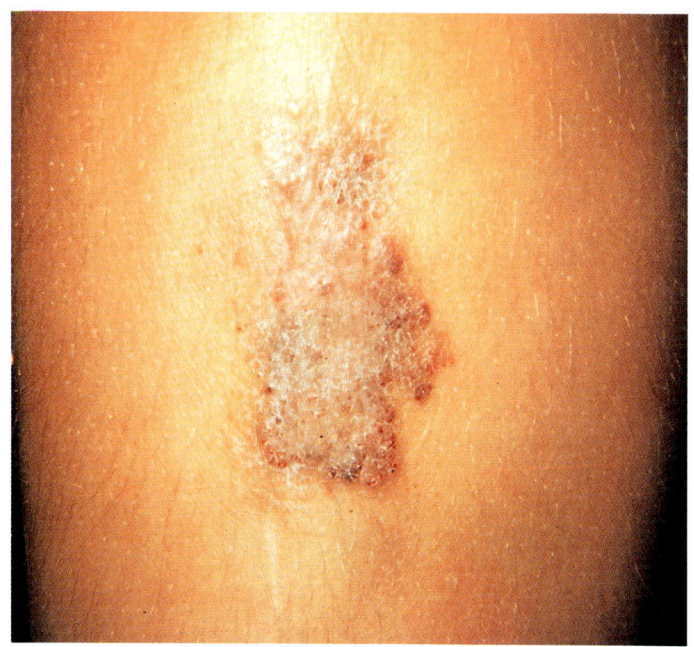

FIG. 5.2-A. Pre-treatment angiofibroma on the anterior tibial area of the leg.

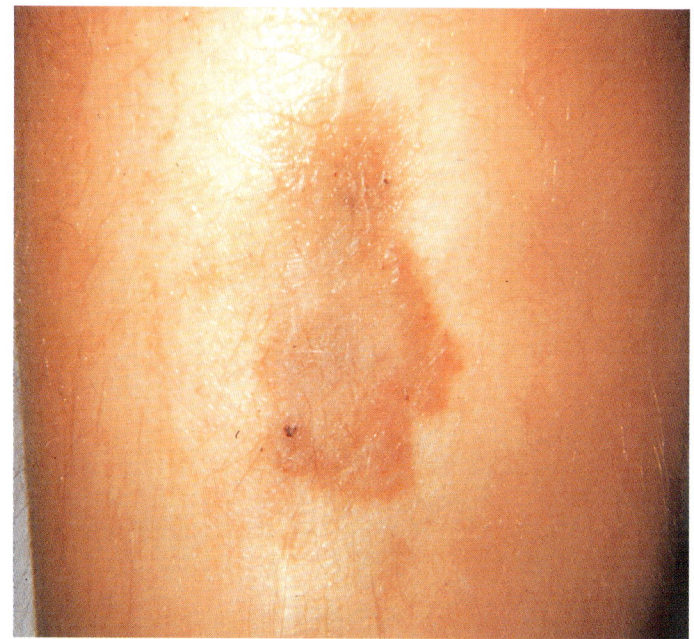

FIG. 5.2-B. Marked blanching of angiofibroma with good epithelial integrity four months following laser treatment.

Case courtesy of *Lovic W. Hobby*, M.D.

CASE 5.3

Angiokeratoma Circumscriptum of the Foot

REVIEW OF CASE. This 2-year-old girl was born with red, irregular spots on the dorsal surface of the left foot. This lesion measured 6 × 3 cm. Over time hyperkeratotic dark brown nodules started to appear. The father of this child had a history of hemangioma on his back during childhood.

CHOICE OF LASER: ARGON. The argon laser was chosen to treat these vascular lesions, confirming its usefulness in the removal of angiokeratomas.

POST-TREATMENT CARE. The patient is instructed to clean the wound every day with soap and water. Bacitracin ointment and bandaging are also used during healing.

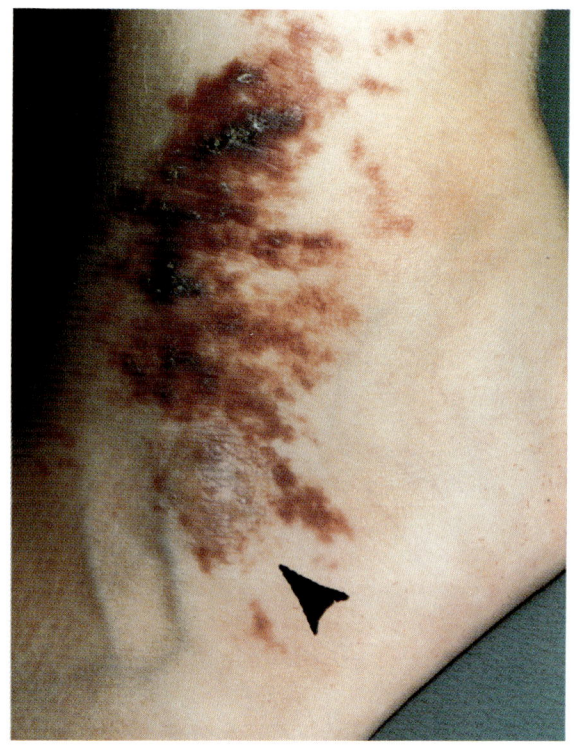

FIG. 5.3-A. Angiokeratoma circumscriptum on the foot in a 2-year-old girl. Arrowhead indicates the good result four months after argon laser test treatment.

Reprinted with permission of Little, Brown and Company.
For literature pertaining to this case see References section.

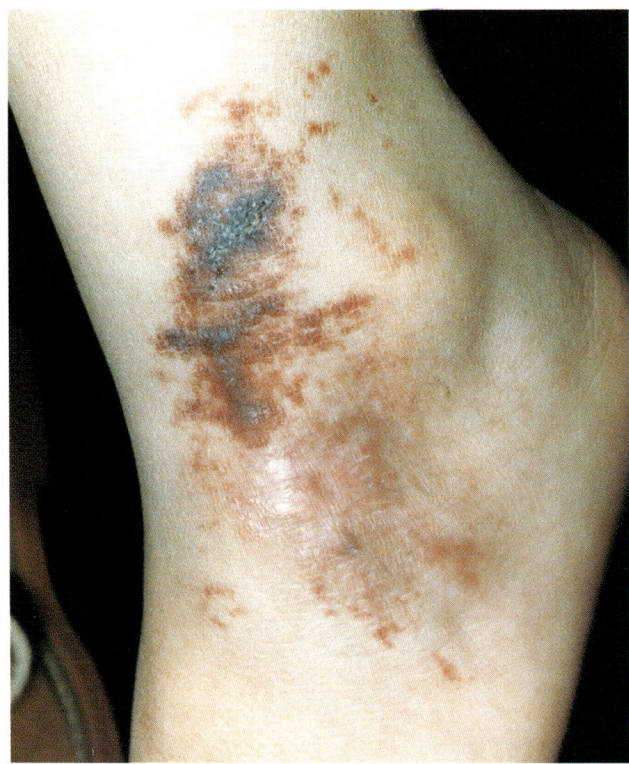

FIG. 5.3-B. Status 3 months after treatment of half the lesion with the argon laser (power 1–1.3 watts, spot size 1 mm, and exposure time 0.2 sec) following local anesthesia with 2% lidocaine without epinephrine.

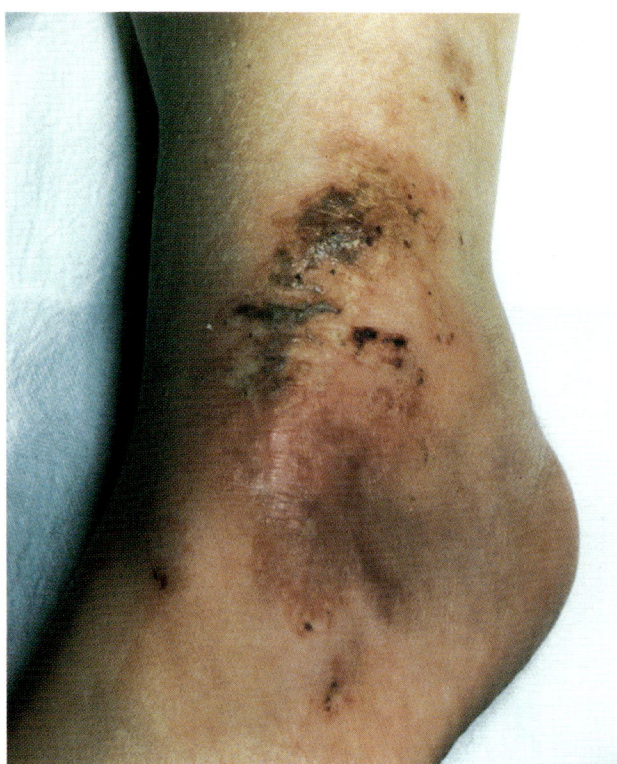

FIG. 5.3-C. Coagulation of the remaining vascular lesions during the last treatment with the argon laser.

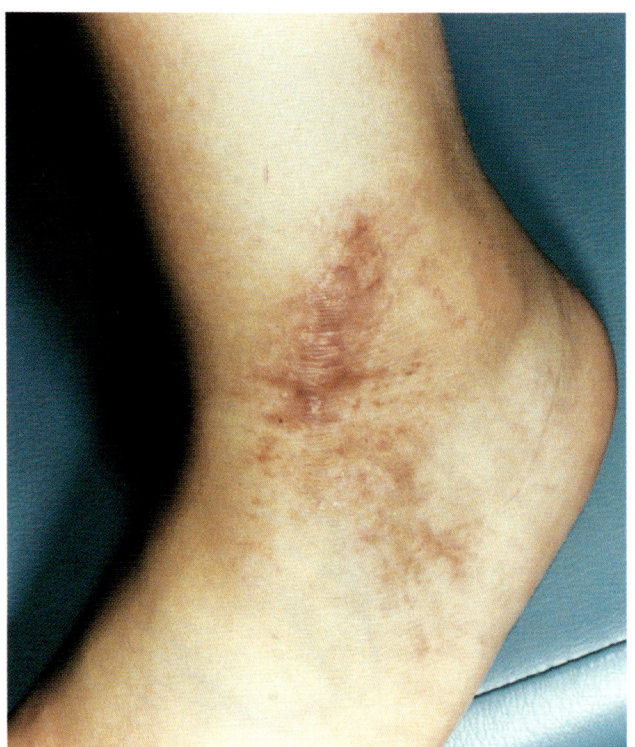

FIG. 5.3-D. Results 6 months after argon laser surgery. During the past 6 years there has been no recurrence of the lesions.

Case courtesy of *Krystyna A. Pasyk*, M.D., Ph.D.

CASE 5.4

Angiokeratoma Circumscriptum of the Thigh

REVIEW OF CASE. This 22-year-old female with semidark skin was born with multiple vascular nodules on her left thigh. The lesions over time became hyperkeratotic. Some of the lesions were excised surgically. The patient was referred to our laser clinic for treatment of the remaining lesions.

CHOICE OF LASER: ARGON. Argon laser energy may coagulate these ectatic blood vessels.

ADDITIONAL INFORMATION. Treatment was performed without local anesthesia. The lesions before and after treatment were cooled with ice cubes.

POST-TREATMENT CARE. Daily cleaning of the lesion with soap and water followed by application of bacitracin ointment, and a dressing. The patient was also cautioned to avoid exposure to the sun of the treated area.

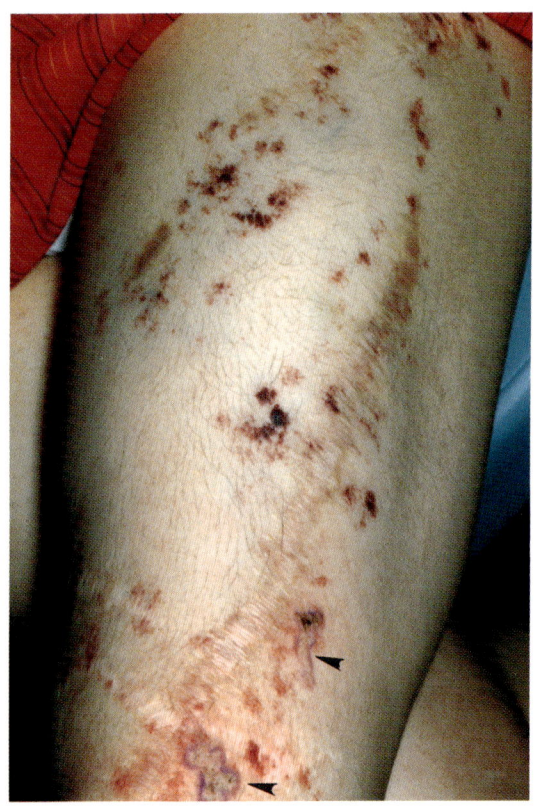

FIG. 5.4-A. Angiokeratoma circumscriptum on the thigh of a 24-year-old female showing a few linear scars after partial surgical excision of the lesions. Arrowheads show the tested areas immediately after irradiation with the argon laser (power 1 watt; spot size 1 mm; exposure time 0.2 sec).

Reprinted with permission of Little, Brown and Company.
For literature pertaining to this case see References section.

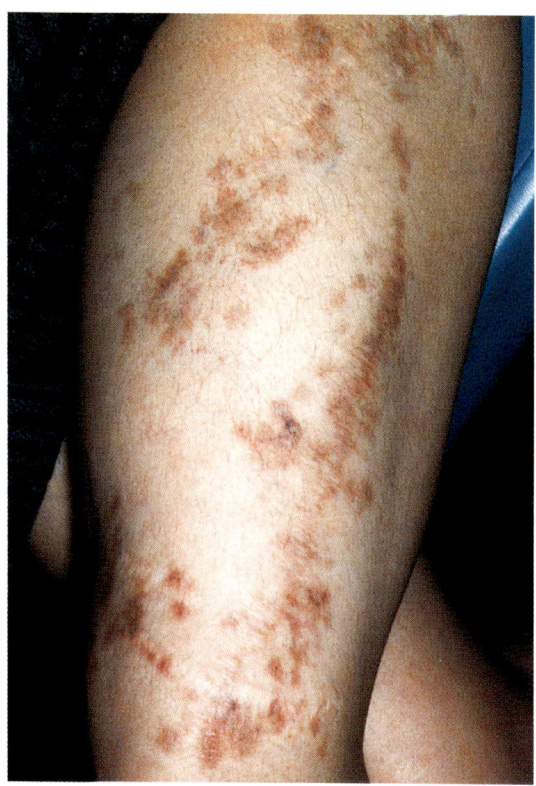

FIG. 5.4-B. Results after a few consecutive treatments with the argon laser using 1–1.7 watts of power, 1 mm spot size, and 0.2 sec exposure time.

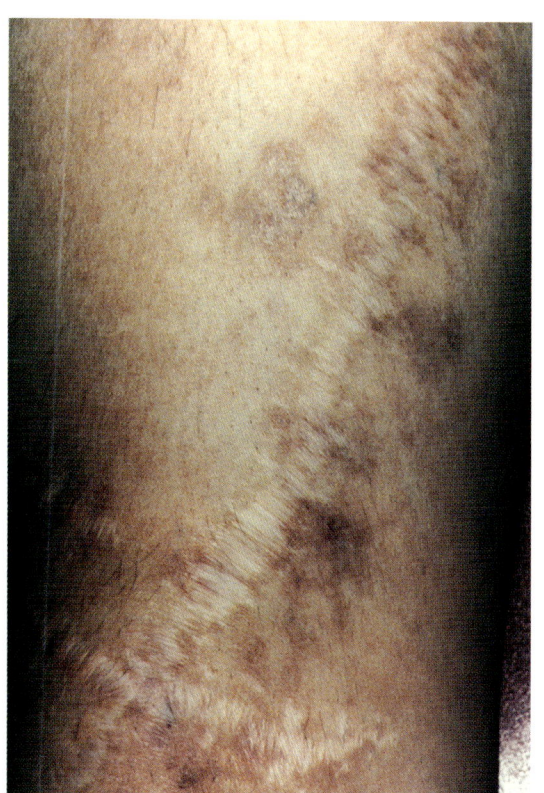

FIG. 5.4-C. Two years after further treatment with the argon laser. Note smooth surface and very little hyperpigmentation in the treated areas.

Case courtesy of *Krystyna A. Pasyk,* M.D., Ph.D.

CASE 5.5
Angiokeratoma of Fordyce

REVIEW OF CASE. Fordyce's angiokeratoma is an uncommon disorder of small venous angiomas of scrotal involvement. It occurs in middle-aged and elderly males and is most prevalent in the Oriental race. Lesions are benign and usually asymptomatic although occasionally pruritus, minor bleeding, and a tingling sensation prior to the eruption of new lesions may occur. The scrotum can be anesthetized by a circumferential field block at the base and sides, thus accomplishing a pudendal/perineal nerve block. Each individual lesion should be coagulated. Multiple treatments may be necessary.

CHOICE OF LASER: ARGON. The argon laser is able to selectively blanch hemoglobin-laden vessels due to the absorption of argon light by hemoglobin. Adjacent tissue is spared. The laser is used with a 1 mm spot size, 0.2 seconds pulse duration, and 0.5–0.8 watts of power.

POST-TREATMENT CARE. The patient may shower daily. The scrotum is lightly coated with a topical antibiotic ointment and protected by 4 × 4 gauze supported by male jockey-type underwear. Intercourse and strenuous physical activity is prohibited until healing is complete (an average of 2 to 3 weeks).

For literature pertaining to this case see References section.

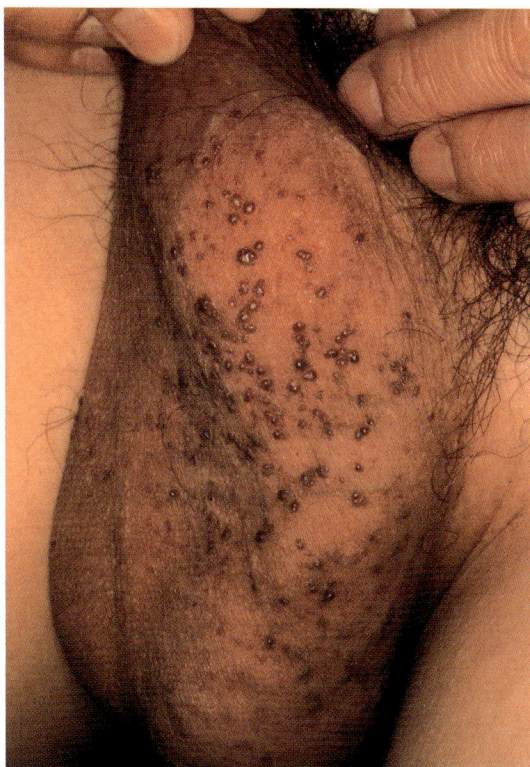

FIG. 5.5-A. Angiokeratoma of Fordyce in the scrotum of an Oriental male.

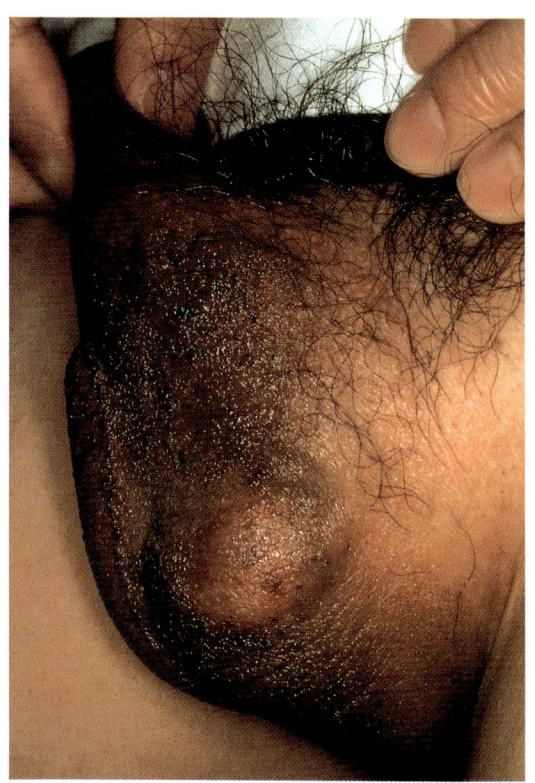

FIG. 5.5-B. Blanching immediately following treatment.

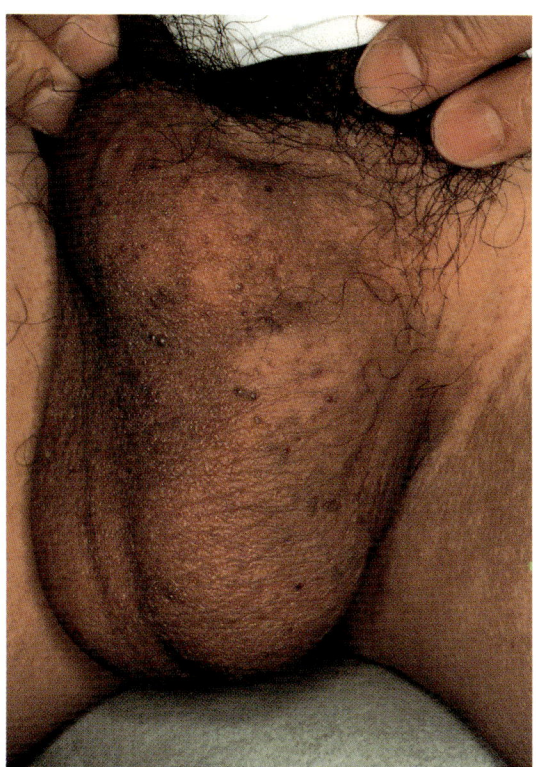

FIG. 5.5-C. Marked clearing of the lesions without scarring.

Case courtesy of *David B. Apfelberg*, M.D.

CASE 5.6

Anogenital/Perineal Strawberry Hemangioma in Infancy

REVIEW OF CASE. This is an 8-week-old infant with the rapid development of multiple perianal, genital, and perineal hemangiomas. Due to soiling of urine and feces from diapers as well as friction, these lesions were chronically ulcerated, frequently bleeding, and partially infected.

CHOICE OF LASER: ARGON. The argon laser produces visible blue-green light between 488–514 nm. Due to the absorption spectrum of hemoglobin and melanin which both absorb light at this wavelength, both vascular and pigmented lesions can be treated. The light is absorbed and converted to heat which has the ability to accomplish thermal photocoagulation to a depth of 1–2 mm of the upper dermis. Adjacent collagen and overlying dermis and epidermis may also be affected by the heat, producing a partial-thickness injury. Dermal appendages such as sweat glands and pilosebaceous glands are relatively resistant to the argon laser energy and aid in the rapid healing of the laser wounds. The laser is most often used with a 1 mm spot size, 0.2 seconds exposure, and a power of 0.8–2 watts.

ADDITIONAL INFORMATION. The laser is hand held perpendicular to the skin at the focal length (2–4 cm from the skin surface) and slowly advanced according to the blanching of the lesion. Fine linear vessels are traced. Local anesthesia without epinephrine is most commonly used for adults, but children require sedation or general anesthesia.

POST-TREATMENT CARE. The wound is treated in an open wound fashion with immediate use of ice compresses, followed by application of an antibiotic ointment. Alternatively, wounds in areas of trauma or in children may necessitate a sterile dressing.

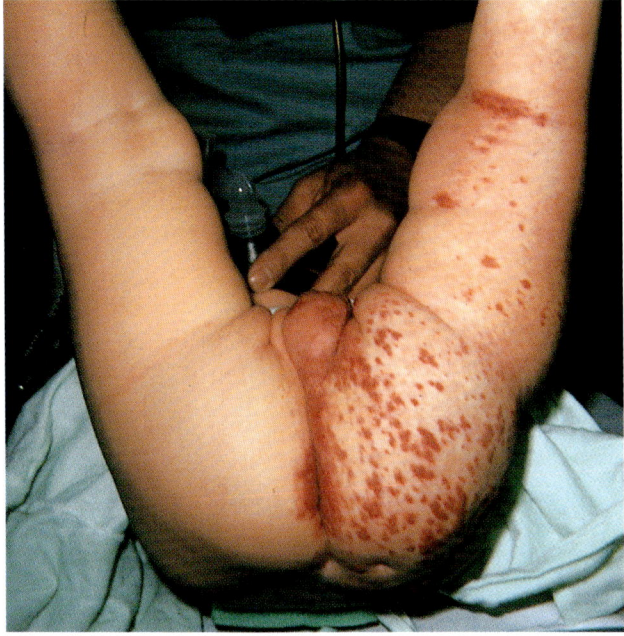

FIG. 5.6-A. Eight-week-old child with ulcerated and bleeding hemangiomas present in many areas of the perianal area, the genital area, and the perineum.

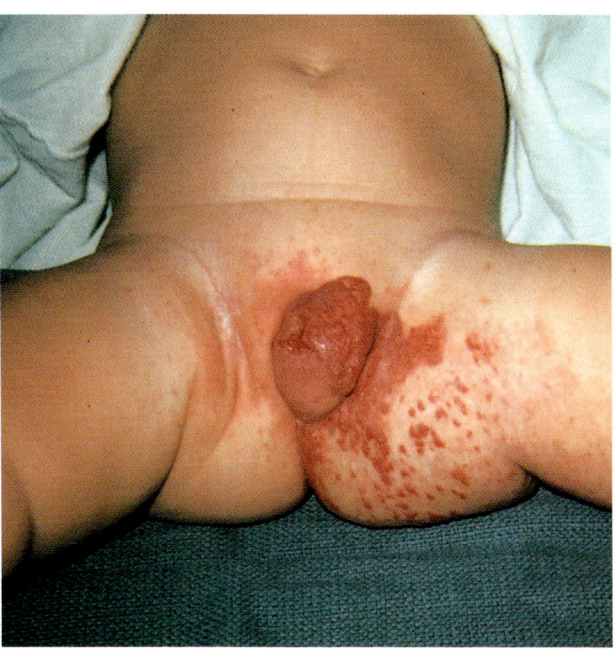

FIG. 5.6-B. Close-up view of the lesions.

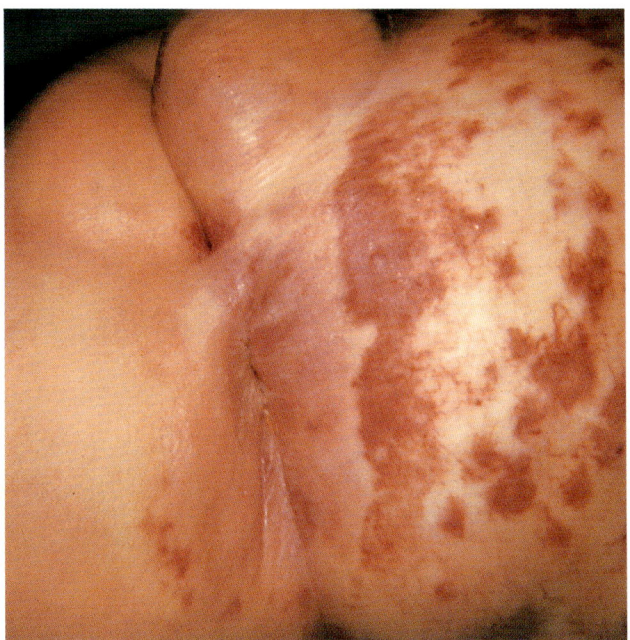

FIG. 5.6-C. Healing of the anal areas four weeks following argon laser photocoagulation.

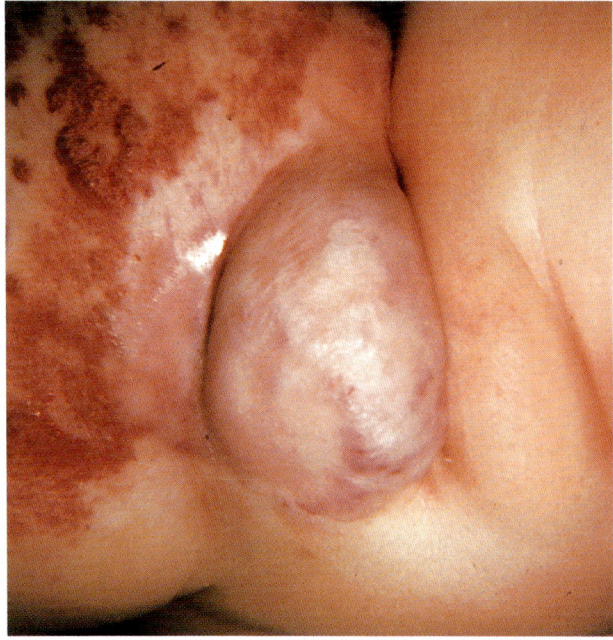

FIG. 5.6-D. Close-up of healing of the perianal and genital areas, but the untreated areas more laterally are beginning to ulcerate and bleed.

Case continues on following page.

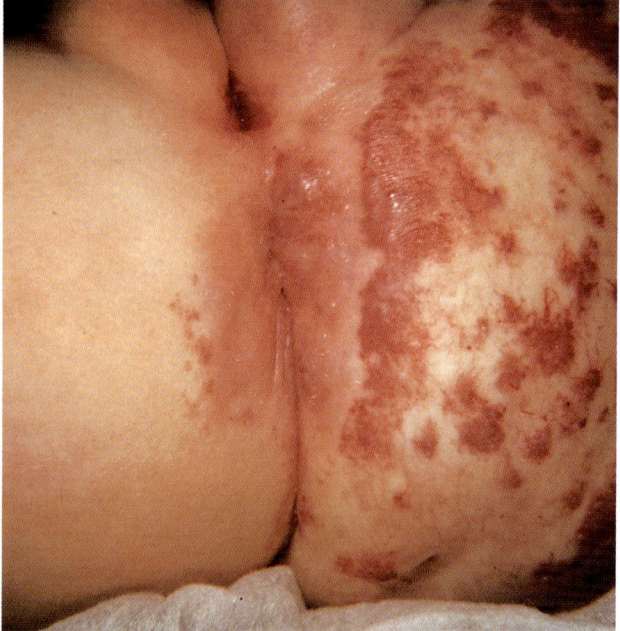

FIG. 5.6-E. Ulceration and bleeding of lateral areas.

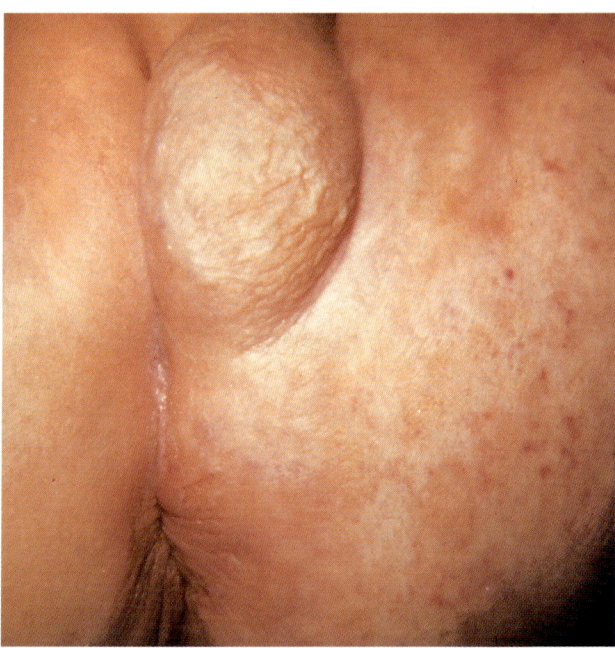

FIG. 5.6-F. Four months post-treatment. All treated areas remain blanched and healed and untreated areas are still unchanged.

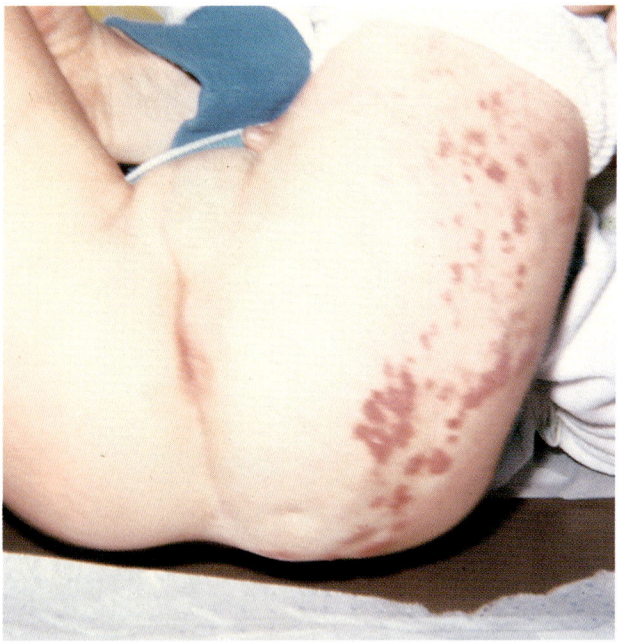

FIG. 5.6-G. Eighteen months following treatment the anal and genital areas are completely blanched and the lesions have disappeared. Lesions in the lateral areas are still present.

Case courtesy of *Lovic W. Hobby,* M.D.

CASE 5.7
Capillary Hemangioma in Infancy

REVIEW OF CASE.   A 7-month-old female infant. Capillary hemangioma appeared on the nose area between the first and second weeks after birth.

CHOISE OF LASER: ARGON.   Argon laser is used widely in treating hemangioma because it is absorbed relatively diathetically by hemoglobin. Capillary hemangioma usually disappears naturally with age. However, irradiation by argon laser has promoted the blanching effect in many cases.

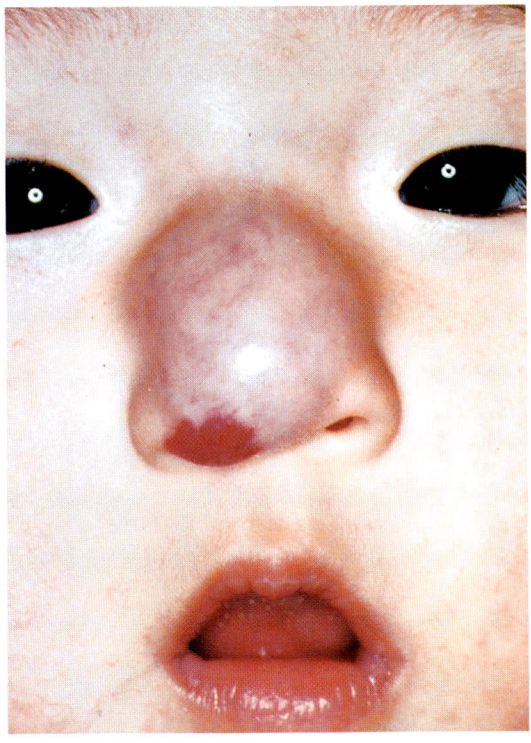

FIG. 5.7-A. Pre-operative view of capillary hemangioma on dorsum nasi.

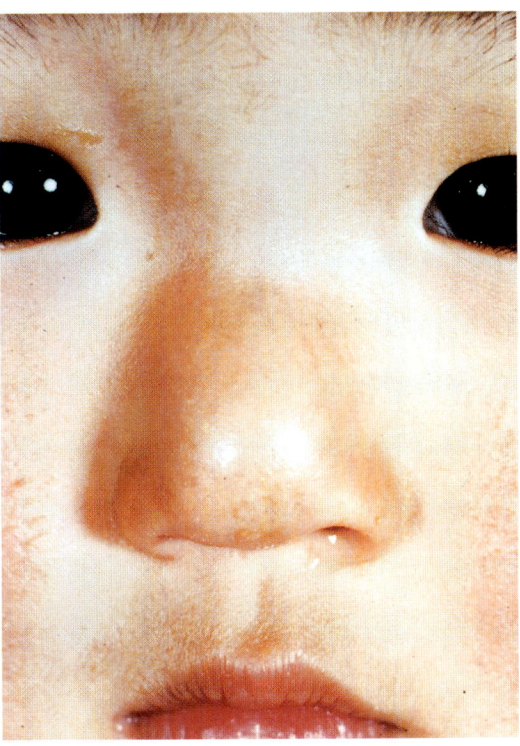

FIG. 5.7-B. Sixteen months after operation. The result is good, without any scars, or deformity of the nose.

Case courtesy of *Taichin Morita*, M.D., *H. Yamada*, M.D., *Muneo Miyasaka*, M.D., *Ryuzaburo Tanino*, M.D., and *Mitsuhiro Osada*, M.D.

CASE 5.8

Capillary and Venous Malformations

REVIEW OF CASE. A 14-year-old girl was referred to the laser clinic for treatment of a purplish discoloration on the right side of her lower lip. Since childhood she has also had slowly enlarging venous malformations on the entire right cheek, right side of the neck, the right hemi tongue, and the soft and hard palate as well the gingiva. She has had no previous treatment. She sought treatment because of concern about her appearance.

CHOICE OF LASER: ARGON. The argon laser, as the best coagulator of blood vessels up to 0.5 mm in diameter, was chosen for treatment of the capillary malformations (a port wine stain type) on the lower lip. A facial Jobst mask was recommended to provide pressure to the vascular lesions on her cheek.

POST-TREATMENT CARE. Daily application of bacitracin ointment on the treated area for approximately 10 days was recommended.

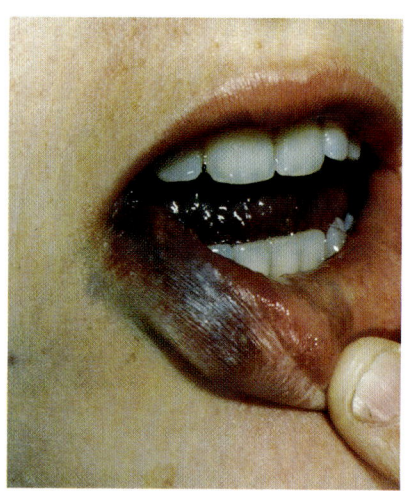

FIG. 5.8-A. Capillary malformations of the lower lip in a 14-year-old female before argon laser surgery. Note the venous malformations on the tongue and right cheek.

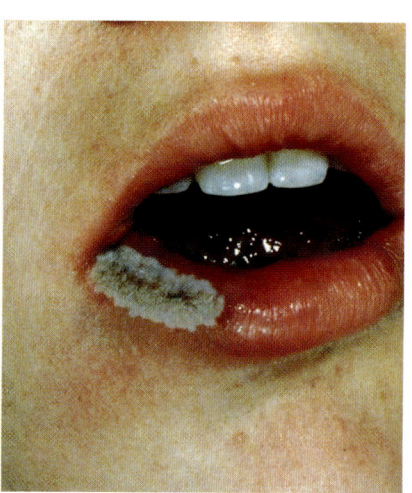

FIG. 5.8-B. The lesion immediately after argon laser irradiation using a power of 1.7 watts, spot size 1 mm, and exposure time 0.2 sec, preceded by local anesthesia with 2% lidocaine without epinephrine.

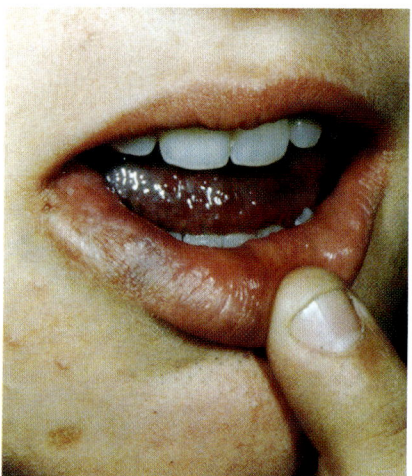

FIG. 5.8-C. Results 4 months after argon laser surgery of the lower lip.

Case courtesy of **Krystyna A. Pasyk**, M.D., Ph.D.

CASE 5.9
Strawberry Type Hemangioma in Growing Phase

REVIEW OF CASE. This 5-month-old infant was born with a pea-sized hemangioma on the buttock that grew slowly to 1.5 cm in diameter. The center of the lesion ulcerated and bled often over a three-week period. She was then referred for laser therapy.

CHOICE OF LASER: ARGON. Argon laser energy is able to coagulate erythrocyte-filled blood vessels up to 0.5 mm in diameter. Because this vascular birthmark consists of small blood vessels, coagulation with the argon laser to a depth of 1 mm will initiate subsequent involution of residual hemangioma.

POST-TREATMENT CARE. During the healing process, clean the lesion with soap and water and apply bacitracin ointment and a dressing.

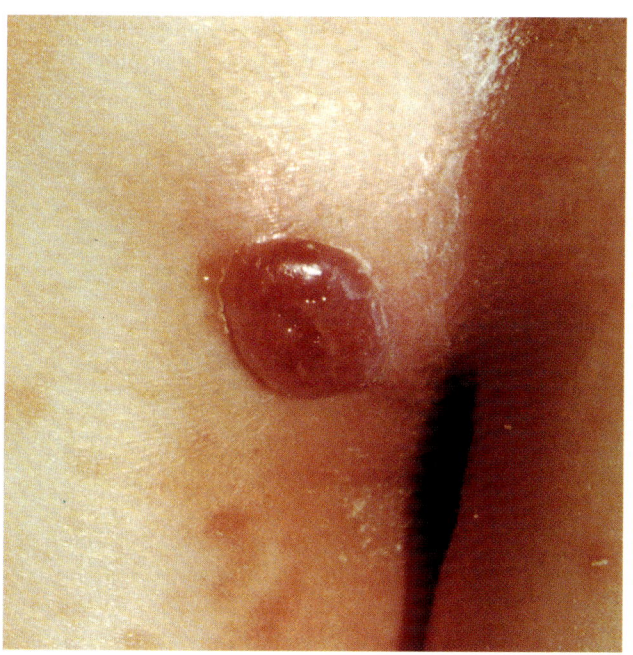

FIG. 5.9-A. Ulcerated hemangioma (strawberry type) on the buttock of 5-month-old infant before treatment with the argon laser.

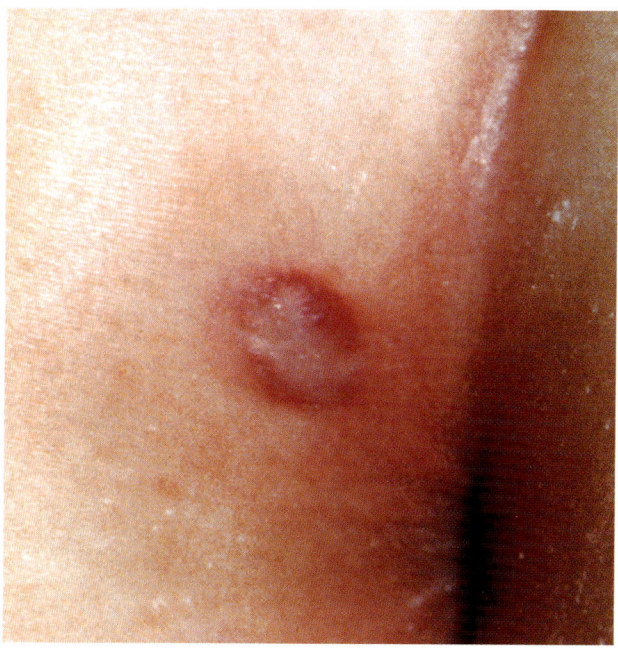

FIG. 5.9-B. Result 3 weeks after exposure to a few beams of argon laser energy (power 2 watts, spot size 1 mm, and exposure time 0.2 sec) without anesthesia. Note disappearance of the center of the lesion and significant shrinkage and flattening in the margin. The residual hemangioma involuted progressively during the 16 month follow-up.

Case courtesy of *Krystyna A. Pasyk*, M.D., Ph.D.

CASE 5.10

Periorbital/Conjunctival Strawberry Hemangioma

REVIEW OF CASE. This is an 8-month-old female with rapidly growing capillary hemangioma present in the left upper eyelid involving the conjunctiva and the superior eyelid. The patient sought treatment upon the recommendation of an ophthalmologist because of the danger of eye closure and deprivation amblyopia. Steroid treatment had not been successful.

CHOICE OF LASER: ARGON. The argon laser produces visible blue-green light between 488–514 nm. Due to the absorption spectrum of hemoglobin and melanin which both absorb light at this wavelength, both vascular and pigmented lesions can be treated. The light is absorbed and converted to heat which has the ability to accomplish thermal photocoagulation to a depth of 1–2 mm of the upper dermis. Adjacent collagen and overlying dermis and epidermis may also be affected by the heat, producing a partial-thickness injury. Dermal appendages such as sweat glands and pilosebaceous glands are relatively resistant to argon laser energy and aid in the rapid healing of the laser wounds. The laser is most often used with a 1 mm spot size, 0.2 seconds exposure, and a power of 0.8–2 watts.

ADDITIONAL INFORMATION. The laser is hand held perpendicular to the skin at the focal length (2–4 cm from the skin surface) and slowly advanced according to the blanching of the lesion. Fine linear vessels are traced. Local anesthesia without epinephrine is most commonly used for adults, but children require sedation or general anesthesia.

POST-TREATMENT CARE. The wound is treated in an open wound fashion with immediate use of ice compresses, followed by application of an antibiotic ointment. Alternatively, wounds in areas of trauma or in children may necessitate a sterile dressing.

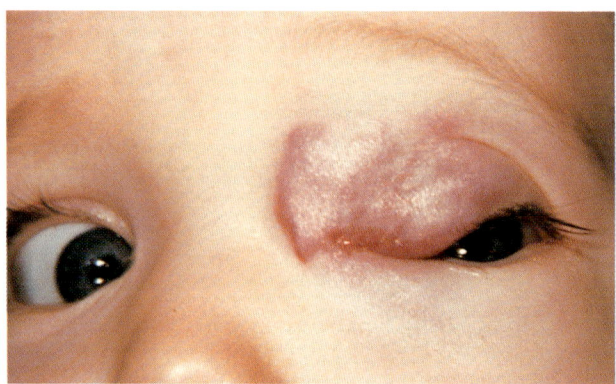

FIG. 5.10-A. Pre-treatment appearance of massive hemangioma of left upper eyelid.

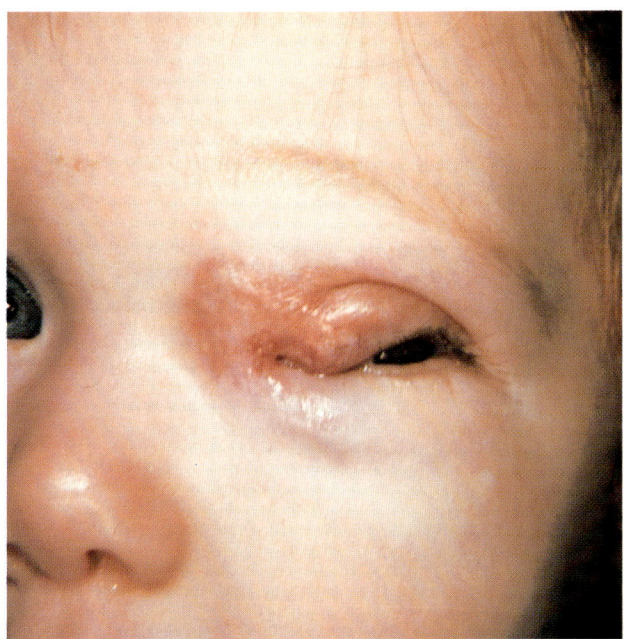

FIG. 5.10-B. Moderate reduction of swelling and size of hemangioma five weeks following treatment, but the threat of deprivation amblyopia is still present.

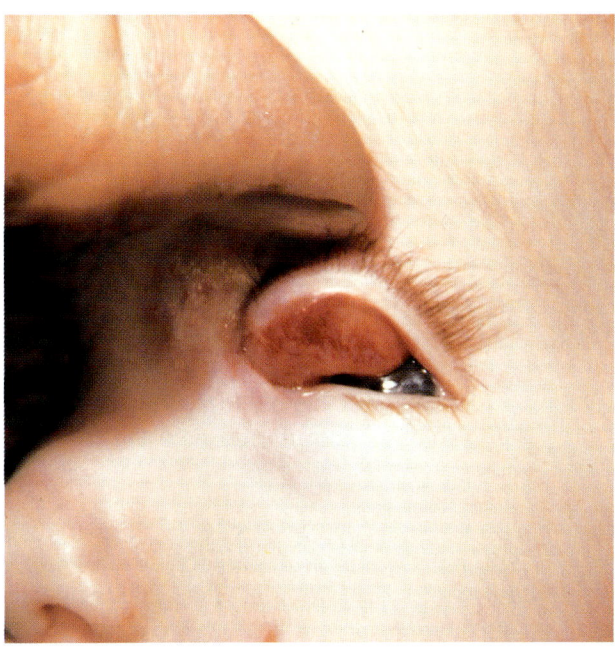

FIG. 5.10-C. Trans-conjunctival extent of hemangioma.

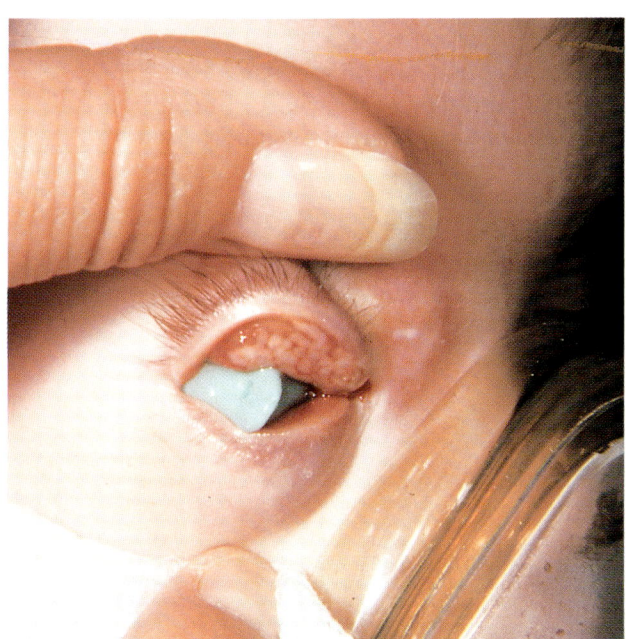

FIG. 5.10-D. Intraoperative view of hemangioma demonstrating the excellent shrinkage and blanching that is achieved in the conjunctival portion with the argon laser.

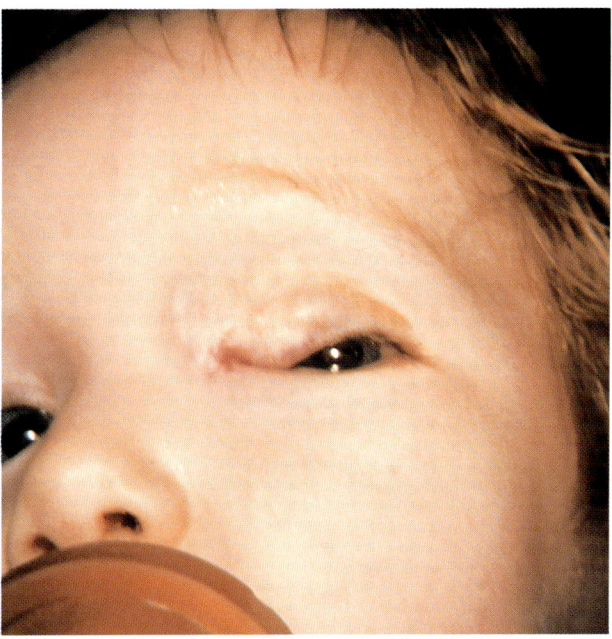

FIG. 5.10-E. Eight weeks following treatment the upper eyelid contour is almost normal, the conjunctival hemangioma has blanched and shrunk considerably, and the patient is able to open the eye without problems.

Case courtesy of *Lovic W. Hobby*, M.D.

CASE 5.11
Hemangioma of Vermilion

REVIEW OF CASE. This is a 43-year-old male with a progressively growing and bulging, blue hemangioma in the left corner of the mouth. This had started approximately 15 years previously and had become more hypertrophic and irregular with a dark blue color. It extended from the oral commissure almost to the midline. The patient requested removal for cosmetic reasons and because of a minor throbbing in the area.

CHOICE OF LASER: ARGON. The argon laser produces visible blue-green light between 488–514 nm. Due to the absorption spectrum of hemoglobin and melanin which both absorb light at this wavelength, both vascular and pigmented lesions can be treated. The light is absorbed and converted to heat which has the ability to accomplish thermal photocoagulation to a depth of 1–2 mm of the upper dermis. Adjacent collagen and overlying dermis and epidermis may also be affected by the heat, producing a partial-thickness injury. Dermal appendages such as sweat glands and pilosebaceous glands are relatively resistant to argon laser energy and aid in the rapid healing of the laser wounds. The laser is most often used with a 1 mm spot size, 0.2 seconds exposure, and a power of 0.8–2 watts.

ADDITIONAL INFORMATION. The laser is hand held perpendicular to the skin at the focal length (2–4 cm from the skin surface) and slowly advanced according to blanching of the lesion. Fine linear vessels are traced. Local anesthesia without epinephrine is most commonly used for adults, but children require sedation or general anesthesia.

POST-TREATMENT CARE. The wound is treated in an open wound fashion with immediate use of ice compresses, followed by application of an antibiotic ointment. Alternatively, wounds in areas of trauma or in children may necessitate a sterile dressing.

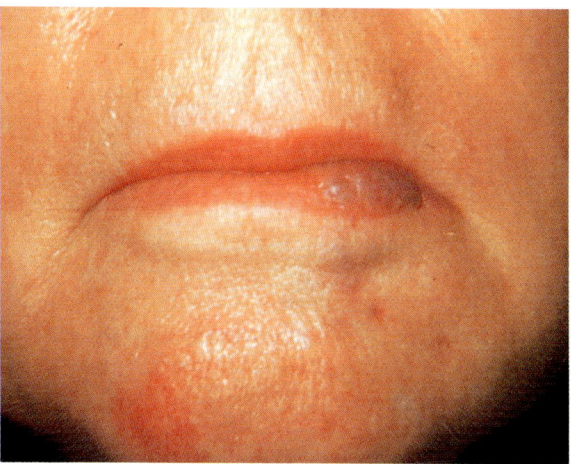

FIG. 5.11-A. Pre-treatment view of vermilion capillary hemangioma. Note port wine stain on chin.

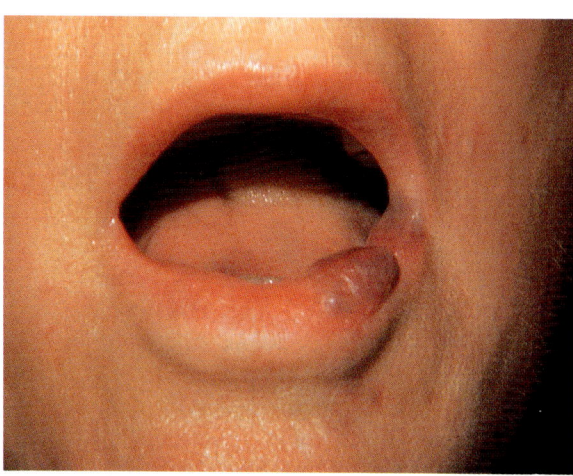

FIG. 5.11-B. The same view as in Fig. A except with mouth open.

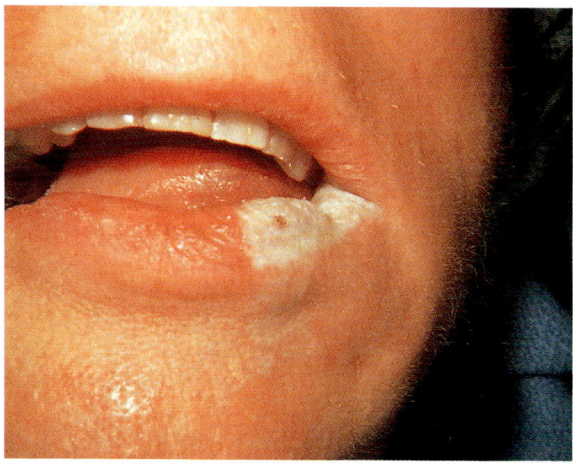

FIG. 5.11-C. Immediately post-argon laser photocoagulation. Note the blanching of the entire lesion.

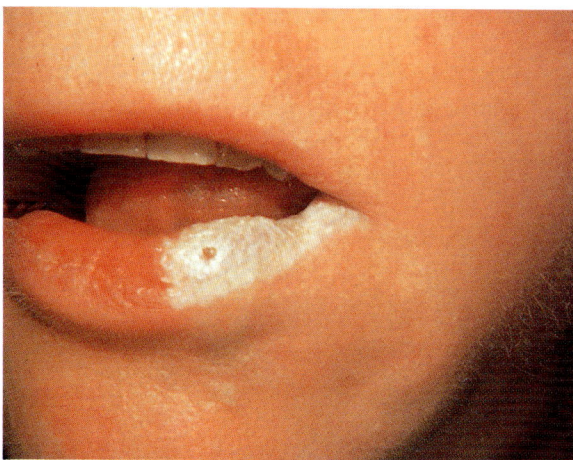

FIG. 5.11-D. Immediately post-argon laser photocoagulation. Note the blanching of the entire lesion.

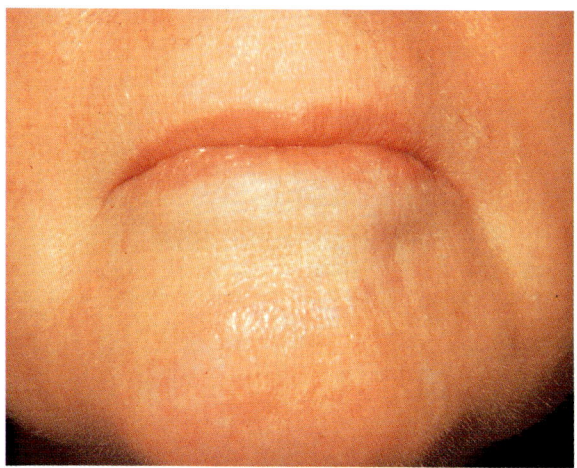

FIG. 5.11-E. Five months post-treatment. There is normal lip contour and normal vermilion color.

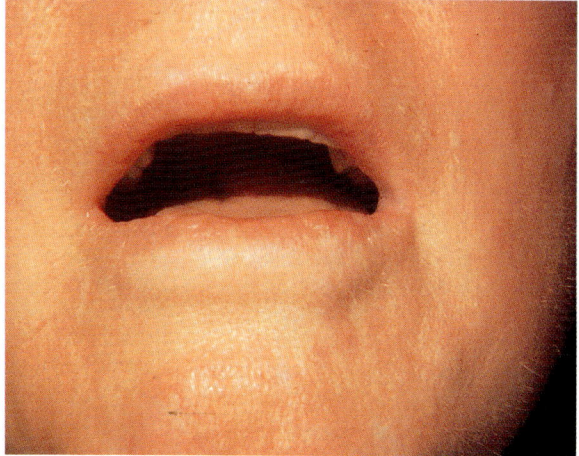

FIG. 5.11-F. Five months post-treatment with mouth open demonstrating excellent contour and color.

Case courtesy of *Lovic W. Hobby*, M.D.

CASE 5.12

Lymphangioma of the Buccal Mucosa

REVIEW OF CASE. This 11-year-old girl had a history of a slowly growing mass inside the right cheek as well as spreading, fine multicystic lesions on the right buccal area, lower lip, and tongue since about 6 months of age. She had undergone a series of incisions of the right cheek tumor; and the tumor reappeared after each excision. The patient was referred to the laser clinic for treatment of the lower lip lesion.

CHOICE OF LASER: ARGON. The argon laser was the only laser available at that time in the laser clinic.

POST-TREATMENT CARE. During the healing process daily washing of the mouth with a hydrogen peroxide solution was recommended.

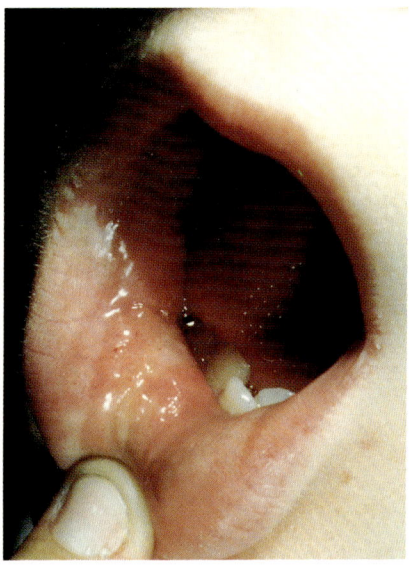

FIG. 5.12-A. Lymphatic malformations of the mouth in an 11-year-old girl before argon laser surgery.

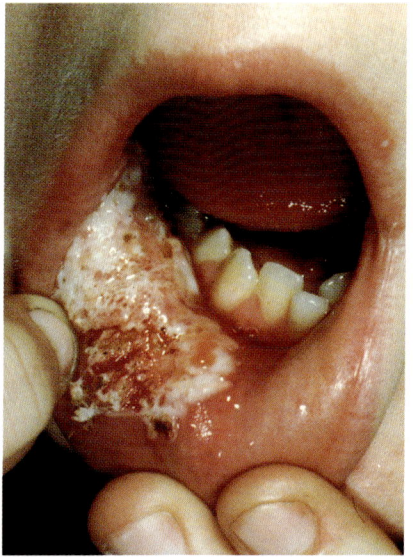

FIG. 5.12-B. Lesions immediately after argon laser irradiation (power 2–2.5 watts; spot size 1 mm; exposure time 0.2 sec). The treatment was performed after local anesthesia with 2% lidocaine without epinephrine.

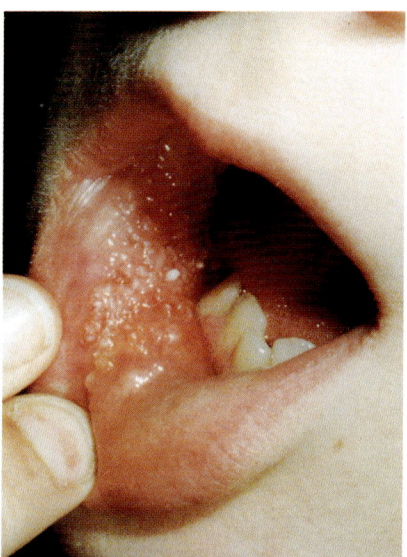

FIG. 5.12-C. Status 6 months after treatment with the argon laser. Note significant improvement in the treated area.

Case courtesy of *Krystyna A. Pasyk, M.D., Ph.D.*

CASE 5.13

Lymphangioma of the Tongue

REVIEW OF CASE. This is a 21-year-old female with a congenital lymphangioma of the tongue which caused macroglossia and recurrent bleeding. The patient was treated previously with embolization of the left lingual artery. After these treatments a marked macroglossia with daily bleeding of the tongue remained.

CHOICE OF LASER: ARGON. The argon laser was chosen in order to obtain tissue shrinkage with a minimal amount of bleeding. A laser power of 5–6 watts, focus diameter of 2 mm, and a pulse time of 1 sec was used. The tongue was treated with the separated spot technique and a total of 10 treatments were given.

ADDITIONAL INFORMATION. The treatments were performed under local anesthesia using a Xylocaine anesthetic spray. There was no special care taken after treatment. The white spots on the tongue caused by laser surgery caused little discomfort and healed within ten days. After the laser treatment the bleeding frequency was remarkably reduced but there was a tendency to recurrence. After the full ten treatment sessions however, bleeding occurred only once a month instead of daily.

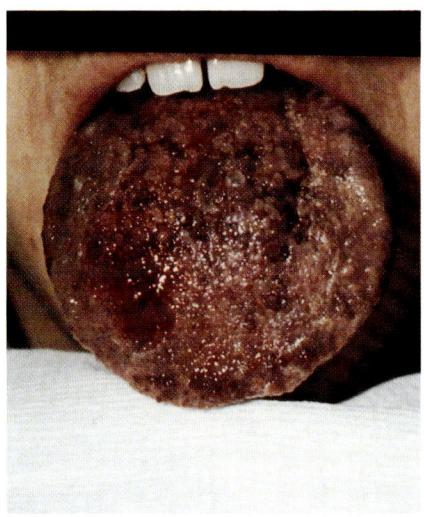

FIG. 5.13-A. Bleeding tongue which bulges out widely before laser treatment.

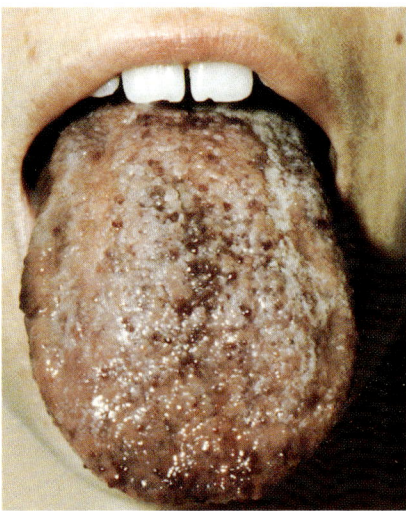

FIG. 5.13-B. The result after three treatments. The color of the tongue is much improved, though small hemangiomas in the middle and on the edges still remain. The tongue is beginning to reach normal proportions.

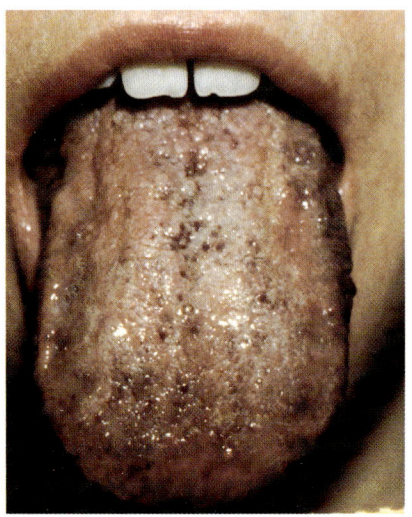

FIG. 5.13-C. The tongue after ten treatments. Note the remarkable improvement of the dimension of the tongue. A small number of hemangiomas still remain.

Case courtesy of *J. P. Hulsbergen Henning*, M.D.

CASE 5.14
Post-Rhinoplasty Red Nose

REVIEW OF CASE. This is a 57-year-old woman who at age 30 underwent a cosmetic rhinoplasty with the removal of a large nasal hump. Pre-operatively no redness of her nasal skin was noted by the patient. Soon after the surgery, the patient's nasal dorsum became diffusely red. She stated that the color varied with environmental temperature fluctuations and emotional state. After the surgery she had experienced a large amount of sun exposure wintering in the Caribbean and summering in New Hampshire. The redness caused her obvious embarrassment.

CHOICE OF LASER: ARGON. The argon laser works very well in treating superficial vascular lesions that involve the nose. The blue-green light in the argon laser is preferentially absorbed by hemoglobin which exists in the superficial ectatic vessels. Light changes to heat, and thermal damage ensues. The patient was treated with the argon laser, receiving 1,503 exposures at 1.6 watts output with a 0.2 second laser pulse duration. A 0.1-cm spot diameter was used. The single pulse irradiance was 120 watts/cm^2 and the energy fluence was 24 J/cm^2.

ADDITIONAL INFORMATION. A complication rarely seen after rhinoplasty is a diffuse "red" blush or telangiectasia, or both, over the dorsum of the nose. Removal of a large nasal hump and wide undermining may predispose to its development. It also has been noted when nasal dorsal implants have been used and is more common after secondary nasal surgery. It is also frequently seen after any nasal trauma including surgery. The dorsal blush may be accompanied by telangiectasias of nostril sill, columella, and alar areas.

2% Xylocaine without epinephrine is used for both anesthesia and to maximize the amount of vasodilatation and to get as many "red" chromophore in place as possible.

POST-TREATMENT CARE. The patient is advised to use soap and water until the wound is healed. In addition she is asked to have absolutely no sun exposure until the wound is healed and then to minimize sun exposure thereafter.

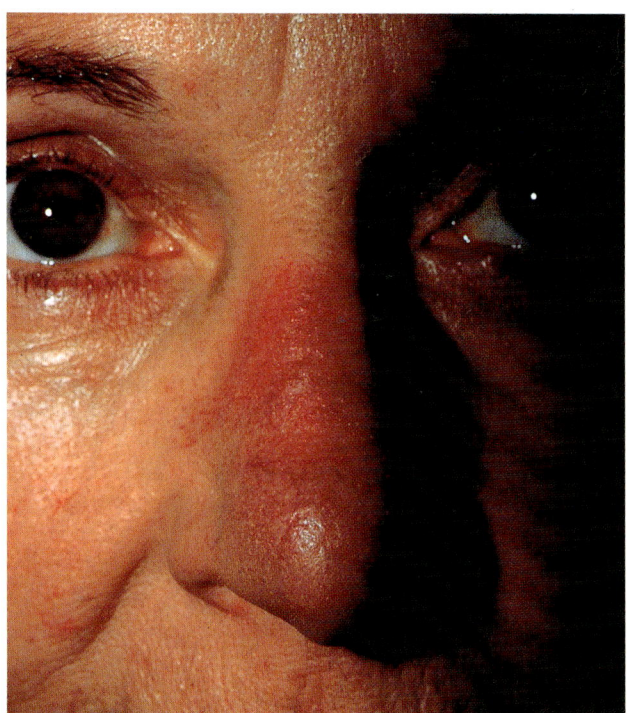

FIG. 5.14-A. Pre-treatment post-rhinoplasty red nose.

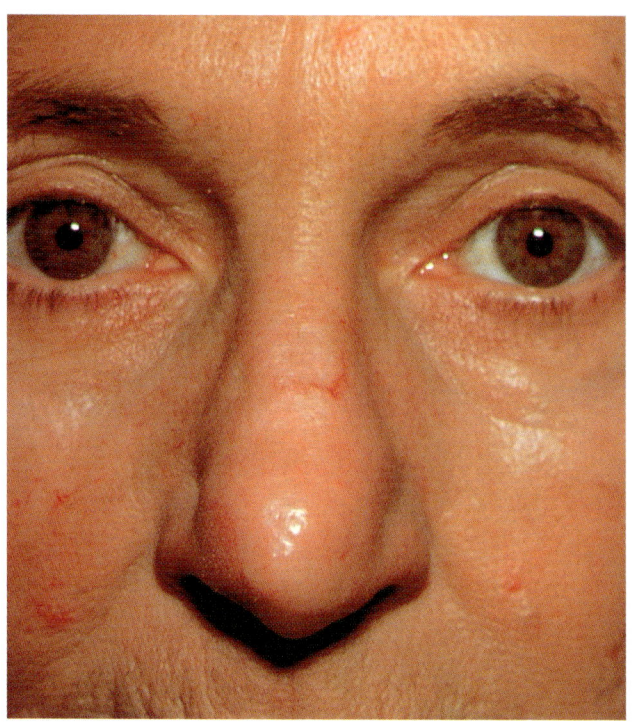

FIG. 5.14-B. After the patient expressed satisfaction with the result of the test area, the remaining area was treated at the same settings.

Case courtesy of *Joel Mark Noe,* M.D.

CASE 5.15

Port Wine Hemangioma of the Face and Neck

REVIEW OF CASE. This 23-year-old female had a congenital port wine hemangioma (nevus flammeus) present on the left face, ear, neck, and mastoid area. She desired removal for cosmetic purposes.

CHOICE OF LASER: ARGON. The argon laser produces visible blue-green light between 488–514 nm. Due to the absorption spectrum of hemoglobin and melanin which both absorb light at this wavelength, both vascular and pigmented lesions can be treated. The light is absorbed and converted to heat which has the ability to accomplish thermal photocoagulation to a depth of 1–2 mm of the upper dermis. Adjacent collagen and overlying dermis and epidermis may also be affected by the heat, producing a partial-thickness injury. Dermal appendages such as sweat glands and pilosebaceous glands are relatively resistant to argon laser energy and aid in the rapid healing of the laser wounds. The laser is most often used with a 1 mm spot size, 0.2 seconds exposure, and a power of 0.8–2 watts.

ADDITIONAL INFORMATION. The laser is hand held perpendicular to the skin at the focal length (2–4 cm from the skin surface) and slowly advanced according to the blanching of the lesion. Fine linear vessels are traced. Local anesthesia without epinephrine is most commonly used for adults, but children require sedation or general anesthesia.

POST-TREATMENT CARE. The wound is treated in an open wound fashion with immediate use of ice compresses, followed by application of antibiotic ointment. Alternatively, wounds in areas of trauma or in children may necessitate a sterile dressing.

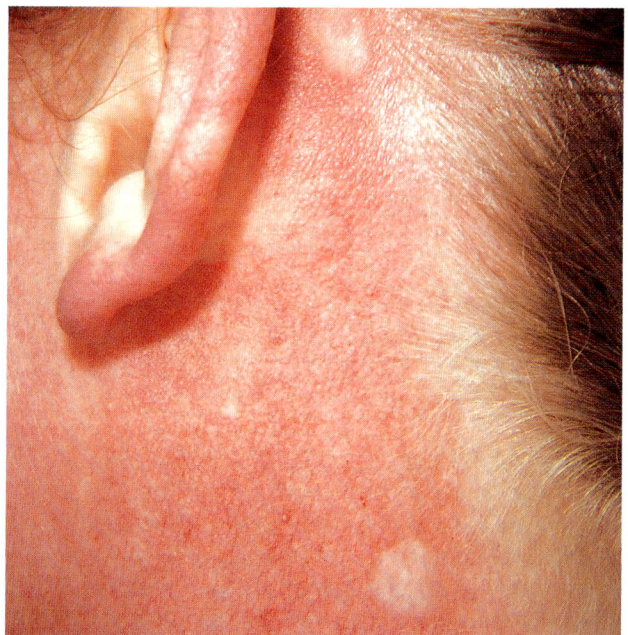

FIG. 5.15-A. Pre-treatment port wine hemangioma. Small clear blanched spot represents a test patch which healed without scarring or residual hemangioma.

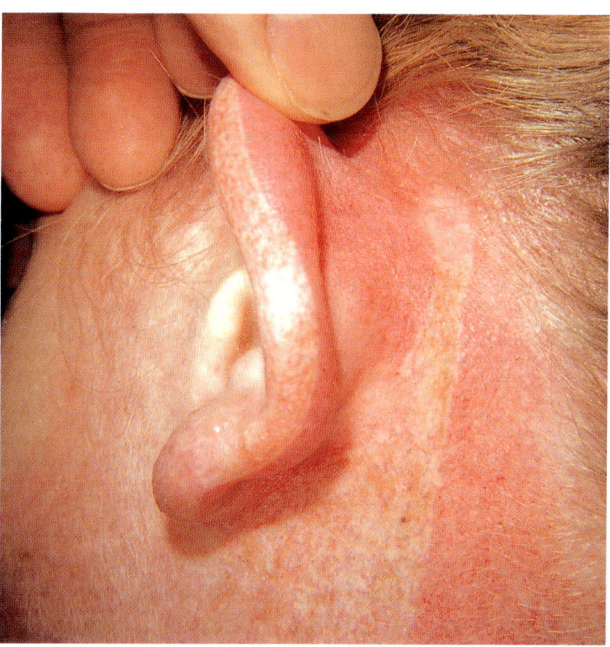

FIG. 5.15-B. Immediate blanching following argon laser photocoagulation done in a continuous manner.

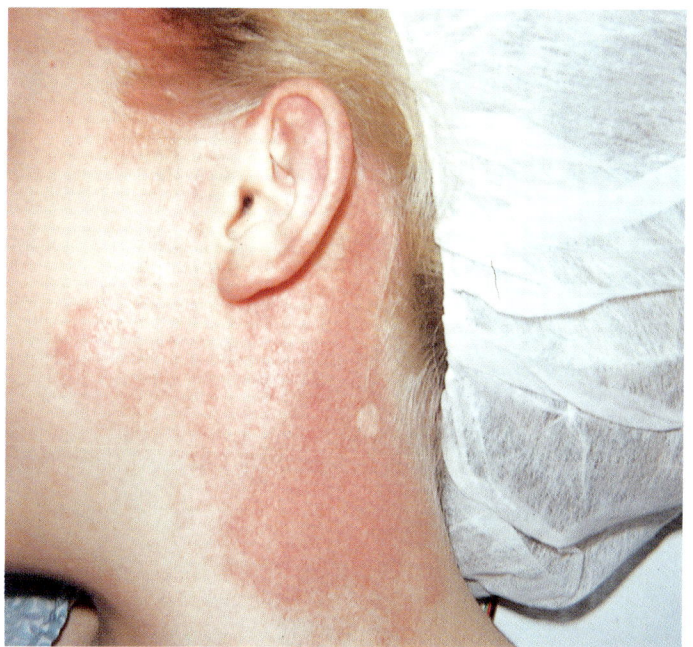

FIG. 5.15-C. Final blanching of hemangioma six months following treatment. Note that there is a 70% to 90% lightening of the lesion without scarring or texture change. Minor residual hemangioma remains.

Case courtesy of *Lovic W. Hobby*, M.D.

CASE 5.16
Port Wine Hemangioma of the Chin and Cheek

REVIEW OF CASE. Hypertrophic hemangioma (nevus flammeus) of chin and cheek in a 47-year-old male. The patient desired removal to improve the cosmetic appearance of the dark color and irregular surface.

CHOICE OF LASER: ARGON. The argon laser produces visible blue-green light between 488–514 nm. Due to the absorption spectrum of hemoglobin and melanin which both absorb light at this wavelength, both vascular and pigmented lesions can be treated. The light is absorbed and converted to heat which has the ability to accomplish thermal photocoagulation to a depth of 1–2 mm of the upper dermis. Adjacent collagen and overlying dermis and epidermis may also be affected by the heat, producing a partial-thickness injury. Dermal appendages such as sweat glands and pilosebaceous glands are relatively resistant to argon laser energy and aid in the rapid healing of the laser wounds. The laser is most often used with a 1 mm spot size, 0.2 seconds exposure, and a power of 0.8–2 watts.

ADDITIONAL INFORMATION. The laser is hand held perpendicular to the skin at the focal length (2–4 cm from the skin surface) and slowly advanced according to the blanching of the lesion. Fine linear vessels are traced. Local anesthesia without epinephrine is most commonly used for adults, but children require sedation or general anesthesia.

POST-TREATMENT CARE. The wound is treated in an open wound fashion with immediate use of ice compresses, followed by application of an antibiotic ointment. Alternatively, wounds in areas of trauma or in children may necessitate a sterile dressing.

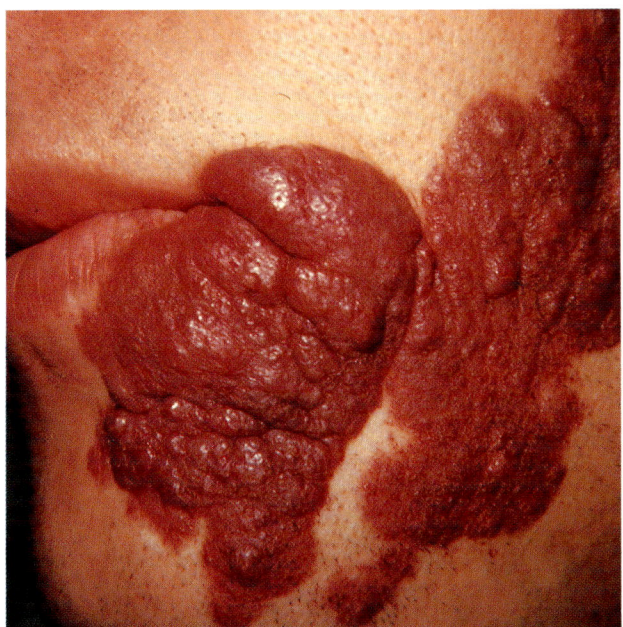

FIG. 5.16-A. Markedly hypertrophic, irregular hemangioma of the cheek and chin in a 47-year-old male. Color is deep purple and the hemangioma surface has become quite irregular with numerous blebs.

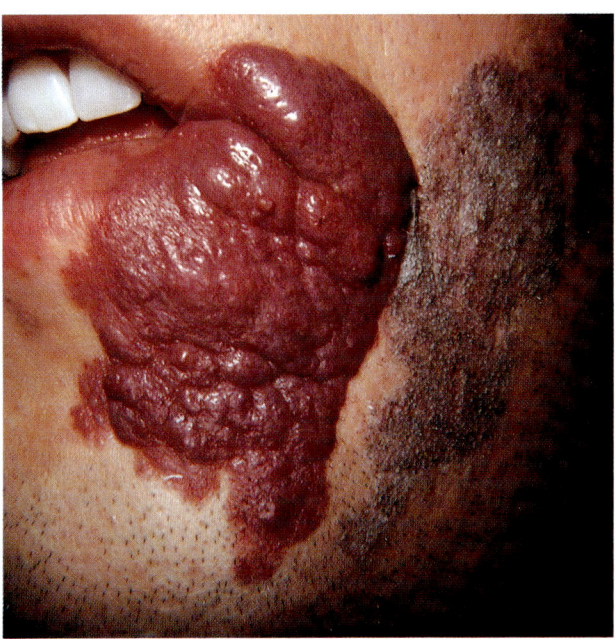

FIG. 5.16-B. Immediately following treatment, the argon laser demonstrating marked blanching and shrinkage of the hemangioma. Dark gray color is quite characteristic of thick hemangiomas immediately following laser treatment.

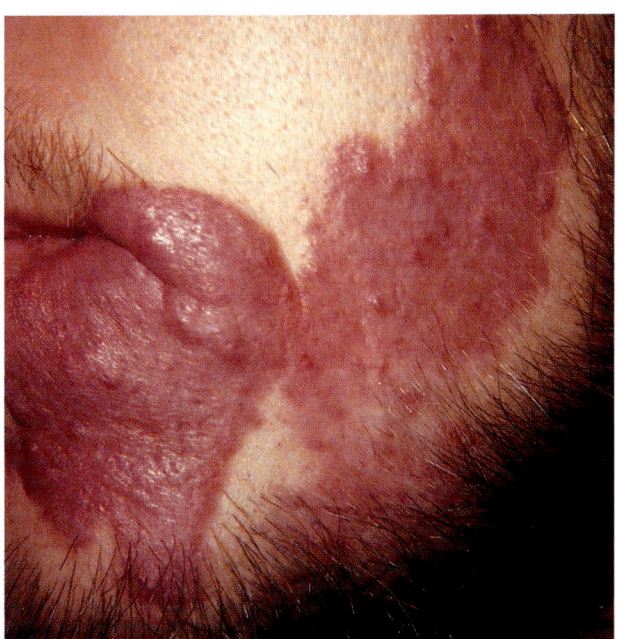

FIG. 5.16-C. Final fading of both areas of hemangioma. There has been a marked smoothening of the surface and both areas are much lighter. There is no scarring.

Case courtesy of *Lovic W. Hobby*, M.D.

CASE 5.17

Port Wine Hemangioma of the Right Face

REVIEW OF CASE. This 30-year-old male patient had a congenital port wine stain hemangioma (nevus flammeus) of his right face since birth. He had been defined as "untreatable" until the advent of the argon laser.

CHOICE OF LASER: ARGON. The blue-green argon laser light will pass through the clear epidermis causing minimal thermal damage with a chance of scarring of less than 2% and is then absorbed by the blood in the abnormal capillary network of the hemangioma in the outer dermis causing thermal damage and thrombosis. It has been shown histologically that the thrombosed "vessel layer" is replaced by colorless fibrous tissue over a period of months with a marked reduction in the color of the hemangioma but the epidermis should return to normal or show very minimal atrophic changes only.

ADDITIONAL INFORMATION. For the performance of both the test patch and treatment "minimal blanching power" is always used. With the beam on "continuous exposure" the power of the laser is gradually increased from 0.4 watts in increments of 0.2 watts until blanching is obtained in the test patch. If the test patch is successful treatment will then be carried out at this power using a focused beam of 1 mm in diameter. In practice a majority of patients in the Wessex laser unit have been treated at power levels between 0.6 and 1.2 watts and the percentage of successful results and the incidence of scarring are comparable to all other series reported in the literature. When treatment is carried out the beam is moved along the normal lines of the skin, although it is often not done directly in straight lines, but in small circles along these skin lines to avoid any linearity or striping of the final result.

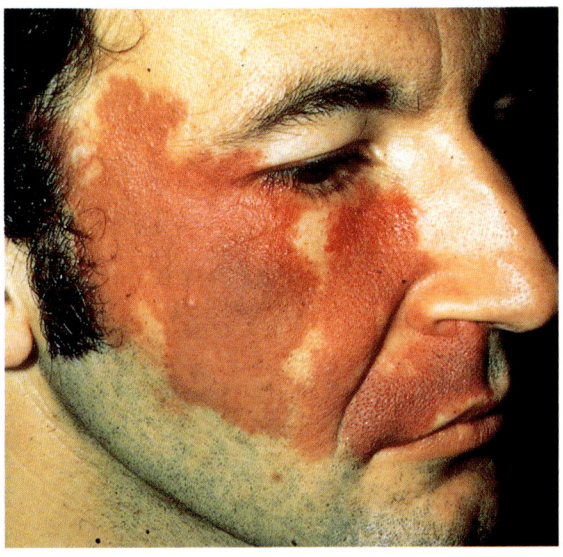

FIG. 5.17-A. Pre-treatment port wine hemangioma of cheek, eyelid, temple, and upper lip.

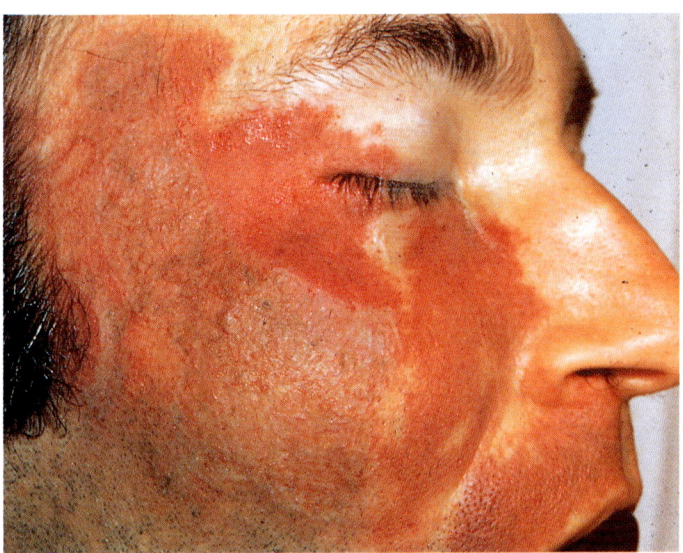

FIG. 5.17-B. The patient at the end of a treatment session which was carried out under a general anesthetic. The slightly gray color of the blanched areas is typical of the color obtained when treating a very dark purple hemangioma.

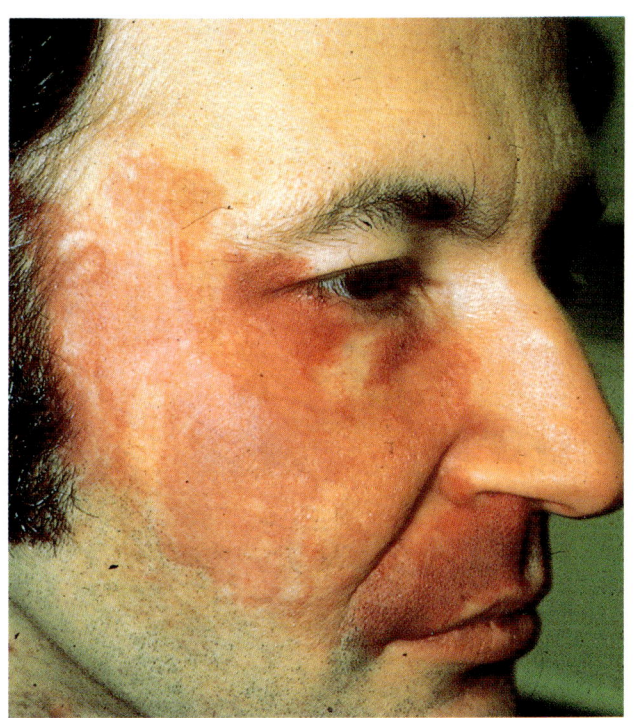

FIG. 5.17-C. The patient at the end of two treatment sessions. The posterior third of the face shows an adequate final blanching, whereas the anterior third shows some post-traumatic hyperpigmentation which is common after treatment with the argon laser and will always resolve after a period of months. It can be seen that a separate test has been carried out on this patient's upper lip. This is routine practice as this area is most prone to hypertrophic scarring, and treatment may well need to be carried out at a power level of 0.2 watts less than that used to treat the cheek. However, with the argon laser there is some significant damage to normal skin pigmentation and treated areas may show permanent hypopigmentation and may not tan normally when exposed to sunlight.

Case courtesy of *J. A. S. Carruth*, F.R.C.S.

CASE 5.18

Port Wine Hemangioma

with Cavernous Component of the Lower Lip

REVIEW OF CASE. This is a forty-year-old male with an extensive facial port wine hemangioma with a cavernous component of the lower lip. In recent years, there has been "bleb" formation in several areas with a sponge-like consistency of the skin. The patient has no associated problems and the family history is negative.

CHOICE OF LASER: ARGON. Considered best at the time of treatment. Test and treatment parameters are as follows: 1 mm spot size, exposure time 0.2 sec for earlier treatments, 20 sec sweep for later treatments; power 1.0–1.4 watts, and total number of seconds 12,256 (8 treatments).

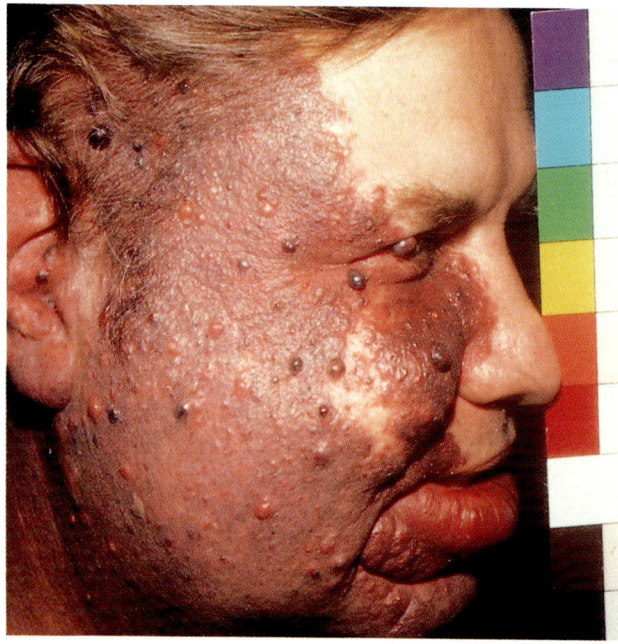

FIG. 5.18-A. Port wine hemangioma with cavernous component of lower lip pre-treatment.

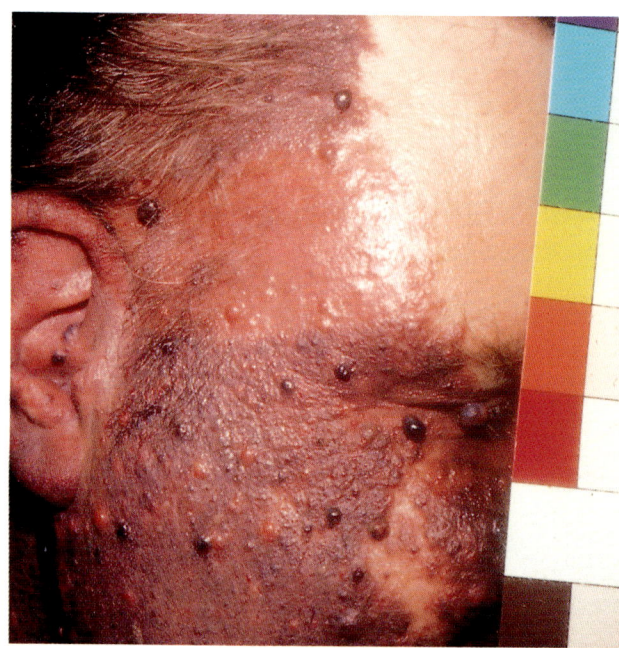

FIG. 5.18-B. Shortly after healing of temporal area.

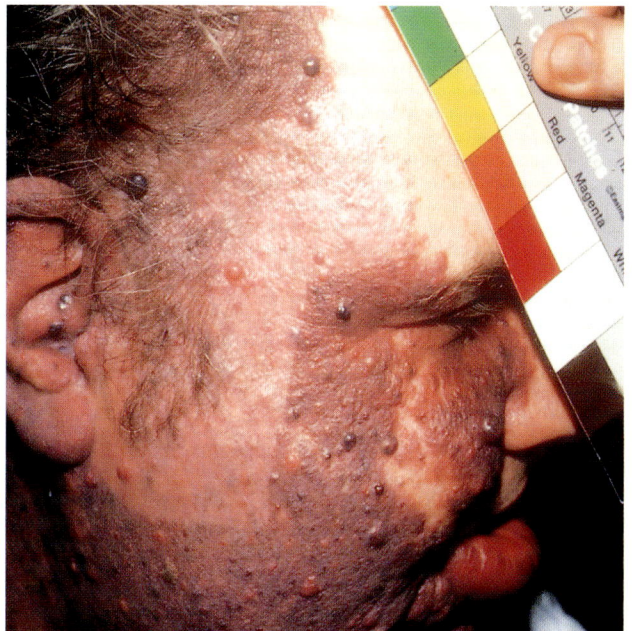

FIG. 5.18-C. Following treatment of preauricular area.

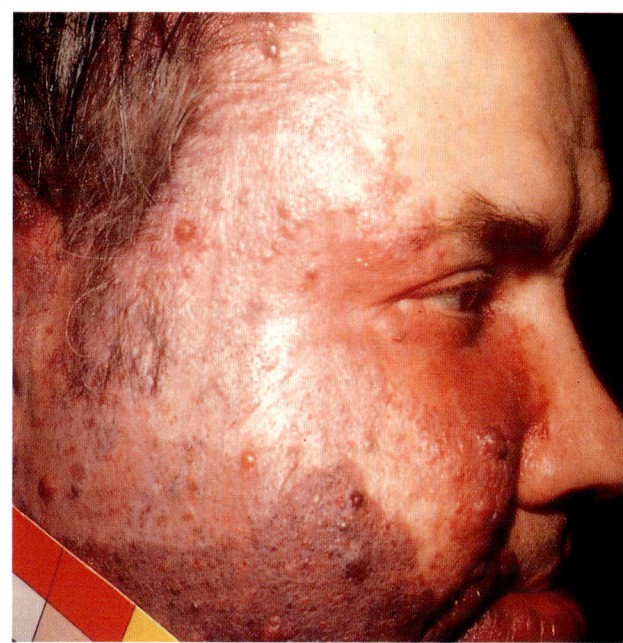

FIG. 5.18-D. Further treatment.

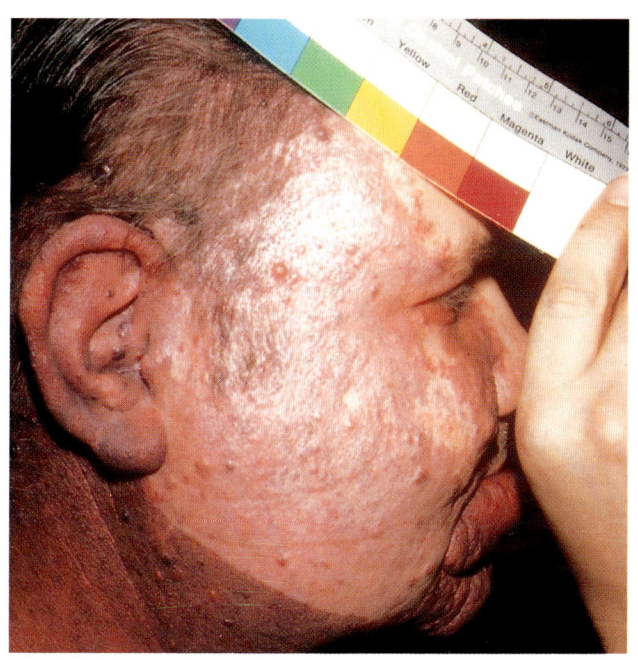

FIG. 5.18-E. Following completion of treatment of right hemi-face (14 month follow-up). Note the dramatic effect that the argon laser treatment has on the darker port wine hemangiomas.

Case courtesy of *Lester Silver*, M.D.

CASE 5.19

Port Wine Hemangioma of the Face

REVIEW OF CASE. This fifty-year-old male presented with a congenital port wine hemangioma (nevus flammeus). No prior treatment has been received. The patient has severely limited vision in the left eye as a result of progressive glaucoma. This probably represents a Sturge-Weber syndrome.

CHOICE OF LASER: ARGON. Considered best at time of treatment. Test and treatment parameters are as follows: 1 mm spot size, 20 sec sweep, 0.8–1.2 watts of power, and 1,695 treatment seconds (2 treatments).

ADDITIONAL INFORMATION. It should be noted that scarring can and does occur as a complication of argon laser photocoagulation as this treatment is a burn. The incidence of scarring is 5–10% (less with a "low dose" technique) and occurs most commonly about the lip/nose area. A lower watt dosage should be used in these areas.

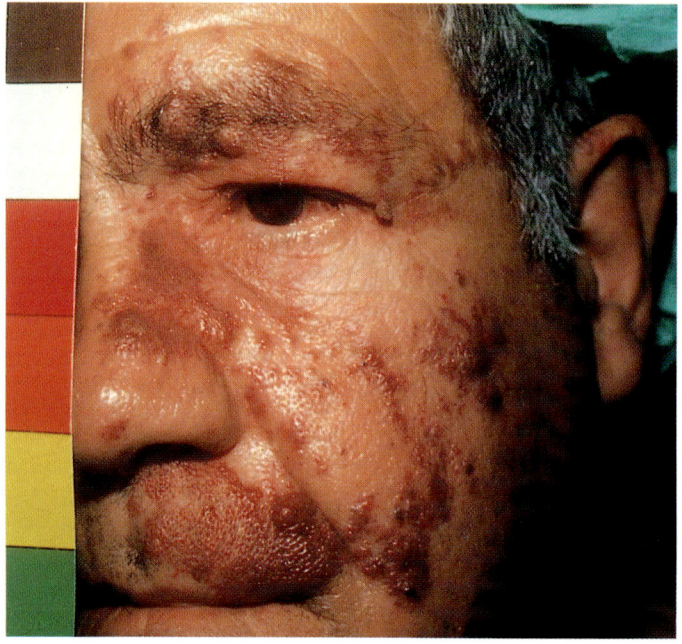

FIG. 5.19-A. Congenital port wine hemangioma pre-treatment.

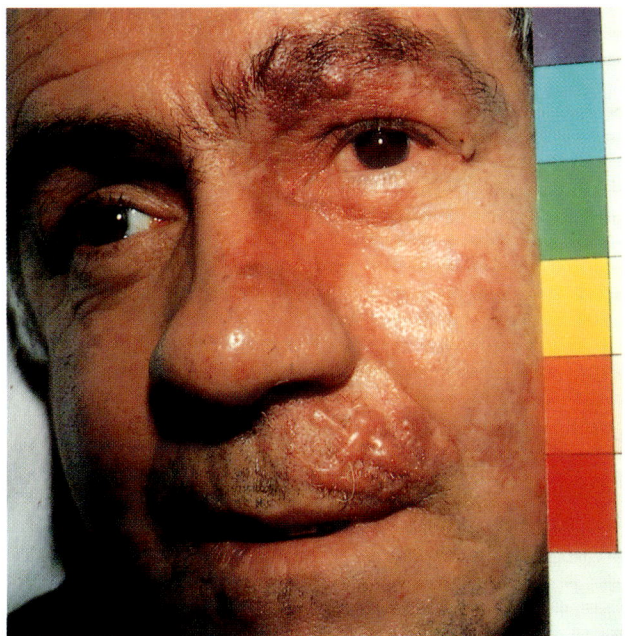

FIG. 5.19-B. Five months following treatment of lip and cheek. One month following treatment of nose. Note lip scar.

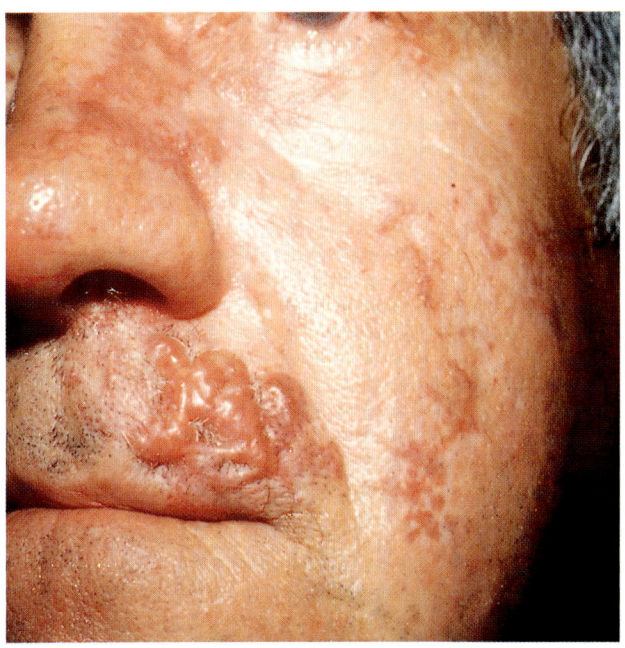

FIG. 5.19-C. Further thickening of lip scar 18 months later despite a course of local steroid injections.

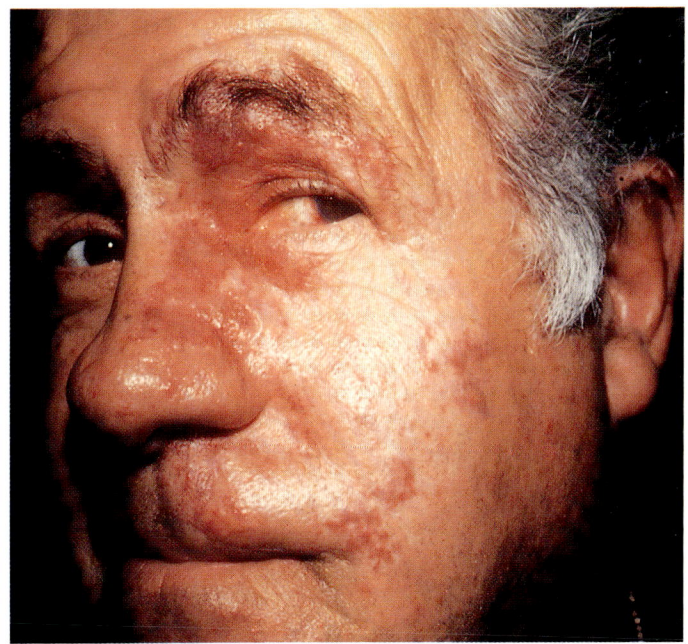

FIG. 5.19-D. Two years following lip scar excision and resurfacing with a nasal-labial flap.

Case courtesy of *Lester Silver*, M.D.

CASE 5.20

Port Wine Hemangioma of the Upper Lip

REVIEW OF CASE. This is a 34-year-old female with a port wine hemangioma (nevus flammeus) present on the upper lip.

CHOICE OF LASER: ARGON. The blue-green argon light at 488–514 nm is selectively absorbed by hemoglobin laden ectatic vessels under the skin. Penetration is down to the upper 1–2 mm of the dermis. The light is converted to heat upon absorption and has the ability to coagulate vessels with lumen diameters of 0.5 mm and smaller. The dermal appendages such as hair follicles and pilosebaceous glands are spared and aid in the rapid healing and epithelialization of the wound. The laser is used with 0.5 watts of power, 0.5 second pulse duration, and 0.2–1 mm spot size.

ADDITIONAL INFORMATION. The peri-oral area, particularly the upper lip, is highly prone to scarring. In an attempt to limit such scarring, the polka dot technique was developed. Areas prone to hypertrophic scarring such as the upper lip, chin, nasolabial fold in the face, trunk, and extremities are now treated with a "polka dot" or "pointillistic" technique. This technique consists of the formation of multiple 1–2 mm dots of blanching produced by minimal power. Each dot is separated from the adjacent one by 1–2 mm. The laser stylus is hand held (perpendicular to the skin) at a focal length of 1–3 cm. Fading as a result of the dots coalescing or the intermediate treatment of non-dotted interspaces in 12 weeks is more modest and slightly more variegated or irregular than the treatment in a single block, but scarring has been quite rare.

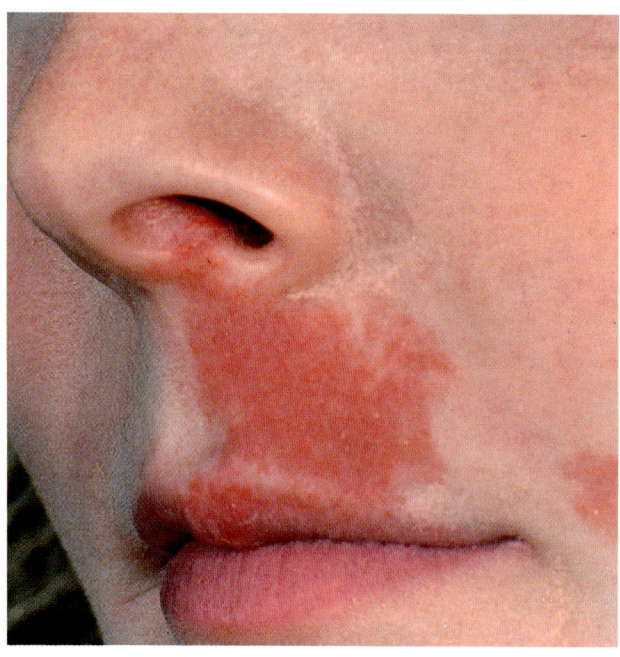

FIG. 5.20-A. Pre-treatment hemangioma of the upper lip.

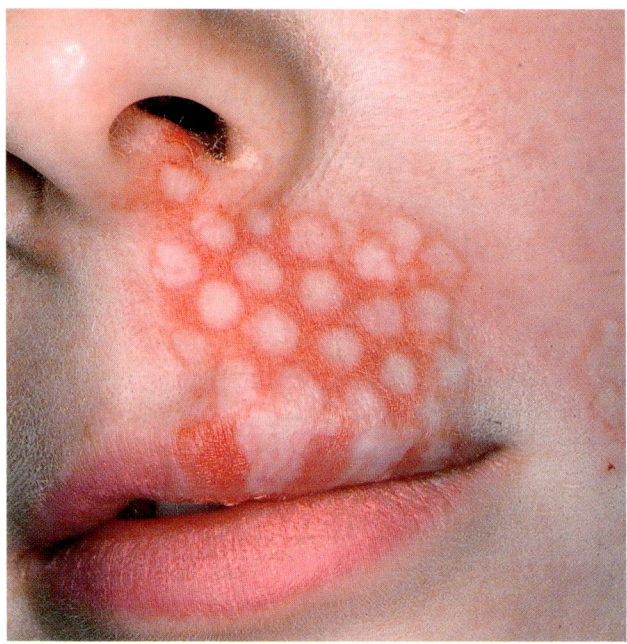

FIG. 5.20-B. Blanching after polka dot application of 1–2 mm spots of laser light leaving interspaces of untreated hemangioma.

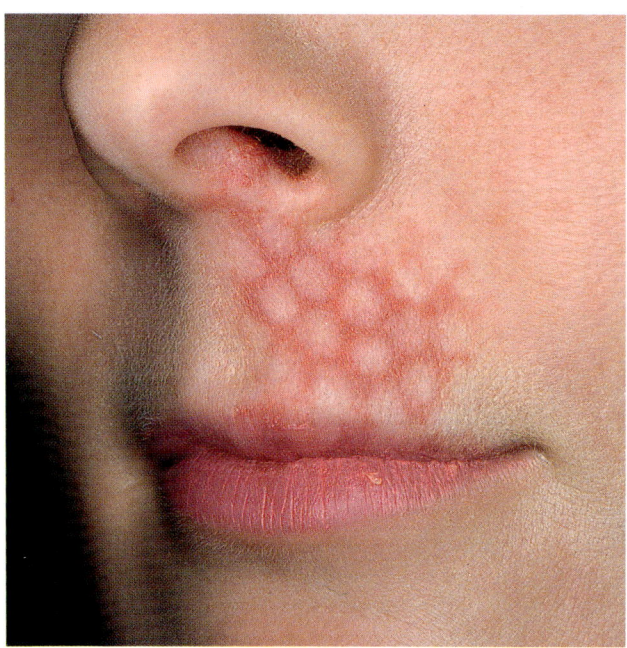

FIG. 5.20-C. Fading of first group of dots.

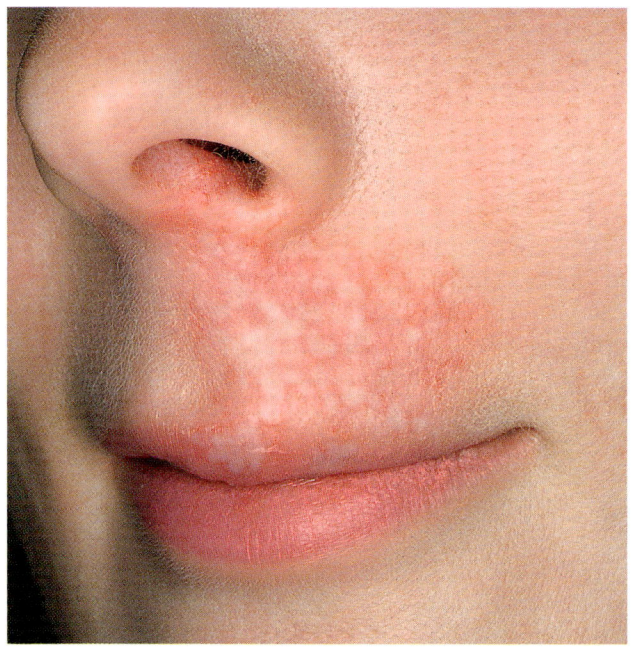

FIG. 5.20-D. Final appearance demonstrating satisfactory fading without scarring and blending together of sequential dot treatments.

Case courtesy of *David B. Apfelberg*, M.D.

For literature pertaining to this case see References section.

CASE 5.21
Strawberry Hemangioma in Infancy
Medial Canthus and Eyelid

REVIEW OF CASE.   This 5-month-old infant presented with a hemangioma involving the right medial canthus and upper eyelid. After rapid growth, she was referred by an ophthalmologist for evaluation and possible laser treatment. There had been no previous treatment.

CHOICE OF LASER: ARGON.   This case was done in 1983 prior to the availability of the pulsed dye laser. The argon laser was chosen due for its specificity to vascular tissue. Although argon laser energy is absorbed superficially, many investigators have noted its ability to induce involution or arrest the growth of a strawberry hemangioma.

ADDITIONAL INFORMATION.   We have found that it is very common to do one or more reconstructive surgical procedures following laser treatment for a complicated strawberry hemangioma. Because of this, we feel it is important to adequately educate the parents at the time of consultation regarding the limitations of laser treatment. Realistic expectations are essential. Families often have very unrealistic expectations since the magic laser is being used.

We have found the healing phase to be the most difficult part of treating infants. Depending on the size of the treated area, 2–3 weeks may be required for complete healing of the laser wound. It may be necessary to use arm restraints to keep infants from disturbing the healing wound. Use of an infant carrier or carseat for sleeping may prevent disruption of the eschar during sleep.

POST-TREATMENT CARE.   Ice pack and elevation of the head is required for the first 24 hours. Bacitracin (ophthalmic) ointment is applied twice daily after cleansing with tepid water. Swelling of the eye is expected for the first 24–48 hours. The lid and lash line is gently cleansed to prevent the eyelash from adhering. Eschar is expected to form; allow it to separate naturally and do not disrupt the scab. The patient is instructed to return to the office at three weeks and to call if he has any questions.

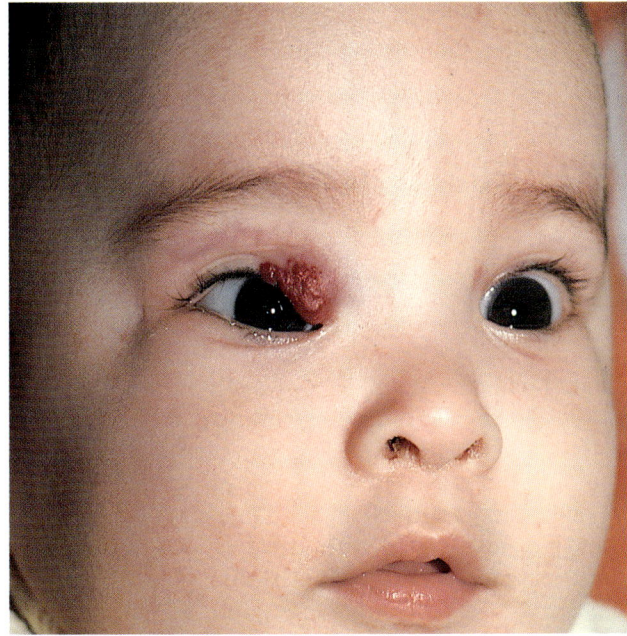

FIG. 5.21-A. Typical bulbous, bright red lesion is documented in the right medial canthal area.

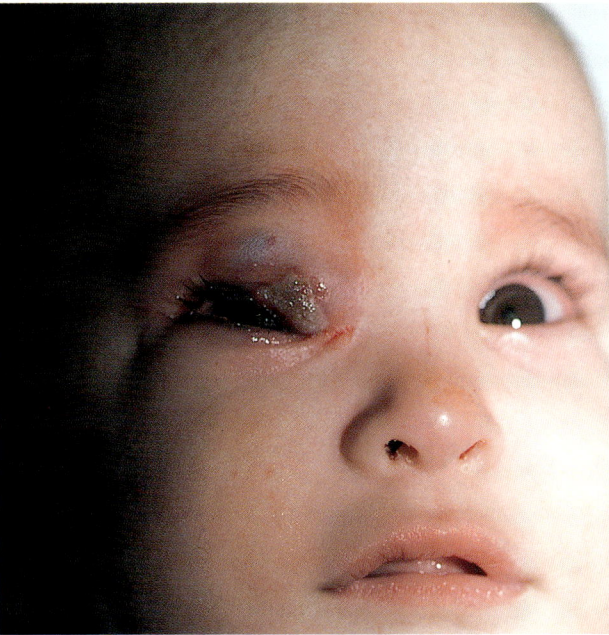

FIG. 5.21-B. Immediately following argon laser treatment, the hemangioma appears blanched. There has been some immediate reduction in the size of the lesion. The swelling noted is from the administration of local anesthetic (1% Xylocaine) prior to treatment.

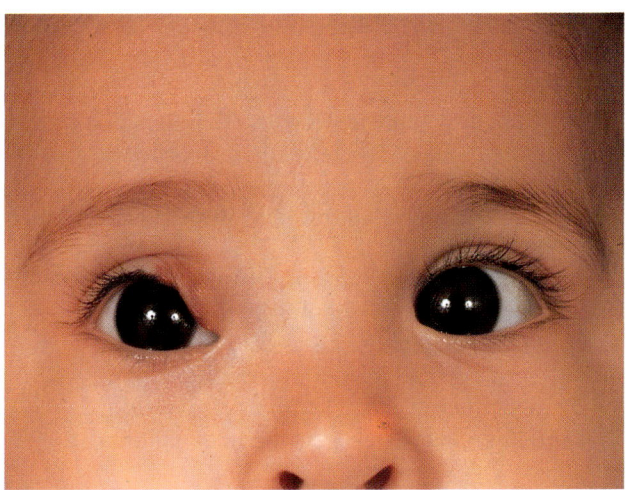

FIG. 5.21-C. Redundant skin and some residual hemangioma are seen two months after the laser treatment.

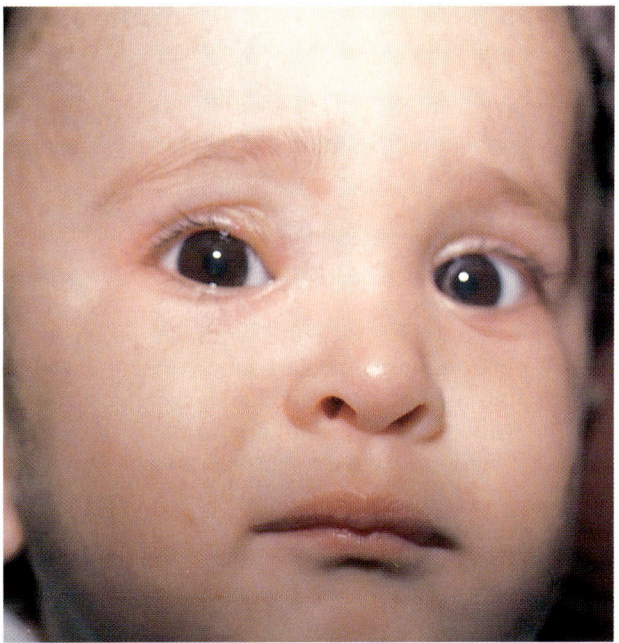

FIG. 5.21-D. Surgical excision of redundant skin and residual hemangioma were accomplished as a bloodless procedure as a result of the prior laser treatment. Result shown is two weeks post-operation.

Case courtesy of *Bruce M. Achauer*, M.D., and *Victoria M. Vander Kam*, R.N.

CASE 5.22

Strawberry Hemangioma in Infancy

Anogenital Region

REVIEW OF CASE. This five-month-old infant presented with an ulcerated, repeatedly infected hemangioma of the anogenital region. A typical history of strawberry hemangioma was related by the parents. A small red spot had been noted on the right labia at birth and grew rapidly in the next few weeks. It became ulcerated at 3 months of age and remained so for eight weeks. At the time of consultation the birthmark was ulcerated and otherwise unchanged. The infant was irritable and the mother reported repeated infection and pain associated with urination and defecation. She was referred by her family doctor and pediatrician for laser treatment. A conservative approach including local wound care over the past eight weeks had been unsuccessful.

CHOICE OF LASER: ARGON. At the time of this treatment the argon laser and Nd:YAG laser were available for the treatment of vascular lesions. Both are specific to vascular tissue with the Nd:YAG laser having a deeper penetration than the argon laser. The argon laser was chosen because it is less likely to produce scarring (1). Although the argon laser is not indicated in the treatment of port wine stain in infancy, we have found it to be useful in the management of ulcerated hemangiomas. Scarring is minimal and the results that are achieved are similar to those seen after the natural involution of a strawberry hemangioma which has become ulcerated or infected (2).

ADDITIONAL INFORMATION. Anesthesia was accomplished by infiltration with 1% lidocaine without epinephrine. The child was restrained in an Olympic papoose. The outpatient procedure involved less than 15 minutes.

In the recovery room ice packs were applied to reduce swelling and antibiotic ointment was applied to the treated area.

We have found that treatment of ulcerated, infected hemangiomas in the anogenital region results in prompt cessation of symptoms. Although healing after treatment may require as long as 3–4 weeks to be complete, with resolution following, symptoms are quickly relieved. The parents reported an immediate improvement in the child's mood, with crying, pain, and irritability minimized. The infant and family were positively impacted by this intervention. The final results (thin, white redundant skin) are the same as those expected when an infected or ulcerated hemangioma is allowed to involute on its own.

POST-TREATMENT CARE. Ice is applied for 24–28 hrs as tolerated. The area is gently cleansed with tepid water and a mild soap at each diaper change, following with an application of antibiotic ointment. The treatment area is left open to air to encourage rapid healing. Blistering and weeping of the skin is expected. Eschar forms in a few days and should not be disrupted. Apply gentle pressure to any bleeding that occurs. If bleeding persists, the doctor must be contacted or the patient taken to the emergency room. The patient's first follow-up appointment should be in three weeks. The parents are instructed to call the office if there are any questions regarding care of the treatment area. Continued resolution of the birthmark is expected over the following months. The parents are instructed to immediately call the office if there is growth of the birthmark.

For literature pertaining to this case see References section.

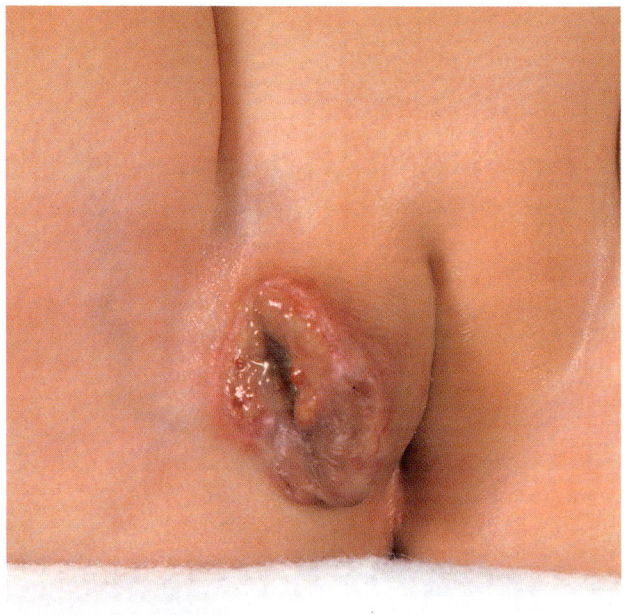

FIG. 5.22-A. Pre-operative view of five-month-old infant with ulcerated hemangioma of the right labia.

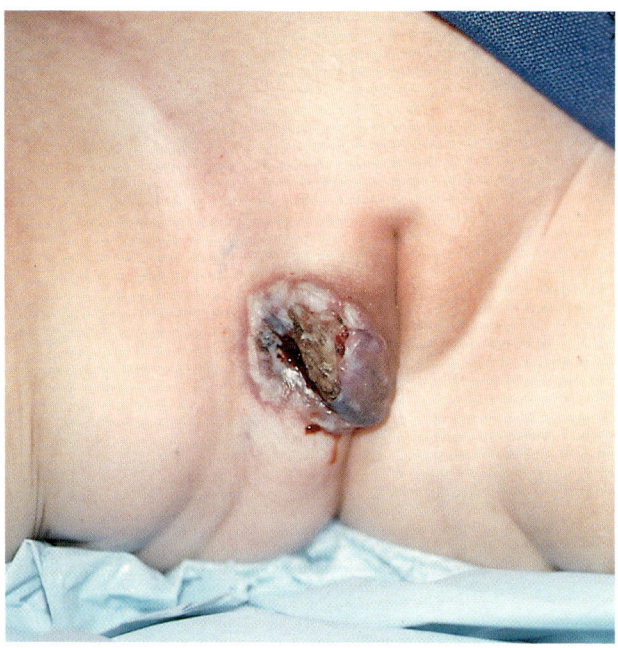

FIG. 5.22-B. Using a 2.0 mm wand, 1.8 watts of power was delivered for 89 seconds. Power was then increased to 2.2 watts for 102 seconds. A paint brush, free hand technique was used. Immediately after treatment note the expected gray/white appearance of the hemangioma. There is some visible shrinkage at the time of treatment.

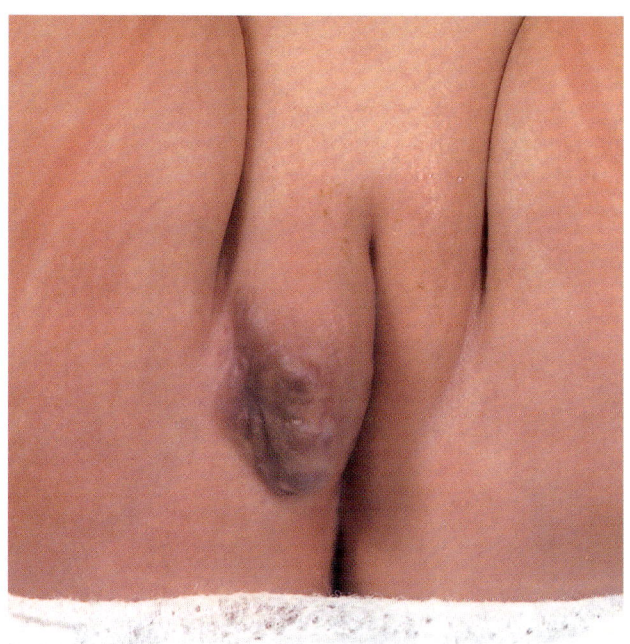

FIG. 5.22-C. Seven weeks following treatment the area is well healed with a noticeable reduction in the size of the hemangioma.

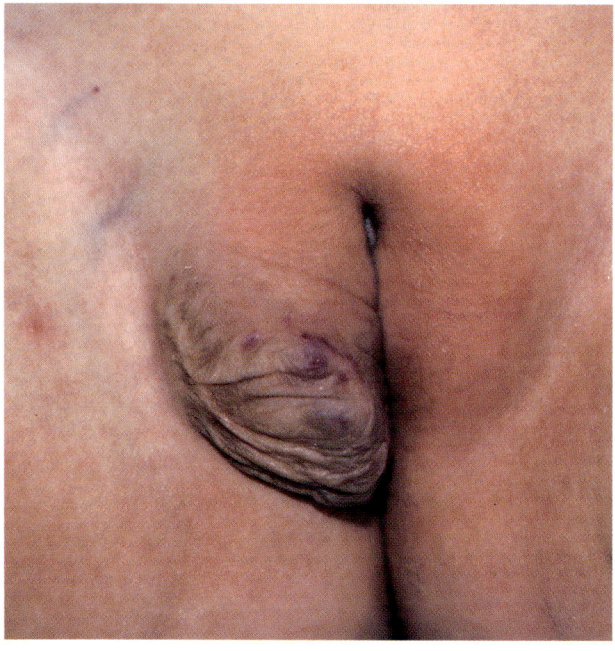

FIG. 5.22-D. Fifteen months after laser treatment there is residual hemangioma and redundant skin noted. Excision and reconstruction may be desired in the future.

Case courtesy of *Bruce M. Achauer, M.D.*, and *Victoria M. Vander Kam, R.N.*

CASE 5.23
Strawberry Hemangioma of the Lip

REVIEW OF CASE. This 4-month-old infant presented with a rapidly growing strawberry hemangioma of the upper lip. This was subject to frequent trauma from nursing and the patient had a chronically irritated bleeding upper lip area.

CHOICE OF LASER: ARGON. The argon laser produces visible blue-green light between 488–514 nm. Due to the absorption spectrum of hemoglobin and melanin which both absorb light at this wavelength, both vascular and pigmented lesions can be treated. The light is absorbed and converted to heat which has the ability to accomplish thermal photocoagulation to a depth of 1–2 mm of the upper dermis. Adjacent collagen and overlying dermis and epidermis may also be affected by the heat, producing a partial-thickness injury. Dermal appendages such as sweat glands and pilosebaceous glands are relatively resistant to the argon laser energy and aid in the rapid healing of the laser wounds. The laser is most often used with a 1 mm spot size, 0.2 seconds exposure, and a power of 0.8–2 watts.

ADDITIONAL INFORMATION. The laser is hand held perpendicular to the skin at the focal length (2–4 cm from the skin surface) and slowly advanced according to the blanching of the lesion. Fine linear vessels are traced. Local anesthesia without epinephrine is most commonly used for adults, but children require sedation or general anesthesia.

POST-TREATMENT CARE. The wound is treated in an open wound fashion with immediate use of ice compresses, followed by application of antibiotic ointment. Alternatively, wounds in areas of trauma or in children may necessitate a sterile dressing.

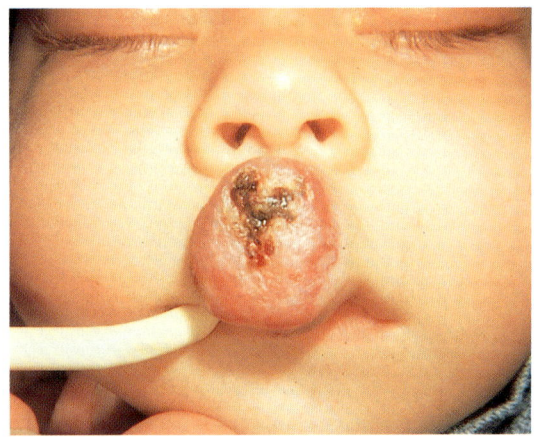

FIG. 5.23-A. Pre-treatment large strawberry hemangioma of upper lip in 4-month-old patient. Note chronic ulceration.

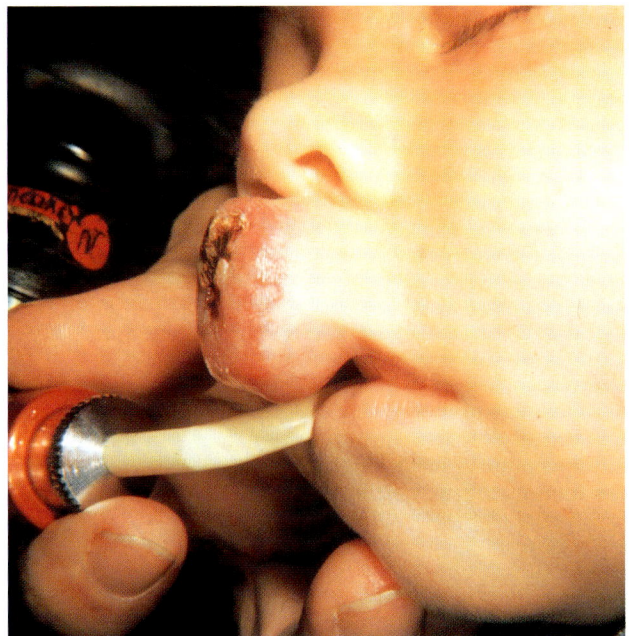

FIG. 5.23-B. Side view.

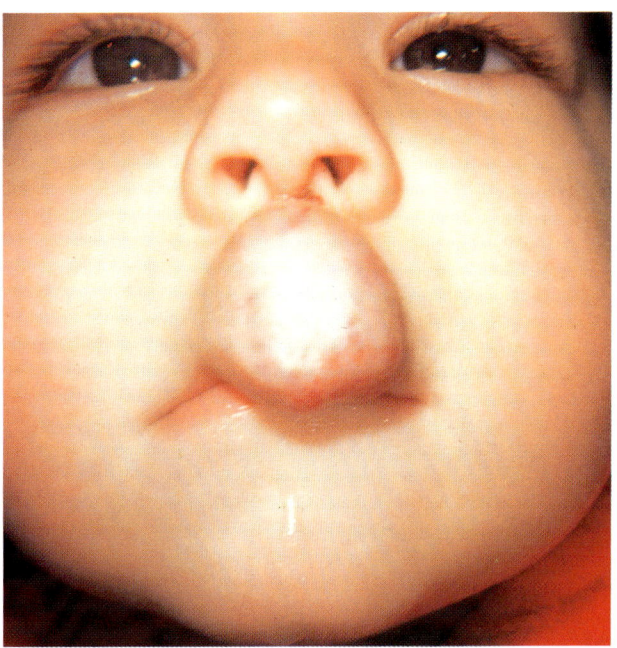

FIG. 5.23-C. Excellent healing of the surface with re-epithelialization and minimal shrinkage six months post-argon laser photocoagulation.

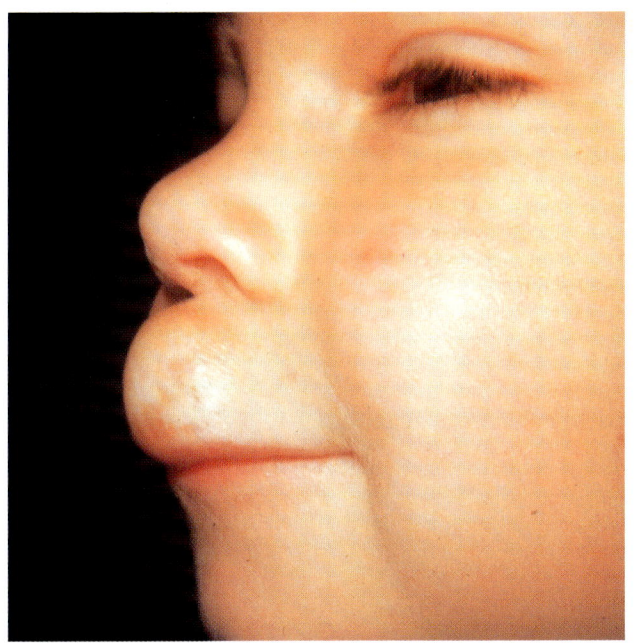

FIG. 5.23-D. Side view of patient six months following treatment.

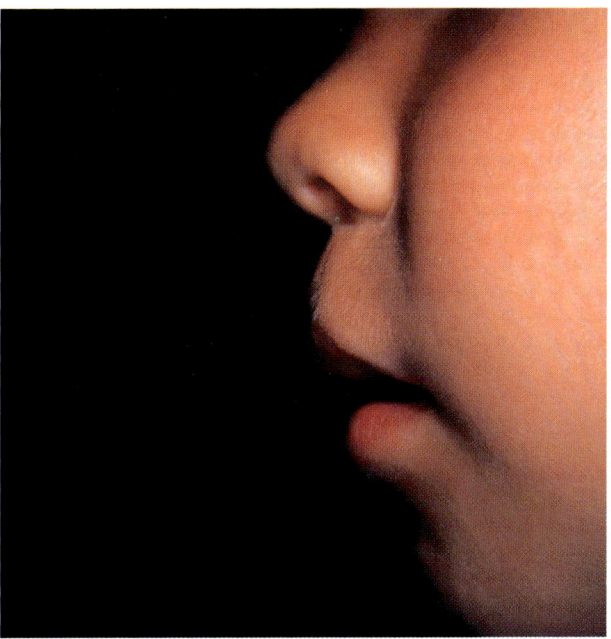

FIG. 5.23-E. Patient at age 5. Residual fibrotic tissue required conventional surgical revision.

Case courtesy of *Lovic W. Hobby*, M.D.

CASE 5.24

Telangiectasia of the Nose and Face

REVIEW OF CASE. This is a 38-year-old white female with a history of excessive sun exposure on the face. She cannot cover these lesions easily with make-up and she wanted treatment for cosmetic reasons.

CHOICE OF LASER: ARGON. It has been shown that the argon laser can absorb red color and cause photocoagulation on blood vessels. Therefore, telangiectasia can be successfully treated using the argon laser.

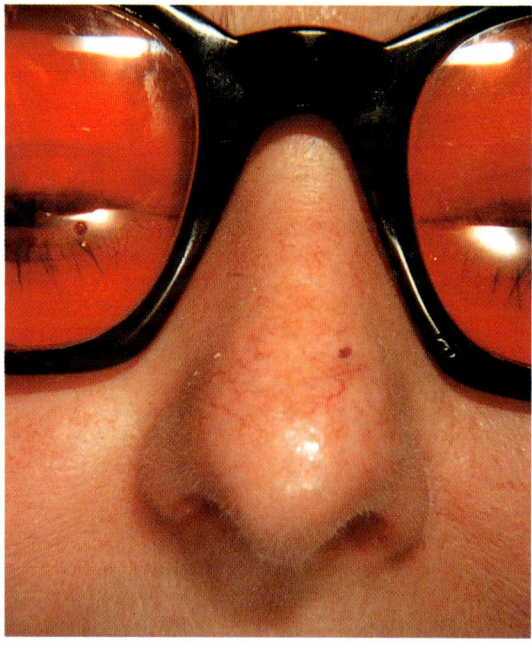

FIG. 5.24-A. Severe telangiectasia on the face, especially on the nose. Argon glasses were used for the patient and staff for eye protection. To obtain blanching 2.9 watts of power, a 0.05 sec exposure time, and repeated mode was used.

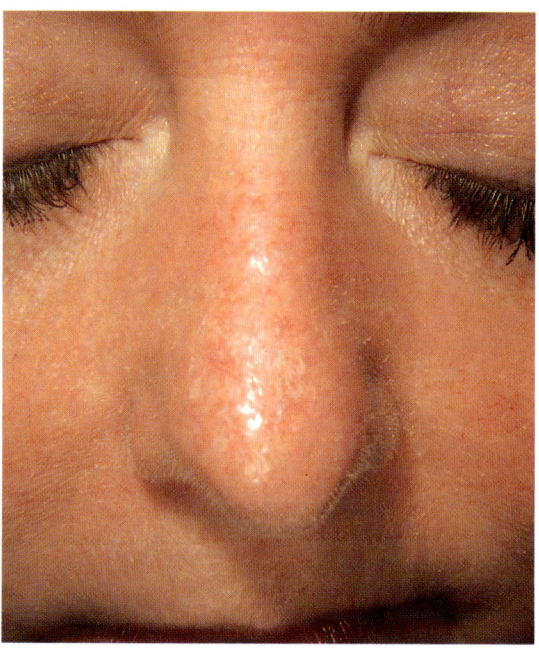

FIG. 5.24-B. Considerable improvement two months after treatment.

Case courtesy of *Syrus Rayhan*, M.D.

CASE 5.25
Telangiectasia of the Nose

REVIEW OF CASE. This is a 33-year-old male who developed telangiectasia on the nose three months after a fall.

CHOICE OF LASER: ARGON. The argon laser was chosen because argon can cause photocoagulation of blood vessels and improve the telangiectasia.

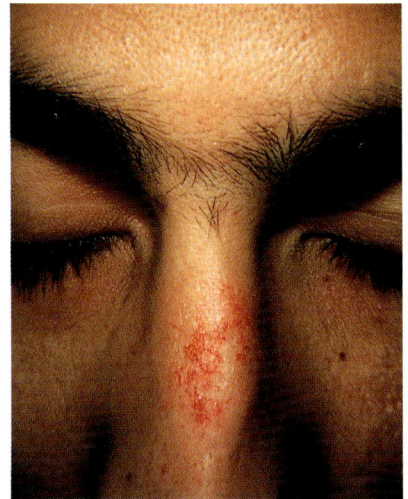

FIG. 5.25-A. Telangiectasia on the nose after an accident.

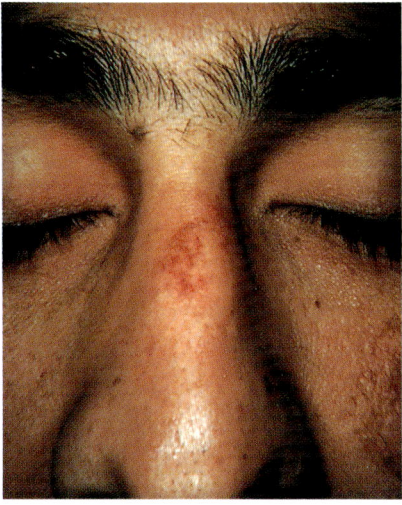

FIG. 5.25-B. One week after argon laser application. To obtain blanching a power of 2.9 watts with a pulse duration of 0.05 seconds, and repeated mode was used.

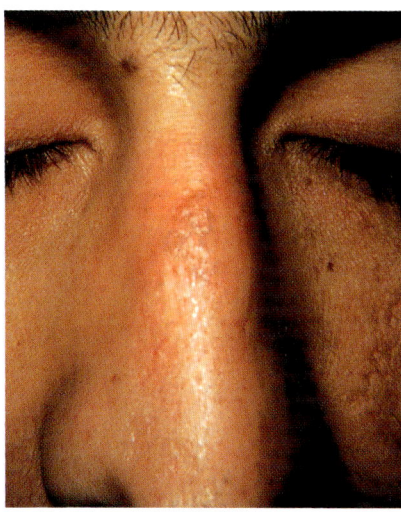

FIG. 5.25-C. Considerable improvement two months after argon laser treatment.

Case courtesy of *Syrus Rayhan, M.D.*

CASE 5.26
Telangiectasia Macularis Erupta Perstans
Urticaria Pigmentosa

REVIEW OF CASE. This 30-year-old woman presented with a generalized form of urticaria pigmentosa. The patient sought treatment because of the cosmetic disturbance and the urticarial reactions occurring on the skin.

CHOICE OF LASER: ARGON. The argon laser was chosen because of the strong telangiectatic factor involved and the patient was treated with a pulse diameter of 2 mm, at 6 watts, and a pulse duration of 0.1 second.

ADDITIONAL INFORMATION. The cosmetic impact as well as the discomfort caused by the macular eruptions was strongly diminished and the patient was very satisfied with the result.

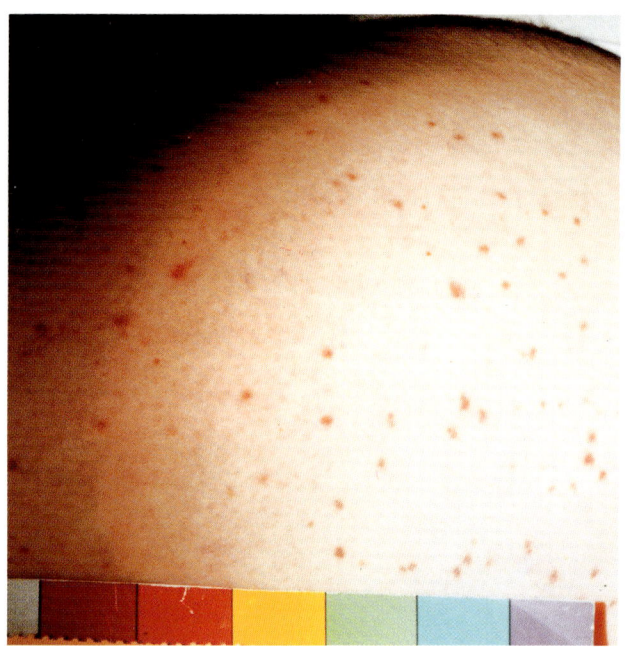

FIG. 5.26-A. Urticaria pigmentosa before treatment.

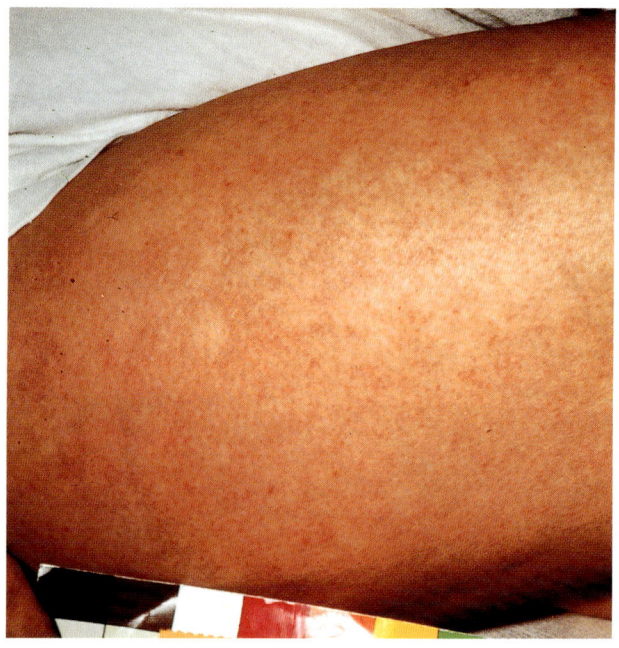

FIG. 5.26-B. Result after laser treatment.

Case courtesy of *J. P. Hulsbergen Henning*, M.D.

CASE 5.27
Venous Lake of the Lower Lip

REVIEW OF CASE. This 46-year-old female had a 6 year history of a dark blue soft nodule on the lower lip. The lesion did not have a history of bleeding.

CHOICE OF LASER: ARGON. The argon laser was used to coagulate and carbonize this vascular lesion as a treatment of choice. Venous lake is composed of dilated blood-filled venules that can be coagulated with argon laser energy.

POST-TREATMENT CARE. The lesion was completely healed after 2 weeks of treatment with bacitracin ointment applied to the scab after eating.

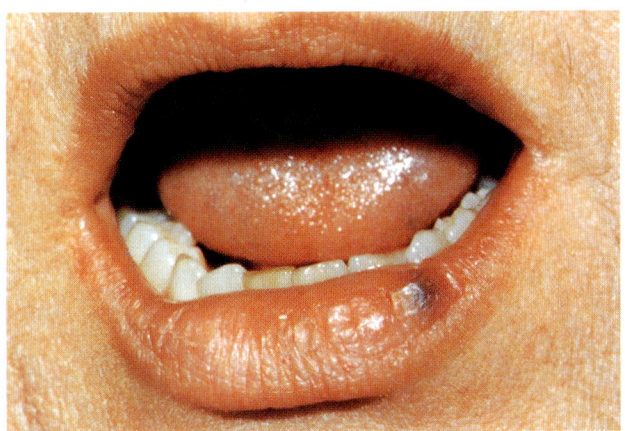

FIG. 5.27-A. Venous lake on the lower lip (0.7 × 0.6 cm in size) in 46-year-old female before treatment.

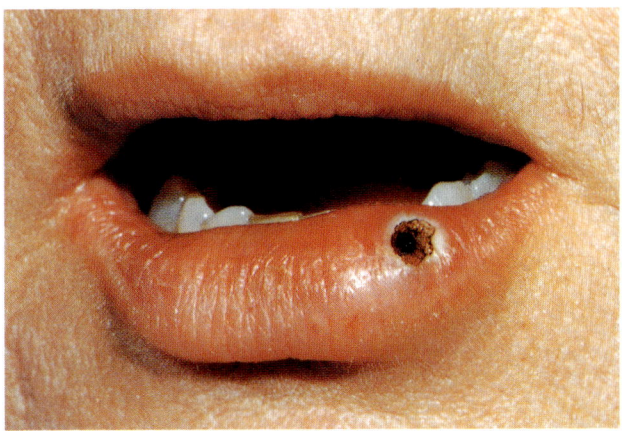

FIG. 5.27-B. The lesion immediately after argon laser irradiation (power 2 watts, spot size 1 mm in continuous mode). Local anesthesia with 2% lidocaine without epinephrine was given before treatment.

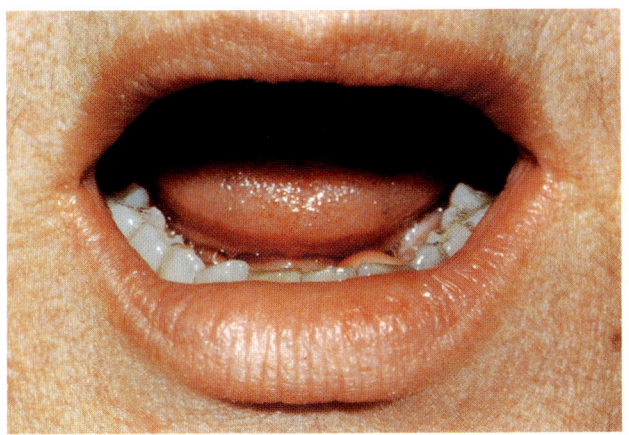

FIG. 5.27-C. Patient 2 months after argon laser treatment.

Case courtesy of *Krystyna A. Pasyk*, M.D., Ph.D.

CASE 5.28
Venous Lake of the Lip

REVIEW OF CASE. This 65-year-old white female developed a venous lake 15 mm in diameter on her lower lip within the past 8 years.

CHOICE OF LASER: ARGON. The energy required was at least 2 watts and the tunable yellow 577 nm wavelength laser could only achieve 1 watt of power. 488–514 nm wavelength was used at 0.5 seconds pulse duration, 2 watts of power, and 3 mm spot size. The 3 mm spot size was used to cause a relatively wide area of tissue damage until a complete collapse, and blanching of the lesion was achieved (Fig. B). A smaller spot size might cause bleeding which would interfere with therapy. The patient underwent a single treatment without recurrence at 6 months.

POST-TREATMENT CARE. The patient was advised to only eat soft, cold food for 48 hours post-treatment and to sleep on two pillows in order to reduce edema formation.

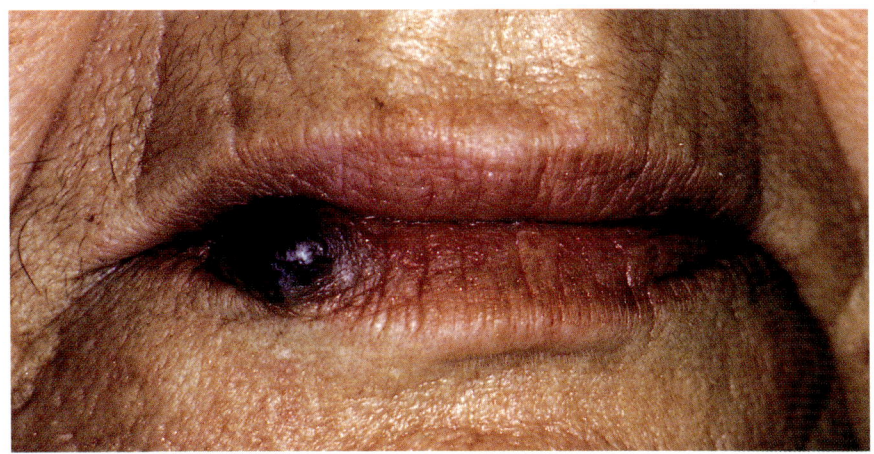

FIG. 5.28-A. Venous lake of the lip.

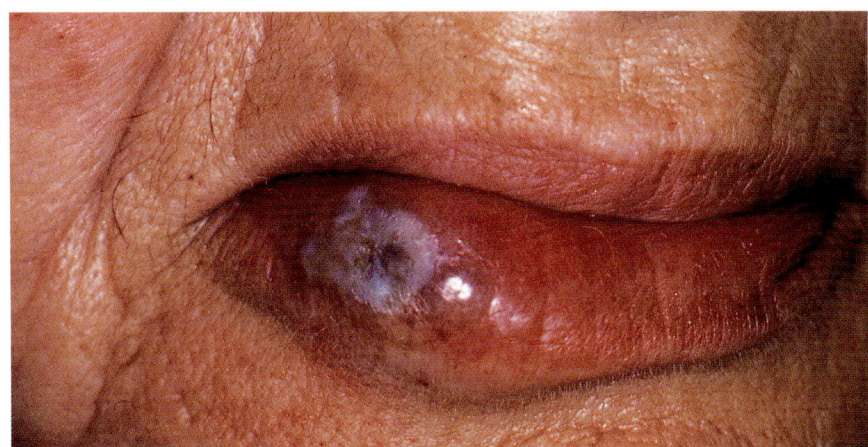

FIG. 5.28-B. Immediately post-treatment.

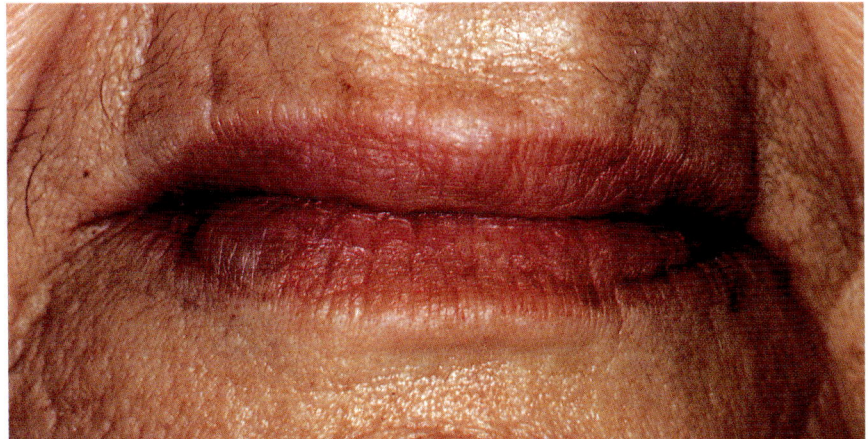

FIG. 5.28-C. Final result, one year post-treatment.

Case courtesy of *Arie Orenstein*, M.D.

CASE 5.29
Venous Malformations

REVIEW OF CASE. This 6-year-old girl was born with vascular lesions on the right corner of her mouth that did not show any tendency to involute. She was referred to the laser clinic for treatment.

CHOICE OF LASER: ARGON. The argon laser, whose energy is selectively absorbed by the hemoglobin in the red blood cells and transformed into heat, was chosen to coagulate these abnormal blood vessels.

POST-TREATMENT CARE. Bacitracin ointment on the corner of the mouth was recommended 4–5 times daily during healing process.

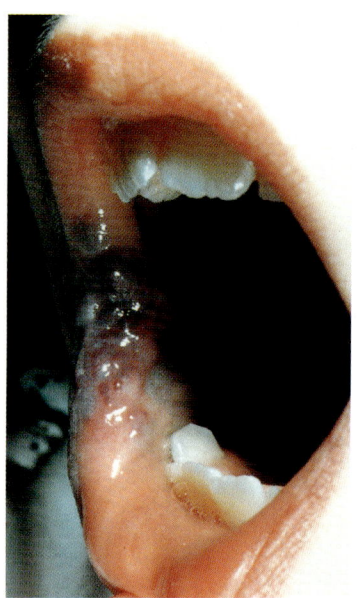

FIG. 5.29-A. Venous malformations in the corner of the mouth in a 6-year-old girl before treatment with the argon laser.

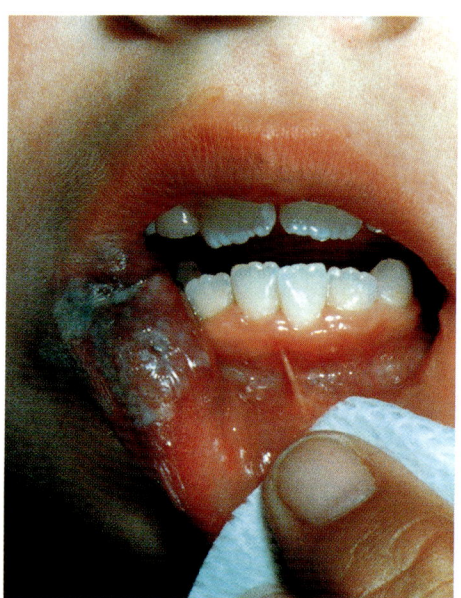

FIG. 5.29-B. Immediately after coagulation of dilated blood vessels the argon laser (power of 2 watts, spot size 1 mm, and exposure time 0.2 sec). Local anesthesia with 2% lidocaine without epinephrine preceded treatment.

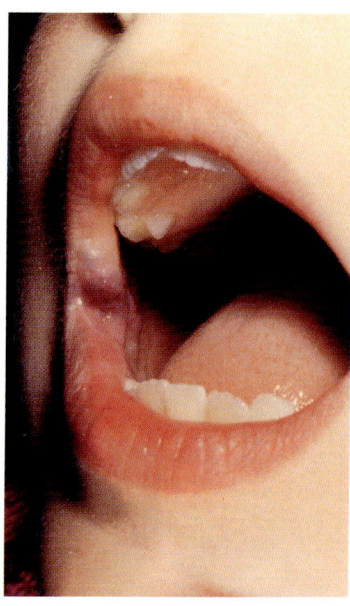

FIG. 5.29-C. Status 6 months after argon laser surgery showing significant improvement. The patient was reexamined at age 9 years and required no further treatment.

Case courtesy of **Krystyna A. Pasyk, M.D., Ph.D.**

CASE 5.30
Verruca Vulgaris of the Finger

REVIEW OF CASE. This 17-year-old female presented with warts on the finger of five years duration. The lesions had been treated with various methods including podophyllin, electrodesiccation and currettage, and cryosurgery. The patient was referred for laser treatment.

CHOICE OF LASER: ARGON. We used the argon laser to vaporize and carbonize the warts knowing that any method of treatment that is employed in warts may be successful because of its psychotherapeutic effects alone.

ADDITIONAL INFORMATION. Vaporization and carbonization of the warts by the argon laser must be done with a smoke evacuator during treatment procedures. The evacuator will remove hazardous particles and papilloma viruses in the smoke, which otherwise could be deposited deep in the respiratory tract.

POST-TREATMENT CARE. Daily cleaning of the treated area with soap and water and application of bacitracin and a dressing was recommended during the healing process.

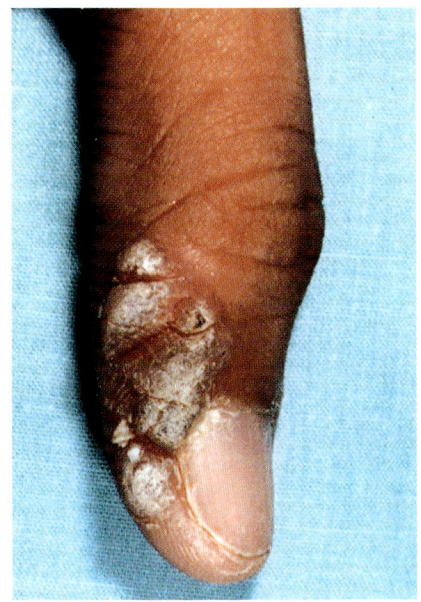

FIG. 5.30-A. Warts on the thumb near the nail margin before laser surgery.

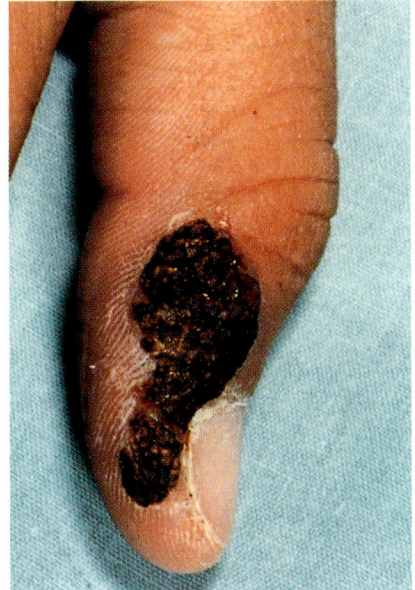

FIG. 5.30-B. Vaporized and carbonized warts immediately after argon laser surgery. Following local anesthesia with 2% lidocaine without epinephrine the lesions were removed using 1,800 laser beams with a power 2.5 watts, spot size 1 mm, and exposure time of 0.2 sec.

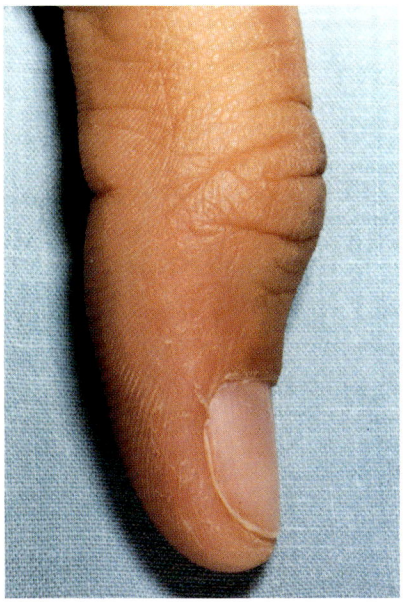

FIG. 5.30-C. No scar was observed 6 months after treatment with the argon laser. The lesions did not recur over a five year follow-up.

Case courtesy of *Krystyna A. Pasyk, M.D., Ph.D.*

CASE 5.31

Decorative Tattoo

Comparison of Argon and CO_2 Lasers

REVIEW OF CASE. This 34-year-old male presented with a professional decorative tattoo on the deltoid area.

CHOICE OF LASER: ARGON AND CARBON DIOXIDE LASERS. Argon laser energy at 488–514 nm is attracted selectively and absorbed by tattoo particles suspended in the upper dermis. The absorbed light is converted to heat and the dye particles regardless of color are expelled in a gaseous form during the localized vaporization of the surrounding cells as part of the laser "plume." An inflammatory wound phase follows with secondary washout of remaining dye particles in the accompanying exudate and subsequent eschar. The result is usually the obliteration of the tattoo pigment, replaced by a shiny, superficial scar or texture change. The argon laser is used with 1 watt of continuous power.

ADDITIONAL INFORMATION. The argon laser is slowly passed over the tattoo until a black vaporization or charring is produced evident at times by an audible "popping" or "snapping." The stylus is focused at the focal length and slowly passed onto new areas. Occasionally, the char is wiped away with saline and a second pass is made with the laser, especially if the tattoo is very deep.

POST-TREATMENT CARE. The wound is treated as an open wound. The patient is instructed to shower daily and apply antibiotic ointment or aloe vera gel until the eschar has separated and the surface epithelializes. If there is evidence of hypertrophy, continuous pressure and cortisone injections are begun.

Reprinted with permission of Little, Brown and Company.
For literature pertaining to this case see References section.

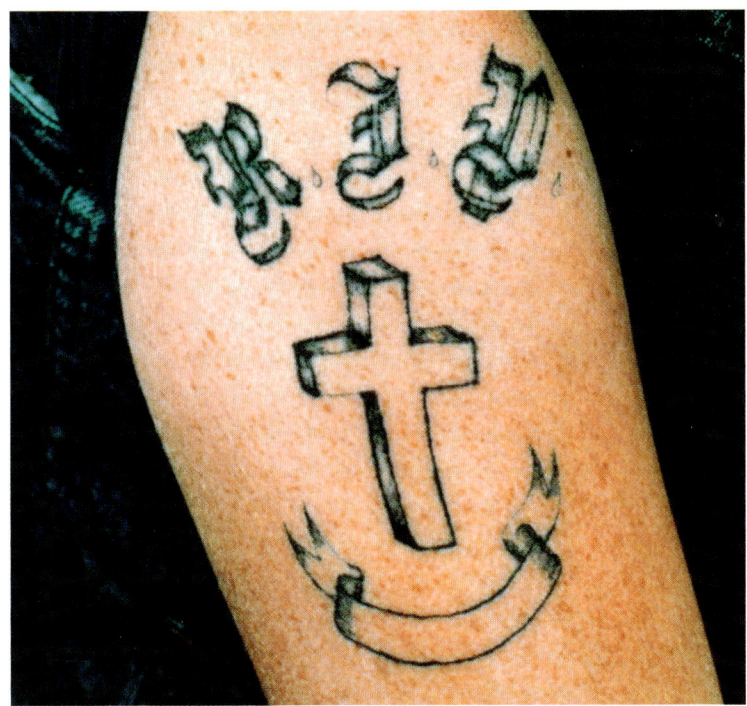

FIG. 5.31-A. Pre-operative view of decorative tattoo of right deltoid area.

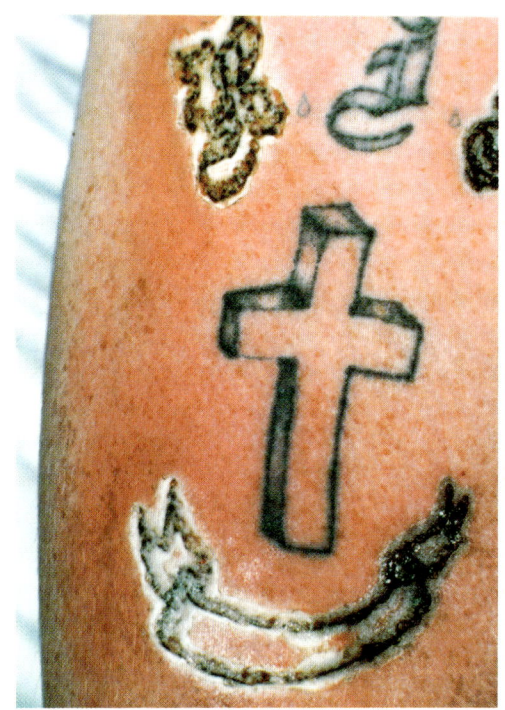

FIG. 5.31-B. The images on the left were treated with the carbon dioxide laser and the images on the right were vaporized with the argon laser.

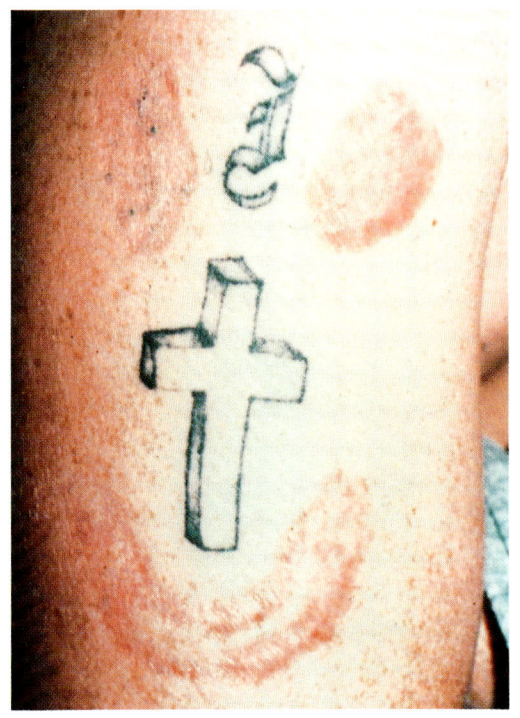

FIG. 5.31-C. Final result 8 weeks after treatment. Left and right sides have an equivalent clinical result.

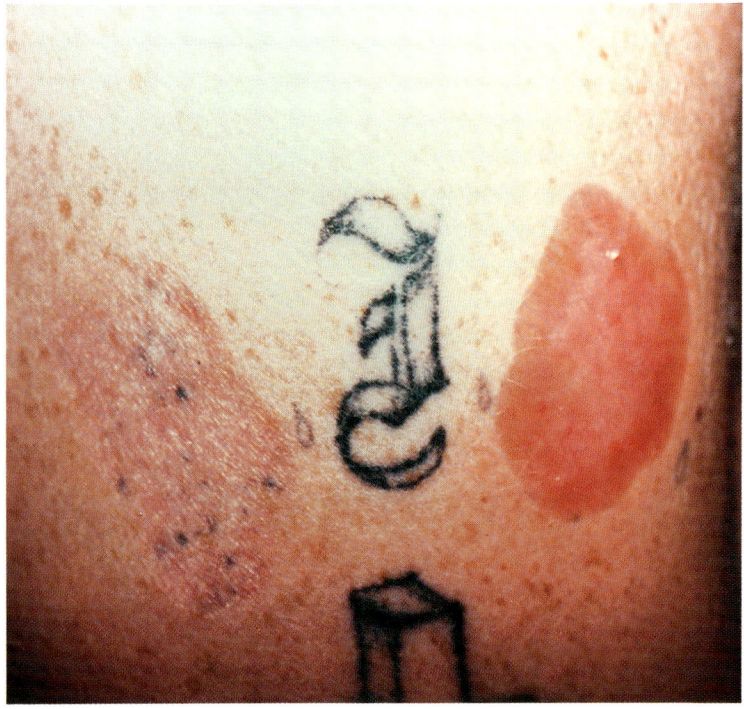

FIG. 5.31-D. Close-up of laser treated areas, left (argon) and right (carbon dioxide).

Case courtesy of *David B. Apfelberg,* M.D.

CASE 5.32

Decorative Tattoo

REVIEW OF CASE. This 25-year-old male desired removal of a colored professional decorative tattoo.

CHOICE OF LASER: ARGON. Argon laser energy at 488–514 nm is attracted selectively and absorbed by tattoo particles suspended in the upper dermis. The absorbed light is converted to heat and the dye particles regardless of color are expelled in a gaseous form during the localized vaporization of the surrounding cells as part of the laser "plume." An inflammatory wound phase follows with secondary washout of remaining dye particles in the accompanying exudate and subsequent eschar. The result is usually the obliteration of the tattoo pigment, replaced by a shiny, superficial scar or texture change. The argon laser is used with 1 watt of continuous power.

ADDITIONAL INFORMATION. The argon laser is slowly passed over the tattoo until a black vaporization or charring is produced evident at times by an audible "popping" or "snapping." The stylus is focused at the focal length and slowly passed onto new areas. Occasionally, the char is wiped away with saline and a second pass is made with the laser, especially if the tattoo is very deep. Care must be taken to disguise or camouflage the original shape and pattern of the tattoo and change it into a geometrical shape (square, oval, etc.). Normal skin adjacent to the tattoo must be vaporized as well, otherwise the original pattern may be discernible.

POST-TREATMENT CARE. The wound is treated as an open wound. The patient is instructed to shower daily and apply antibiotic ointment or aloe vera gel until the eschar has separated and the surface epithelializes. If there is evidence of hypertrophy, continuous pressure and cortisone injections are started.

For literature pertaining to this case see References section.

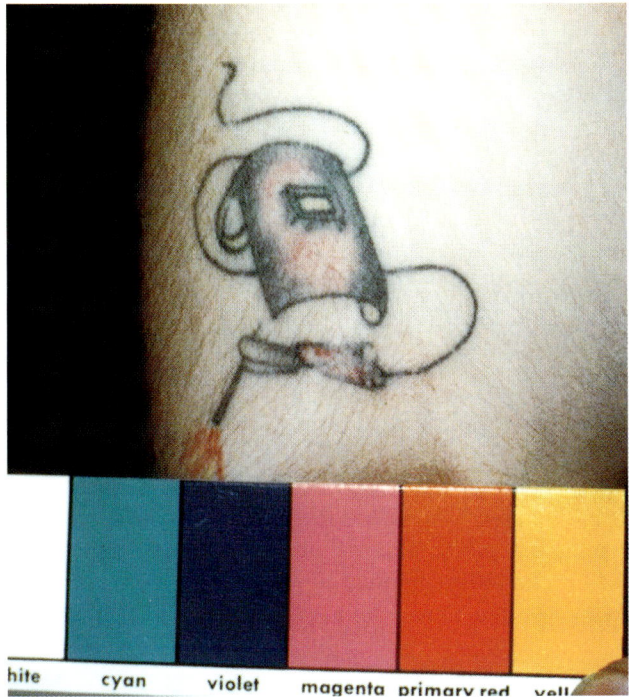

FIG. 5.32-A. Professional tattoo of right deltoid area showing welder's mask and torch.

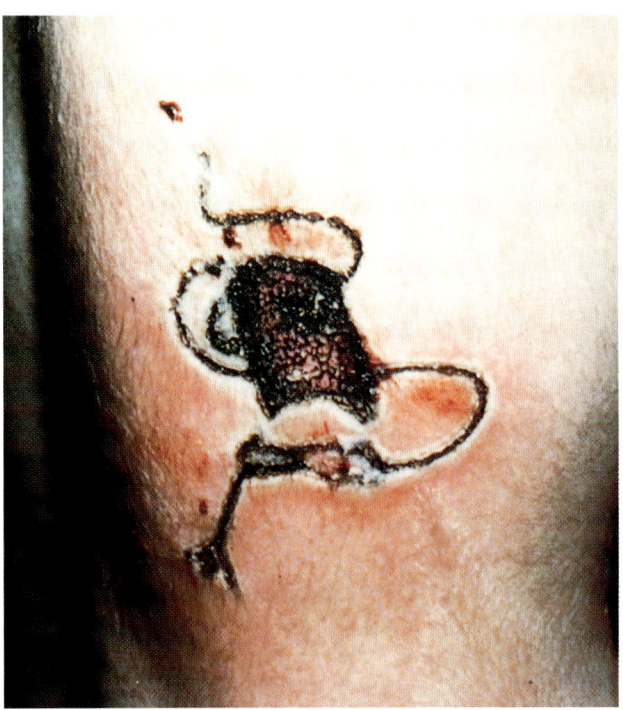

FIG. 5.32-B. Immediately following vaporization of pigment by argon laser.

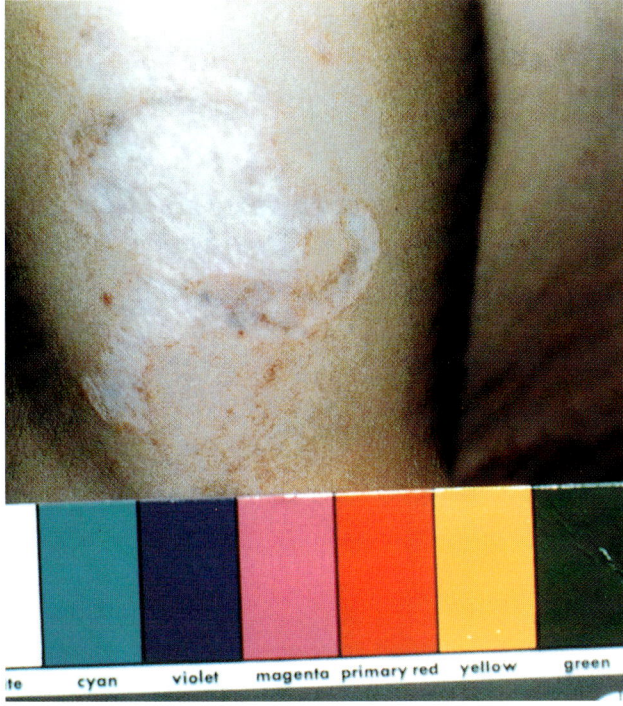

FIG. 5.32-C. Final result demonstrating obliteration of pigment with residual texture change of skin.

Case courtesy of *David B. Apfelberg*, M.D.

CASE 5.33
Decorative Tattoo

REVIEW OF CASE. This 27-year-old female had an India ink home-made tattoo. She desired removal for cosmetic purposes.

CHOICE OF LASER: ARGON. Argon laser energy at 488–514 nm is attracted selectively and absorbed by tattoo particles suspended in the upper dermis. The absorbed light is converted to heat and the dye particles regardless of color are expelled in a gaseous form during the localized vaporization of the surrounding cells as part of the laser "plume." An inflammatory wound phase follows with secondary washout of remaining dye particles in the accompanying exudate and subsequent eschar. The result is usually the obliteration of the tattoo pigment, replaced by a shiny, superficial scar or texture change. The argon laser is most often used with a 1 mm spot size, 0.2 seconds exposure, and a power of 0.8 to 2 watts.

ADDITIONAL INFORMATION. The laser is hand held perpendicular to the skin at the focal length (2–4 cm from the skin surface) and slowly advanced according to blanching of the lesion. Fine linear vessels are traced. Local anesthesia without epinephrine is most commonly used for adults, but children require sedation or general anesthesia.

POST-TREATMENT CARE. The wound is treated in an open wound fashion with immediate use of ice compresses, followed by application of an antibiotic ointment. Alternatively, wounds in areas of trauma or in children may necessitate a sterile dressing.

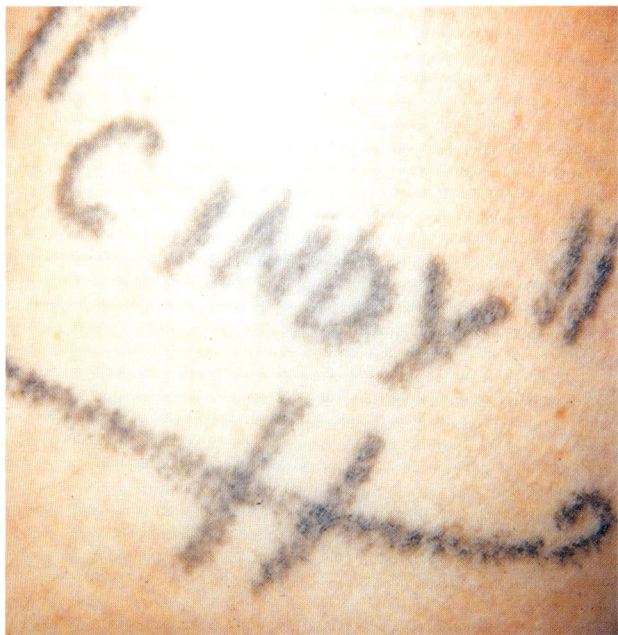

FIG. 5.33-A. Tattoo of left upper outer arm prior to treatment demonstrating home-made amateur tattoo.

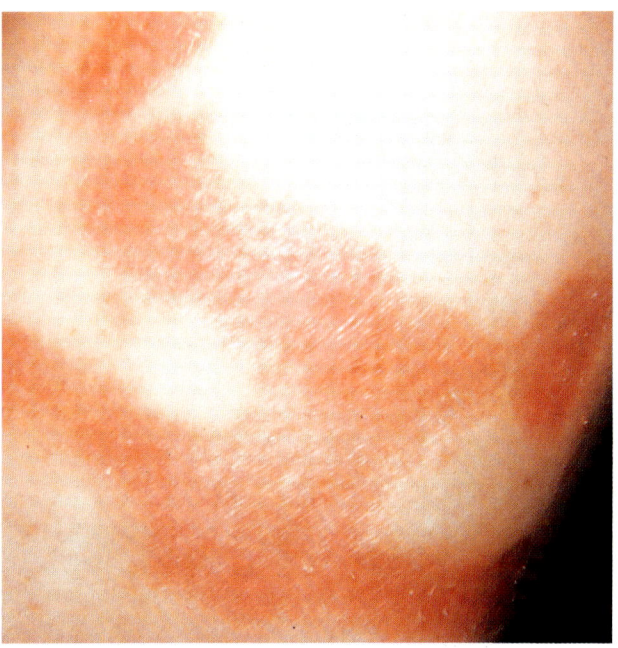

FIG. 5.33-B. Two months following laser treatment. Note significant erythema and induration.

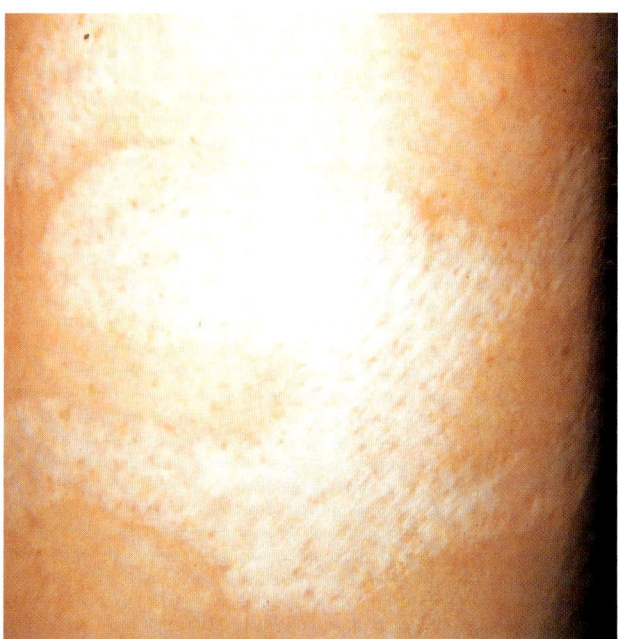

FIG. 5.33-C. Eight months post-treatment. Satisfactory elimination of all tattoo pigment without residual, but with mild skin texture change and slight hypopigmentation.

Case courtesy of *Lovic W. Hobby*, M.D.

CASE 5.34
Adenoma Sebaceum

REVIEW OF CASE. This 23-year-old young woman presented with the classical stigmata of tuberous sclerosis. Her face showed multiple small and large angiofibromas. She has significant mental retardation, and it is necessary for her to take dilantin for her seizure state. The lesions would on occasion spontaneously bleed and she found her facial lesions cosmetically embarrassing.

CHOICE OF LASER: ARGON. The argon laser was chosen for treatment because of the considerable success I have had in treating other patients in a similar fashion. This laser was initially chosen because of the prominent vascular component seen in some patients' lesions. Argon light absorption by vessels within the angiofibroma leads to nonspecific thermal destruction of the entire polypoid lesion. Under local anesthesia the laser was used on continuous wave for a sufficient period of time to induce the whitening of thermal effect on epidermis with coincident lesion flattening. The distance from handpiece to skin varied from 2–4 cm and the average meter setting was 1.2 watts.

ADDITIONAL INFORMATION. Either the argon laser or CO_2 laser may be used with considerable success in treating the lesions of adenoma sebaceum (2). The effect of the argon laser is primarily nonspecific thermal photocoagulation, and that is identical to the mechanism of action of the CO_2 laser as well. This patient was later treated with the CO_2 laser, 5 watts CW defocused, with the same local effects and same degree of success as previously. Small lesions may be treated without local anesthesia, particularly if using the argon laser.

POST-TREATMENT CARE. The patient need only apply topical antibiotic ointments with or without a nonocclusive dressing.

For literature pertaining to this case see References section.

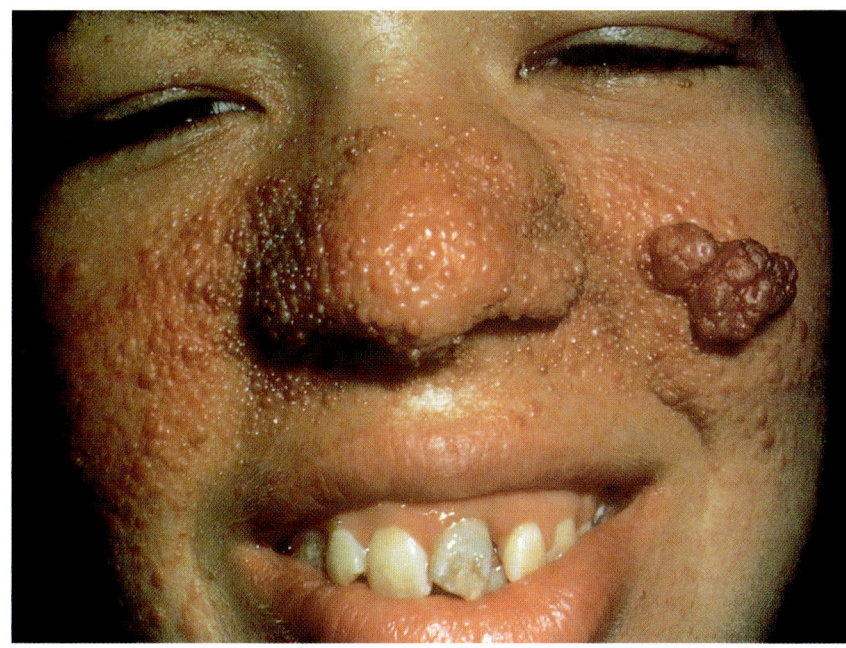

FIG. 5.34-A. Pre-operative prominent flesh colored and erythematous angiofibromas.

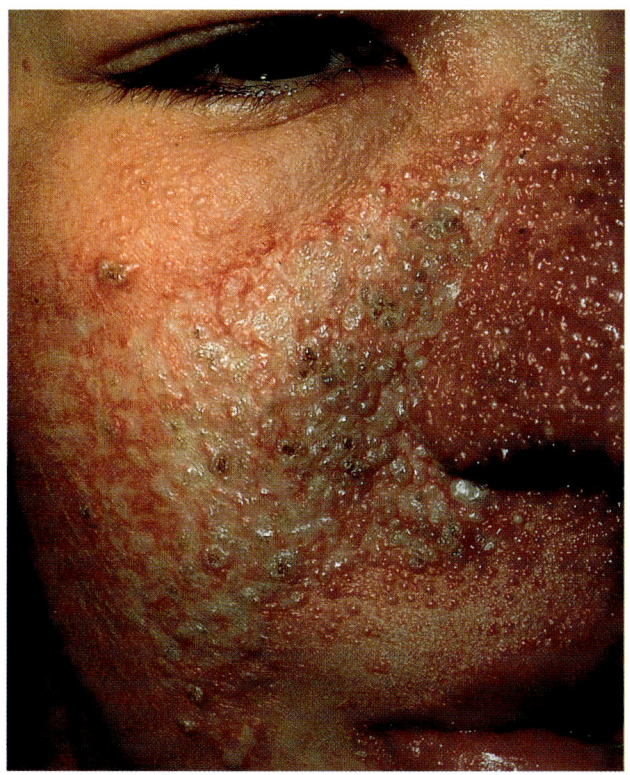

FIG. 5.34-B. Immediately post-operative, note discrete whitening effects caused by the argon laser on the right cheek lesions.

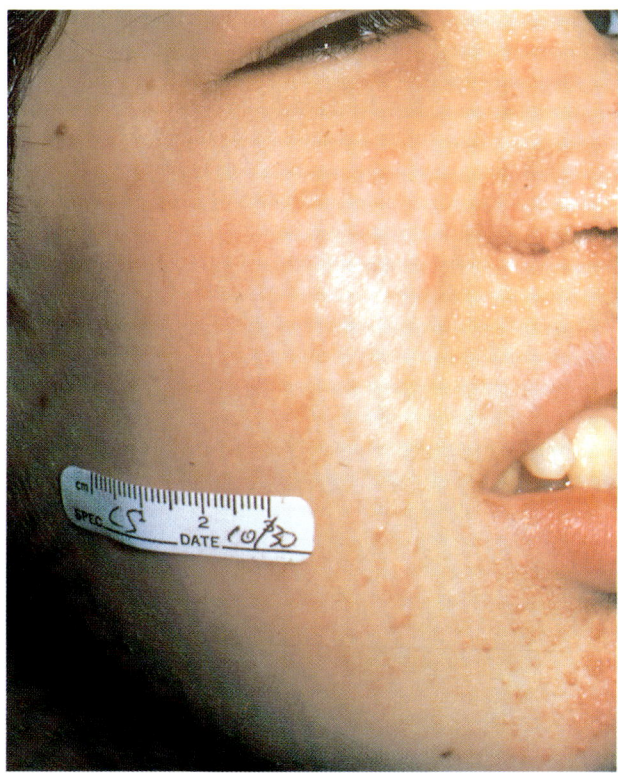

FIG. 5.34-C. Treated site five months after argon laser surgery.

Case courtesy of *Kenneth A. Arndt, M.D.*

CASE 5.35

Angiofibromas

In a Patient with Tuberous Sclerosis

REVIEW OF CASE. This 19-year-old female with the diagnosis of tuberous sclerosis entered our laser clinic for removal of pea-sized tumors located in the nasolabial folds and numerous pinhead reddish papules disseminated over her face. All these lesions had increased in number and size during the past ten years. The patient has had epileptic seizures since age 12.

CHOICE OF LASER: ARGON. Angiofibromas are small, reddish papules containing numerous dilated, erythrocyte-filled blood vessels that are a target tissue for argon laser energy.

POST-TREATMENT CARE. After daily cleaning of the face with soap and water, bacitracin ointment was used for approximately 2 weeks.

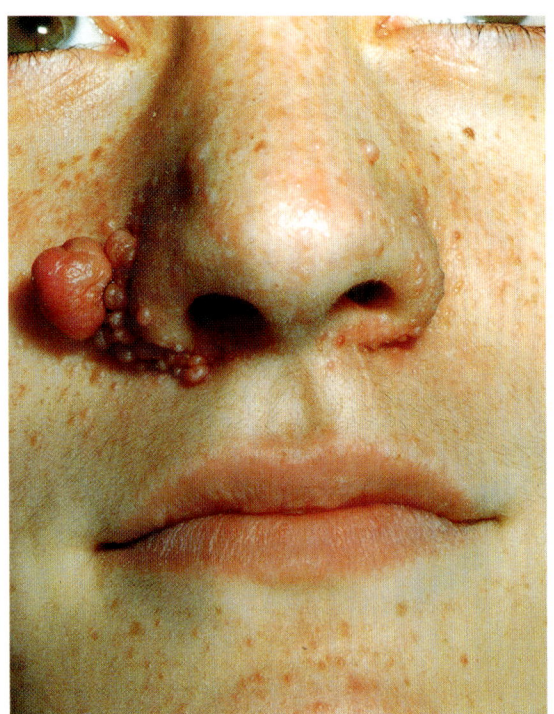 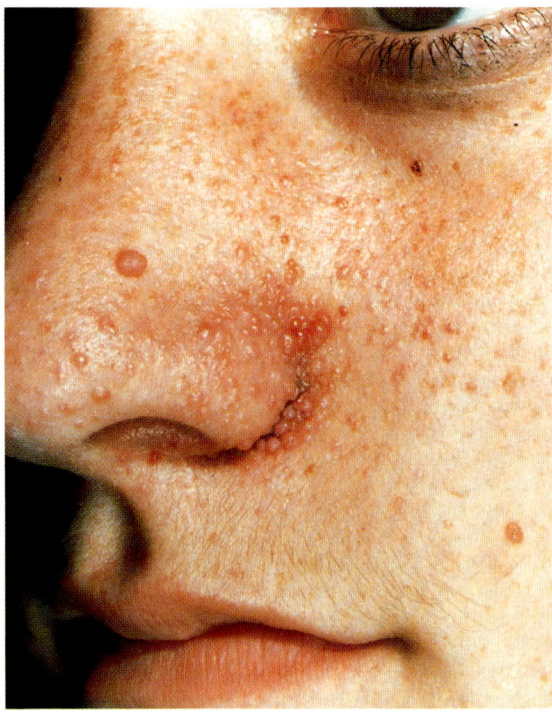

FIG. 5.35-A, B. Multiple angiofibromas on the face of a 19-year-old female with tuberous sclerosis before argon laser surgery.

Reprinted with permission of Little, Brown and Company.
For literature pertaining to this case see References section.

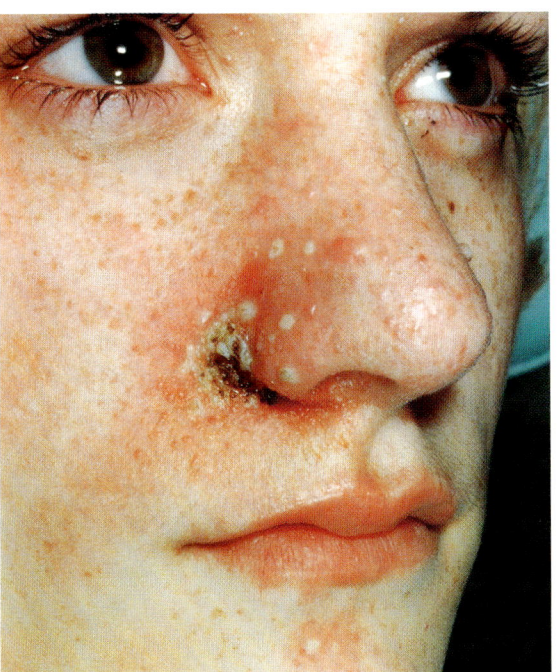 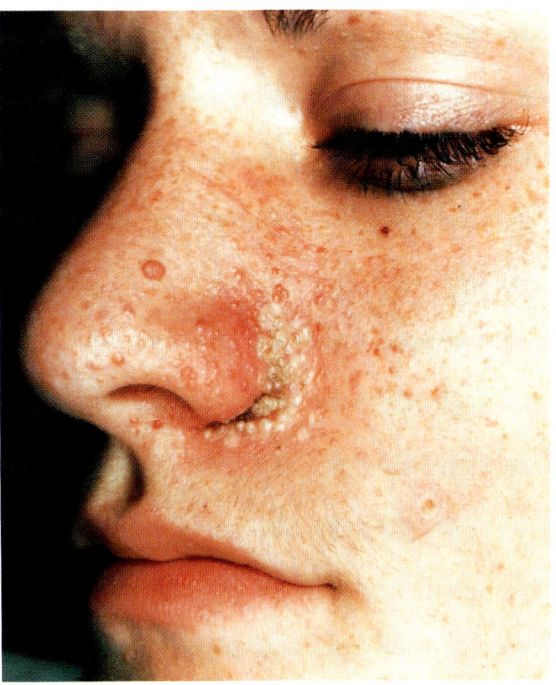

FIG. 5.35-C, D. Immediately after carbonization and coagulation of part of the lesions. Following local anesthesia with 2% lidocaine without epinephrine, tumors from the nasolabial folds were removed with the argon laser; power 2.0–2.5 watts, spot size 1 mm, and exposure time 0.2 sec. The small, reddish papules were coagulated with a power of 1.5–1.7 watts, spot size 0.1 cm, and exposure time 0.2 sec.

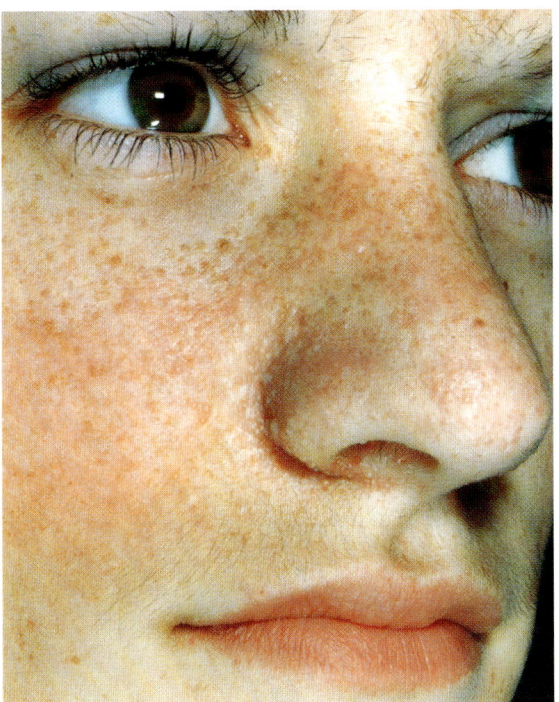 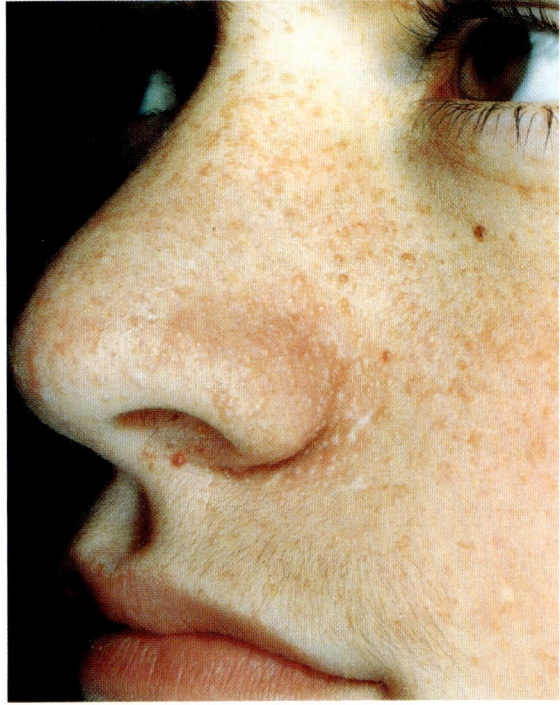

FIG. 5.35-E, F. Result 10 months after completion of surgery. The tumors were removed during four sessions, with three weeks between each treatment. The reddish papules were coagulated during another seven sessions. The areas exposed to laser energy healed in two to three weeks. There was no regrowth during a five-year follow-up period.

Case courtesy of ***Krystyna A. Pasyk***, M.D., Ph.D.

CASE 5.36
Hypertrophic Surgical Scar

REVIEW OF CASE. This is a 44-year-old lady with a hypertrophic mid sternotomy scar from open heart surgery three years before. She attempted to wear Jobst compression garments, had multiple injections of steroids, and was unresponsive to steroid tapes. The scar was painful and uncomfortable because of irritation by her bra, clothes, and jewelry.

CHOICE OF LASER: ARGON. The argon laser was chosen to treat this patient in 1981 because it was felt at that time, to be the only laser effective for treating hypertrophic scars. The CO_2 laser has been found to work equally well and is actually quite a bit easier to use.

ADDITIONAL INFORMATION. The entire area should be chilled for at least 10 minutes with crushed ice in a sterile plastic bag prior to treatment. The smallest possible hole should be drilled into the scar with the laser, holding the hand as steady as possible and at the proper distance to achieve the smallest spot. This will leave an area of vaporization surrounded by an area of thermal damage. The CO_2 laser is technically easier to use, inasmuch as the time interval only needs to be 0.1 seconds. The spot size of the CO_2 laser is 0.1–0.2 mm. The argon laser requires a time interval of one second, which makes it more difficult to hold the hand steady. The spot size of the argon laser is 0.2 mm. These holes should be drilled approximately 3 to 4 mm apart. It is absolutely imperative that perfectly normal skin be present between the two adjacent areas of thermal damage. The resultant wound will show a small vaporized spot, a white halo of thermal damage, and then normal tissue. If the vaporization is not achieved, the result will be compromised. If the areas of thermal damage coalesce one upon the other, an even worse scar might occur.

There is no bleeding following the use of the argon laser. With the CO_2 laser, small blood vessels are sometimes encountered with blood coming from the wound. This can be controlled with pressure and ice.

At the end of the procedure, the entire area is injected with triamcinolone. No further injections of triamcinolone are made unless the patient develops a recurrence.

Hypertrophic scars, both surgical and post-thermal, represent a "temporary" imbalance in collagen synthesis–collagen lysis. In our experience, burn scars respond approximately 90% of the time to laser impaction while hypertrophic surgical scars respond approximately 65% of the time. If they do respond to this treatment, no further subsequent injections of steroids are needed as they are in keloid scars. It is extremely rare to have a recurrence of a hypertrophic scar.

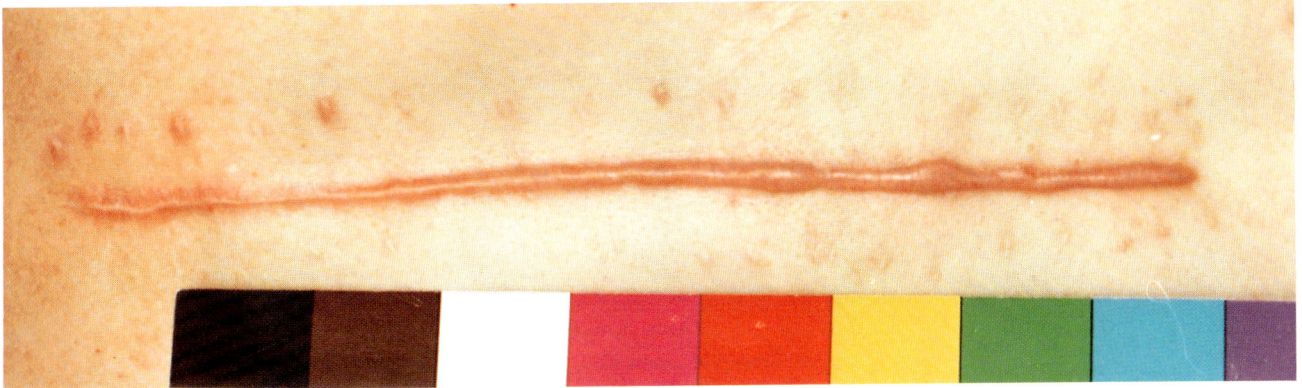

FIG. 5.36-A. A thick, ropy hypertrophic scar of three years duration.

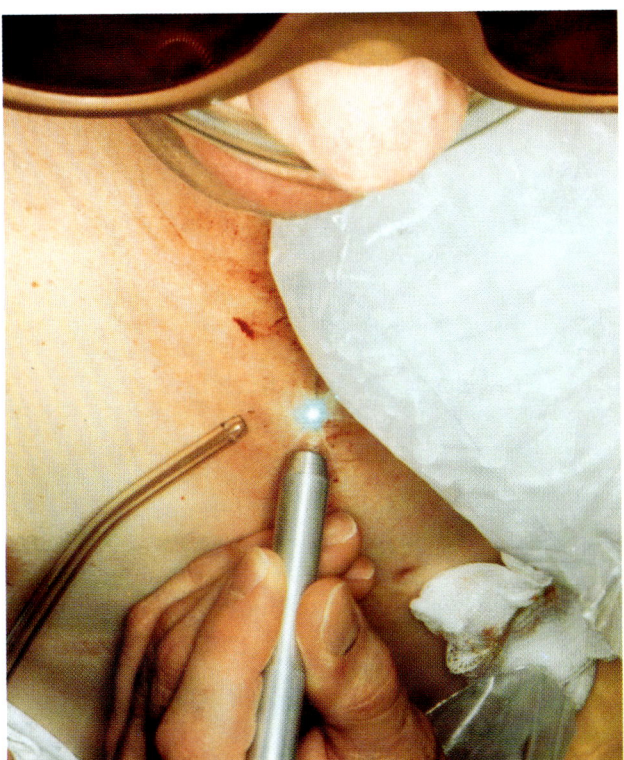

FIG. 5.36-B. Note the ice bag in place and the argon laser being held at a 90° angle to the skin. Alternate areas of the scar are treated and the entire scar is chilled before, during, and after treatment. Under no circumstances is the scar allowed to be heated by the laser.

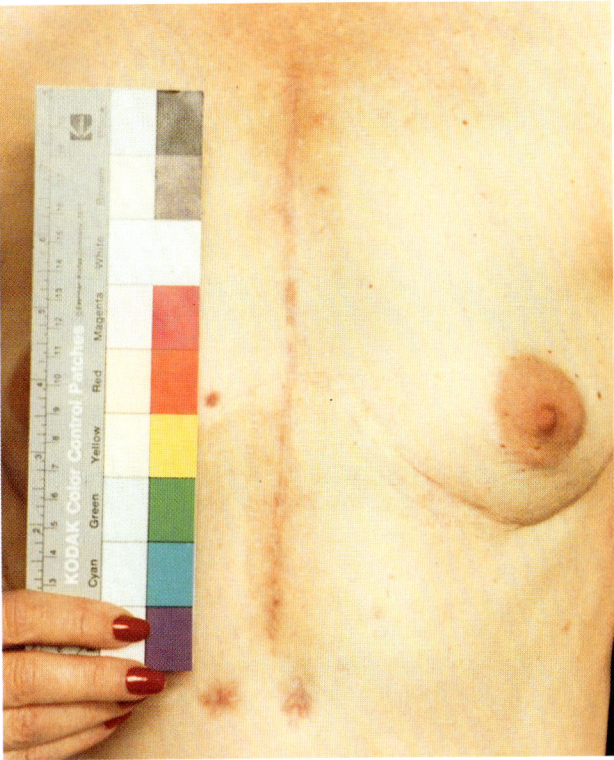

FIG. 5.36-C. Note marked reduction of the scar with no evidence of scar hypertrophy 2½ years later.

Case courtesy of *Darrell L. Henderson*, M.D.

ARGON LASER   271

CASE 5.37

Keloid of the Earlobe

REVIEW OF CASE. This is a 28-year-old female with a firm, hard keloid, dumbbell configuration, occupying all of the anterior aspect of the earlobe and all of the posterior aspect. The keloid itself is 1½ cm in diameter and 1 cm thick. It goes down to a small stalk of approximately 0.5 cm. This area had been injected with triamcinolone (40 mg/cc) on multiple occasions without result and had also been surgically excised on two separate occasions. Each time the keloid came back larger.

CHOICE OF LASER: ARGON. An argon laser was chosen to treat this lesion in 1983, mainly because at that time I felt only the argon laser was useful. While the parameters do change, the CO_2 or the Nd: YAG laser can be used with equal success.

ADDITIONAL INFORMATION. The keloid is transected from the underlying earlobe at a level with the skin. No effort is made to remove all of the keloid, and many times parts of the keloid are left in place. General anesthesia is preferred so as to prevent additional needle sticks in the normal skin inasmuch as these sticks may cause keloid formation. If local anesthesia must be used, the needle sticks must be kept as close to the keloid as possible to lessen the chance of new keloids.

The entire area is cooled with crushed ice placed in a sterile plastic bag so as to eliminate, as much as possible, the unwanted heat associated with a subsequent laser impaction.

The base of the wound is impacted with the laser, with the impact points at 2 mm centers. The spots should be made at random and iced or cooled very frequently to prevent heat. We are now using running iced saline over the area through an IV tube and lasering through the iced saline so as to lessen the heat. The prevention of heat buildup is extremely critical, in my opinion, in all laser surgery.

After both sides have been impacted and the area again chilled with ice, triamcinolone (40 mg/cc) is instilled throughout the area on both sides of the ear.

No attempt is made to suture or close the wound, as additional suture marks will probably lead to additional keloid formation.

The ear is coated with triamcinolone ointment, and the patient is instructed to keep this ointment on continuously.

The patient should be re-injected with triamcinolone every four to six months, indefinitely. If the keloid begins to come back, earlier injection may be necessary. For injection, we use triamcinolone (40 mg/cc) and equal parts of 1% Xylocaine with epinephrine. Approximately ¼ cc of this mixture is used in the front part of the ear and ¼ cc in the back of the ear.

Keloids represent an uncontrollable imbalance in the collagen synthesis-collagen lysis balance of the body. Collagen synthesis is overwhelming as compared to collagen lysis. The above method of treatment will temporarily abate this collagen synthesis-lysis imbalance from four to sixty months, but, if subsequent triamcinolone injections are not intermittently made, this imbalance will occur again with a resultant reformation of the keloid. It appears that removal of the keloid and the use of the laser temporarily slows wound healing and, probably more importantly, sensitizes the patient to the injections of triamcinolone. If the keloid is allowed to regrow to a mature status, triamcinolone usually will not work.

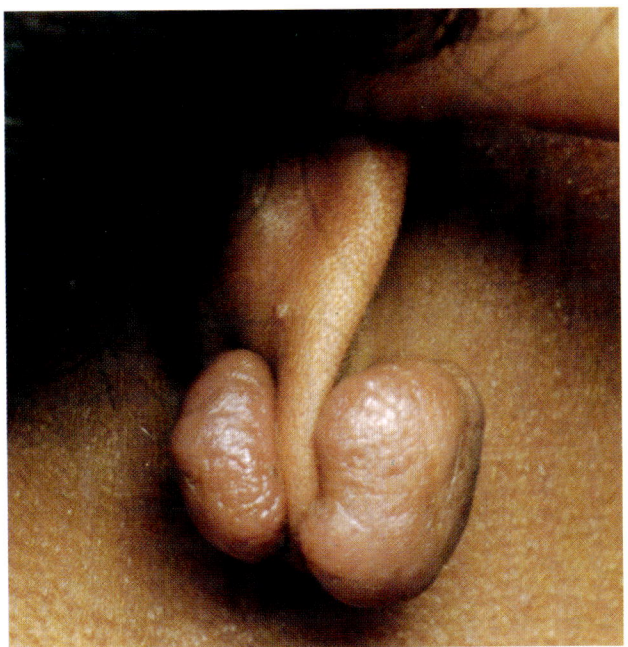

FIG. 5.37-A. Example of a typical dumbbell keloid that has been treated many times and by many different methods.

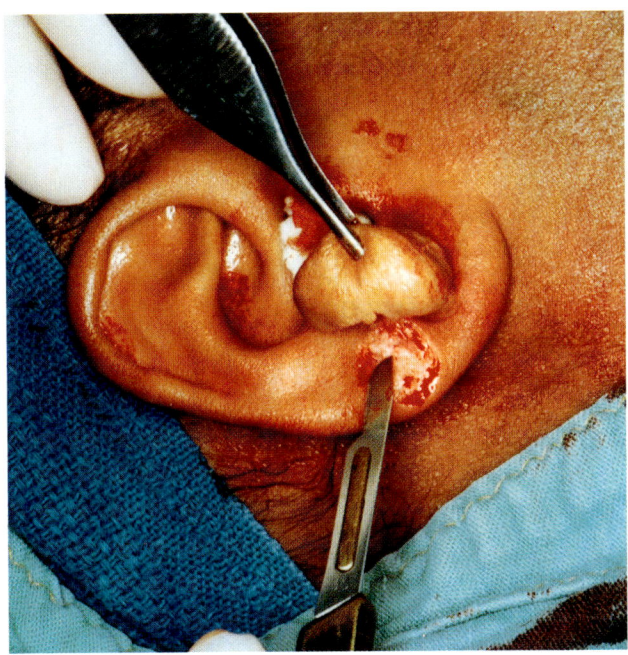

FIG. 5.37-B. The keloid is resected at the level of the skin with a sharp scalpel under general anesthesia.

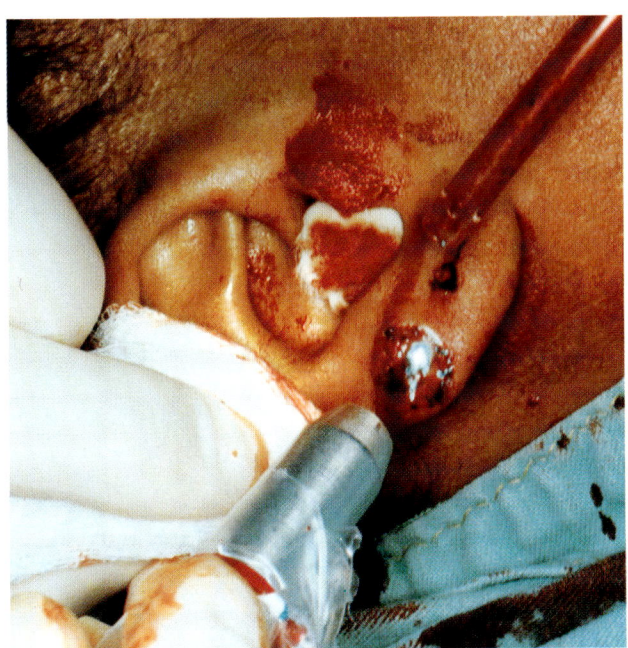

FIG. 5.37-C. After thoroughly chilling the ear with crushed ice and even running saline water, the laser is sterilely wrapped and the base on both sides of the ear are thoroughly impacted. Care should be taken that there is still living tissue between the areas that are impacted. The base must *not* be charred.

Case continues on following page.

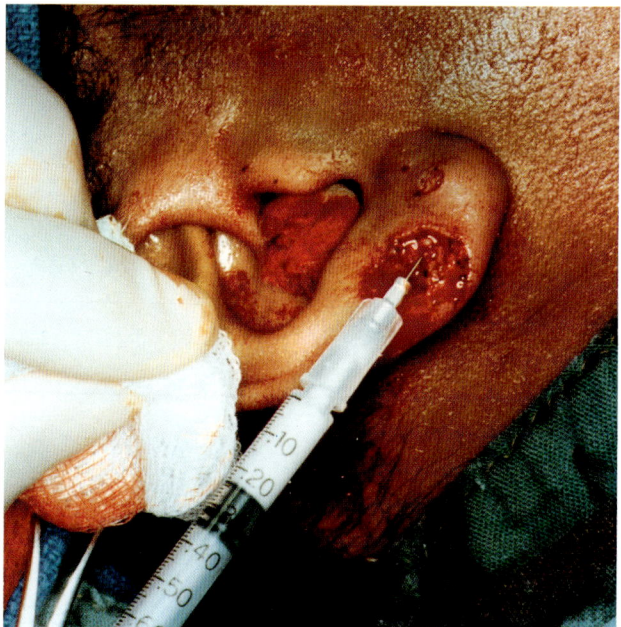

FIG. 5.37-D. ¼ cc of triamcinolone (40 mg/cc) is instilled in front of the ear and ¼ cc in back of the ear. The needle is injected through the lasered area. Note the laser impact points and the normal red tissue between the laser impact points.

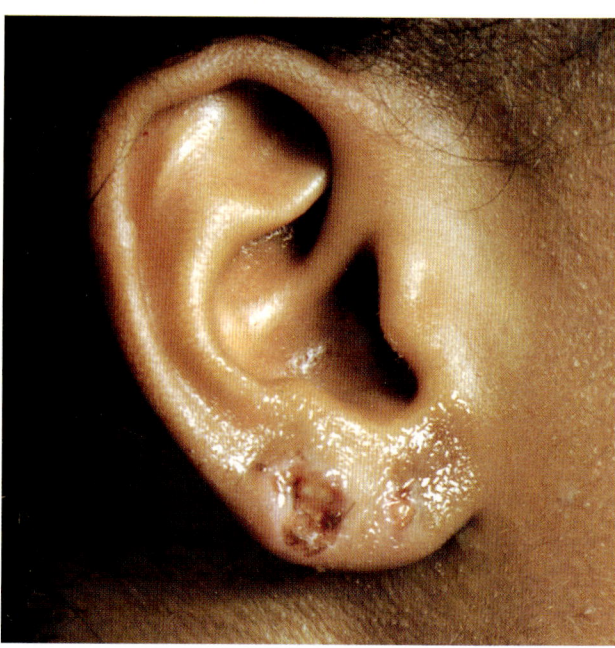

FIG. 5.37-E. Healing wound coated with triamcinolone ointment one week after treatment.

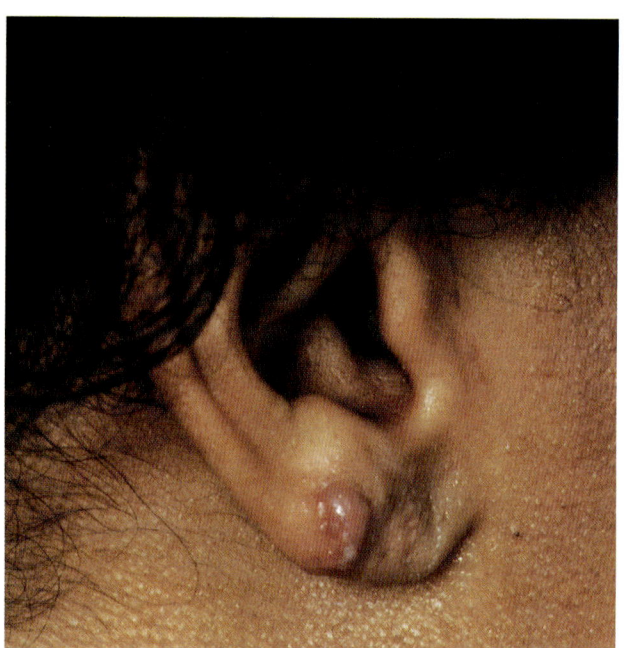

FIG. 5.37-F. Ear five years after treatment. Notice the relatively flat scar, which represents the abated keloid which is under control but which still has the capability of returning if injections are discontinued.

Case courtesy of *Darrell L. Henderson*, M.D.

CASE 5.38
Keloid of the Pubic Area

REVIEW OF CASE. Keloid on the pubic area of a 40-year-old black female present for the past 4 years. It grew very close to a cesarean section scar and was painful to touch.

CHOICE OF LASER: ARGON. The argon laser was chosen for treatment. It may also successfully vaporize and carbonize keloids.

POST-TREATMENT CARE. Immediately after laser surgery and at 4–6 week intervals, the base of the treated area is injected with triamcinolone acetonide (Kenalog, 40 mg/ml) a total of five times. The patient is instructed to clean the treated area two times daily with soap and water and to cover it with gauze and bacitracin ointment during the healing process.

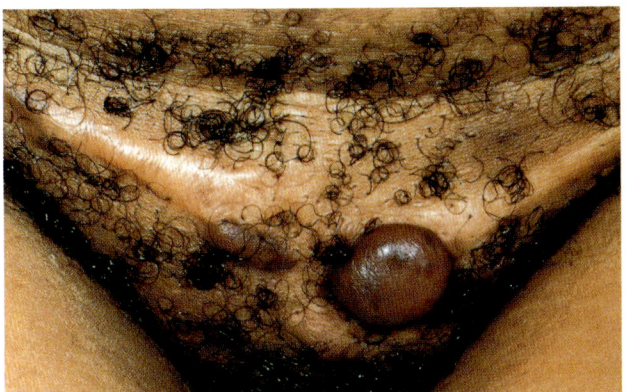

FIG. 5.38-A. Keloid of the pubic region in 40-year-old black female before argon laser surgery.

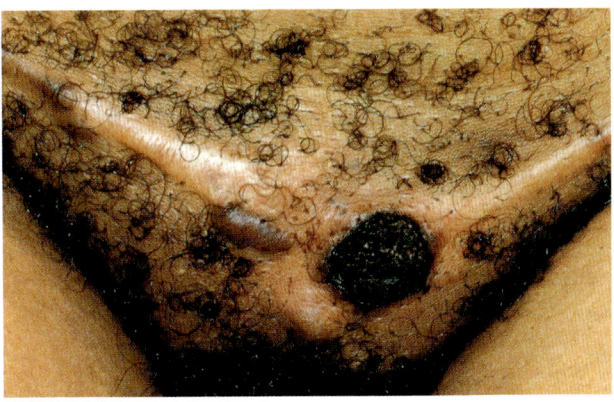

FIG. 5.38-B. Immediately after vaporization and carbonization of keloid with the argon laser (power 3 watts, spot size 1 mm, in continuous mode). Local anesthesia with 2% lidocaine without epinephrine was done prior to argon laser surgery.

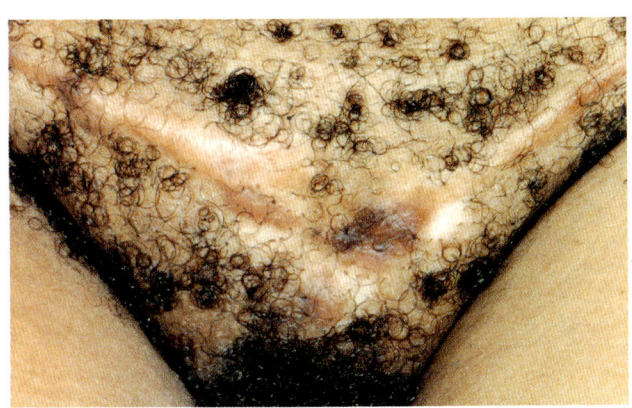

FIG. 5.38-C. Result eight months after argon laser surgery. No regrowth was observed during three years of follow-up.

Case courtesy of **Krystyna A. Pasyk,** M.D., Ph.D.

CASE 5.39
Linear Hyperkeratotic Nevus

REVIEW OF CASE. A 36-year-old man had pinkish-brown rough papules arranged in a linear plaque on his forearm since childhood. These lesions were treated unsuccessfully with dermabrasion and he was referred for surgical excision.

CHOICE OF LASER: ARGON. The argon laser was chosen to try to remove these lesions instead of surgical excision.

ADDITIONAL INFORMATION. Treatment with the argon laser was done after local anesthesia with 2% lidocaine without epinephrine and with the use of a magnifying glass.

POST-TREATMENT CARE. The patient is instructed to wash the treated areas with water and soap and apply bacitracin ointment with a dressing until the lesions are healed completely. Sun exposure to the treated area should be avoided for 6 months after irradiation.

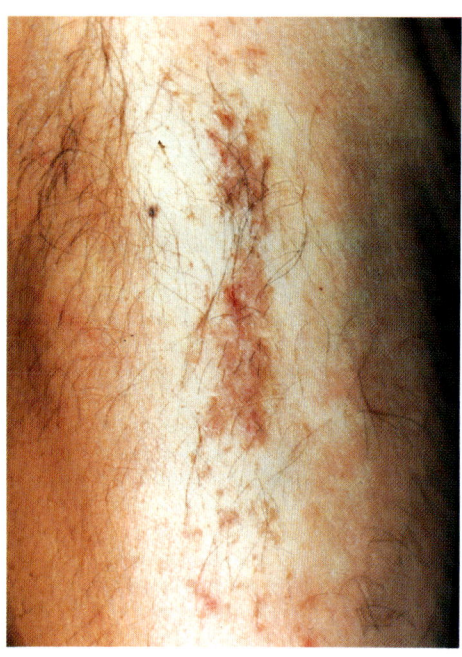

FIG. 5.39-A. Linear, hyperkeratotic nevus on the forearm in a 36-year-old male before treatment.

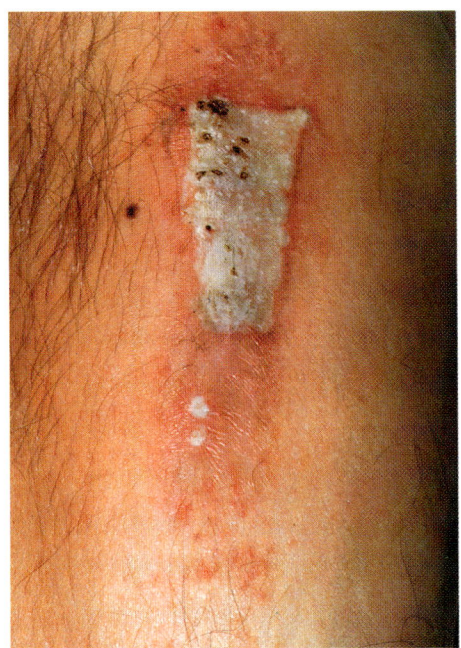

FIG. 5.39-B. Immediately after second, consecutive irradiation with the argon laser (power 1.7 watts, spot size 1 mm, exposure time 0.2 sec). Note carbonized areas and flat scar after first treatment.

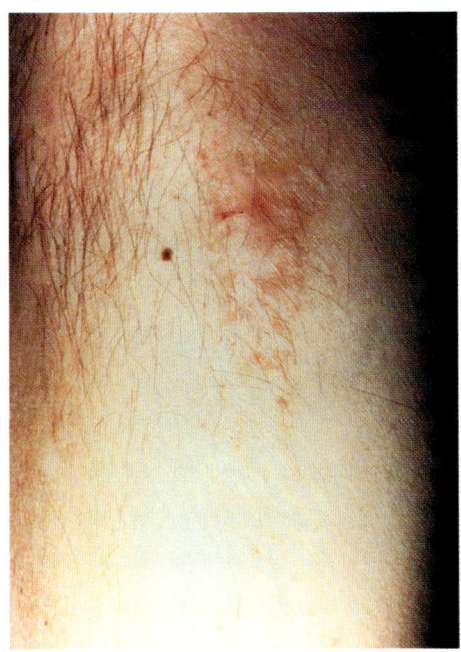

FIG. 5.39-C. Status 6 months after finishing treatment with the argon laser. Note flat scar but disappearance of the rough papules.

Case courtesy of ***Krystyna A. Pasyk,*** M.D., Ph.D.

CASE 5.40
Nevus of Ota

REVIEW OF CASE. This 32-year-old female presented with a dark gray-black pigmentation in the left forehead, cheek, and eyelid. The patient has one parent who is Oriental. The discoloration was only mildly noticeable at birth but became more definite and prominent during the late teen years.

CHOICE OF LASER: ARGON. The blue-green argon light at 488–514 nm is selectively absorbed by pigment particles of melanin present in the upper dermis. The light is converted to heat which vaporizes and fragments these pigment cells. Subsequent inflammatory reaction phagocytizes the cells and produces a partial-thickness injury of the epidermis and upper dermis. Dermal appendages such as hair follicles and pilosebaceous glands are spared and aid in the healing and epithelialization of the wound. A 0.2–1 mm spot size is used at 0.5–1.5 watts of power pulsed at 1–2 seconds.

ADDITIONAL INFORMATION. The eyelids respond best to argon laser treatment of nevus of Ota. The remainder of the face is usually treated with snowy dry ice plus epithelial peeling. These treatments must be repeated monthly for 6–10 months. The eyelid skin is not treated with snowy ice because of its delicacy, thinner character, and proximity to the eye.

For literature pertaining to this case see References section.

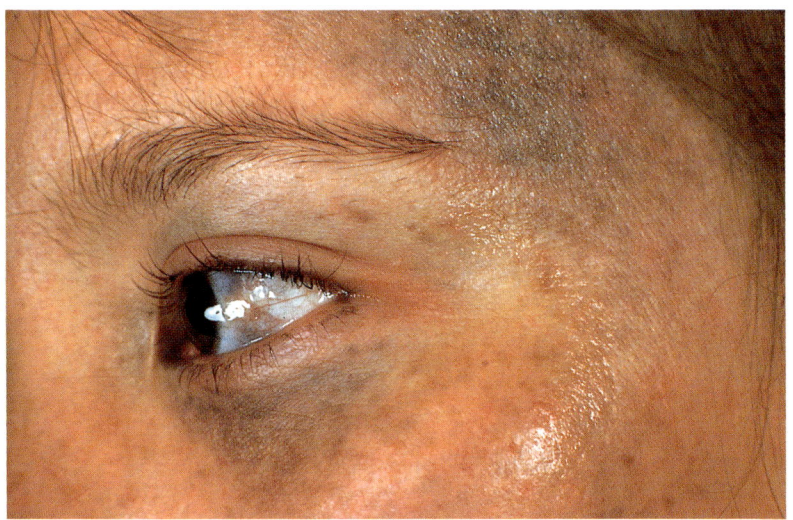

FIG. 5.40-A. Pre-treatment nevus of Ota present on forehead, eyelid, and cheek.

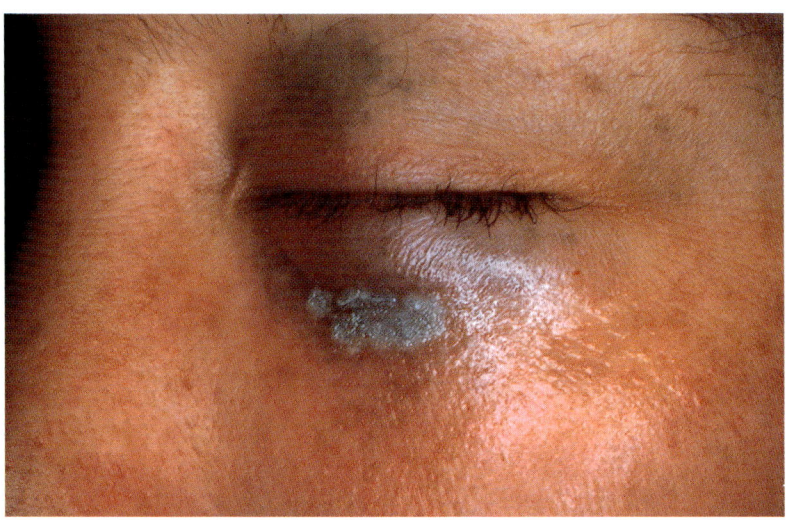

FIG. 5.40-B. Immediately after argon laser photocoagulation of eyelid demonstrating marked blanching.

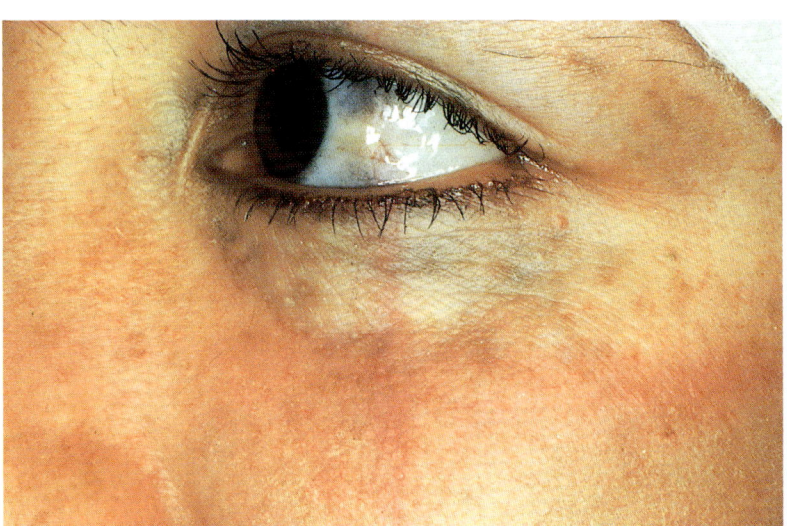

FIG. 5.40-C. Final appearance of eyelid with marked lightening of dark pigment without scarring.

Case courtesy of *David B. Apfelberg*, M.D.

ARGON LASER 279

CASE 5.41
Nevus Sebaceum

REVIEW OF CASE. This 15-year-old boy presented with nevus sebaceum on the face. The patient desired removal because of the cosmetic appearance.

CHOICE OF LASER: ARGON. The argon laser was chosen instead of the CO_2 laser because of the easier handling and increased accuracy necessary when working on a lesion of this type. The power was varied between 5 and 6 watts, and a 1–2 focus diameter was used with pulse time varying from 0.1 to 0.5 second.

POST-TREATMENT CARE. The lesion is treated as an open wound with the use of a topical antibiotic.

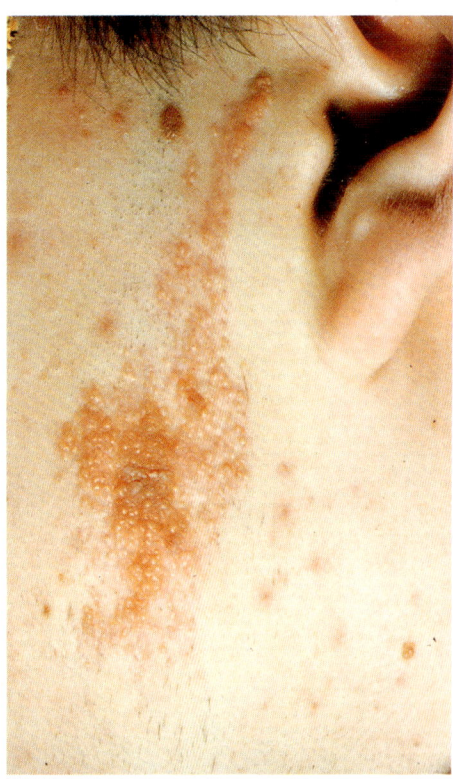

FIG. 5.41-A. Nevus prior to treatment.

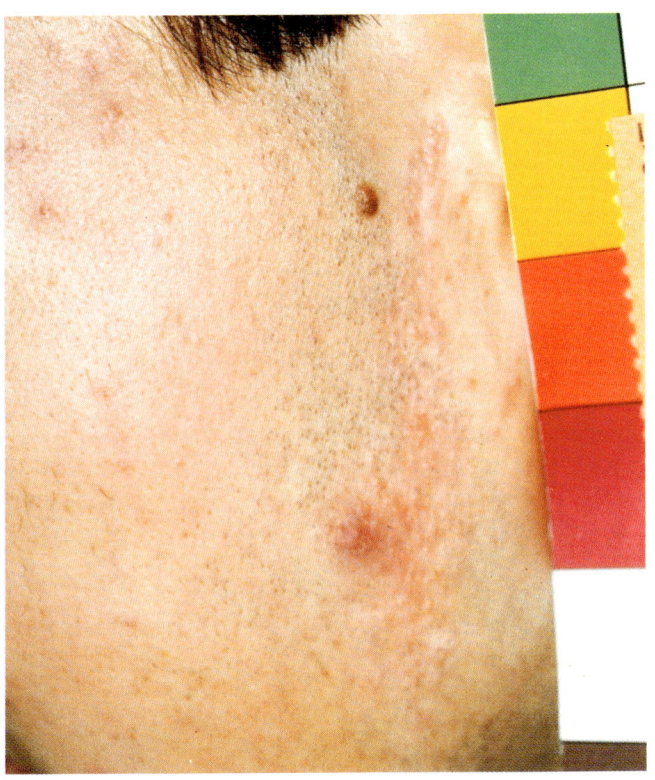

FIG. 5.41-B. After three treatments. The upper part of the lesion was treated with cryosurgery (*stripes*). Response was poor and this area was re-treated with the laser.

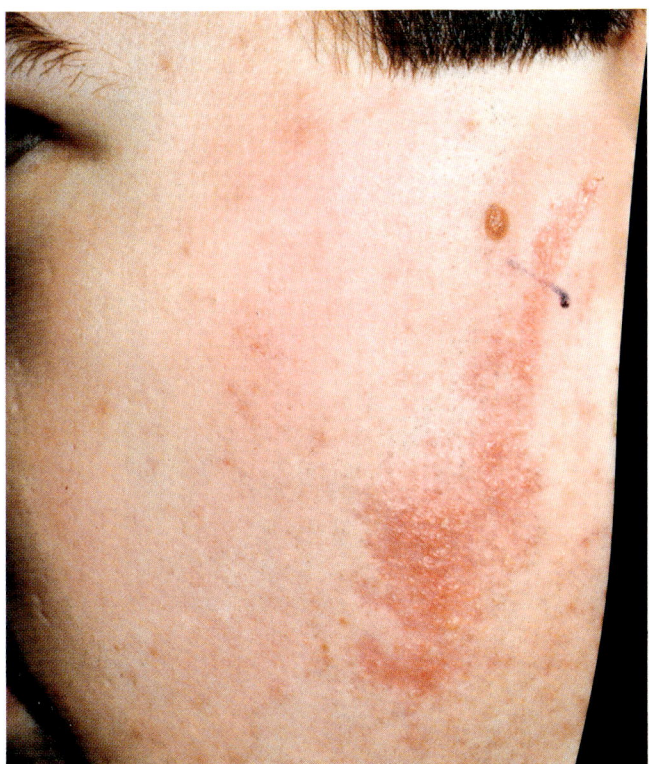

FIG. 5.41-C. Result after 5 laser treatments.

Case courtesy of *J. P. Hulsbergen Henning*, M.D.

CASE 5.42
Nevus Unilateralis

REVIEW OF CASE.   This 21-year-old female presented with a congenital nevus unilateralis, previously treated with cryosurgery without a satisfying result.

CHOICE OF LASER: ARGON.   The argon laser was used at 8 watts, focus diameter 3 mm, with pulse time varying in the beginning from 0.02 to 15 and 20 μsec. The short pulse times were chosen to refine the treatment result after the thickening of the lesion had disappeared. Short pulses can be used in order to treat the color differences.

POST-TREATMENT CARE.   The patient was instructed to keep the lesion dry. Local antibacterial tincture was only to be applied in case of excoriation of the skin.

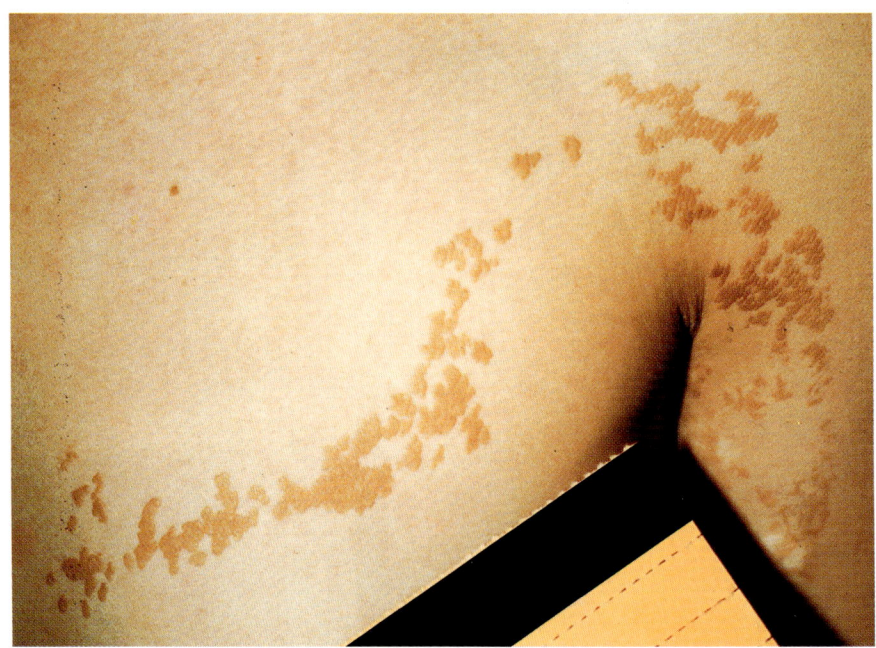

FIG. 5.42-A. Nevus prior to treatment.

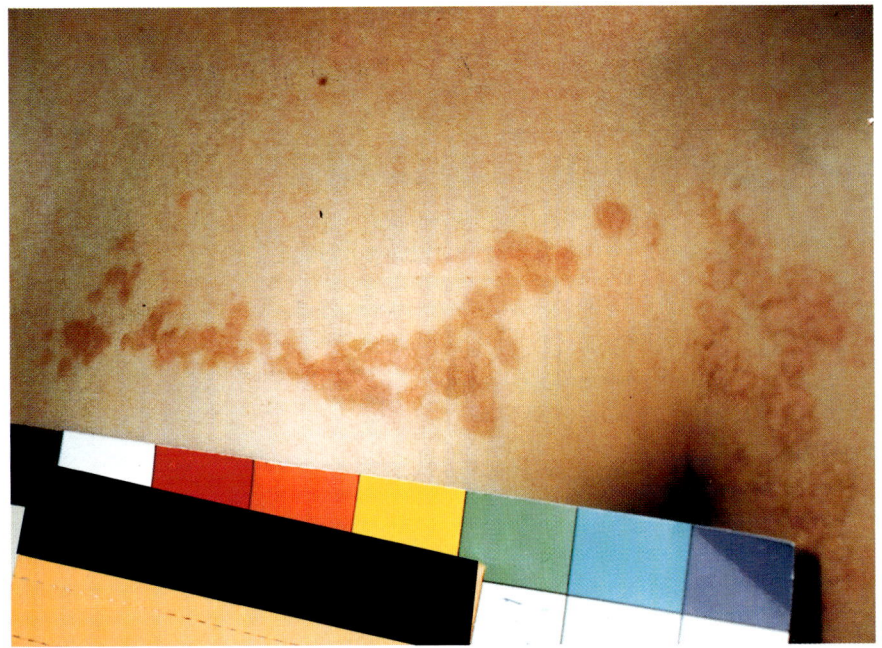

FIG. 5.42-B. Nevus after 5 treatments of 10 μsec pulses of 8 watts and a 2 mm focus diameter.

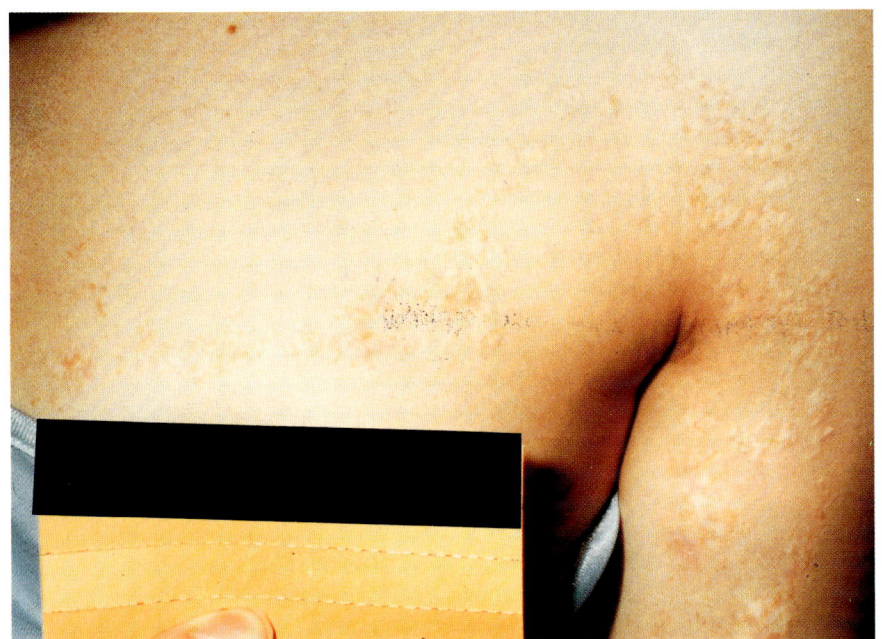

FIG. 5.42-C. Follow-up treatment with 7 watts, 2 mm diameter, and 15–20 μsec pulses.

Case courtesy of *J. P. Hulsbergen Henning*, M.D.

CASE 5.43

Papillomatosis of the Lip

In a Patient with EEC Syndrome

REVIEW OF CASE. This 15-year-old boy presented with EEC syndrome (ectrodactyly-ectodermal dysplasia-clefting syndrome) and was referred to the laser clinic for treatment of papillomatous lesions on his lower lip that had been noted in childhood. The patient was born with split feet and hands of the "lobster-claw" type, bilateral cleft lip and cleft palate, and various ectodermal anomalies including hypodontia, defective nails and hypotrichosis. The patient has undergone numerous surgical procedures.

CHOICE OF LASER: ARGON. These papillomatous lesions are rich in ectatic, blood-filled vessels that are target tissues for argon laser energy. The results of treatment of these lesions indicate that the argon laser can be safely used repeatedly for re-treatment of lip papillomatosis.

POST-TREATMENT CARE. The patient is instructed to apply bacitracin ointment on the treated surface 4–5 times daily.

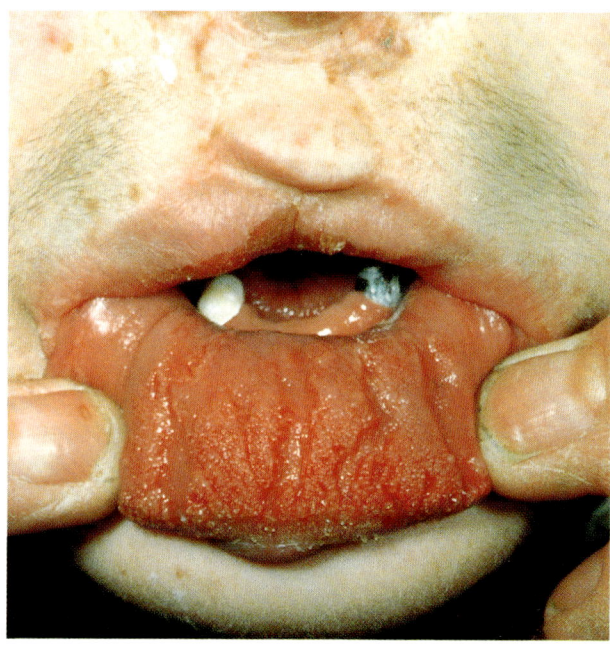

FIG. 5.43-A. Papillomatosis of the lip in 17-year-old male with EEC syndrome before treatment.

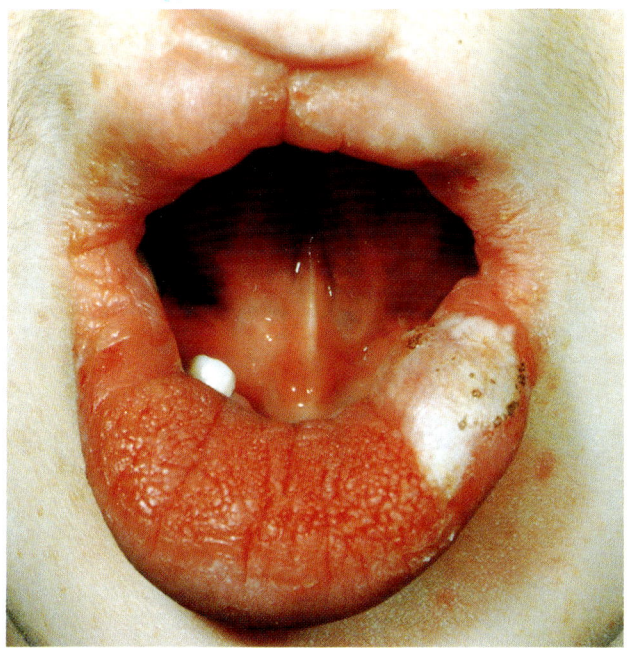

FIG. 5.43-B. Immediately after argon laser test treatment using 1.7 watts of power, 1 mm spot size, and 0.2 sec exposure time.

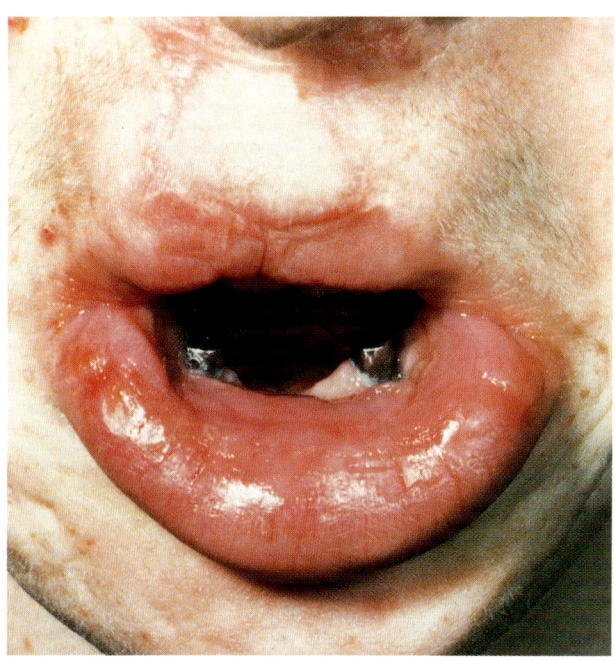

FIG. 5.43-C. Result 1 year after argon laser surgery (power 1.7–2 watts, spot size 1 mm, exposure time 0.2 sec). During the next 3 years there was no recurrence of these lesions.

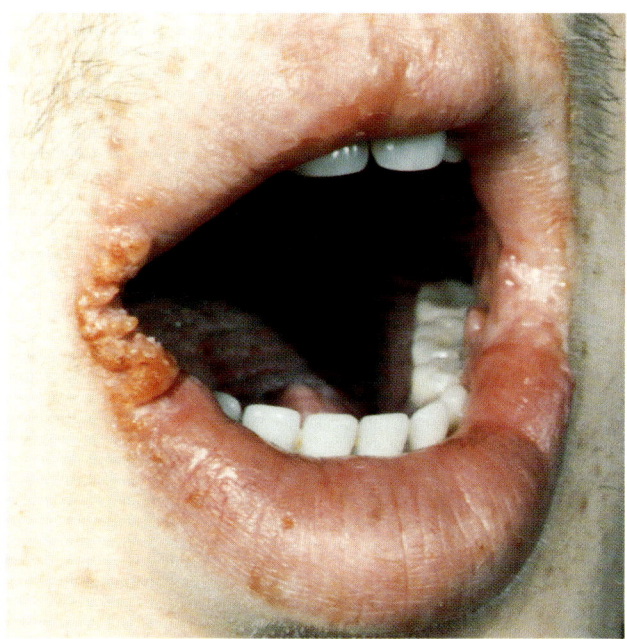

FIG. 5.43-D. The same patient aged 18 years with recurrent papillomatous lesions in the right corner of the mouth.

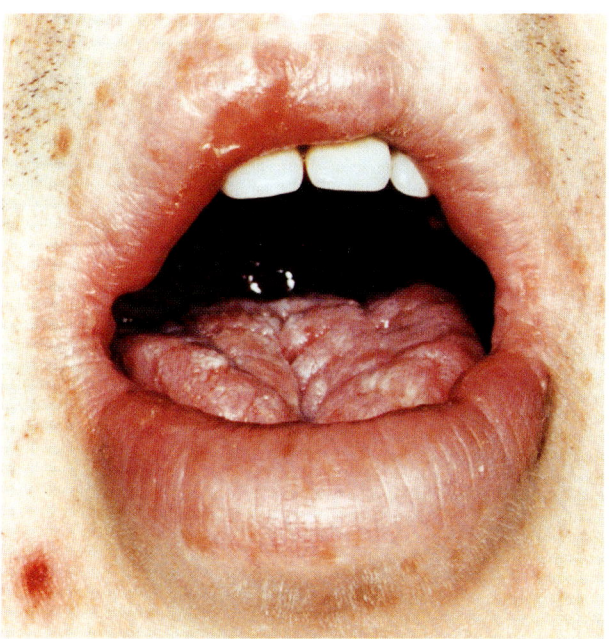

FIG. 5.43-E. Results 2 months after re-treatment of papillomatosis with the argon laser. During the past 4 years there has been no regrowth of the lesions.

Case courtesy of *Krystyna A. Pasyk*, M.D., Ph.D.

CASE 5.44
Seborrheic Keratosis

REVIEW OF CASE. This 52-year-old female had a brown, hyperkeratotic spot on her forehead present for the past 4 years. She was referred for laser treatment.

CHOICE OF LASER: ARGON. The argon laser was chosen to carbonize this lesion. It has been shown that the argon laser is also able to successfully treat pigmented lesions by absorption of the laser energy by the pigment.

POST-TREATMENT CARE. Application of bacitracin ointment was recommended during the healing process.

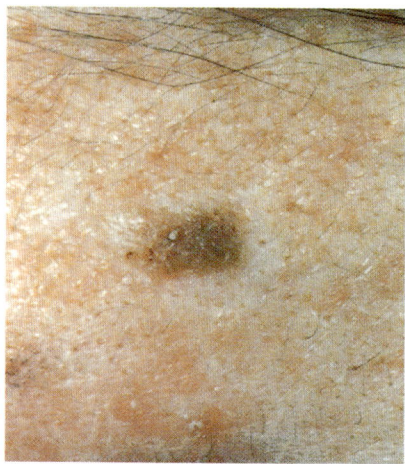

FIG. 5.44-A. Seborrheic keratosis on the temple area in a 52-year-old female before treatment.

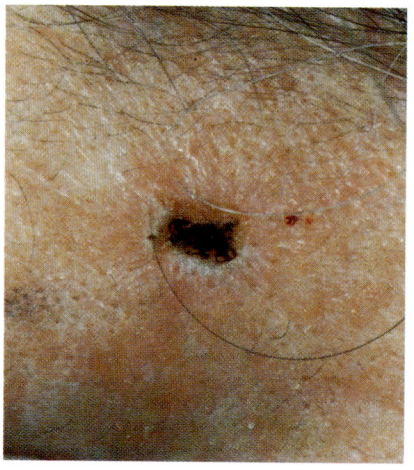

FIG. 5.44-B. Result immediately after argon laser surgery using a power of 1.7 watts, spot size 1 mm, and exposure time of 0.2 sec. The treatment was performed without local anesthesia.

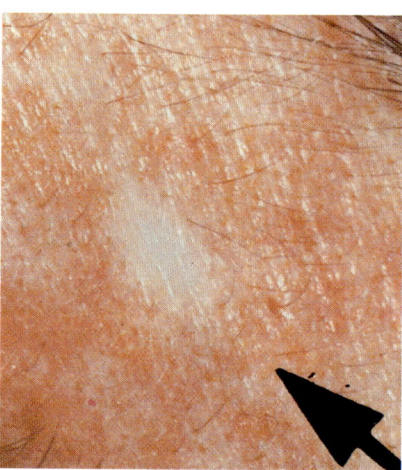

FIG. 5.44-C. Results 4 months after argon laser surgery. Note slight hypopigmentation of treated area.

Case courtesy of *Krystyna A. Pasyk, M.D., Ph.D.*

CASE 5.45

Port Wine Hemangioma

Dot/Pointillistic Technique

REVIEW OF CASE. This 27-year-old presented with a port wine hemangioma on the upper lip, side of nose, cheek, and eyelid.

CHOICE OF LASER: ARGON. The blue-green argon light at 488–514 nm is selectively absorbed by hemoglobin-laden ectatic vessels under the skin. Penetration is down to the upper 1–2 mm of the dermis. The light is converted to heat upon absorption and has the ability to coagulate vessels with lumen diameters of 0.5 mm and smaller. The dermal appendages such as hair follicles and pilosebaceous glands are spared and aid in the rapid healing and epithelialization of the wound. The laser is used with 0.5 watts of power, 0.5 second pulse duration, and 0.2–1 mm spot size.

ADDITIONAL INFORMATION. The peri-oral and nasolabial area, particularly the upper lip, are highly prone to scarring. In an attempt to limit such scarring, the polka dot technique was developed. Areas prone to hypertrophic scarring such as the upper lip, chin, and the nasolabial fold in the face; and trunk, and extremities are now treated with a "polka dot" or "pointillistic" technique. This technique consists of the formation of multiple 1–2 mm dots of blanching produced by minimal power. Each dot is separated from the adjacent one by 1–2 mm. The laser stylus is hand held (perpendicular to the skin) at a focal length of 1–3 cm. Fading as a result of the dots coalescing or the intermediate treatment of non-dotted interspaces in 12 weeks is more modest and slightly more variegated or irregular than the treatment in a single block, but scarring is quite rare.

POST-TREATMENT CARE. Immediate use of ice compresses and open wound treatment with topical antibiotic or aloe vera gel is used following laser treatment.

Case continues on following page.

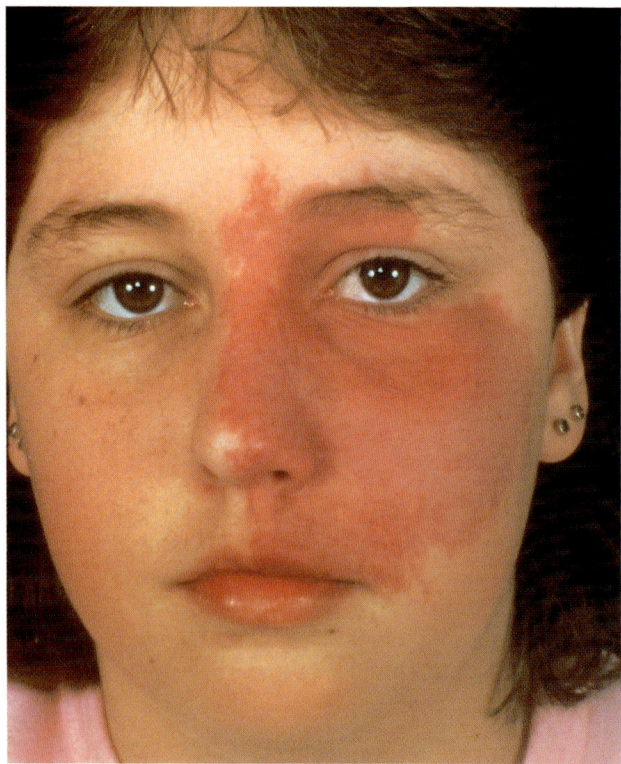

FIG. 5.45-A. Pre-treatment port wine hemangioma of left cheek, eyelid, upper lip, and side of nose.

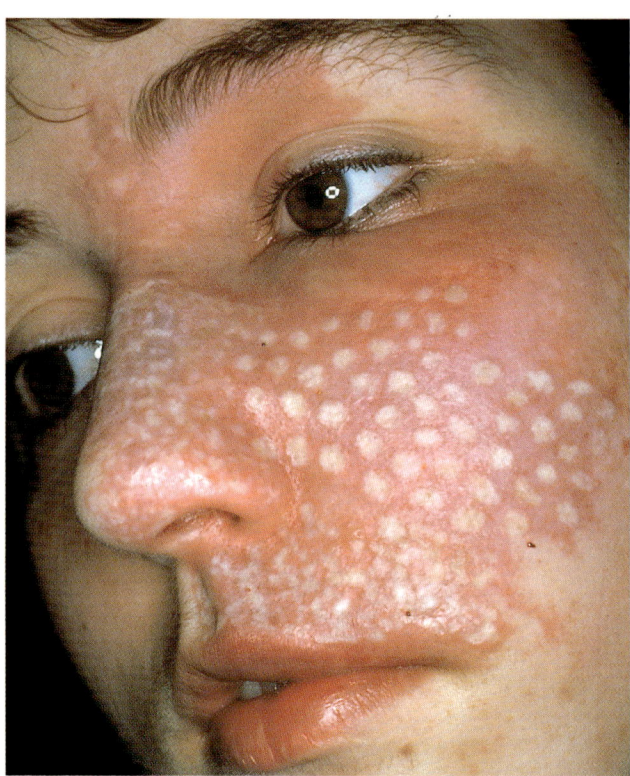

FIG. 5.45-B. Blanching after polka dot application of 1–2 mm spots of laser light leaving interspaces of untreated hemangioma.

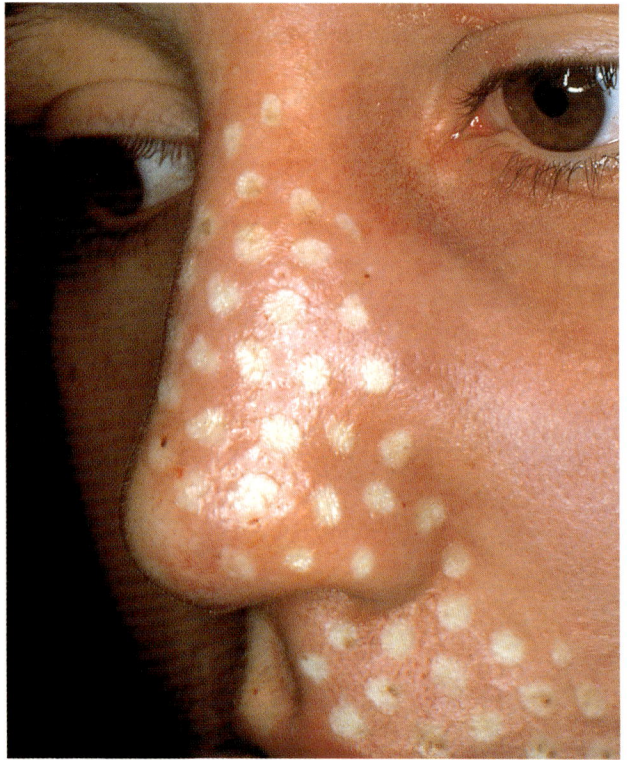

FIG. 5.45-C. Close-up of side of nose.

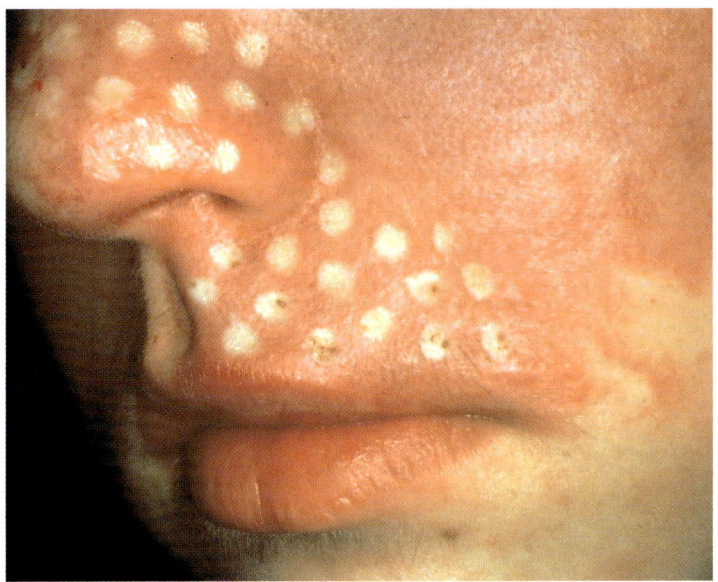

FIG. 5.45-D. Close-up of upper lip.

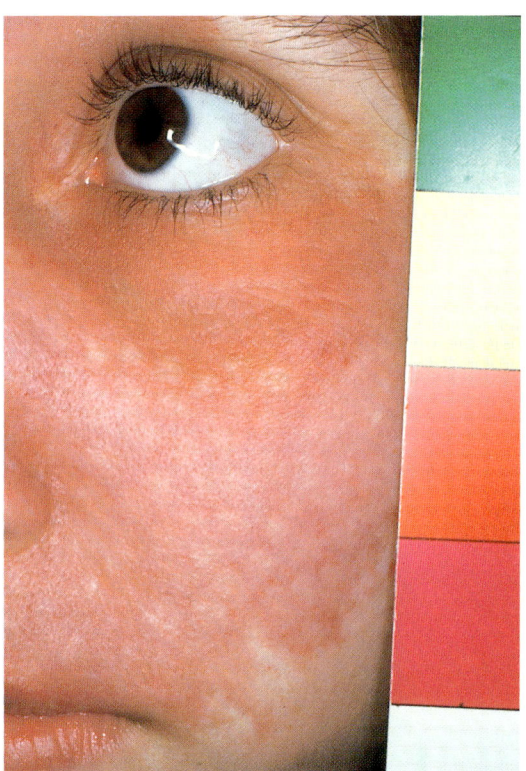

FIG. 5.45-E. Fading without scarring, cheek and upper lip, six months post-treatment.

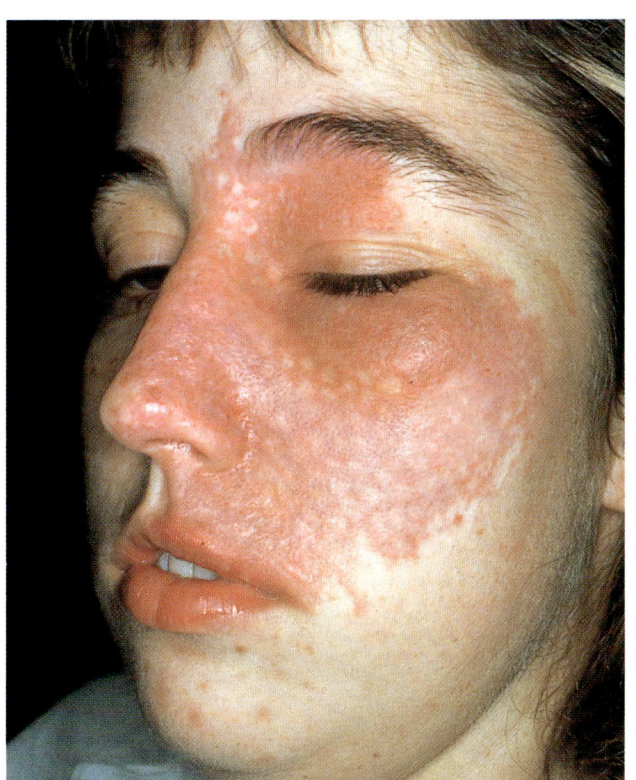

FIG. 5.45-F. Overall fading of area without scarring.

Case courtesy of *David B. Apfelberg*, M.D.

6

YAG LASER

VASCULAR AND RELATED LESIONS
6.1 Arteriovenous malformation of the right third finger
6.2 Cavernous capillary hemangioma: strawberry hemangioma
6.3 Cavernous hemangioma of the oral buccal mucosa
6.4 Cavernous hemangioma of the lip
6.5 Port wine stain of the mid-forehead
6.6 Port wine nevus
6.7 Port wine hemangioma of the face
6.8 Port wine hemangioma
6.9 Strawberry hemangioma of the eyelid
6.10 Strawberry hemangioma in infancy

MALIGNANT AND PREMALIGNANT LESIONS
6.11 Kaposi's sarcoma: upper eyelid

TATTOO
6.12 Decorative tattoo (thigh)
6.13 Decorative tattoo (shoulder)

MISCELLANEOUS
6.14 Keloid post-traumatic wound
6.15 Keloid scarring post acne

SURGICAL PROCEDURES
6.16 Cavernous hemangioma of the face
6.17 Cavernous hemangioma of the left chest
6.18 Cavernous hemangioma of the left cheek
6.19 Capillary/cavernous hemangioma of the forehead and eyelid
6.20 Capillary/cavernous hemangioma of the cheek
6.21 Deep burn excisions
6.22 Ulcerated capillary hemangioma of the vulva/perineum
6.23 Ulcerated oral capillary/cavernous hemangioma
6.24 Infiltrating Ductal Carcinoma of the Breast

CASE 6.1.

Arteriovenous Malformation of the Right Third Finger

REVIEW OF CASE. This patient first seen in 1985 was a 24-year-old dentist from Mexico with a history of two failed attempts at surgical ligation of the lesion at the base of the finger.

The patient was treated on 6/85, 9/85, 1/89, and 7/89. The involution of this lesion is palliative with new areas appearing after a few years. The patient has been treated as an outpatient with local anesthesia and does not wish to undergo surgery that might compromise the use of this finger on his dominant hand.

CHOICE OF LASER: Nd:YAG. The Nd:YAG laser was used because of the minimal surface damage and the ability to treat thick, deep, relatively high-flow lesions. After the first treatment/test evaluation, 50–55 watts and 0.1 sec exposure with the tip of the unfocused fiber 1 cm from the skin surface was considered optimal.

ADDITIONAL INFORMATION. Large blood vessels (greater than 2 mm) may have damage to the superficial walls, resulting in active bleeding and possibly requiring hemostatic suture. This occurred during the patient's first treatment.

POST-TREATMENT CARE. Elevation of the hand 30 degrees or more and the application of a topical antibiotic (Polysporin ointment) if blistering occurs.

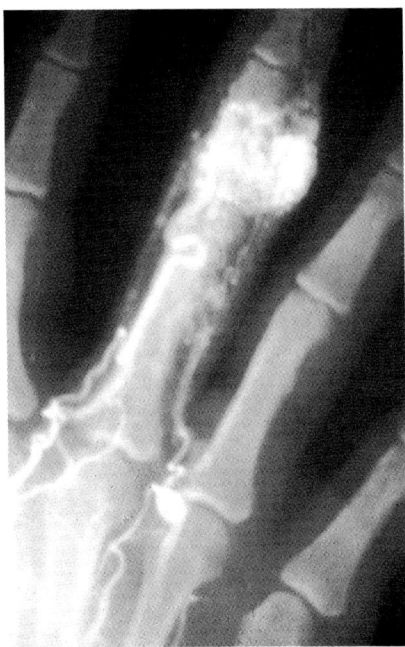

FIG. 6.1-A. Arteriogram of arteriovenous malformation of the right third finger.

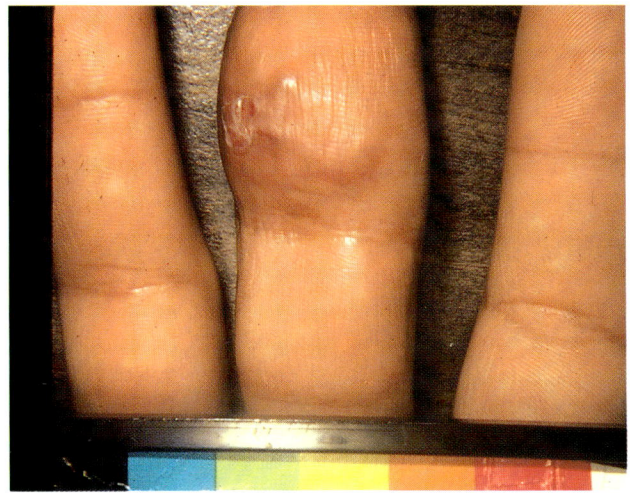

FIG. 6.1-B. Pre-treatment volar view of lesion.

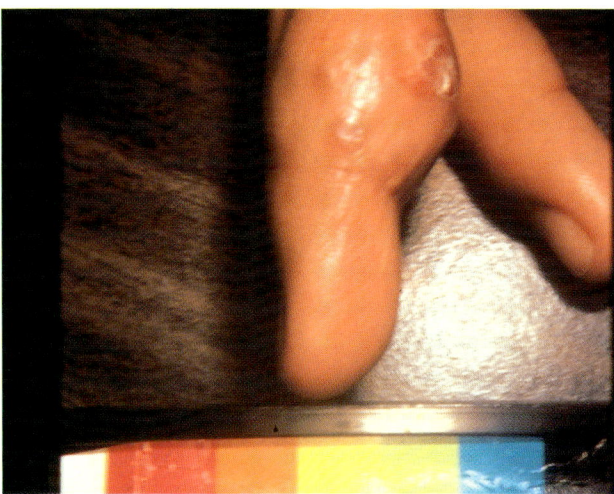

FIG. 6.1-C. Pre-treatment lateral view of lesion.

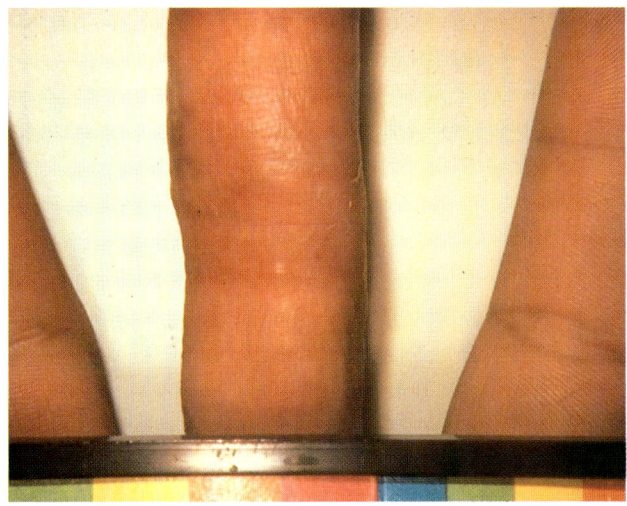

FIG. 6.1-D. Six months post-treatment; note preservation of normal skin appearance.

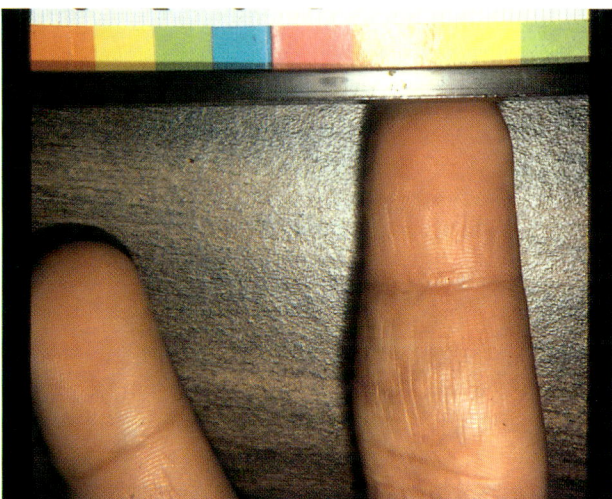

FIG. 6.1-E. Fifteen months post-treatment with fullness suggestive of recurrence. Note the normal surface architecture.

Case courtesy of *Harold L. Rosenfeld,* M.D.

CASE 6.2
Cavernous Capillary Hemangioma
Strawberry Hemangioma

REVIEW OF CASE. This patient developed hemangioma involving the head and neck shortly after birth with progressive obstruction of the right ear canal causing chronic superficial draining otitis externa.

CHOICE OF LASER: Nd:YAG. The Nd:YAG causes little surface damage while allowing for treatment of deep and/or thick blood vessels by heating them from the inside out. Nd:YAG is used with a no focusing lens at 0.1 second intervals for exposure, with the fiber tip 1 cm from the skin surface. Because of the child's age and extent of the lesion, all procedures were done under general anesthesia. The patient had two one-hour treatment sessions on 4/85 and 7/85 with resection of redundant tissue on 3/86.

ADDITIONAL INFORMATION. Because of the deep penetration of this wavelength, stainless steel scleral shields are used when working around the eyes. Although there is an immediate blanching visible, this is partially due to vasospasm, the actual permanent involution of the lesion starts to occur 3 months after treatment and may progress for as long as 1 year.

POST-TREATMENT CARE. Elevation of the head and neck 30 degrees or more and application of topical antibiotic (Polysporin ointment) if blistering occurs. Sun exposure is limited using sunscreens, clothing, or avoidance until all redness from the treatment has subsided.

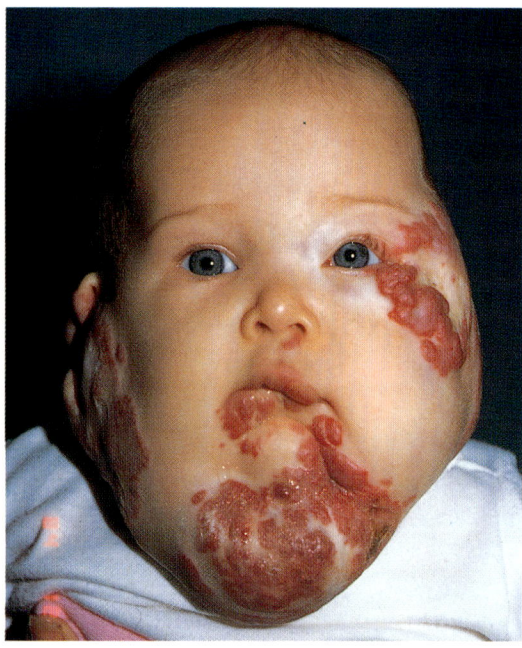

FIG. 6.2-A. Pre-treatment cutaneous and subcutaneous mass.

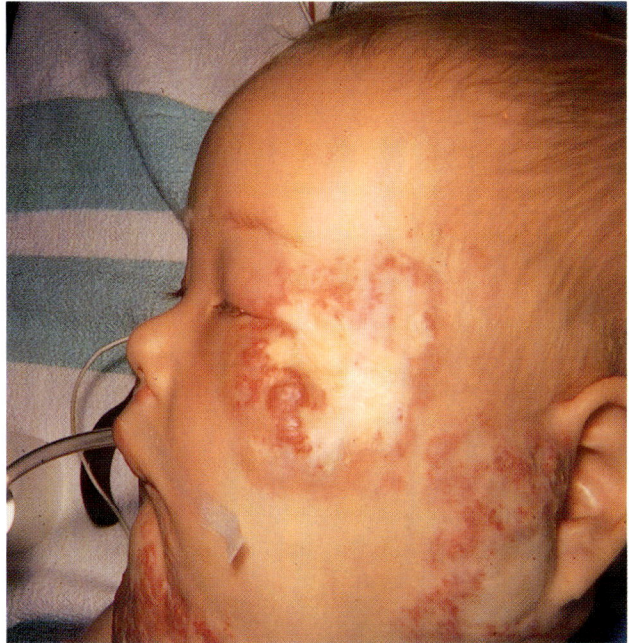

FIG. 6.2-B. Three months post-initial treatment with some spotty regrowth of cutaneous vessels as well as remaining bulk.

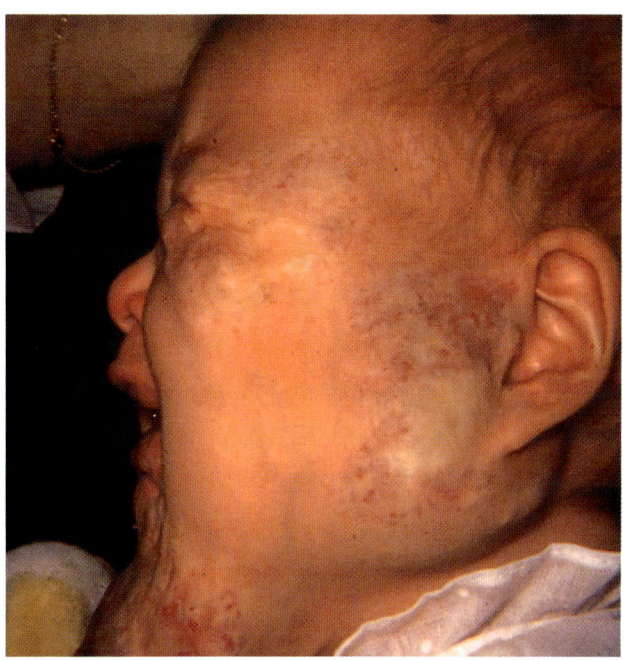

FIG. 6.2-C. Three months post-second treatment.

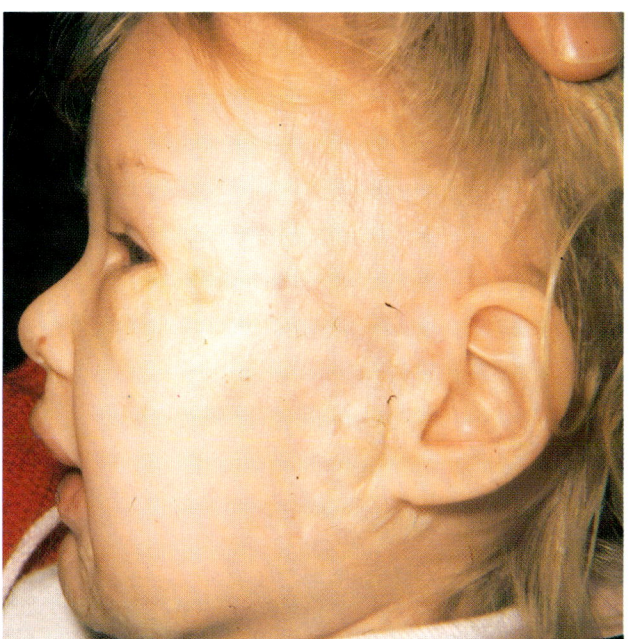

FIG. 6.2-D. Eighteen months post-second treatment. Nine months after resection of involuted redundant tissue.

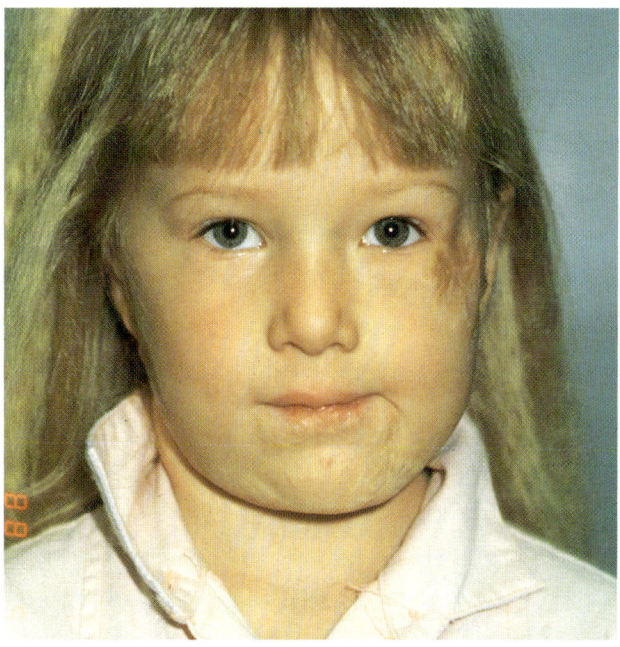

FIG. 6.2-E. 2-½ years post-surgical resection of redundant tissue. No signs of recurrence are present.

Case courtesy of *Harold L. Rosenfeld*, M.D.

CASE 6.3

Cavernous Hemangioma of the Oral Buccal Mucosa

REVIEW OF CASE. This 25-year-old female presented with a rapidly growing congenital hemangioma of the right upper lip, buccal sulcus, and mucosa. The lesion occasionally swells and hurts with exercise, motion, or extremes of heat and cold.

CHOICE OF LASER: Nd:YAG. The Nd:YAG laser is able to photocoagulate to a depth of 5–7 mm in the dermis. It was felt that the argon laser, which penetrates only the upper 1 mm of the dermis, would not be able to penetrate the entire depth of this hemangioma. The CO_2 laser would have to photovaporize the entire area or have to be used for excision. Therefore, deep photocoagulation as the mechanism of action for the Nd:YAG laser was chosen. In addition, the oral cavity heals well.

The use of the Nd:YAG laser for the treatment of thick hemangiomatous lesions of the oral cavity is ideally suited. Deep coagulation necrosis heals well in this area and the hemangiomas can be resolved.

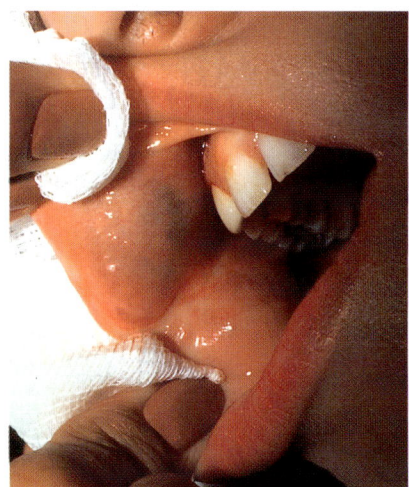

FIG. 6.3-A. Pre-treatment cavernous hemangioma of the oral buccal mucosa. The deep blue hypertrophic hemangioma is apparent under the mucosa.

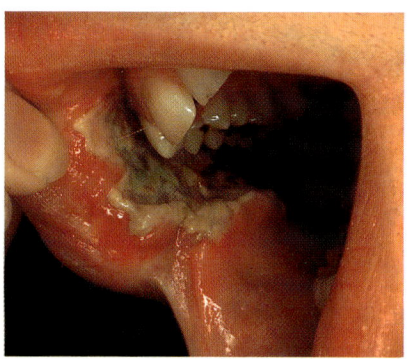

FIG. 6.3-B. Four days following photocoagulation of the area. There is a diffuse mucosal full-thickness necrosis.

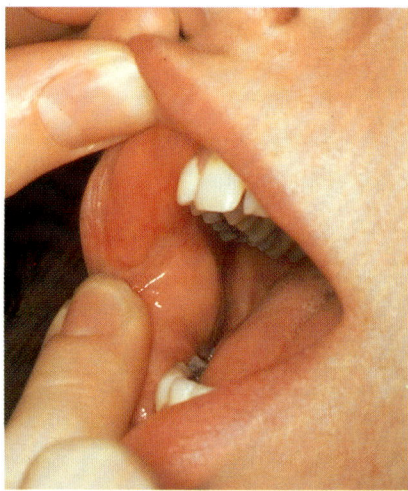

FIG. 6.3-C. Final healing shows the mucosalization of the oral cavity. The area was smoothed without residual hemangioma or bulging.

Case courtesy of *David B. Apfelberg*, M.D.

CASE 6.4
Cavernous Hemangioma of the Lip

REVIEW OF CASE. This 52-year-old male presented with a lifelong history of a progressively enlarging cavernous hemangioma of the lower lip. The patient was highly desirous of having this lesion removed, as it was chronically irritated, at times, bleeding and generally deforming in appearance.

CHOICE OF LASER: Nd:YAG. The lesion was treated with the Nd:YAG laser administered through a focusing handpiece. The Nd:YAG laser was chosen due to the fact that cavernous hemangiomas are composed mostly of blood-filled spaces, and the coagulation effect of the Nd:YAG laser was utilized and maximized.

ADDITIONAL INFORMATION. A conservative approach and multiple treatment plan was designed. Topical ice and peripheral infiltration with 1% Xylocaine with 1:100,000 epinephrine was utilized for anesthesia. Progressing in a very conservative manner the lesion was ablated over four treatments with power settings never exceeding 18 watts at 0.5 seconds application. The cosmetic result noted in Fig. C is very acceptable for the patient. He is left with just a small amount of scabbing on the lower aspect of the right lower lip, which has subsequently resolved.

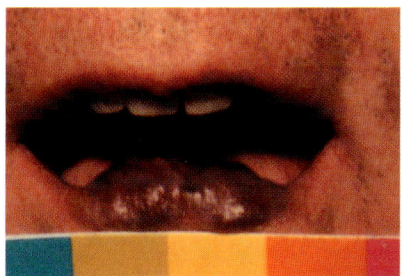

FIG. 6.4-A. Pre-treatment cavernous hemangioma of lower lip demonstrating bulky hypertrophy, irregular surface, and chronic ulceration.

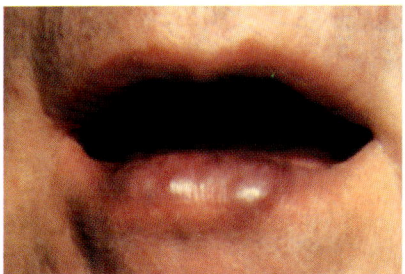

FIG. 6.4-B. After second treatment, note marked blanching and shrinkage of lesion with improvement of lip contour.

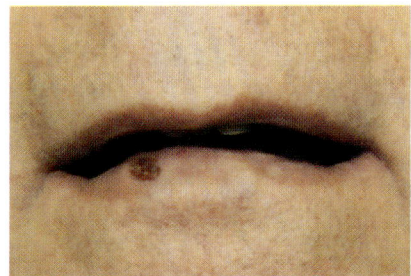

FIG. 6.4-C. Final appearance showing satisfactory resolution of hemangioma after three treatments. Lip contour and color are almost normal.

Case courtesy of *Ronald Allen Kirschner*, D.O.

CASE 6.5

Port Wine Stain of the Mid-Forehead

REVIEW OF CASE. This patient is a dark-skinned Latin female seen for the first time at age 24 with a port wine stain (nevus flammeus) of the mid-forehead. The test area was done on 12/85 varying from 20–35 watts at 0.1 seconds. Under local anesthetic, she was treated on 5/86 with 20 watts for 0.1 seconds and on 1/87 and 9/87 with 35 watts for 0.1 seconds.

CHOICE OF LASER: Nd:YAG. The Nd:YAG laser causes little surface damage while allowing for treatment of deep and/or thick blood vessels by heating them from the inside out. The Nd:YAG laser is used with a no focusing lens at 0.1 second intervals for exposure with the fiber tip 1 cm from the skin surface.

ADDITIONAL INFORMATION. Because of the deep penetration of this wavelength, stainless steel scleral shields are used when working around the eyes. Although there is an immediate blanching visible, this is partially due to vasospasm, the actual permanent involution of the lesion starts to occur 3 months after treatment and may progress for as long as 1 year.

Hyperpigmentation has appeared in other dark-skinned patients after similar treatment and has gone away spontaneously in as long as 2 years or somewhat sooner if topical hydroquinones are used.

POST-TREATMENT CARE. Elevation of the head 30 degrees or more and application of topical antibiotic (Polysporin ointment) if blistering occurs. Sun exposure is limited using sunscreens, clothing, or avoidance until all redness from the treatment has subsided.

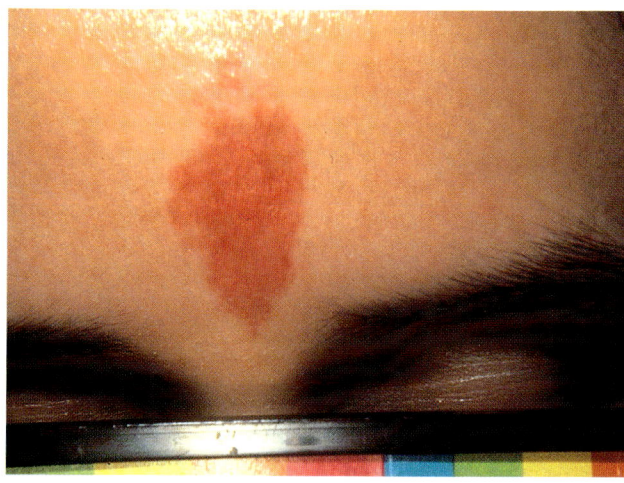

FIG. 6.5-A. Pre-treatment port wine stain of mid-forehead on dark-skinned female patient.

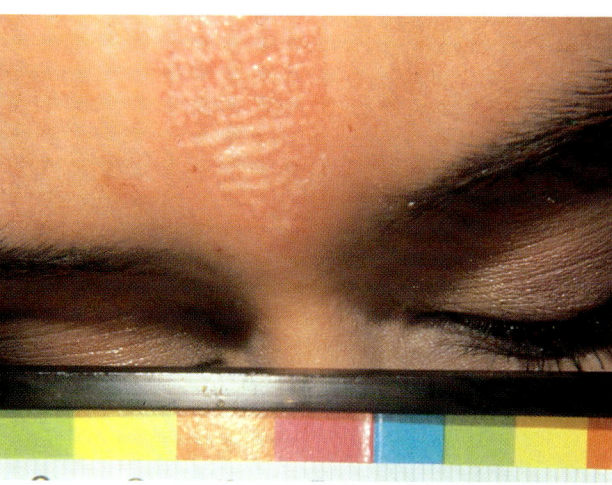

FIG. 6.5-B. Immediately post-treatment, note blanching.

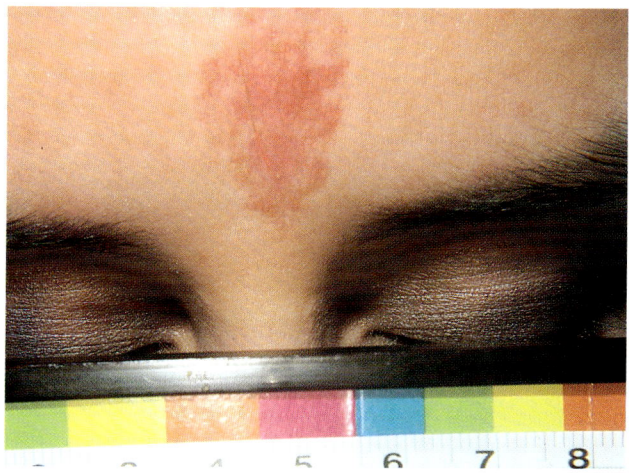

FIG. 6.5-C. Three months post-treatment, some involution evident.

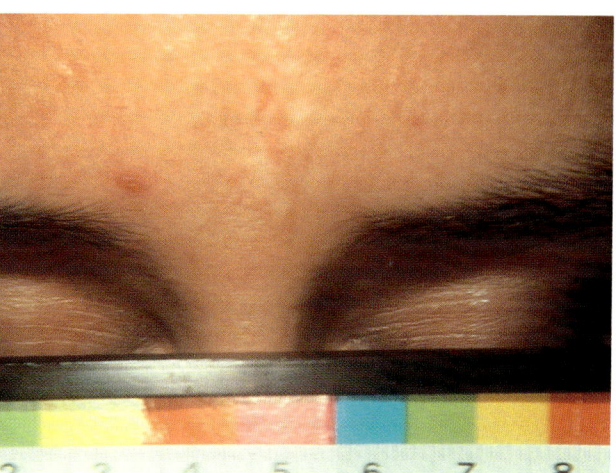

FIG. 6.5-D. Three years post-treatment with essentially complete involution of lesion with no signs of recurrence. There is slight hypopigmentation present.

Case courtesy of *Harold L. Rosenfeld*, M.D.

CASE 6.6
Port Wine Nevus

REVIEW OF CASE. This 48-year-old man presented with a port wine nevus on the right side of the face with areas that are distinctly representative of a cavernous hemangiomata.

CHOICE OF LASER: Nd:YAG. The Nd:YAG laser was chosen because of the mixed elements of the hemangioma and because of the laser's coagulation capabilities. The large areas were treated with a focusing lens and power settings of 13 to 15 watts at maximum level of duration of application of 0.5 seconds. The smaller capillary areas were treated individually utilizing the Nd:YAG laser and a contact tip. In this mode the setting was a maximum application of 18 watts with very short exposure times averaging 0.2 seconds.

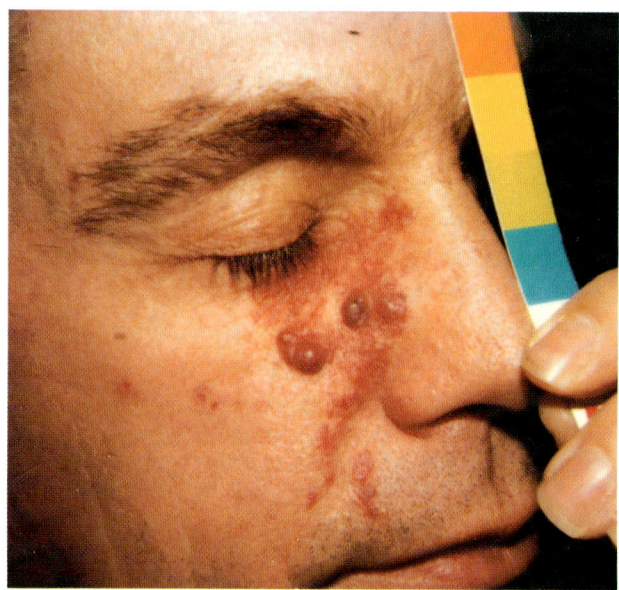

FIG. 6.6-A. Pre-treatment port wine nevus of right side of face demonstrating hypertrophic blebs and surface irregularities.

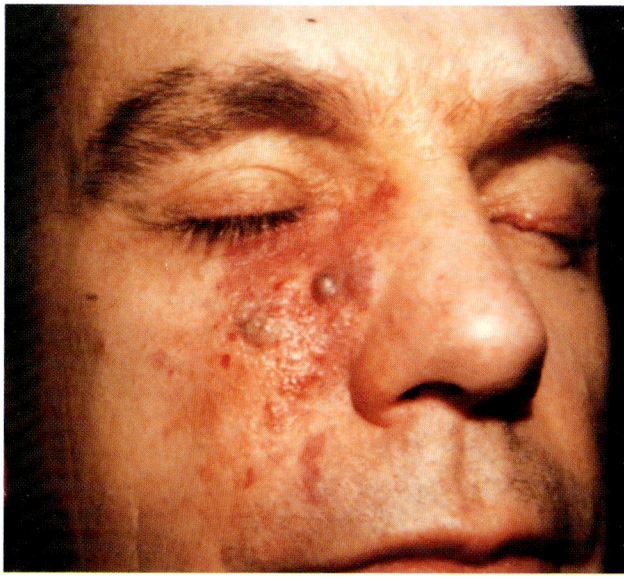

FIG. 6.6-B. Immediately after first treatment showing blanching and shrinkage of hypertrophic areas.

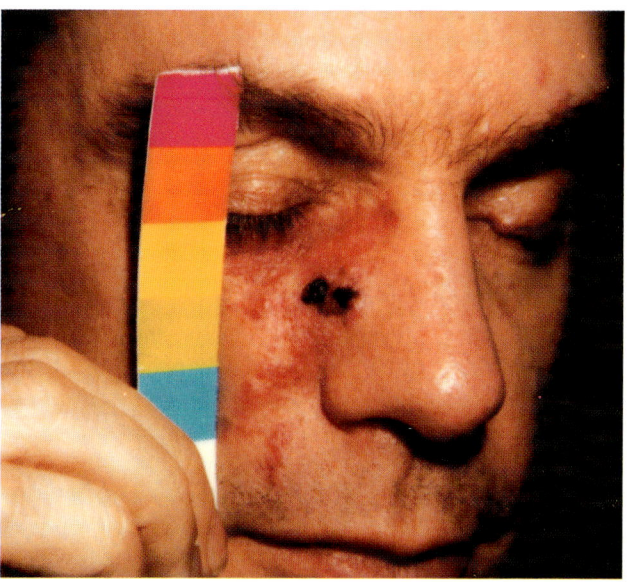

FIG. 6.6-C. Char from first treatment after 5 days.

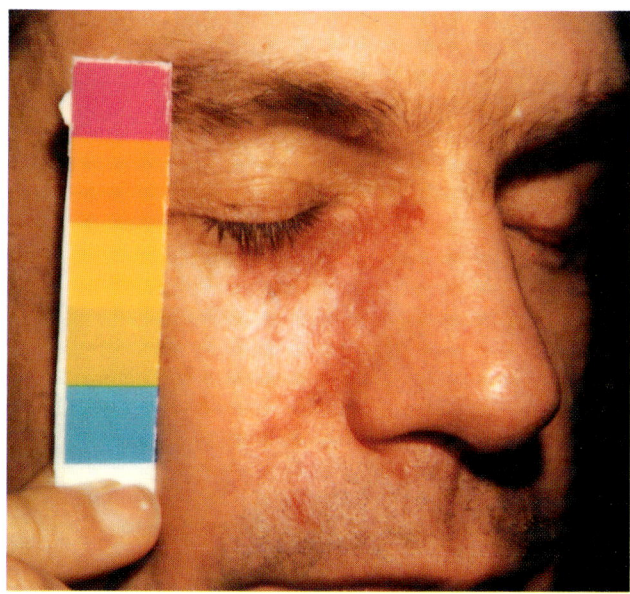

FIG. 6.6-D. Marked blanching with shrinkage and smoothening of surface after 7 months. Additional touch-up is necessary in the lower lid and nasolabial fold.

Case courtesy of *Ronald Allen Kirschner,* D.O.

YAG LASER   301

CASE 6.7
Port Wine Hemangioma of the Face

REVIEW OF CASE.   This 55-year-old male presented with a diffuse port wine hemangioma on his face. Over the past 5 years, the patient had had numerous argon laser treatments which have partially but incompletely blanched the hemangioma. Irregularity of the skin surface was also present.

CHOICE OF LASER: Nd:YAG.   The Nd:YAG laser is able to photocoagulate hemangioma to a depth of 5–7 mm in the dermis. The previous argon laser treatment had failed to completely blanch or shrink the hemangioma. Therefore, it was felt that the greater depth of the Nd:YAG laser could improve upon the initial argon result.

ADDITIONAL INFORMATION.   Due to the diffuse and deep photocoagulation of the Nd:YAG laser, it is safer to treat in a "polka dot" manner. One mm spots of Nd:YAG laser photocoagulation are interspersed with normal hemangioma, varying the spots by about one mm. The untreated and unburned skin aids in the healing of the photocoagulated spots. The untreated interstices can then be re-treated 8 to 12 weeks following treatment.

POST-TREATMENT CARE.   Iced compresses and antibiotic ointment are used topically.

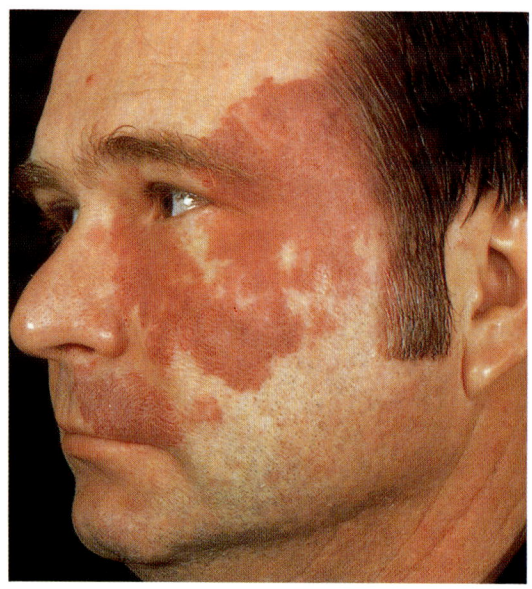

FIG. 6.7-A. Patient before laser treatment.

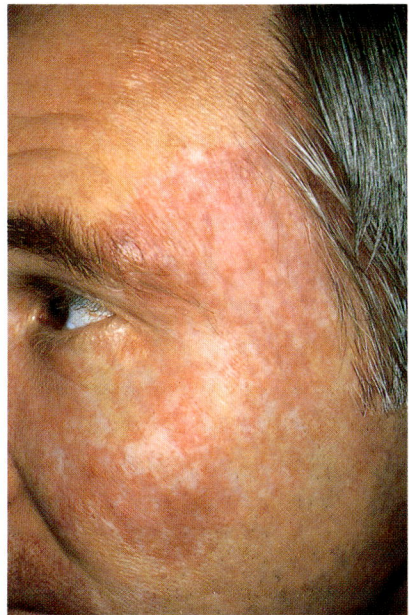

FIG. 6.7-B. Patient following argon laser treatment. Note marked blanching which is incomplete and skin surface irregularities.

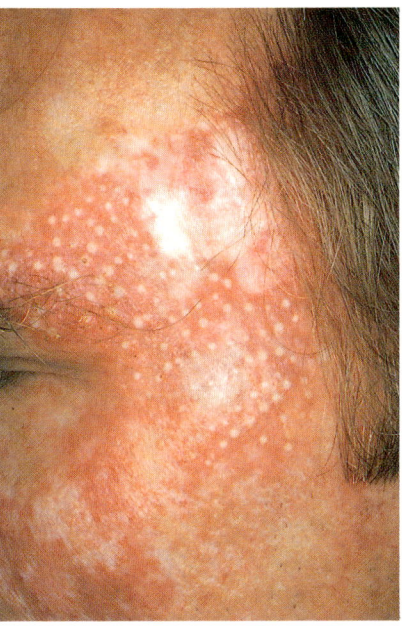

FIG. 6.7-C. "Polka dot" pattern of Nd:YAG laser photocoagulation on temple and cheek.

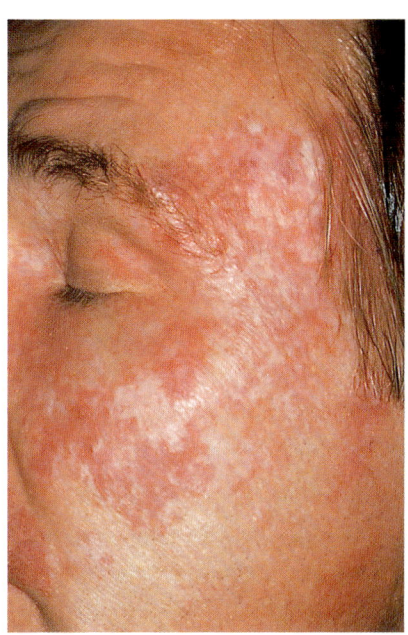

FIG. 6.7-D. Result after healing, showing improved blanching and good surface contour.

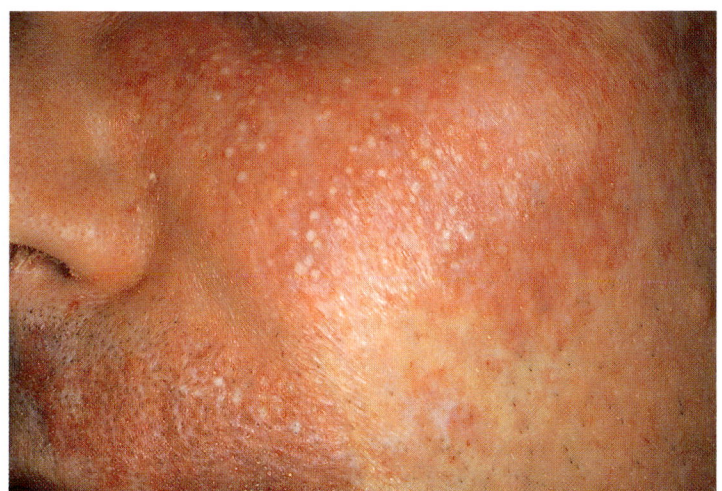

FIG. 6.7-E. Result after further "polka dot" Nd:YAG laser treatments on cheek and upper lip.

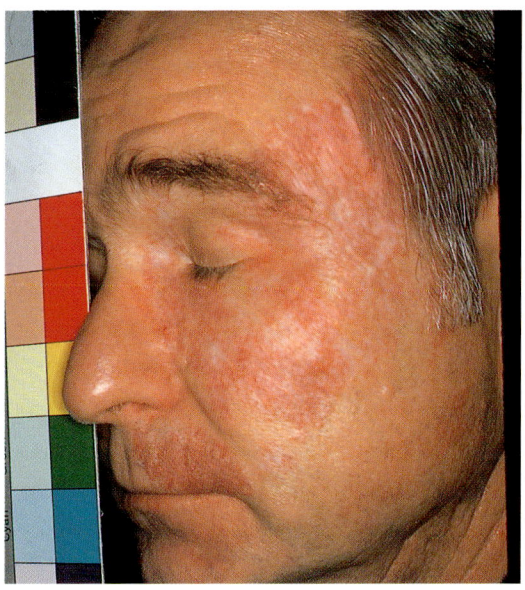

FIG. 6.7-F. Further blanching, fading, and smoothening of the lesion.

Case courtesy of *David B. Apfelberg,* M.D.

CASE 6.8
Port Wine Hemangioma

REVIEW OF CASE.   This 33-year-old female presented with a diffuse port wine hemangioma of the cheek, lower lip, and oral lingual mucosa. At approximately age 25 through 30 she was treated numerous times with the argon laser with good but incomplete fading. She continued to have marked hypertrophy and irregularity of the lower lip, chin, and the lower labial mucosa.

CHOICE OF LASER: Nd:YAG.   The Nd:YAG laser is able to photocoagulate hemangioma to a depth of 5–7 mm in the dermis. The previous argon laser treatment had failed to completely blanch or shrink the hemangioma. Therefore, it was felt that the greater depth of the Nd:YAG laser could improve upon the initial argon laser result.

ADDITIONAL INFORMATION.   Due to the diffuse and deep photocoagulation of the Nd:YAG laser, it is safer to treat in a "polka dot" manner. One mm spots of Nd:YAG laser photocoagulation are interspersed with normal hemangioma, varying the spots by about one mm. The untreated and unburned skin aids in the healing of the photocoagulated spots. The untreated interstices can then be re-treated 8 to 12 weeks following treatment.

POST-TREATMENT CARE.   Iced compresses and antibiotic ointment are used topically.

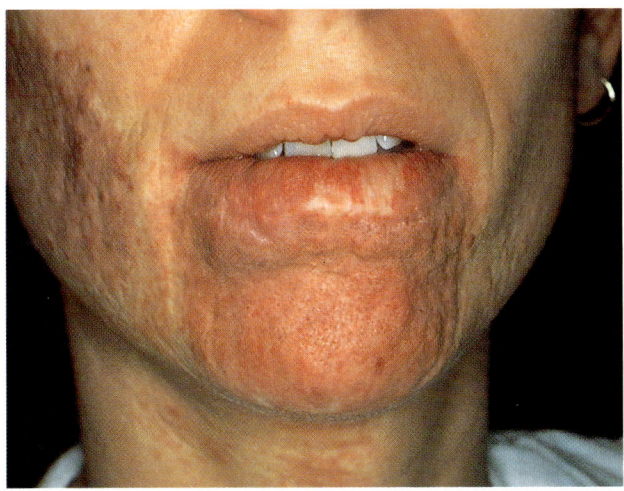

FIG. 6.8-A. Port wine hemangioma of lower lip and chin prior to treatment. Previous argon treatment had blanched the hemangioma and contoured it as much as possible.

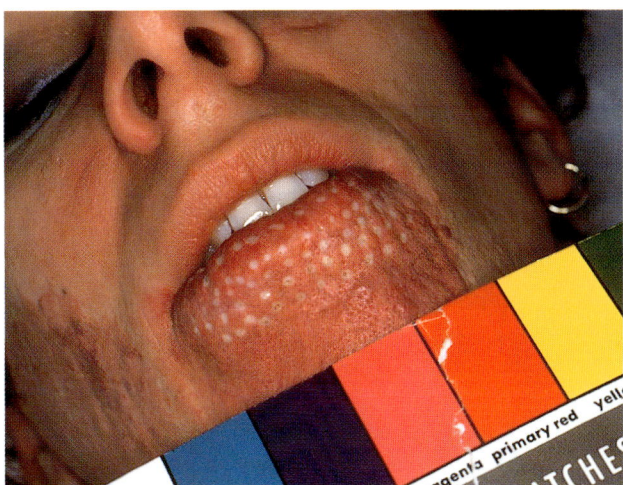

FIG. 6.8-B. "Polka dot" technique with the Nd:YAG laser. One mm spots of photocoagulation are utilized, leaving at least one to two mm of normal hemangioma untreated in the interspaces.

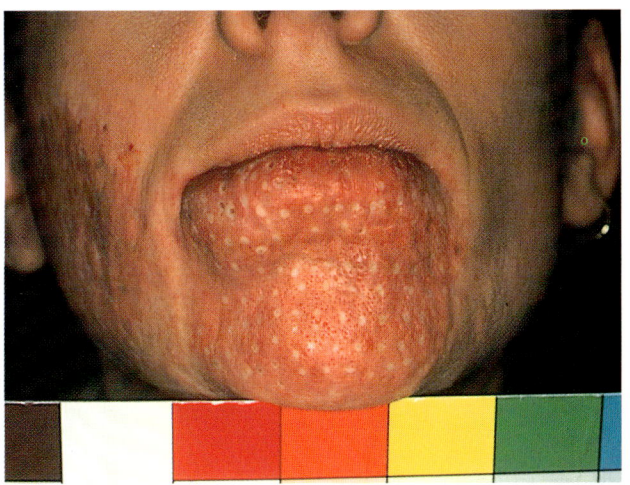

FIG. 6.8-C. Same as Fig. 6.8-B.

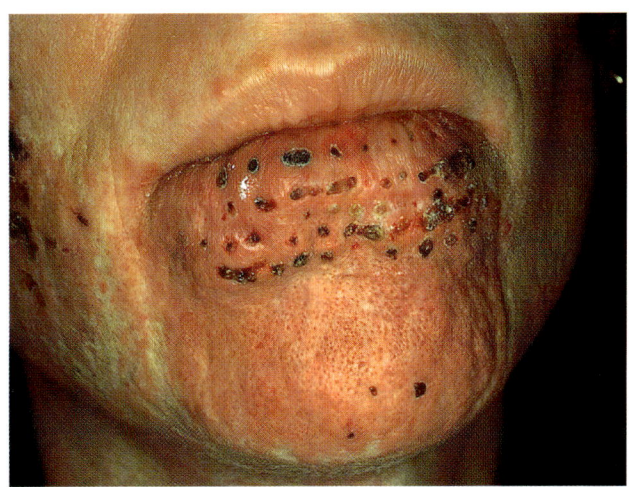

FIG. 6.8-D. Healing of "polka dots" two weeks post-treatment.

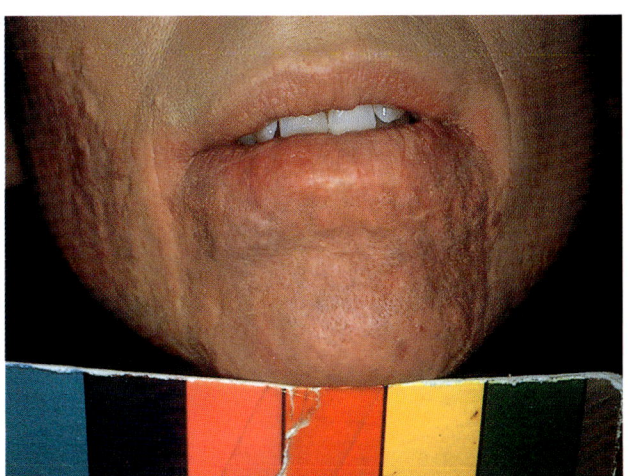

FIG. 6.8-E. Final appearance eight weeks following Nd:YAG photocoagulation, note marked improvement in contour and blanching of color.

Case courtesy of *David B. Apfelberg*, M.D.

CASE 6.9
Strawberry Hemangioma of the Eyelid

REVIEW OF CASE. This patient was examined at two months of age with a strawberry hemangioma on the right upper eyelid. There was no obstruction of vision at that time. She was observed for three months and was also examined by an ophthalmalic plastic surgeon. The recommendation at that time was that as long as there was no obstruction of vision or any symptoms or signs of amblyopia or strabismus intervention, treatment was to be deferred. After another three months of observation, the lesion had quickly grown and was causing obstruction of vision. At that time, the mother wanted treatment and the plan was to do Nd:YAG laser surgery followed by reconstructive surgery. The result of the laser surgery alone was quite acceptable to the mother and no reconstructive surgery was performed.

CHOICE OF LASER: Nd:YAG. The Nd:YAG laser was chosen because it has been shown that Nd:YAG can treat thick hemangiomas successfully. It penetrates a few millimeters deep in tissue and coagulates the blood vessels.

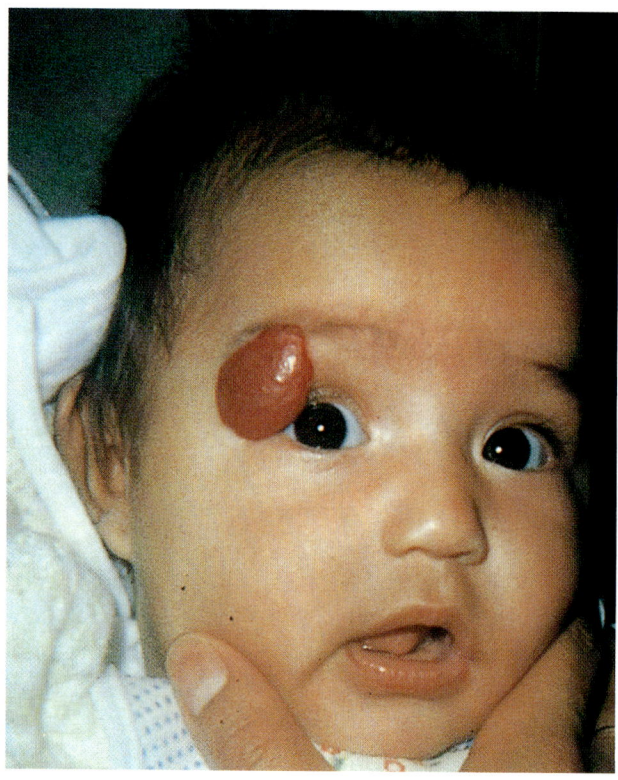

FIG. 6.9-A. Strawberry hemangioma involving the right upper eyelid extending to the eyebrow. Size 2.5 × 2.2 cm.

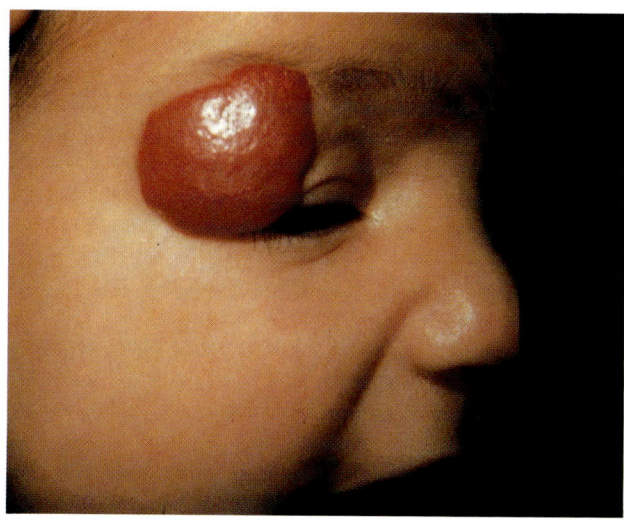

FIG. 6.9-B. Three months after initial treatment, the lesion is 3.4 × 2.7 cm. Since the lesion was rapidly growing the patient's mother consented to laser therapy.

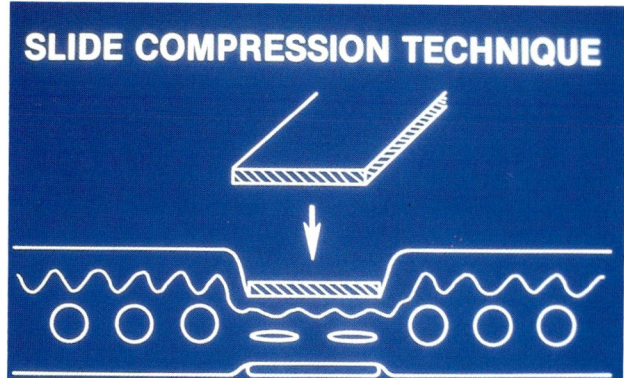

FIG. 6.9-C. Slide compression technique for thick hemangioma. A glass slide is placed on the lesion and pressure is applied to make the lesion thinner. The Nd:YAG is then focused through the glass in order for the beam to reach the whole thickness of the lesion. (Courtesy of Lawrence David, M.D.)

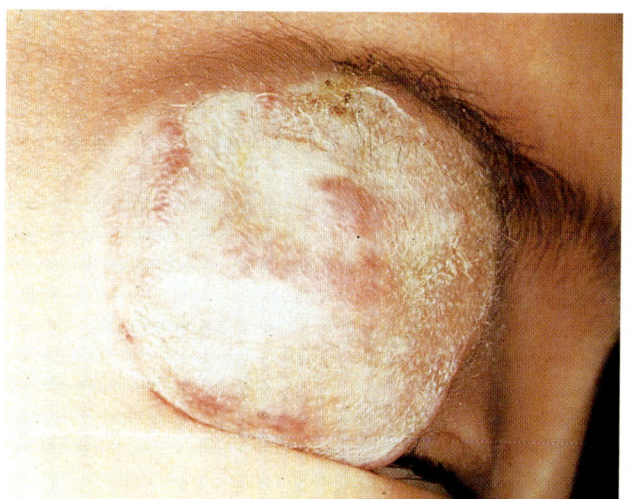

FIG. 6.9-D. Immediately post-Nd:YAG: therapy. Note blanching that is required to obtain a result. Under general anesthesia, a focused Nd:YAG laser was used with power of 30 watts. 0.1 mm spot size, in a polka dot manner to photocoagulate the entire surface of the hemangioma. She received dexamethasone to reduce swelling and erythromycin for antibiotic therapy. An eye shield was not used, however, using an eye shield under the eyelid is a safer method.

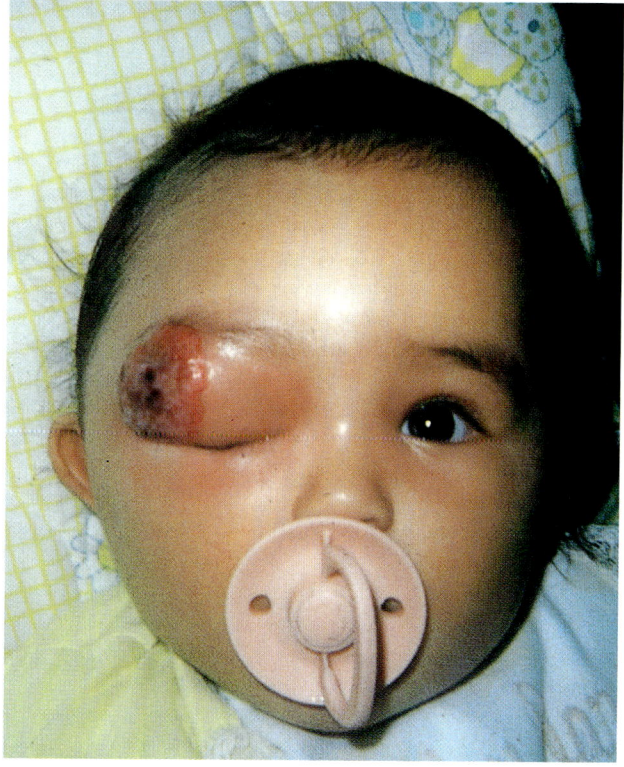

FIG. 6.9-E. A few days after therapy with some swelling of the eyelid.

Case continues on following page.

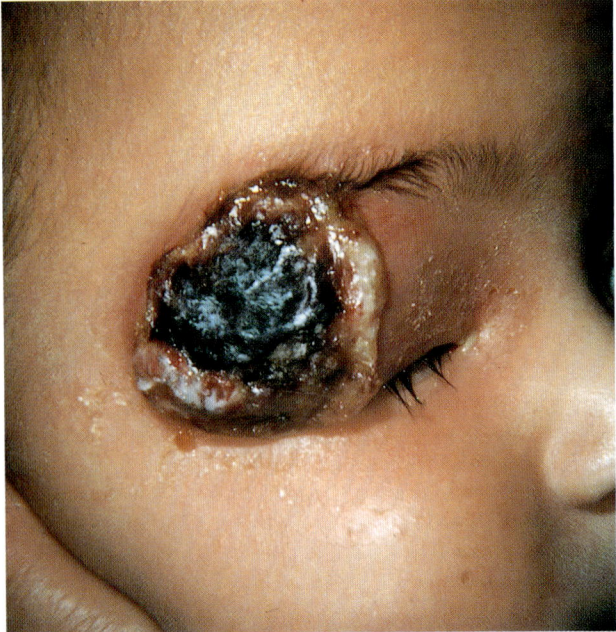

FIG. 6.9-F. Two weeks after treatment. The area is healing but a localized *Staphylococcus aureus* infection is present. Cephalosporin antibiotic therapy was initiated to treat the infection.

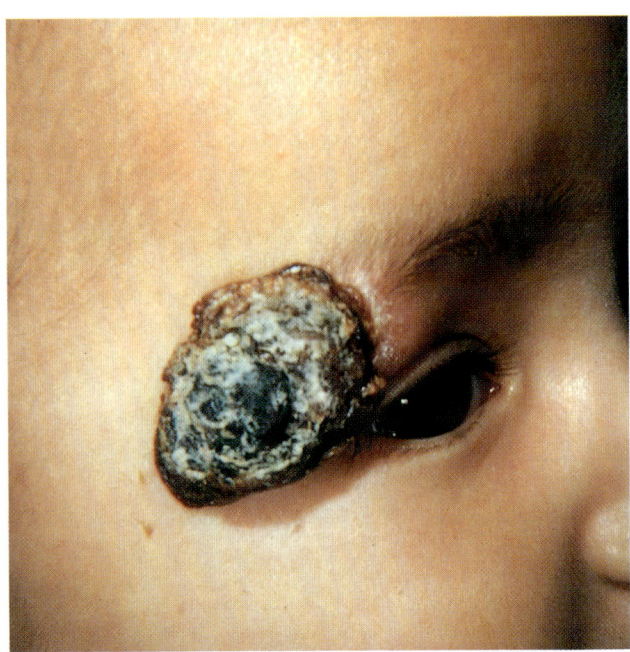

FIG. 6.9-G. Healing with scab formation.

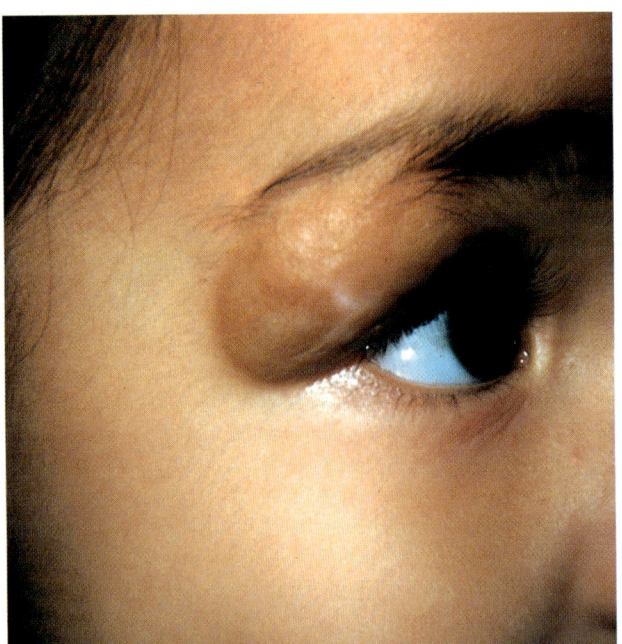

FIG. 6.9-H. After the scab fell off, the lesion healed with minor scarring.

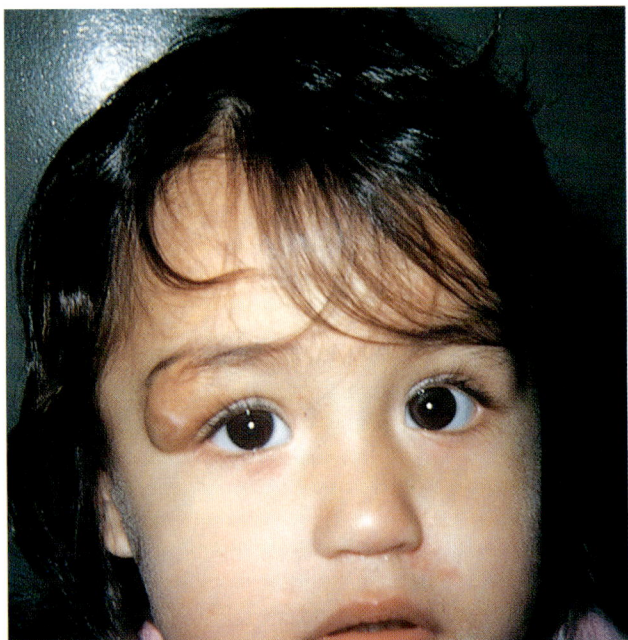

FIG. 6.9-I. Three months after laser therapy. Her mother chose not to do any reconstructive surgery since the result of the Nd:YAG laser was quite satisfactory. The ophthalmic plastic surgeon reported normal eyes.

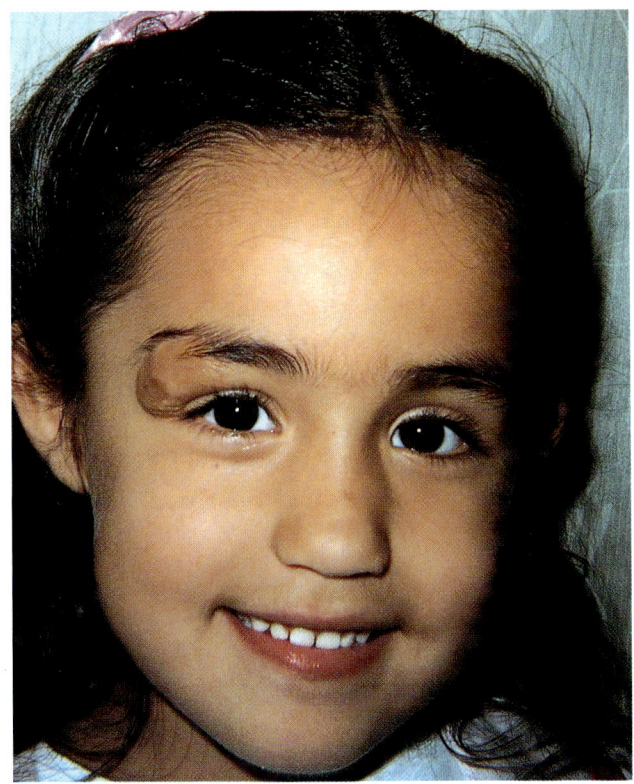

FIG. 6.9-J. Five years later. Color has improved. The patient's mother did not want any reconstructive surgery because the results were quite satisfactory to her.

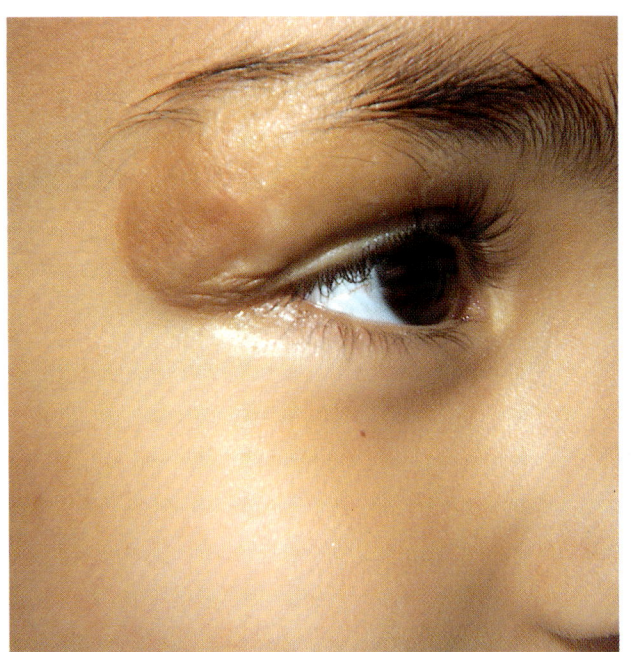

FIG. 6.9-K. Close-up of the right upper eyelid.

Case courtesy of *Syrus Rayhan*, M.D.

CASE 6.10
Strawberry Hemangioma in Infancy

REVIEW OF CASE. This 7-month-old infant was referred by her pediatrician due to an ulcerated, non-healing hemangioma of the right flank. There had been repeated episodes of ulceration. The child was almost constantly crying and irritable.

CHOICE OF LASER: Nd:YAG. At the time of this treatment, both the argon laser and Nd:YAG lasers were available. The Nd:YAG laser was chosen because of the depth of the birthmark. Both the argon and Nd:YAG lasers are useful for treating vascular lesions; however, the Nd:YAG will penetrate more deeply.

ADDITIONAL INFORMATION. Ice packs in the recovery room and for 24 hours as tolerated are helpful in reducing swelling and erythema following treatment. It is not necessary to treat every square centimeter of the birthmark. Using a polka-dot technique, the entire birthmark can be impacted without actually exposing all of it. A comparison of the argon and Nd:YAG lasers for treatment of this condition concluded that the argon was most suitable due to the increased risk of scarring and other complications (such as post-operative bleeding) when using the Nd:YAG. We believe that the Nd:YAG laser should be reserved for very large or deep hemangiomas. The Nd:YAG is also useful when delivered via sapphire tip for excision of large hemangiomas.

POST-TREATMENT CARE. Ice for 24–48 hours as tolerated. Antibiotic ointment should be applied several times daily. The area should be gently cleansed with tepid water and mild soap. Over the first 24–72 hours blistering and weeping of the skin are expected, and some skin may peel away. This is normal and within a few days, eschar will form. Eschar should not be disrupted and should be allowed to separate on its own. Parents are instructed to watch for bleeding. If bleeding occurs gentle pressure should be applied. If bleeding persists, the doctor must be contacted or the patient taken to the emergency room. A follow-up appointment is scheduled for three weeks.

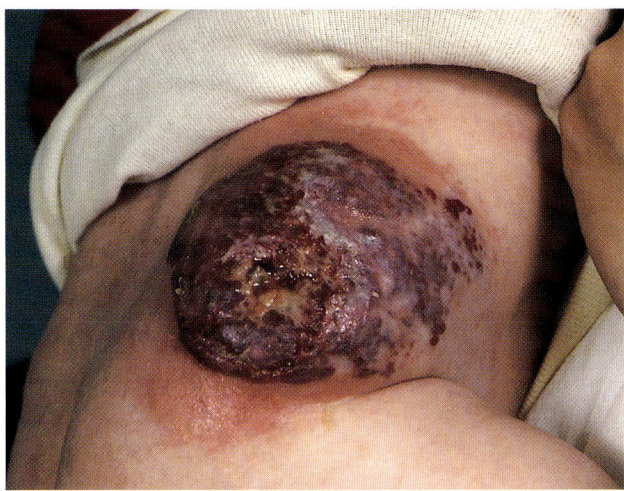

FIG. 6.10-A. Pre-operatively, a large, ulcerated hemangioma that is symptomatic.

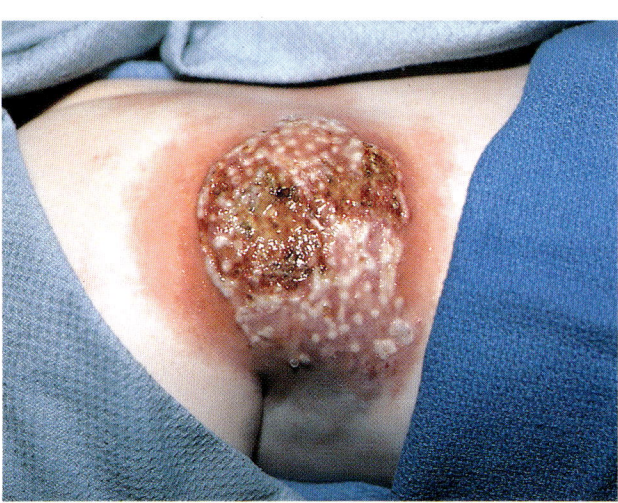

FIG. 6.10-B. Immediately following treatment. Note the polka-dot pattern over the entire hemangioma. In addition to blanching, some shrinkage of the hemangioma is noted during treatment. A profound erythema is noted around the periphery of the birthmark.

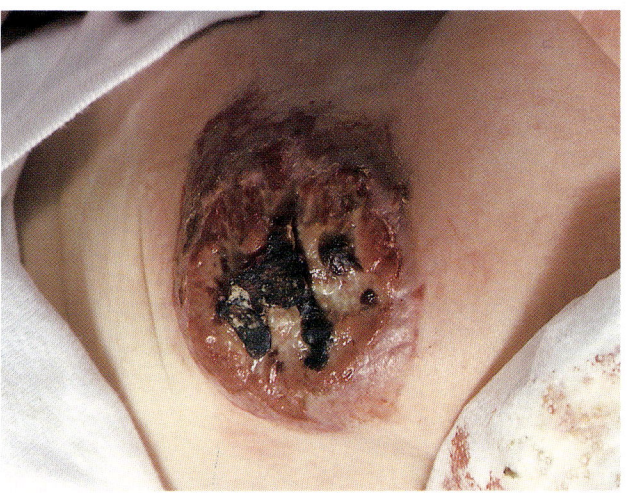

FIG. 6.10-C. At three weeks eschar is present. It is important to note that symptoms of this birthmark were relieved within a day of the treatment.

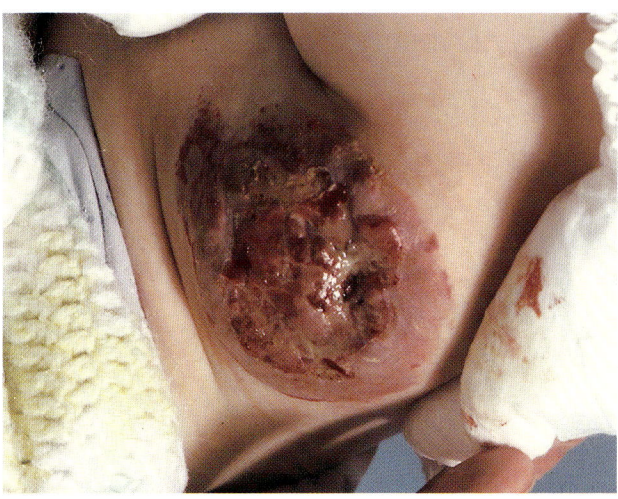

FIG. 6.10-D. At six weeks, eschar has separated and healing is still taking place.

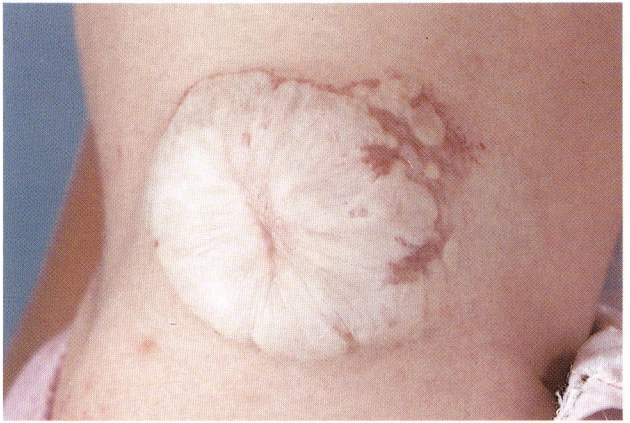

FIG. 6.10-E. Result at 18 months. Scarring and skin texture changes are noted. There is residual hemangioma peripherally. The mother reported that complete healing took 7–8 weeks, and that the symptoms were immediately relieved. She was grateful for the treatment and pleased with the outcome. The value of surgical excision in the future was discussed.

Case courtesy of **Bruce M. Achauer,** M.D., and **Victoria M. Vander Kam,** R.N.

CASE 6.11

Kaposi's Sarcoma: Upper Eyelid

REVIEW OF CASE. A 76-year-old Latin male with systemic Kaposi's sarcoma was referred for treatment of an eyelid lesion that was irritating the globe. This area was treated once in 1987 under local anesthesia as an outpatient. The remaining lesions were treated successfully with systemic chemotherapy.

CHOICE OF LASER: Nd:YAG. The Nd:YAG laser was chosen because of its ability to treat thick lesions. The Nd:YAG laser was calibrated to 55 watts and the exposure duration was 0.1 seconds. 217 pulses were used to deliver 1,313 joules of energy.

Stainless steel scleral shields are used when treating around the eyelids. The Nd:YAG laser in this power range causes epidermal disruption (second-degree burns).

POST-TREATMENT CARE. Ophthalmic neosporin ointment is applied until the epidermis heals.

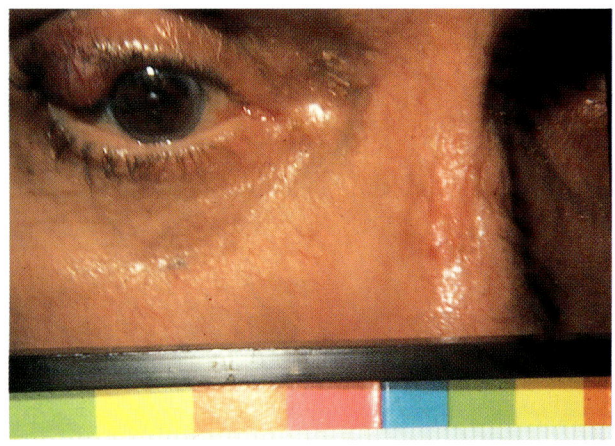

FIG. 6.11-A. Pre-treatment Kaposi's sarcoma impinging on palpabral fissure.

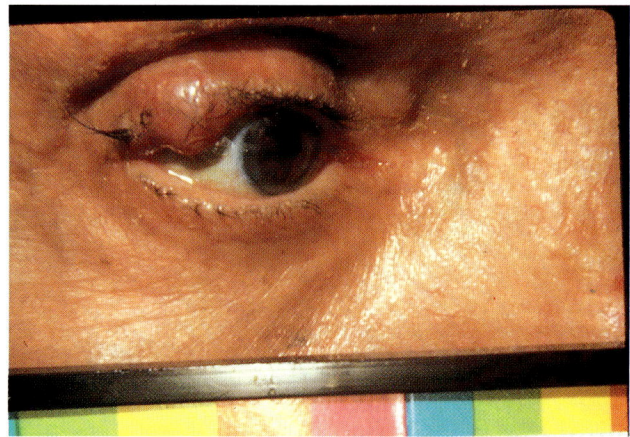

FIG. 6.11-B. Pre-treatment Kaposi's sarcoma lateral view.

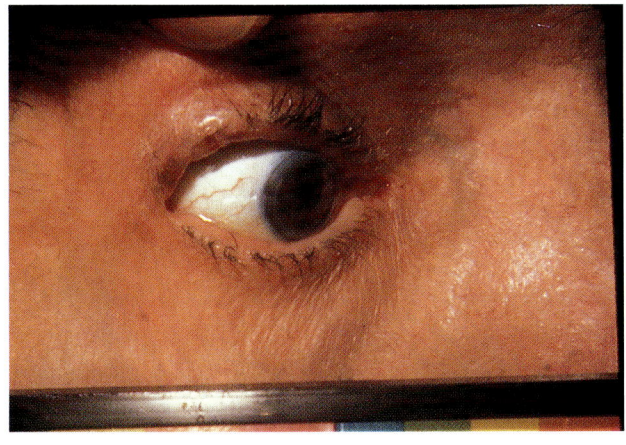

FIG. 6.11-C. Kaposi's sarcoma four weeks post-treatment.

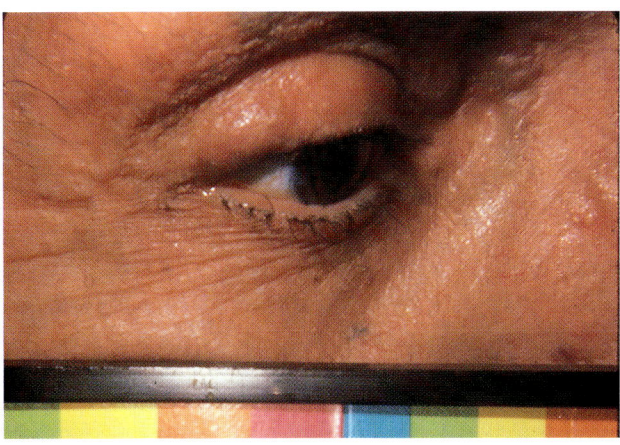

FIG. 6.11-D. Kaposi's sarcoma six weeks post-treatment.

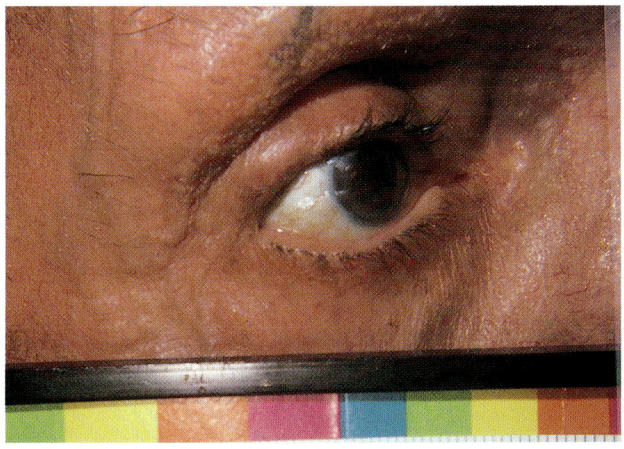

FIG. 6.11-E. Kaposi's sarcoma 3 months post-treatment. Note the continued involution of the treated lesion.

Case courtesy of *Harold L. Rosenfeld*, M.D.

CASE 6.12
Decorative Tattoo

REVIEW OF CASE. This 22-year-old female presented with a 5 year history of decorative tattoo. The patient felt the tattoo was a social liability and desired removal.

CHOICE OF LASER: Nd:YAG. The Nd:YAG laser was chosen because of its "facultative absorption by dark colors" and minimal absorption by normally colored skin. Power settings were 18 watts at a maximum duration of 0.5 seconds.

ADDITIONAL INFORMATION. After the test spot healed satisfactorily, a multistage procedure was planned. 1% Xylocaine with 1:100,000 epinephrine was used for anesthesia. The patient cleaned the wound with hydrogen peroxide and was debrided in the office 5 days post-operatively.

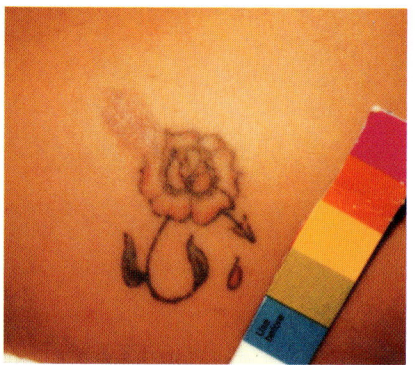

FIG. 6.12-A. Three months after initial test spot.

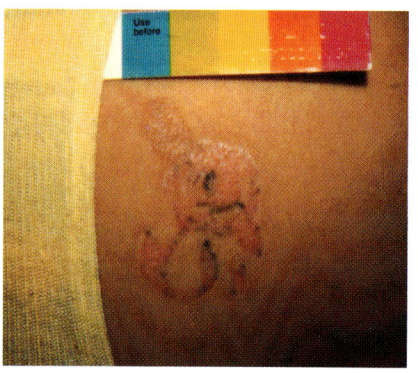

FIG. 6.12-B. Slight residuum left after several treatments.

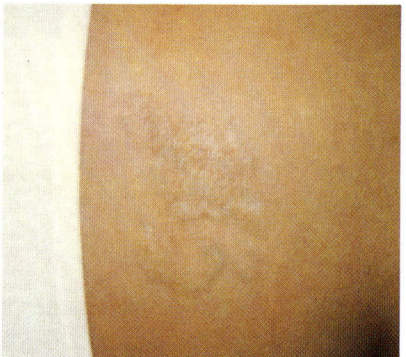

FIG. 6.12-C. Final result after one year. Most of pigment is removed and minimal texture change is present. There is minimal surface irregularity with acceptable ghosting (slightly discernible outline of the tattoo).

Case courtesy of *Ronald Allen Kirschner, D.O.*

CASE 6.13

Decorative Tattoo

REVIEW OF CASE. This 29-year-old female presented with a 10 year history of a decorative tattoo.

CHOICE OF LASER: Nd:YAG. The Nd:YAG laser was chosen to remove this tattoo because of its "facultative absorption by dark colors" and minimal absorption by normally colored skin.

ADDITIONAL INFORMATION. The laser radiation was administered through a quartz fiberoptic to a focusing handpiece. At each step of the removal the pigment was exposed by transmitting energy to the pigment with subsequent loss of external layers of skin. The patient removed the pigment with hydrogen peroxide and cotton-tipped applicators at home. This lesion was removed over three separate sessions as we have found that smaller areas that are treated in difficult to heal areas seem to heal better.

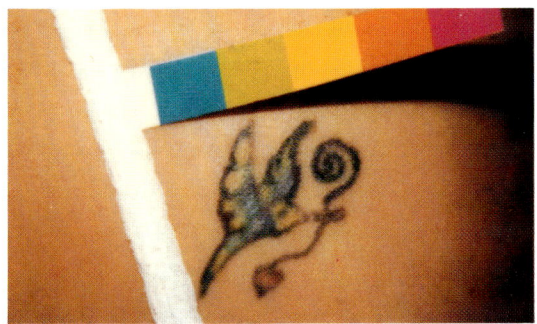

FIG. 6.13-A. Pre-treatment tattoo on left shoulder.

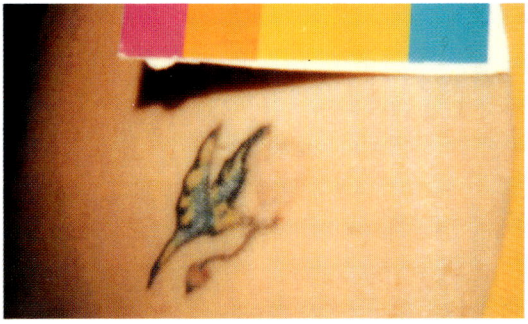

FIG. 6.13-B. Satisfactory test spot 3 months after treatment.

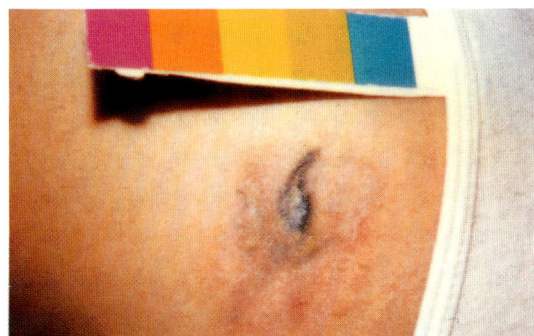

FIG. 6.13-C. Sequential removal of various segments of tattoo.

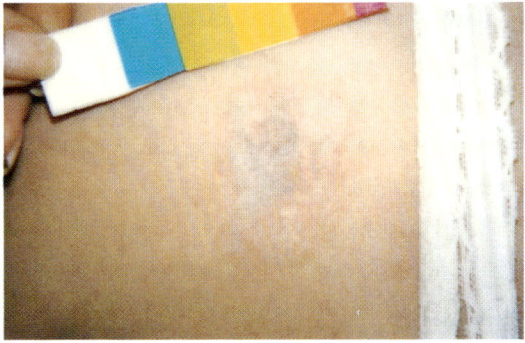

FIG. 6.13-D. Final result 4 months after treatment demonstrating satisfactory removal of tattoo pigment with minor skin texture change. Slight ghosting and a small bit of residual pigment are present.

Case courtesy of ***Ronald Allen Kirschner,*** D.O.

CASE 6.14
Keloid Post-Traumatic Wound

REVIEW OF CASE. This 43-year-old black female presented with a keloid on the vortex of the forearm. She previously had steroid injections to the area with no relief of symptoms.

CHOICE OF LASER: Nd:YAG. The Nd:YAG laser seems to inhibit collagen production by fibroblasts. This patient was treated with 0.3 seconds exposure at 40 watts using a bare (unfocused) fiber tip, 1 cm from the surface of the skin for 340 pulses to deliver 4,032 joules.

ADDITIONAL INFORMATION. Commonly when treating unpigmented lesions under local anesthesia patients will complain of pain which may be due to the absence of a chromophore blocking exposure to the laser of the deeper sensory nerves.

POST-TREATMENT CARE. The patient is instructed to wash with soap and water and apply Polysporin ointment. Sun exposure is avoided until treated areas return to normal color.

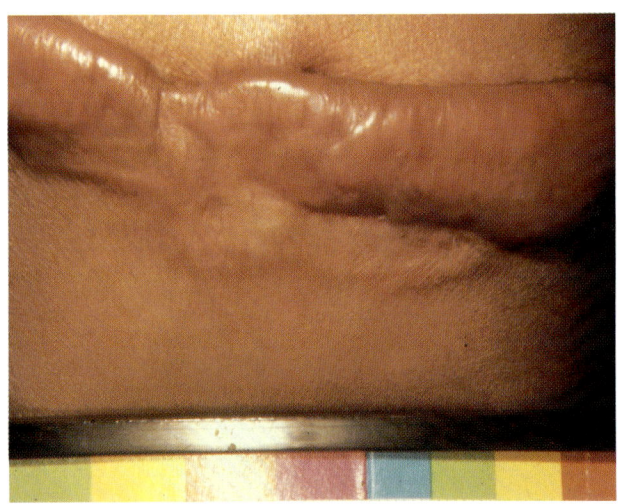

FIG. 6.14-A. Post-traumatic keloid of volar forearm.

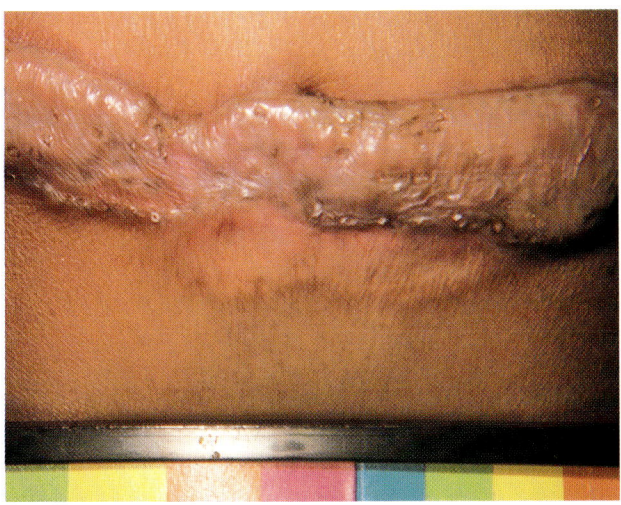

FIG. 6.14-B. Immediately after treatment, note blanching and punctate pattern caused by individual exposure sites. Note also the absence of char.

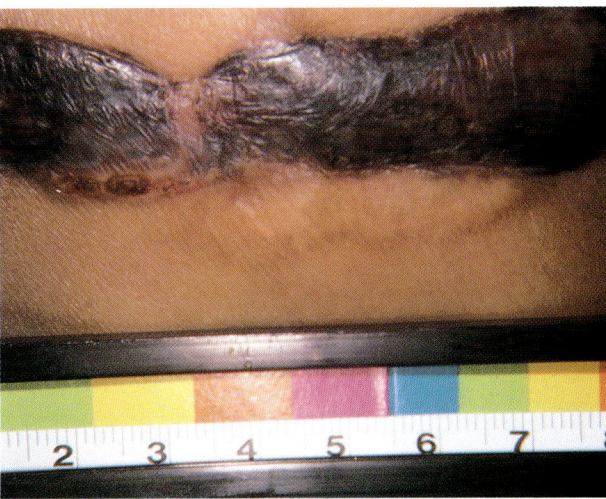

FIG. 6.14-C. One week post-treatment, dry eschar of scar surface from vascular infarction.

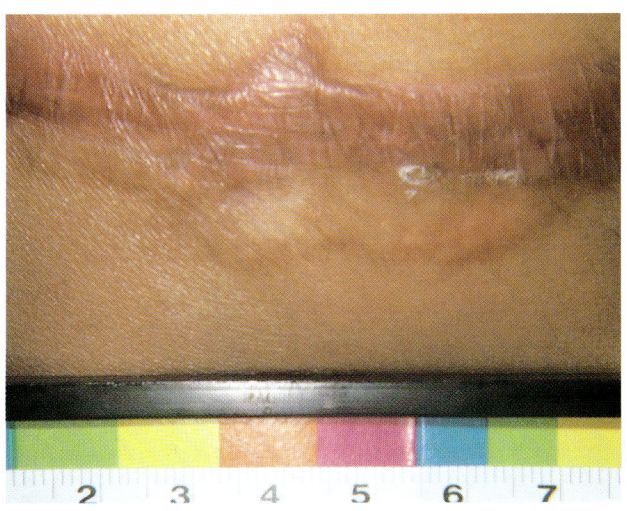

FIG. 6.14-D. Four months post-treatment, note flattening of scar.

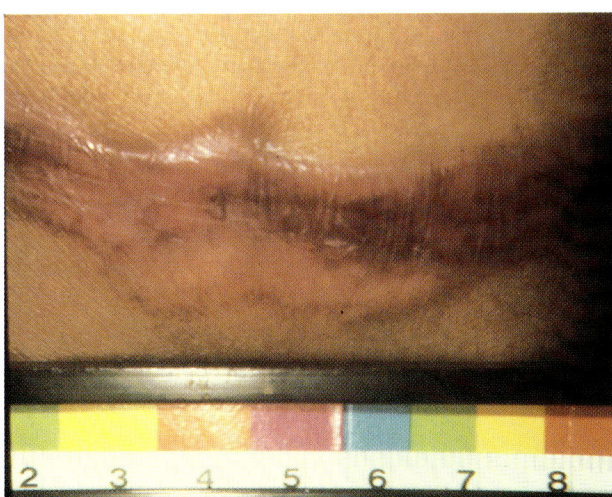

FIG. 6.14-E. Five months post-treatment. There is a suggestion of regrowth which has not progressed in the subsequent three years. The patient continues to have relief of pruritis and pain in the lesion.

Case courtesy of *Harold L. Rosenfeld*, M.D.

CASE 6.15
Keloid Scarring Post Acne

REVIEW OF CASE.   This 15-year-old dark complected male of Italian descent presented with multiple keloids. Intralesional steroid injections were unsuccessful treatments for this patient in the past.

CHOICE OF LASER: Nd:YAG.   The Nd:YAG laser is said to inhibit collagen production by fibroblasts. The laser was calibrated to 0.1 seconds at 70 watts with the unfocused fiber tip held 0.5–1 cm from the skin surface.

ADDITIONAL INFORMATION.   The initial blanching indicates treated areas are vascular, but at these energy levels the entire field will necrose and commonly, as in this patient's case, heal over without further hypertrophy.

Because the necrosis is due to infarction of the vessels and is sterile, separation of the wound by autolysis takes about two weeks. Even in only partially successful treatments there is symptomatic relief of burning and puritis which commonly drives patients to seek treatment.

POST-TREATMENT CARE.   The patient is instructed to wash the area with soap and water and apply Polysporin ointment. Sun exposure is avoided until treated areas return to normal color.

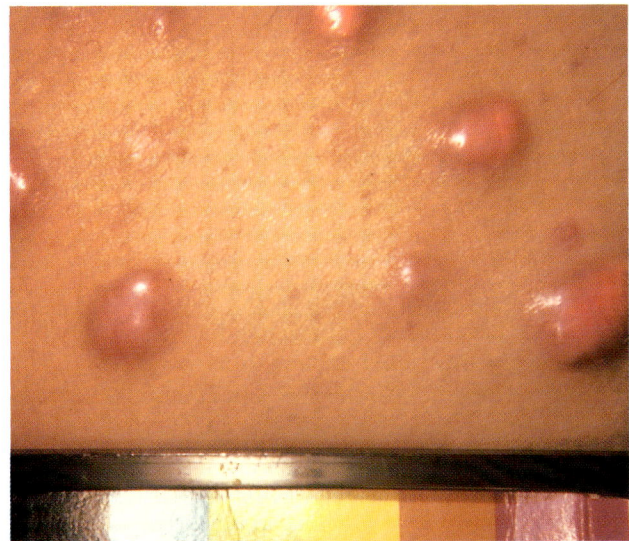

FIG. 6.15-A. Keloids on the back from acne vulgaris.

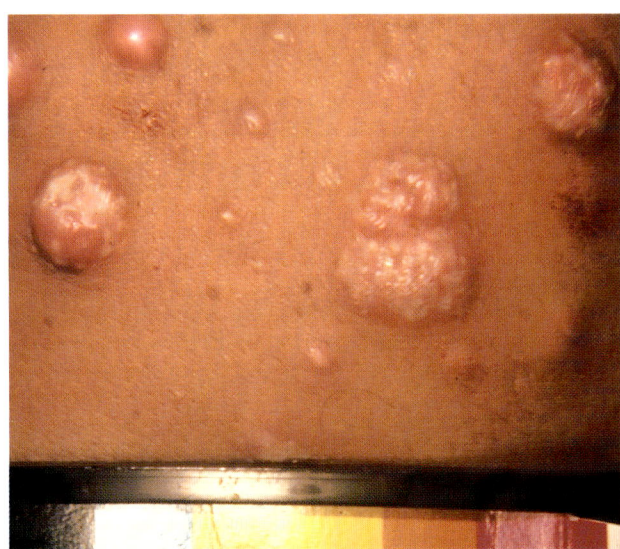

FIG. 6.15-B. Immediately after treatment: cutaneous blanching indicates the sites of treatment lesions.

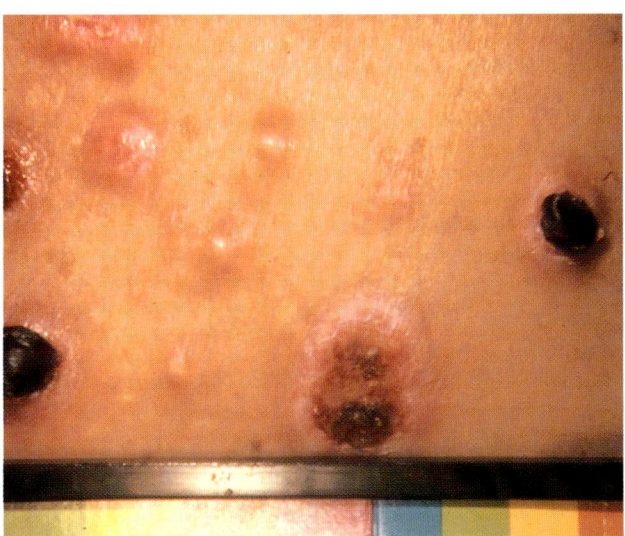

FIG. 6.15-C. Two weeks post-treatment: dry eschar sloughing by autolysis.

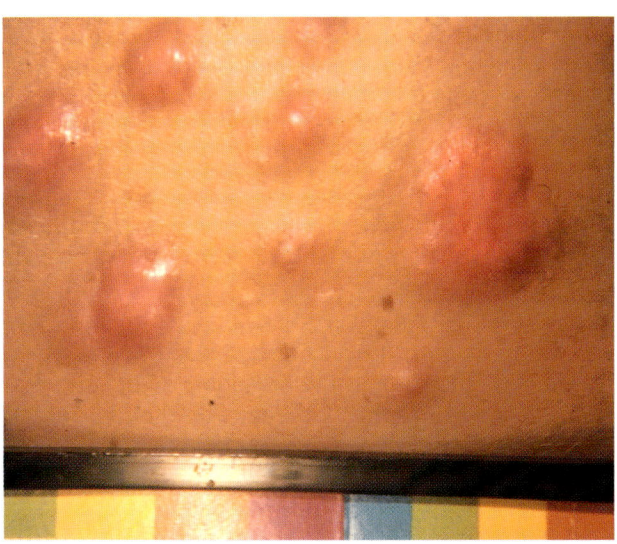

FIG. 6.15-D. Six weeks post-treatment: early involution with re-epithelization.

Case courtesy of *Harold L. Rosenfeld*, M.D.

CASE 6.16
Cavernous Hemangioma of the Face

REVIEW OF CASE. This 19-month-old female presented with a large capillary/cavernous hemangioma on the left mandible, cervical, and cheek area. This was present at birth and had grown significantly for the first 11 months without evidence of regression. Initial examination revealed a 6 × 8 cm hemangiomatous mass present on the left cheek and mandible area. The patient initially had a Nd:YAG laser photocoagulation with direct steroid injection that stopped the growth of the hemangioma and caused a 25% shrinkage. Five months following this procedure, the Nd:YAG laser with sapphire scalpel was used to resect the hemangioma completely. The resection was accomplished with only 75 cc of blood loss and the hemangioma resection was total.

CHOICE OF LASER: Nd:YAG. The Nd:YAG laser is able to be used in direct contact with tissue through the development of synthetic sapphire scalpel tips. These scalpel tips concentrate the laser energy to a small, limited area, providing excellent incision with hemostasis. The Nd:YAG laser is not limited by its absorption spectrum to any particular type of tissue and is the best possible thermocoagulator. Blood loss studies with sapphire scalpels show significantly less bleeding and the ability to balance cutting and coagulation. Very little smoke is produced by contact scalpels compared to the non-contact technique and the amount of adjacent tissue necrosis is limited.

ADDITIONAL INFORMATION. The laser produces a zone of thermal necrosis on the skin edge which must be resected prior to closure, otherwise wound healing problems may ensue. Approximately 1 mm of skin and subcutaneous tissue must be resected to get back to good non-thermally damaged tissue. When there is a great deal of excess skin hypertrophy over a hemangioma which needs to be resected, it is warranted to cut skin with the laser. There will be much less bleeding at the beginning of the operation in this case. Following total resection of the hemangioma, the skin edge can then be resected prior to closure. Alternatively, if excess skin is not present for resection, then the skin can be cut with the regular scalpel and the laser used only in the subcutaneous tissue. Unfortunately, since most skin over a hemangioma is involved with the hemangioma, this means that blood loss will begin during the initial incision.

The arteriography is usually performed 24 hours prior to the laser resection. Diagnostic angiography is performed first with superselective embolization usually following in the same session. The embolization is accomplished with Gel foam slurry. The addition of arteriography with superselective embolization has rendered the subsequent laser surgery easier to complete with limited blood loss.

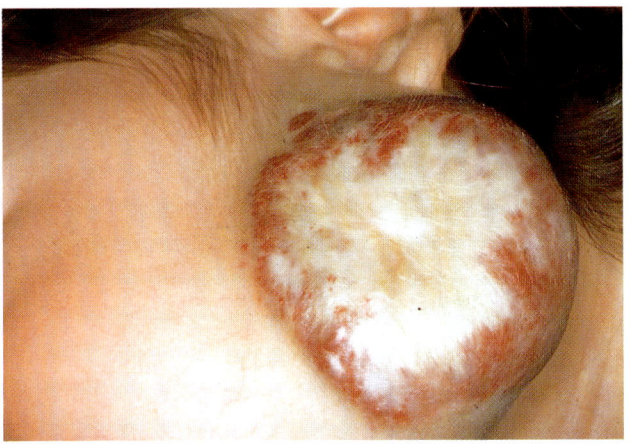

FIG. 6.16-A. Capillary/cavernous hemangioma of the left cheek, mandible, and neck area prior to treatment.

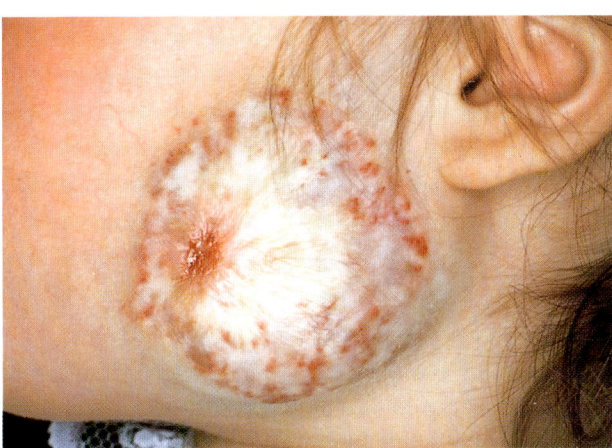

FIG. 6.16-B. Lesion following Nd:YAG laser photocoagulation and steroid injection demonstrating marked blanching and partial shrinkage of the hemangioma.

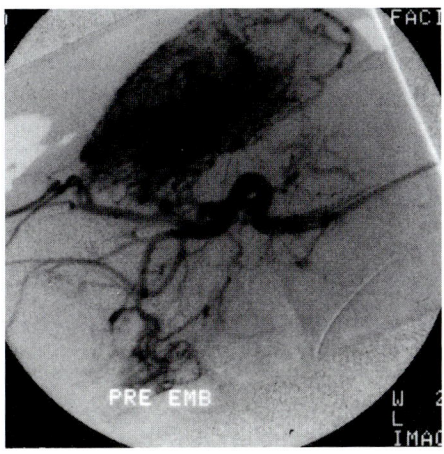

FIG. 6.16-C. Pre-operative arteriogram demonstrating numerous afferent vessels coming from the external maxillary and external carotid vessels.

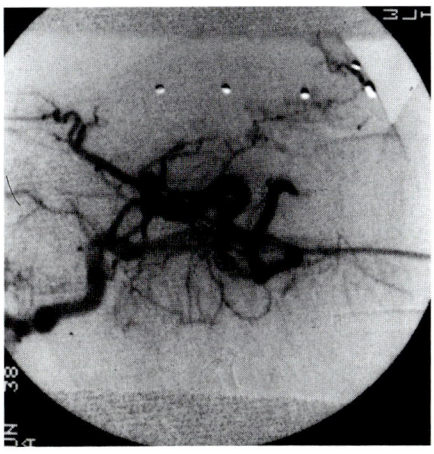

FIG. 6.16-D. Post-embolization arteriogram demonstrating occlusion of afferent vessels.

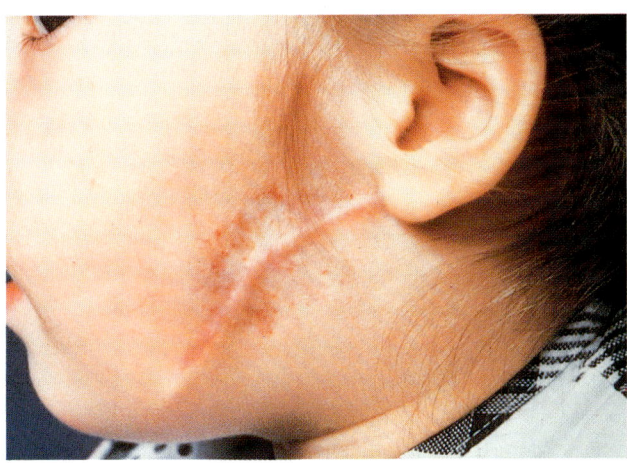

FIG. 6.16-E. Final appearance of healed lesion six months following resection.

Case courtesy of *David B. Apfelberg*, M.D.

CASE 6.17
Cavernous Hemangioma of the Left Chest

REVIEW OF CASE. This 4-year-old female presented with congenital hemangioma of the left thorax and anterior chest wall. This was present at birth and grew rapidly for the first 9 months and has not regressed. The dimensions at pre-operative examination were 9 to 10 cm in width and about 8 cm in height from the chest wall. The lesion interfered with left arm motion and had potential for distortion of the breast tissue area.

CHOICE OF LASER: Nd:YAG. The Nd:YAG laser is able to be used in direct contact with tissue through the development of synthetic sapphire scalpel tips. These scalpel tips concentrate the laser energy to a small limited area, providing excellent incision with hemostasis. The Nd:YAG laser is not limited by its absorption spectrum to any particular type of tissue and is the best possible thermocoagulator. Blood loss studies with sapphire scalpels show significantly less bleeding and the ability to balance cutting and coagulation. Very little smoke is produced by contact scalpels in distinction to the non-contact technique and the amount of adjacent tissue necrosis is limited.

ADDITIONAL INFORMATION. The laser produces a zone of thermal necrosis on the skin edge which must be resected prior to closure, otherwise wound healing problems may ensue. Approximately 1 mm of skin and subcutaneous tissue must be resected to get back to good non-thermally damaged tissue. When there is a great deal of excess skin hypertrophy over a hemangioma which needs to be resected, it is warranted to cut skin with the laser. There will be much less bleeding at the beginning of the operation in this case. Following total resection of the hemangioma, the skin edge can then be resected prior to closure. Alternatively, if excess skin is not present for resection, then the skin can be cut with the regular scalpel and the laser used only in the subcutaneous tissue. Unfortunately, since most skin over a hemangioma is involved with the hemangioma, this means that blood loss will begin during the initial incision.

The arteriography is usually performed 24 hours prior to the laser resection. Diagnostic angiography is performed first with superselective embolization usually following in the same session. The embolization is accomplished with Gel foam slurry. The addition of arteriography with superselective embolization has rendered the subsequent laser surgery easier to complete with limited blood loss.

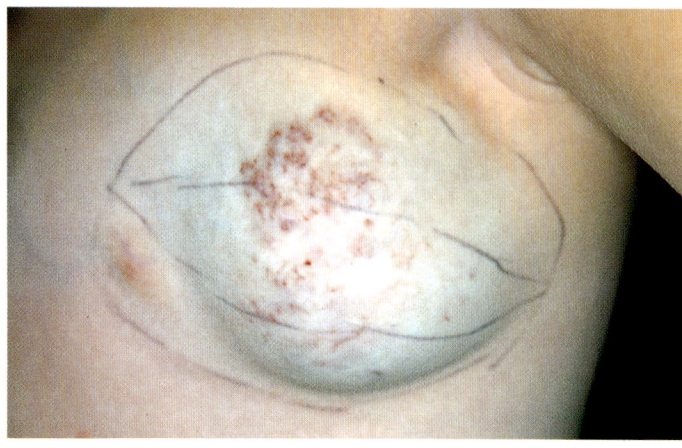

FIG. 6.17-A. Pre-operative massive hemangioma of left chest and thorax.

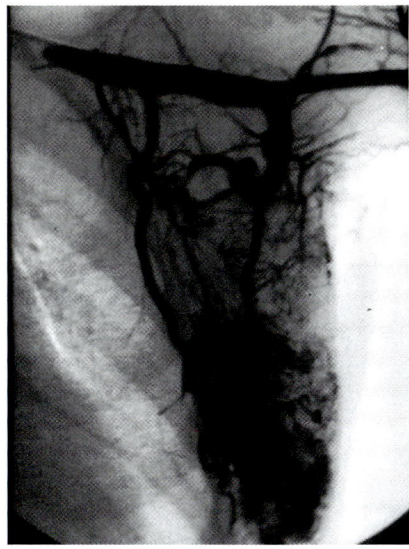

FIG. 6.17-B. Pre-operative arteriogram demonstrating major afferent feeding vessels from the left internal thoracic and axillary vessels.

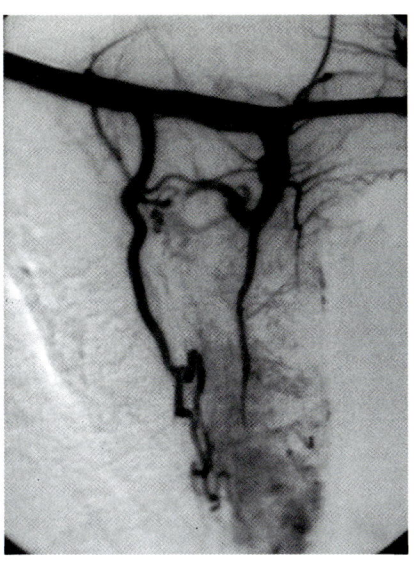

FIG. 6.17-C. Post-embolization film demonstrating obliteration of afferent blood vessels.

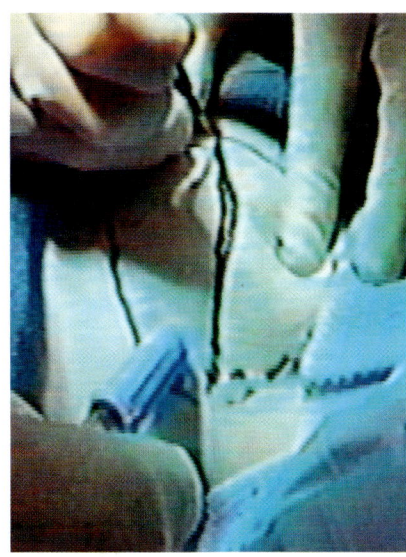

FIG. 6.17-D. Incision of skin over hemangioma with Nd:YAG laser with sapphire contact tip.

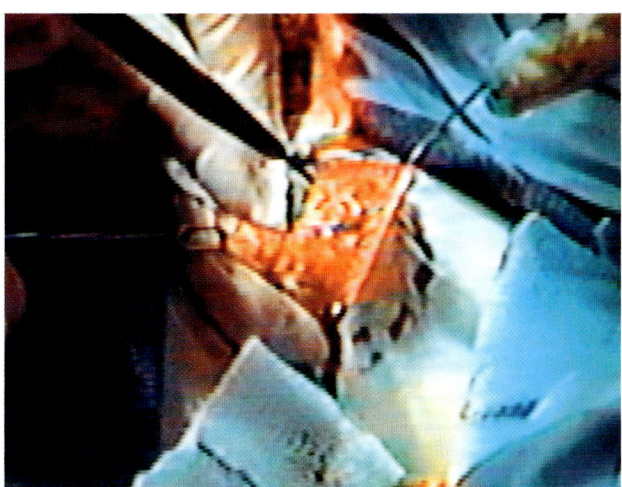

FIG. 6.17-E. Dissection of right lateral flap.

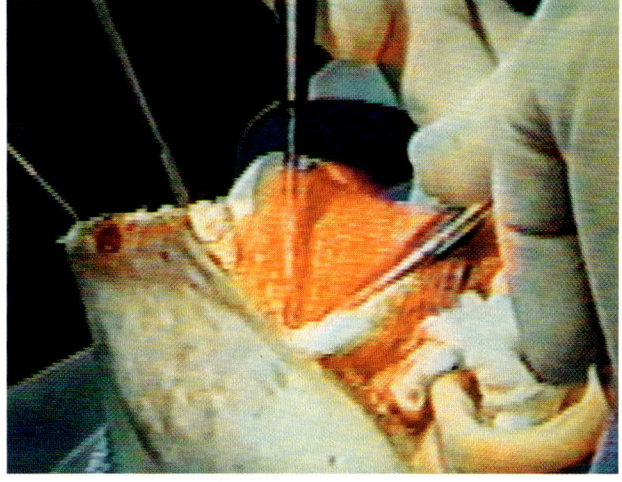

FIG. 6.17-F. Close-up of left flap dissection.

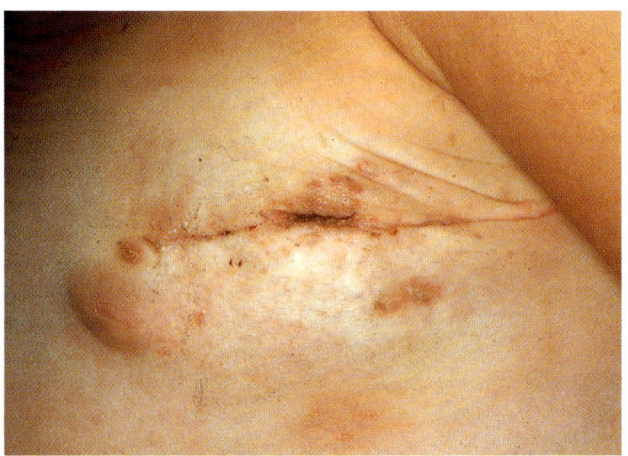

FIG. 6.17-G. Completely healed resection three months following surgery.

Case courtesy of *David B. Apfelberg*, M.D.

CASE 6.18

Cavernous Hemangioma of the Left Cheek

REVIEW OF CASE. This 12-year-old male presented with a massive hemangioma involving the left face. Previous surgeries including ligation of both external carotid arteries and minor excisions were unsuccessful. He has had several bleeding episodes from his lip. Physical examination revealed a diffuse hemangioma deformity in the entire left face with sagging of the left corner of the mouth.

CHOICE OF LASER: Nd:YAG. The Nd:YAG laser is the only current laser able to be used in direct contact with tissue through the development of synthetic sapphire probes and scalpels. The laser energy is concentrated to a small, limited area producing excellent incisions with hemostatic action. The traditional tissue contact is more comfortable for the surgeon than a non-touch technique. Sapphire scalpels create a well-defined localized region of high power density right at the tip of the probe which is placed precisely against the target tissue. No focusing is required. The Nd:YAG laser is the best possible thermal coagulator. Blood loss is markedly reduced and very little smoke is produced by the contact scalpels. Tissue necrosis secondary to the heat of the scalpel is approximately 5.5 mm.

ADDITIONAL INFORMATION. The high heat produced by the Nd:YAG laser causes thermal necrosis of the skin edge. Therefore, it is necessary to cut back 1 mm of thermally damaged skin edge for good wound healing. Failure to do this may result in delayed wound healing, dehiscence, or increased scars.

POST-TREATMENT CARE. The wound is treated as any other surgical wound with compression and cold compresses.

For literature pertaining to this case see References section.

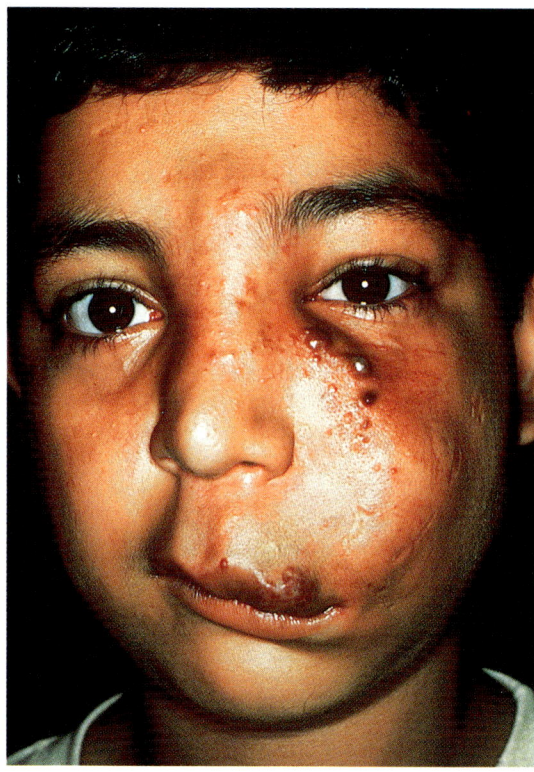

FIG. 6.18-A. Thirteen-year-old male with massive cavernous hemangioma of the left cheek.

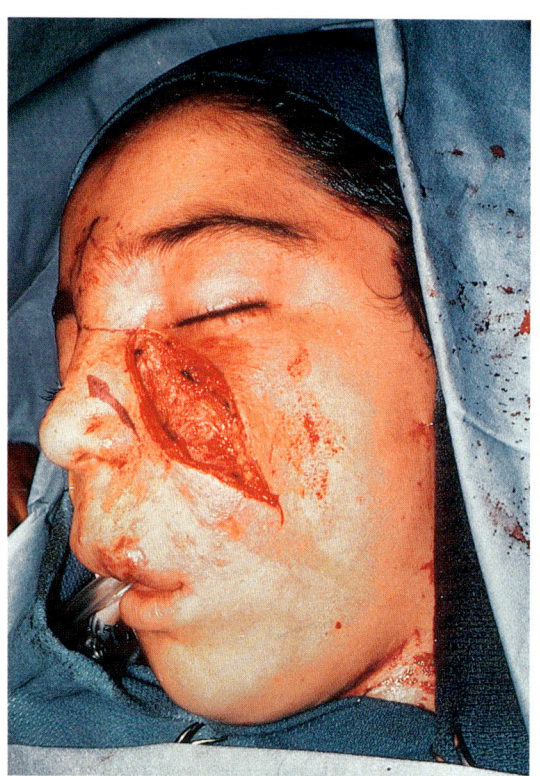

FIG. 6.18-B. Intraoperative excision in the left nasolabial fold. Note absence of any major bleeding.

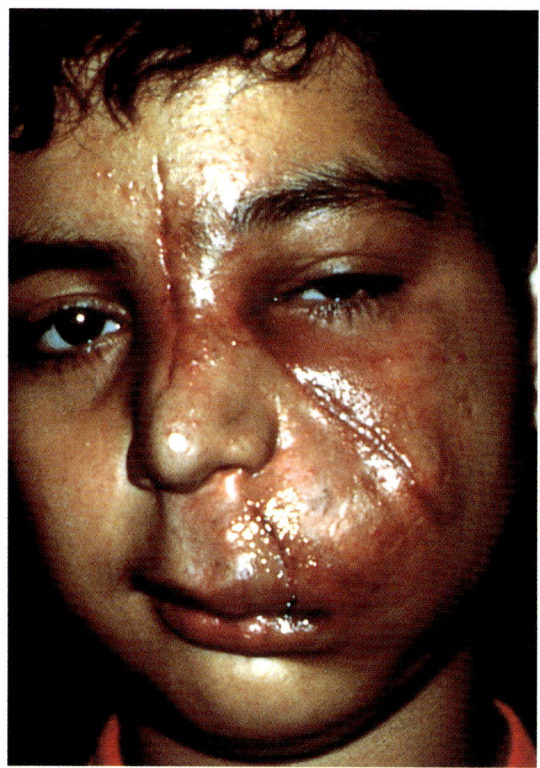

FIG. 6.18-C. Post-operative lesion demonstrating partial excision and better symmetry of the face with excellent wound healing.

Case courtesy of *David B. Apfelberg*, M.D., and *Morton R. Maser*, M.D.

CASE 6.19

Capillary/Cavernous Hemangioma of the Forehead and Eyelid

REVIEW OF CASE. This 4-month-old male presented with a rapidly enlarging hemangioma of the right upper eyelid and forehead totally obstructing the vision. Despite oral prednisone, the eye has remained closed. Deprivation amblyopia as well as astigmatism is a definite danger. The eye has been closed for 1½ months.

CHOICE OF LASER: Nd:YAG. The Nd:YAG laser is able to penetrate a hemangioma to a depth of 5–7 mm. This photocoagulation has the effect of not only blanching the hemangioma but also causing an approximately 25% shrinkage. It is thought that the laser institutes the thrombogenesis potential of the hemangiomas. The Nd:YAG laser photocoagulation is used in combination with direct injection of steroids. Treatment is done as an outpatient under sedation or anesthesia. The Nd:YAG laser is used with 30 watts of power, 1 mm spot size, and 0.5 second pulse duration.

ADDITIONAL INFORMATION. The hemangioma is compressed as narrowly as possible with a glass slide to reduce the height of the hemangioma to 7 mm or less, which is the thermocoagulation necrosis depth of the Nd:YAG laser. The laser is hand held at its focal length (2–4 cm) perpendicular to the surface and focused on the hemangioma in a "polka dot pattern," alternating 1 mm dots of treatment with 1 mm of normal untreated hemangioma. An instant blanching and noticeable tissue shrinkage are readily observed. Proper eye and skin protection for the patient and all personnel in the room are important. Immediately following laser treatment a short-acting and long-acting steroid are directly injected into the lesion in multiple sites. The amount of steroid depends on the size of the hemangioma. Owing to the vascular nature of the spongy hemangiomas, there may be brisk oozing from the puncture sites, which easily and promptly stops with 3 to 5 minutes of pressure.

POST-TREATMENT CARE. Antibiotic ointment and iced saline compresses are used following the procedure.

For literature pertaining to this case see References section.

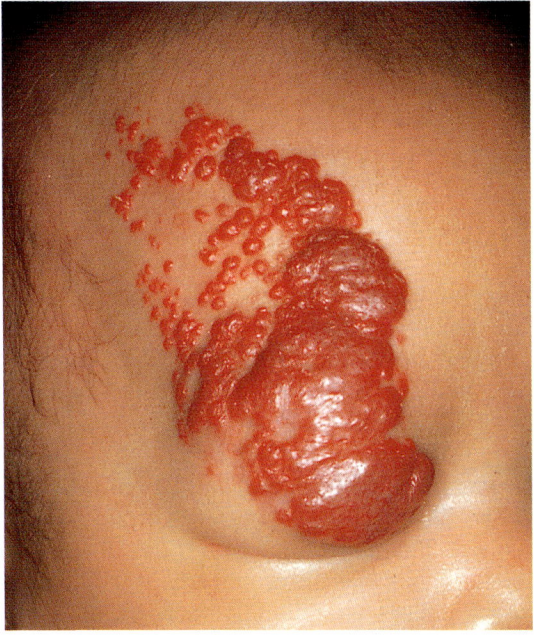

FIG. 6.19-A. Capillary/cavernous hemangioma of right forehead and upper eyelid, totally closing and obstructing the eye and blocking the vision.

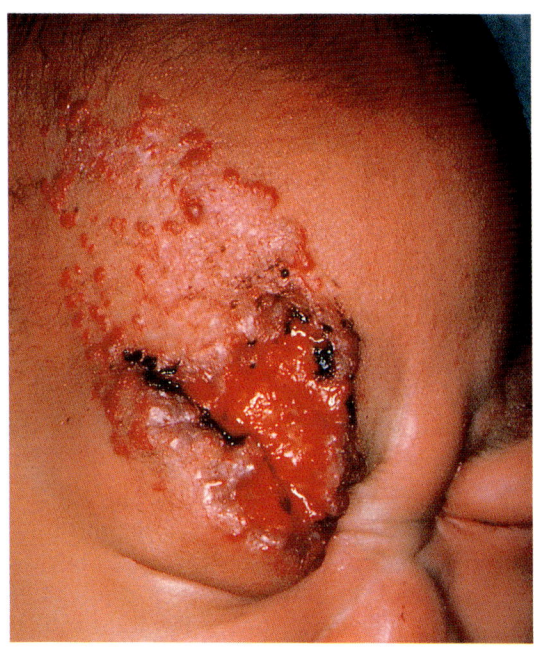

FIG. 6.19-B. Ten days following treatment showing marked shrinkage of hemangioma with ulcerated surface.

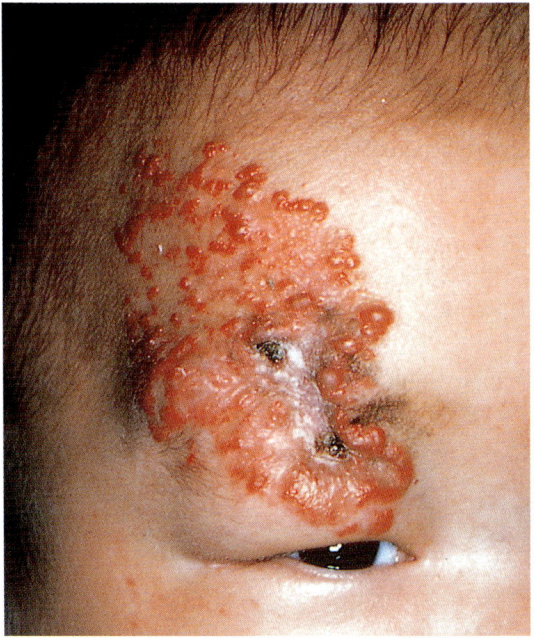

FIG. 6.19-C. Six weeks following treatment the eye is opened and there has been fibrosis of the hemangioma.

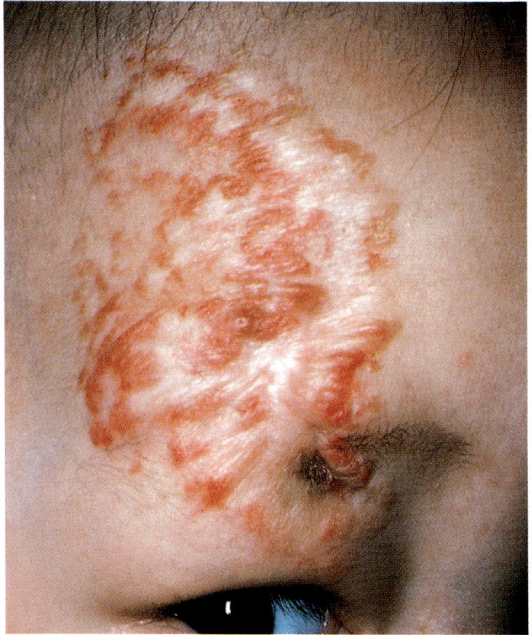

FIG. 6.19-D. Further blanching and shrinkage of the hemangioma with continued opening of the eye.

Case courtesy of *David B. Apfelberg*, M.D.

CASE 6.20

Capillary/Cavernous Hemangioma of the Cheek

REVIEW OF CASE. This 13-month-old female presented with a rapidly enlarging capillary/cavernous hemangioma of the left cheek and upper lip which was distorting the cheek and upper lip. The hemangioma appeared 3 weeks after birth and had grown steadily. It had bled twice and was partially obstructing the left nostril and depressing and distorting the corner of the mouth.

CHOICE OF LASER: Nd:YAG. The Nd:YAG laser was used because of its ability to produce photocoagulation of tissue to a depth of 5–7 mm. The Nd:YAG laser produces a continuous wave power output at 1064 nm (near infrared, invisible). This laser light penetrates to a depth of 5–7 mm into the dermis as a result of back scatter, forward scatter, and absorption. This scattering effect transforms the light into heat, which causes coagulation necrosis with hemostasis over a large volume (5–7 mm) of tissue without its removal.

ADDITIONAL INFORMATION. Under general anesthesia, the hemangioma is compressed as narrowly as possible with a cold or iced glass slide to reduce the height of the hemangioma to 7 mm or less if possible. This depth is chosen because the thermal coagulation necrosis of the Nd:YAG laser is known to extend approximately 5 to 7 mm. The laser is hand held at its focal length (2–4 cm) perpendicular to the surface and focused on the hemangioma in a polka-dotted pattern, alternating 1 mm dots of treatment with 1 mm of normal untreated hemangioma. An instant white blanching and notable tissue shrinkage is readily and immediately observed.

Proper eye and skin protection for the patient, anesthesiologist, and treating personnel precede instigation of the procedures. These include the wearing of safety glasses or the use of protective moist gauze pads over the eyes and draping the adjacent wound edges with moist gauze. Suction evacuation of the laser plume is important as well.

Immediately following laser treatment, Celestone (betamethasone sodium phosphate, betamethasone acetate 6 mg/ml) 1–3 cc and triamcinolone hexacetonide (40 mg/ml) 1–3 cc are injected directly into the lesion in multiple sites with a 3 cc syringe and 25 gauge ¾ inch needle. The amount of steroid depends on the size of the hemangioma. Because of the vascular nature of these spongy hemangiomas, there may be brisk oozing from the puncture sites that easily and promptly stops with 3 to 5 minutes of pressure.

POST-TREATMENT CARE. Continuous ice compresses for 48 hours and topical antibiotic ointment are used for treatment.

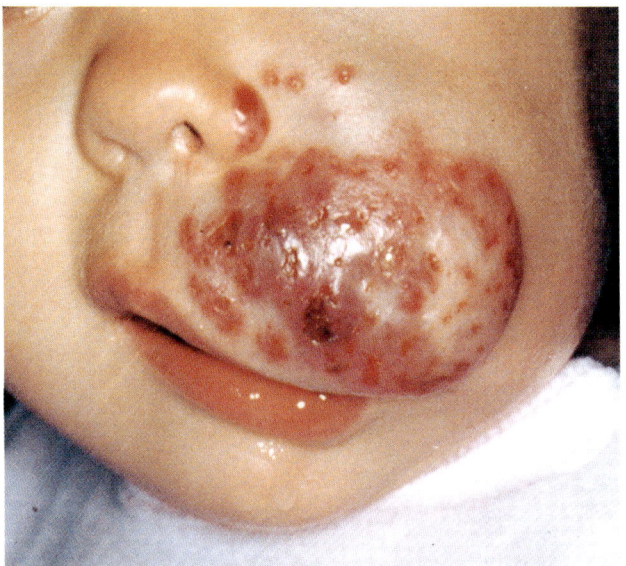

FIG. 6.20-A. Preoperative appearance of patient.

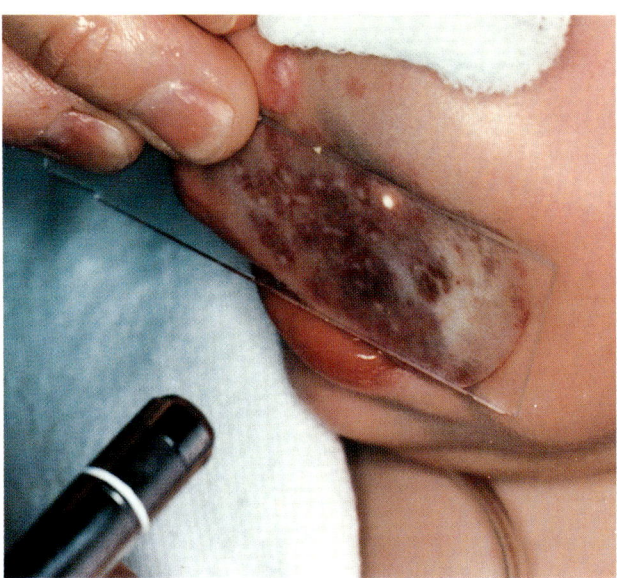

FIG. 6.20-B. Nd:YAG laser photocoagulation through a glass slide compression of the hemangioma to 5–7 mm (the depth of Nd:YAG laser photocoagulation). Note the patient's eye protection with gauzes.

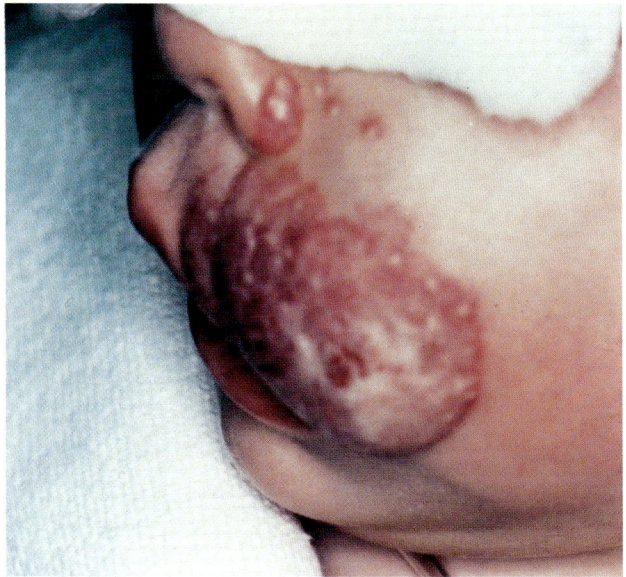

FIG. 6.20-C. Result Nd:YAG laser photocoagulation in a polka dot pattern.

Case continues on following page.

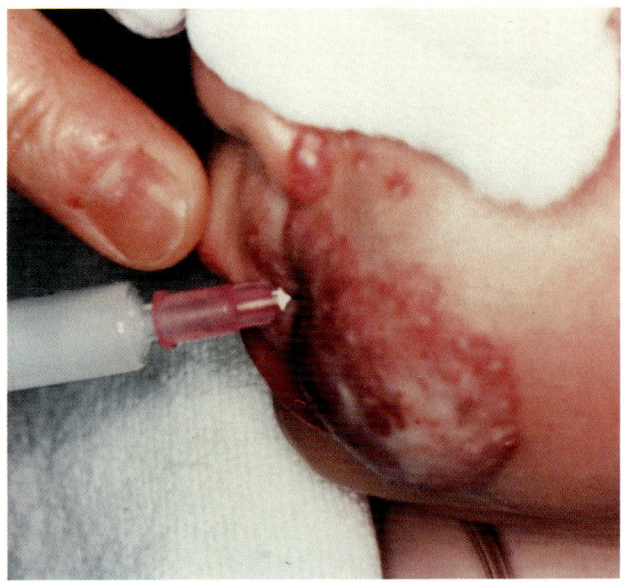

FIG. 6.20-D. Injection of steroids.

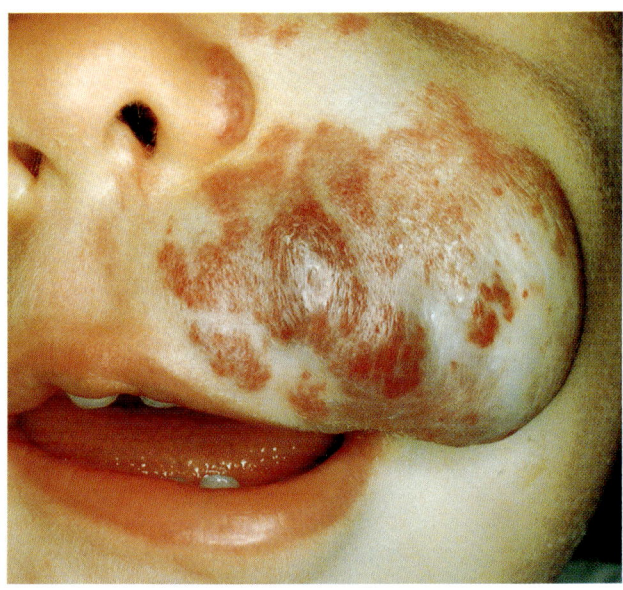

FIG. 6.20-E. Appearance eight weeks following treatment.

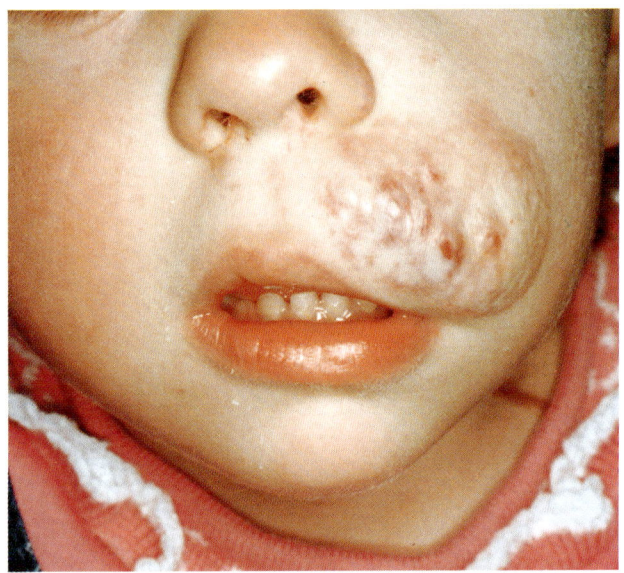

FIG. 6.20-F. Final result, demonstrating marked shrinkage and blanching of hemangioma six months post-treatment.

Case courtesy of *David B. Apfelberg*, M.D.

CASE 6.21
Deep Burn Excisions

REVIEW OF CASE. We have operated on several deep burn injuries of different sizes using the contact Nd:YAG laser, and compared the results with those obtained by using steel scalpel. The age of the patients varied from 36 to 71 years with full-thickness burns covering 4–28% of the body surface on the trunk and/or extremities.

CHOICE OF LASER: Nd:YAG. The Nd:YAG laser was chosen for the following reasons:

(i) Bleeding is one of the major problems in burn surgery especially in connection with tangential (sequential) excision. Because excisions through fat are known to bleed more than those carried out on the fascial plane many surgeons prefer fascial excision. This is also a factor in cases where some of the subcutaneous tissue could be spared. However, in full-thickness burns non-sequential complete excision has proved superior to fascial excision as far as functional and aesthetic results are concerned. Therefore, methods other than steel scalpel, electrocautery, or dermatomes are searched for.

(ii) Blood loss from the excision area diminished by 44% using the contact method as compared with the steel scalpel. Capillary bleeding did not occur after the use of the contact Nd:YAG laser. After excision the operating field remained "dry" and there were no signs of diffuse bleeding or oozing afterwards. When the right technique was learned, most moderate size blood vessels were coagulated. Larger vessels, like the saphenous veins in the forearm, were preferably treated by ligation.

(iii) The greatest disadvantage of the contact laser method in burn surgery is a twofold (1.7–2.5×) prolongation of the operating time. No speed can be gained by forcing the contact scalpel through tissues as this may lead to permanent damage to the scalpel and increased bleeding. An increase in power did not seem to have much effect on incisional speed either. The slow speed of incision is of no major importance when the area to be operated on is small, as in the upper extremities, where the advantages of a relatively dry field can be achieved by the contact laser method.

(iv) An SLT contact Nd:YAG laser (Model CL 60, Surgical Laser Technologies, Inc., Malvern, PA) was used. The contact Nd:YAG laser was employed at average 15 watt power using 0.8–1.0 mm scalpels. The laser beam was passed through a 400 µm flexible glass fiber enclosed in a 2.2 mm polyethylene cannula, which also served as a conduit for coaxial CO_2 gas. The fiber was connected to a handpiece (SLT) equipped with an artificial sapphire scalpel with frosted end.

ADDITIONAL INFORMATION. We have operated on most of the patients using "nonsequential complete" excision, removing all skin and damaged underlying fat in one layer to the level of healthy tissue in an attempt to spare as much intact fat as possible. We believe sparing the intact fat leads to better functional and aesthetic results without significantly impairing graft take. Only in cases where that procedure has not been possible, we have performed fascial excision.

The use of the contact Nd:YAG laser even with the thinnest scalpel has resulted in a delay in graft take and epithelialization near the skin margins. Because of this, we have used an ordinary surgical knife instead of a contact scalpel in all skin incisions.

Slight tension to the tissues was kept constant and excision was continued in healthy fat tissue using the contact Nd:YAG laser. Too much tension resulted in diminished hemostatic capabilities while dividing the vessels. Identification of the healthy tissue level was guided by known parameters, like thrombosed vessels and edema layer. Small vessels were divided without delay, whereas larger vessels needed a zig-zag movement with the contact scalpel prior to cutting in order to prevent bleeding. If too much tension was maintained, some vessels kept bleeding in spite of this procedure. These vessels were coagulated by a local touch with the contact scalpel. Larger blood vessels required ligation. Diathermy was seldom needed during excision procedure using the contact laser. All skin incisions were done with steel scalpel.

Many of the blood vessels are coagulated during the procedure by the touch of the contact scalpel. If the vessel continues to bleed after a few attempts for hemostasis with the contact scalpel, the vessels should be ligated. Failure to do so may lead to unnecessarily deep local necrosis and graft loss.

Excision through dry fat with the contact scalpel (after resolution of the edema) is likely to produce more damage to the fat. Early excision (3–5 days) is recommended.

For literature pertaining to this case see References section.

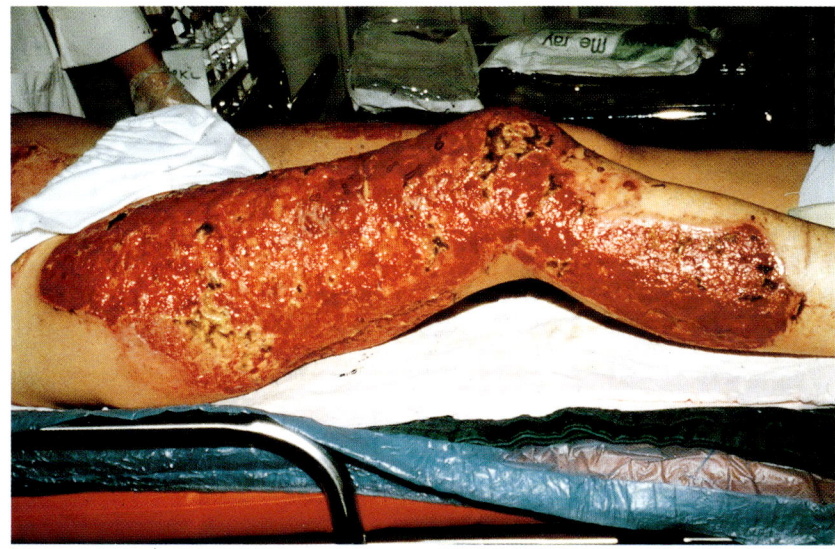

FIG. 6.21-A. A female patient with full-thickness burn injury operated on 2 weeks earlier in another hospital. Too superficial excision has resulted in total graft loss and severe pseudomonas infection.

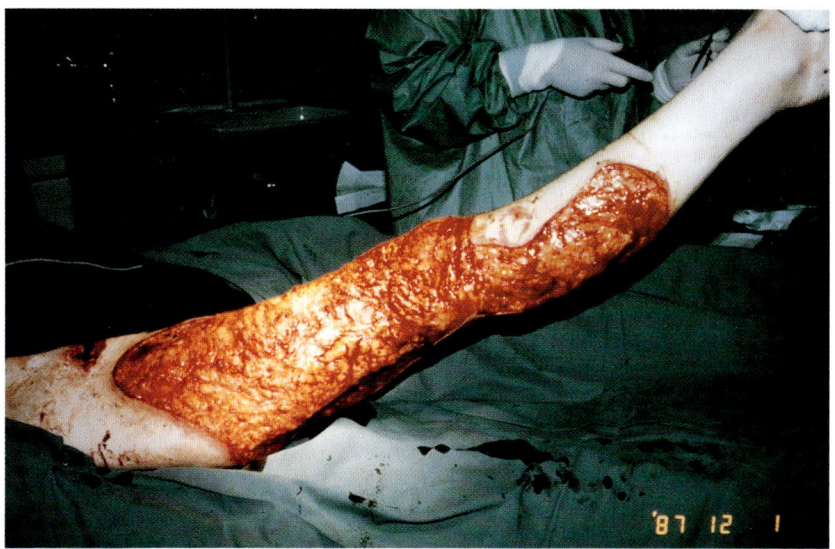

FIG. 6.21-B. The same patient as in Fig. A. The upper thigh has been operated on with the contact Nd:YAG laser using non-sequential complete excision. A considerable thickness of subcutaneous fat was spared. The lower thigh as well as the area around the knee were operated on with steel scalpel and electrocautery for comparison.

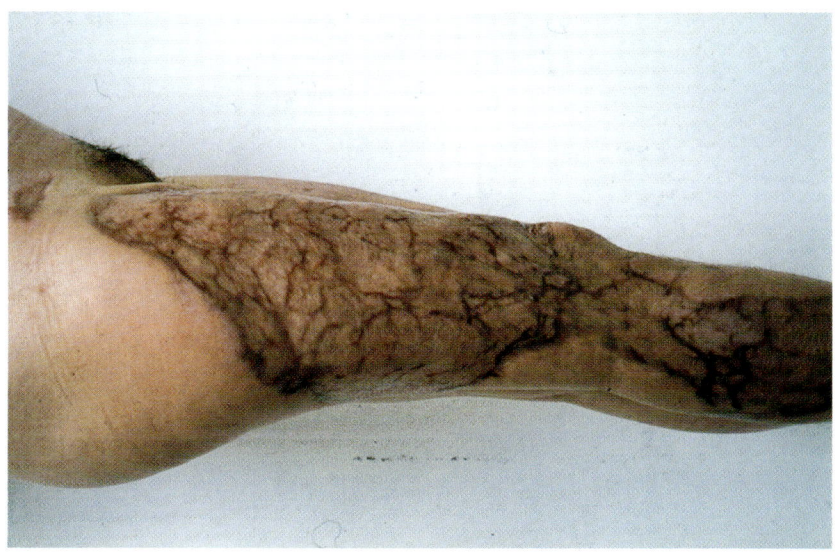

FIG. 6.21-C. Three months after surgery. Graft take has been equal. No difference in the appearance of scars can be observed. However, the laser-operated area remains dryer than the reference area for several months.

Case continues on following page.

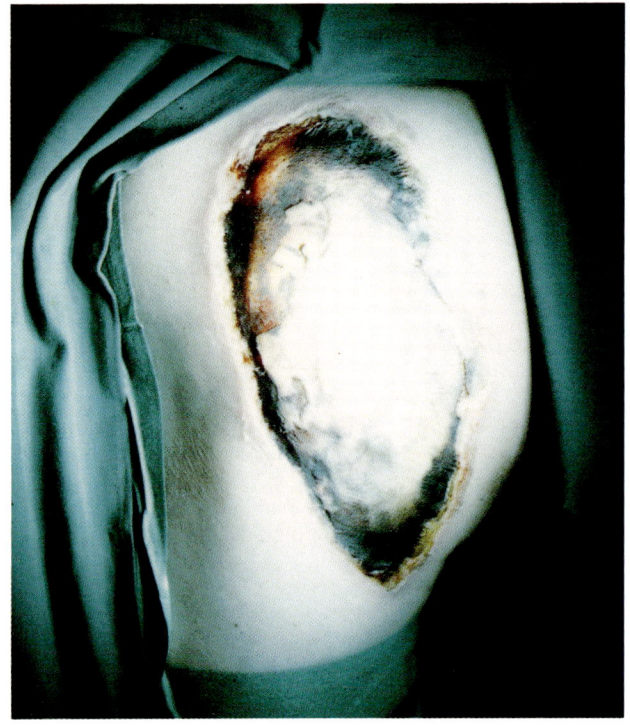

FIG. 6.21-D. A male patient with a deep contact burn in left buttock.

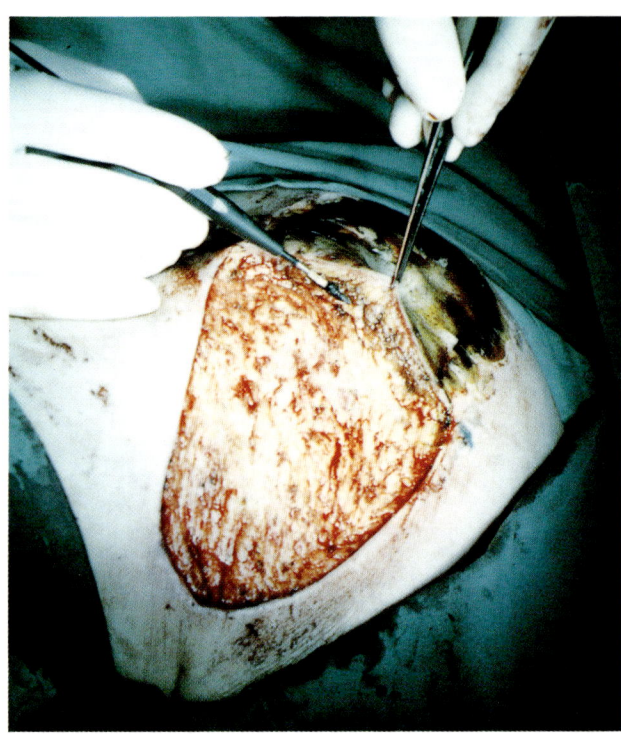

FIG. 6-21-E. Operation performed with contact Nd:YAG laser. Skin margins were incised with steel scalpel. Slight tension is kept using forceps.

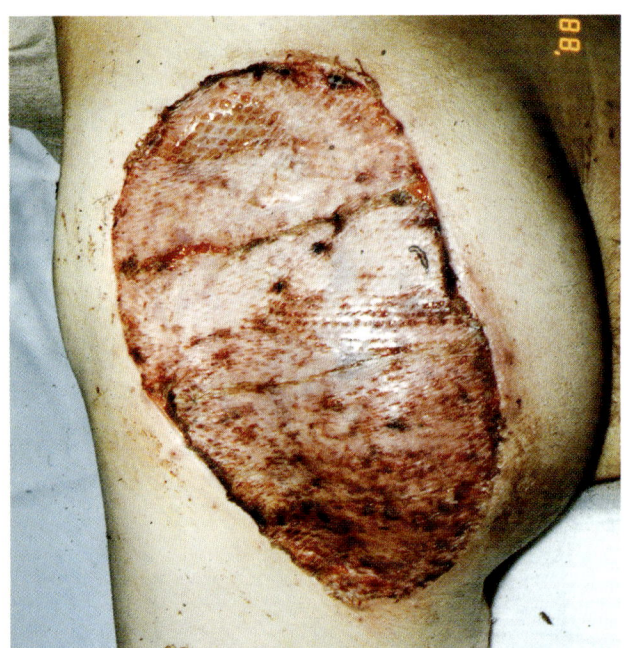

FIG. 6.21-F. Area ten days post-operation.

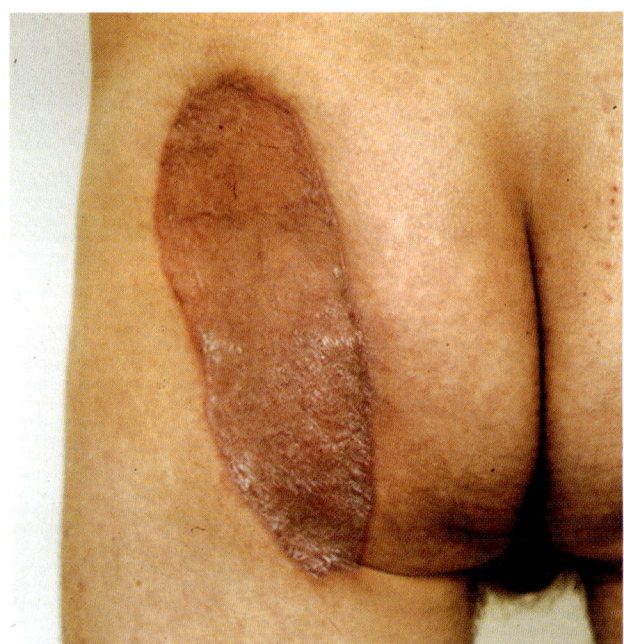

FIG. 6.21-G. Six months postoperation.

Case courtesy of *Tom Schroder,* M.D., *and Jyri J. Hukki,* M.D.

CASE 6.22

Ulcerated Capillary Hemangioma of the Vulva/Perineum

REVIEW OF CASE. This is an 11-month-old female with a chronically infected and ulcerated capillary/cavernous hemangioma of the left vulva, vagina, and perineum. The hemangioma was not present at birth but appeared as a small red dot about 7 to 12 days postpartum and gradually enlarged into a massive hemangioma. The area has been raw and ulcerated chronically with numerous episodes of bleeding, pain, and infection. Local and systemic antibiotics and topical treatment have been unsuccessful in healing the lesion.

CHOICE OF LASER: Nd:YAG. The Nd:YAG laser is able to penetrate a hemangioma to a depth of 5–7 mm. This photocoagulation has the effect of not only blanching the hemangioma but also causing an approximately 25% shrinkage. It is thought that the laser institutes the thrombogenesis potential of the hemangiomas. The Nd:YAG laser photocoagulation is used in combination with direct injection of steroids. Treatment is done as an outpatient under sedation or anesthesia. The Nd:YAG laser is used with 30 watts of power, 1 mm spot size, and 0.5 second pulse duration.

ADDITIONAL INFORMATION. The hemangioma is compressed as narrowly as possible with a glass slide to reduce the height of the hemangioma to 7 mm or less, which is the thermocoagulation necrosis depth of the Nd:YAG laser. The laser is hand held at its focal length (2–4 cm) perpendicular to the surface and focused on the hemangioma in a "polka dot pattern," alternating 1 mm dots of treatment with 1 mm of normal untreated hemangioma. An instant blanching and noticeable tissue shrinkage are readily observed. Proper eye and skin protection for the patient and all personnel in the room are important. Immediately following laser treatment a short-acting and long-acting steroid are directly injected into the lesion in multiple sites. The amount of steroid depends on the size of the hemangioma. Owing to the vascular nature of the spongy hemangiomas, there may be brisk oozing from the puncture sites, which easily and promptly stops with 3 to 5 minutes of pressure.

For literature pertaining to this case see References section.

Case continues on following page.

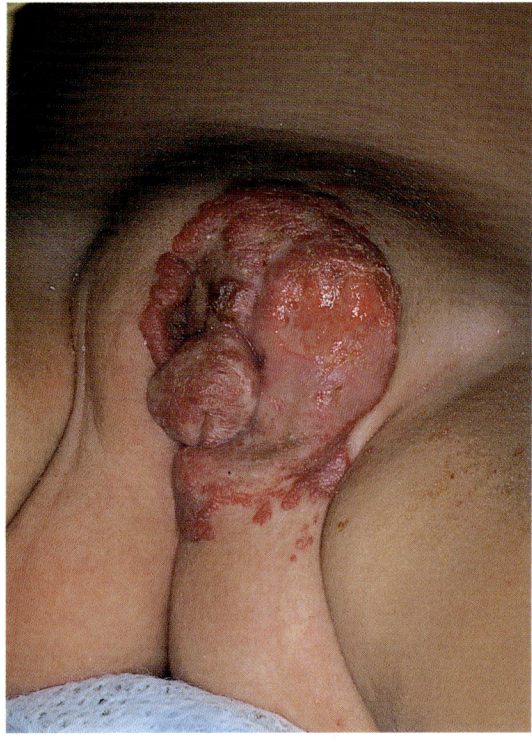

FIG. 6.22-A. Chronically ulcerated, infected nonhealing capillary hemangioma of the vulva and perineum prior to treatment.

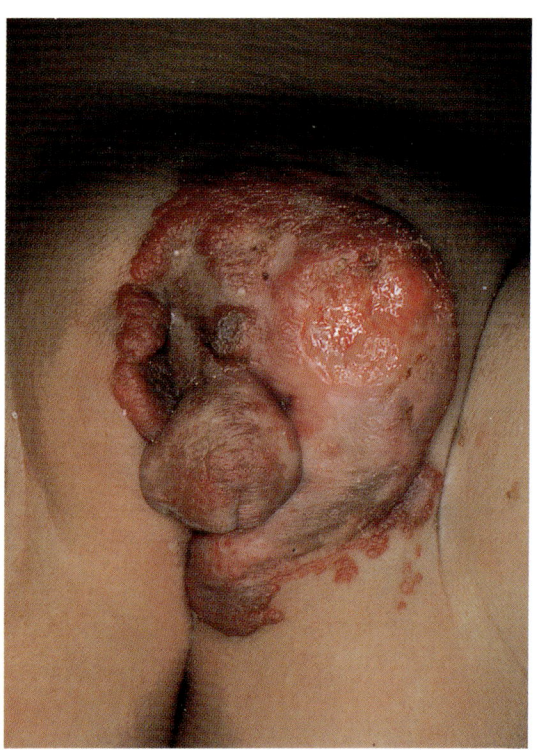

FIG. 6.22-B. Close-up view.

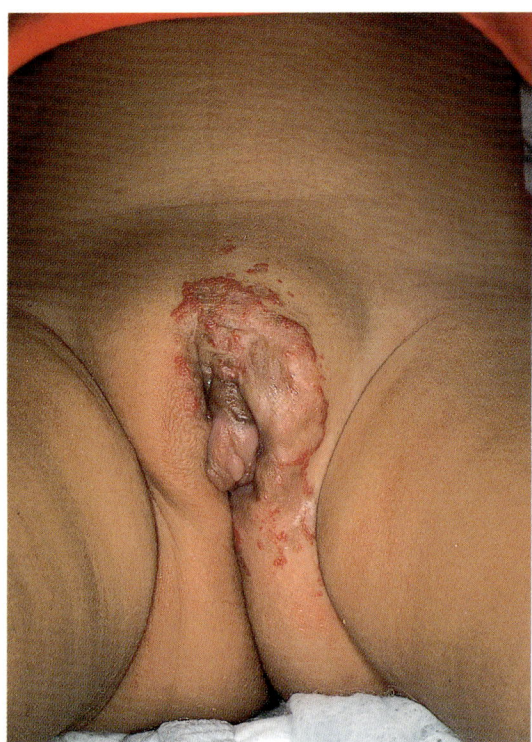

FIG. 6.22-C. Healed lesion 8 weeks post-treatment demonstrating complete healing and epithelialization, marked blanching, and shrinkage.

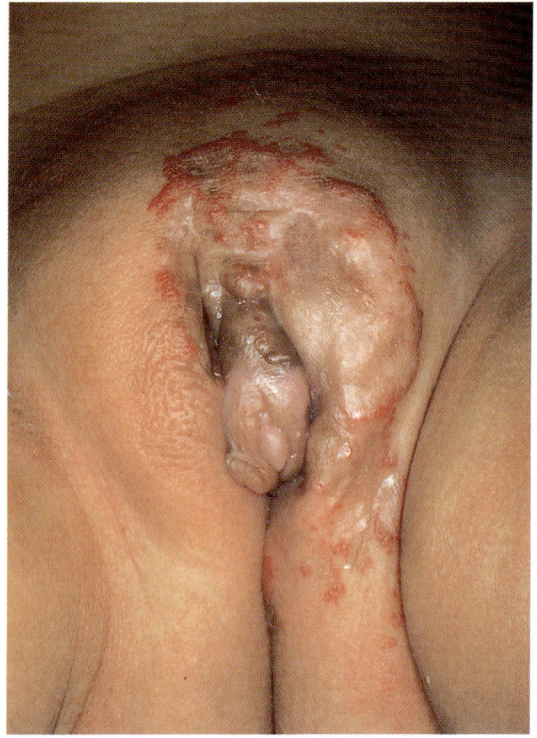

FIG. 6.22-D. Close-up view.

Case courtesy of *David B. Apfelberg*, M.D.

CASE 6.23

Ulcerated Oral Capillary/Cavernous Hemangioma

REVIEW OF CASE. This is an 8-month-old male who has a capillary/cavernous hemangioma that is distorting the upper lip. It has been chronically ulcerated and traumatized with frequent bleeding. Examination revealed a 2 × 3 cm ulcerated capillary/cavernous hemangioma of the upper lip occupying the vermilion as well as the skin of the upper lip. The hemangioma extended through-and-through the lip and could be seen in the labial mucosa.

CHOICE OF LASER: Nd:YAG. The Nd:YAG laser was chosen because it produces a continuous wave output power at 1064 nm (near infrared, invisible). This laser light penetrates to a depth of 5–7 mm into the dermis as a result of back scatter, forward scatter, and absorption. This scattering effect transforms the light into heat which causes coagulation necrosis with hemostasis over a large volume (5–7 mm) of tissue without its removal. The laser is hand held at its focal length (2–4 cm) perpendicular to the surface and focused on the hemangioma in a "polka dot pattern," alternating 1 mm dots of treatment with 1 mm of normal untreated hemangioma. An instant white blanching and noticeable tissue shrinkage is rapidly and immediately observed. Pulse duration of 0.5 seconds, spot size of 1 mm, and power of 30 watts is used.

ADDITIONAL INFORMATION. The combination of Nd:YAG laser photocoagulation plus direct steroid injection has been useful in causing blanching and shrinkage of capillary/cavernous hemangiomas. Approximately 1 cc of a short-acting and 1 cc of a long-acting steroid are injected for each cm of hemangioma.

POST-TREATMENT CARE. Iced saline compresses and topical antibiotic complete the procedure.

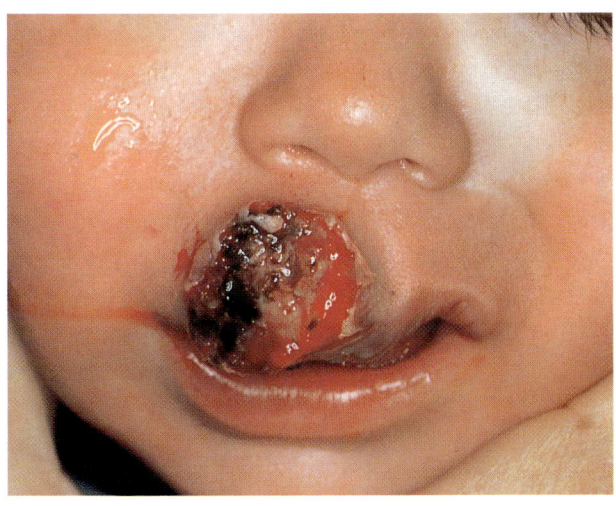

FIG. 6.23-A. Ulcerated capillary/cavernous hemangioma of upper lip.

For literature pertaining to this case see References section.

Case continues on following page.

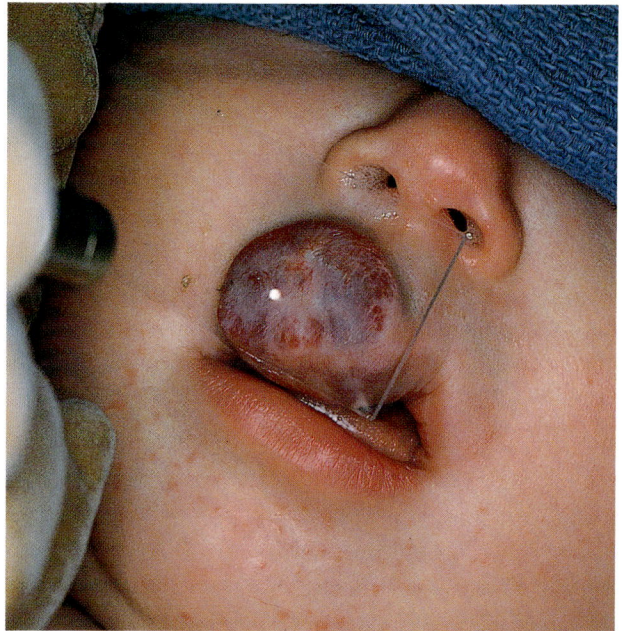

FIG. 6.23-B. Nd:YAG laser photocoagulation through a glass slide in a polka dot manner.

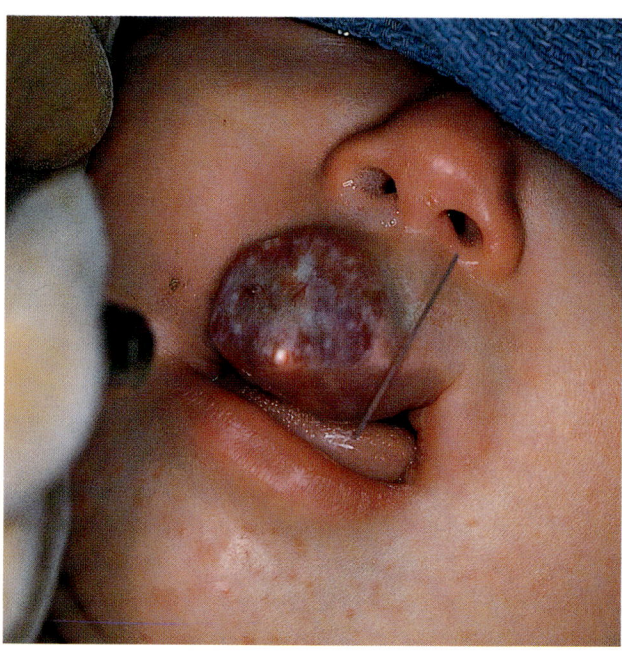

FIG. 6.23-C. Nd:YAG laser photocoagulation through a glass slide in a polka dot manner.

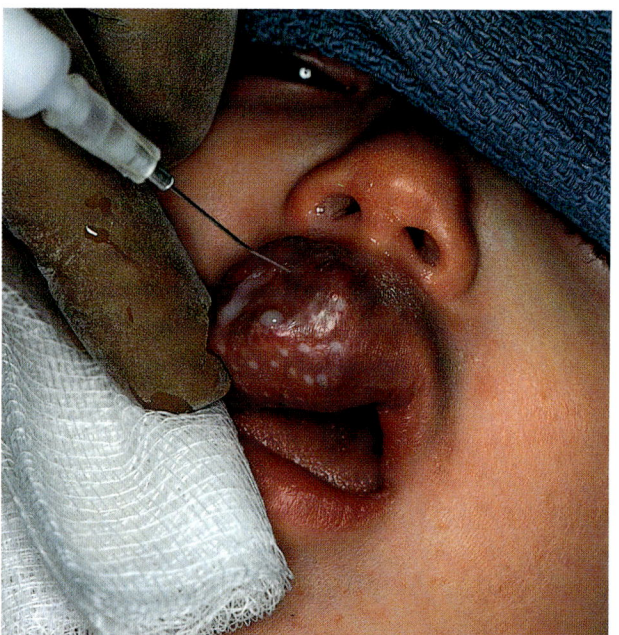

FIG. 6.23-D. Direct injection of steroids.

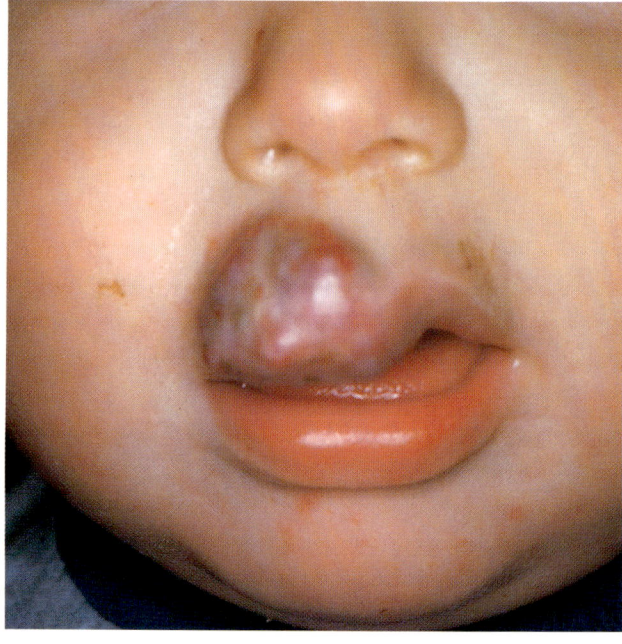

FIG. 6.23-E. Marked blanching and shrinkage of hemangioma with good epithelialization approximately four weeks following treatment.

Case courtesy of *David B. Apfelberg*, M.D.

CASE 6.24

Infiltrating Ductal Carcinoma of the Breast

Treated by Modified Radical Mastectomy

REVIEW OF CASE. This patient is a 48-year-old white female with a left breast biopsy done 24 hours previously, indicating infiltrating ductal carcinoma. The lesion was nonpainful, mobile, and 1.5 cm in size.

CHOICE OF LASER: Nd:YAG. The Nd:YAG laser was chosen in association with the artificial sapphire contact scalpel because of the need for precision and control of penetration during the axillary dissection. It was chosen instead of the CO_2 laser because the contact method tends to produce less smoke plume and does not cause overheating of liquified fat.

ADDITIONAL INFORMATION. The most precision needed in this surgery is in the axilla. Here the contact fibers should dissect along the edge of the tubular structure (blood vessel or nerve) to avoid iatrogenic injury. Do not dissect over the top of the structure.

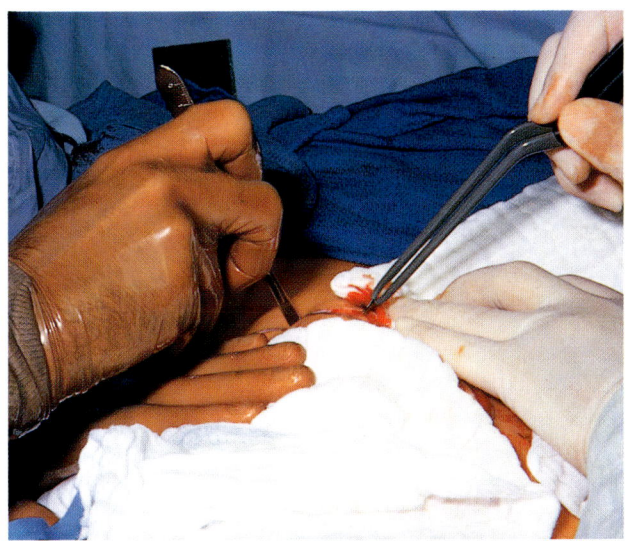

FIG. 6.24-A. Skin incisions are made with regular scalpel and cautery, except where very thin skin is present which allows rapid use of the contact scalpel at 15 watts without significant lateral heat absorption.

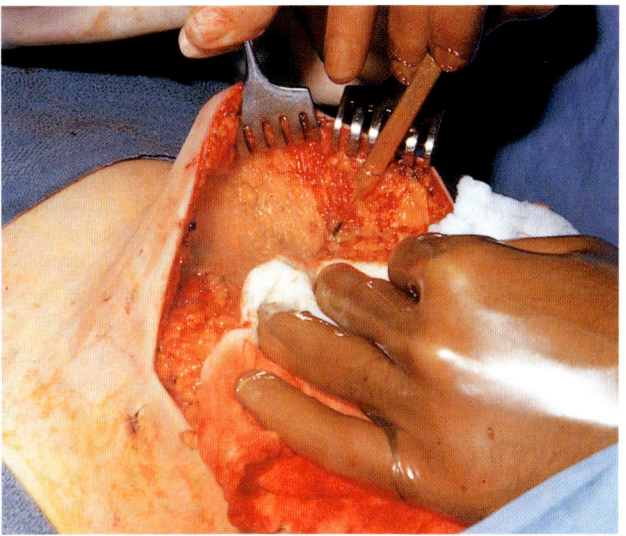

FIG. 6.24-B. Skin flaps are developed in the usual manner, with the laser set at 15 to 20 watts. A 0.8 to 1.0 mm frosted scalpel is used. Current technology would allow use of a 600 or 1,000 microcontoured laser contact fiber at the same wattage.

Case continues on following page.

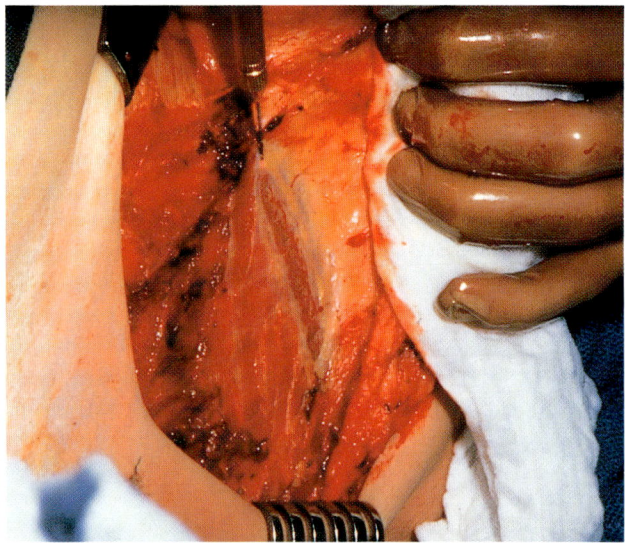

FIG. 6.24-C. The breast and pectoral fascia is dissected off at 12 watts, with the procedure progressing toward the left axilla.

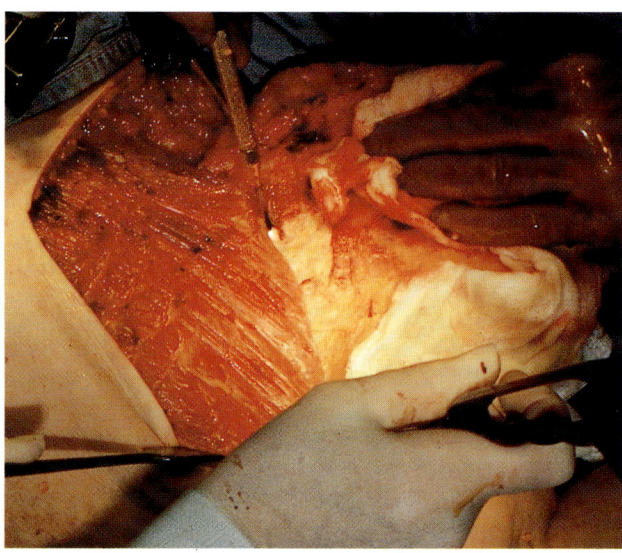

FIG. 6.24-D. Dissection continues along the serratus anterior muscle.

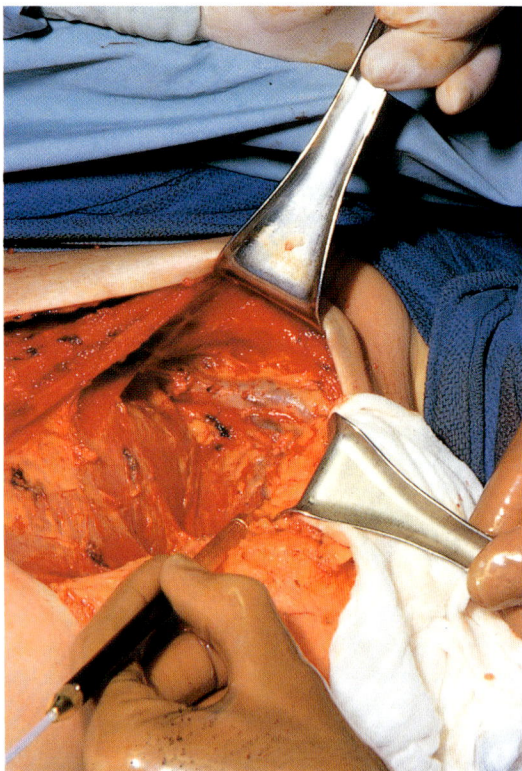

FIG. 6.24-E. The axillary compartment is dissected at 10 to 12 watts, taking care to dissect along the edge of tubular structures such as the axillary vein and adjacent nerves. Branches of the vein are still clamped, divided, and tied.

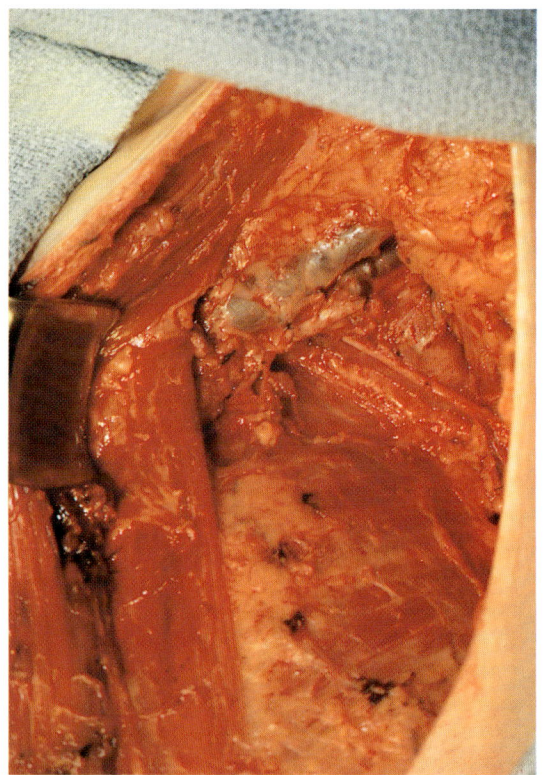

FIG. 6.24-F. Axillary dissection is completed. Note cautery char, denoting that cautery is still occasionally required for hemostasis.

Case courtesy of *Leonard S. Schultz,* M.D.

7

TUNABLE DYE LASER

VASCULAR MALFORMATIONS
7.1 Capillary hemangioma
7.2 Diffuse angiokeratoma
7.3 Cherry angioma
7.4 Cherry hemangioma
7.5 Hemangioma: superficial/capillary
7.6 Large telangiectasias
7.7 Mat telangiectasias secondary to CRST syndrome
7.8 Mat telangiectasias
7.9 Nevus araneus
7.10 Port wine stain
7.11 Port wine stain: vascular malformation
7.12 Port wine stain hemangioma of the right face
7.13 Port wine stain hemangioma
7.14 Port wine stain: macular vascular malformation
7.15 Port wine stain hemangioma (chest)
7.16 Port wine stain with hypertrophy
7.17 Port wine stain of the left cheek
7.18 Port wine stain of the upper lip
7.19 Port wine stain birthmark with prior dermal tattoo
7.20 Spider angioma
7.21 Spider hemangioma
7.22 Adult onset telangiectasia
7.23 Essential telangiectasia
7.24 Essential facial telangiectasia
7.25 Facial telangiectasia (lower face)
7.26 Facial telangiectasia (check)
7.27 Nasal venous telangiectasia
7.28 Telangiectatic congenital vascular malformation
7.29 Telangiectatic leg vein/telangiectatic matting
7.30 Telangiectasia on the ali nasi
7.31 Venous lake
7.32 Venous lake of the lower lip

CASE 7.1
Capillary Hemangioma

REVIEW OF CASE. This seven-week-old infant female was referred for rapid enlarging hemangioma of the right pre-auricular area, cheek, lip, chin, and anterior neck. There is no history of stridor, ulceration, or clotting abnormalities.

CHOICE OF LASER: TUNABLE DYE. Capillary hemangiomas are composed of proliferating endothelial cells and red blood cells. These lesions undergo rapid proliferation shortly after birth and may grow until the infant is 9 months of age. This is followed by gradual involution which may take several years. Generally 50% of capillary hemangiomas have completely involuted by five years, 70% by seven years, and 90% by nine years. Only 2 to 3% of hemangiomas require any intervention, be it for hemorrhage, infection, or disseminated intravascular coagulation (Kassabach-Merritt syndrome). The standard of therapy accepted by most pediatricians is to watch and wait for involution. If the lesion requires intervention, corticosteroids by injection or parenterally is the usual treatment. The Candela dye laser has been shown to ablate port wine stains in children and more recently to have an impact on the growth of capillary hemangiomas. As the dye laser has a depth of penetration of 1.8 mm, it is best used on lesions that are slightly raised off the surface of the skin. Therefore the earlier treatment can be instituted on smaller thin hemangiomas, the greater the improvement will be. There is a minimal risk of scarring when port wine stains are treated (5%), so the risk of scarring from treating hemangiomas should also be small. The Candela flashlamp pulsed tunable dye laser is based on the process of selective photothermolysis. It is by selectively targeting the chromophore hemoglobin with the yellow wavelength of 585 nm and by limiting the thermal injury to blood vessels with a pulse duration of 400 μsec that ablation can be achieved without any scarring.

Several treatments at two to four week intervals may be necessary to completely ablate a hemangioma. However, if the goal is to simply induce involution, fewer treatments are necessary.

ADDITIONAL INFORMATION. The treatment of vascular areas with the candela dye laser is relatively painless. Adults and older children compare it to a hot rubber band snap on the skin. Because the pain is minimal, treatment of hemangiomas in infants can be performed without any anesthesia or with intralesional Xylocaine. The heat and itching that is felt post-operatively for 5–10 minutes can be immediately reduced by placing a cool wet cloth over the treatment site.

The patient should have their eyes shielded with appropriate laser goggles or with gauze pads placed over the eyes. The parents may hold the child during the treatment or a papoose board may be used. A bottle should be near by for when the treatment is completed.

In most cases, an energy density of 5.5 J/cm^2 appears to achieve the same results as 6.0 J/cm^2 with reduced pain and scarring. If there is no change with a treatment of 5.5 J/cm^2, then the energy density may be increased by 0.5 J/cm^2 increments. Proliferating hemangiomas may be treated in 2–4 week intervals, while treatment intervals may be prolonged for older lesions.

POST-TREATMENT CARE. Bacitracin should be applied two or three times a day. A telfa dressing can be used if the infant tolerates it. Be sure that the adhesive tape does not touch the treated area. As the treatment area heals the patient should be cautioned not to remove any scabs or crusting that may form because of the profound cosmetic impact.

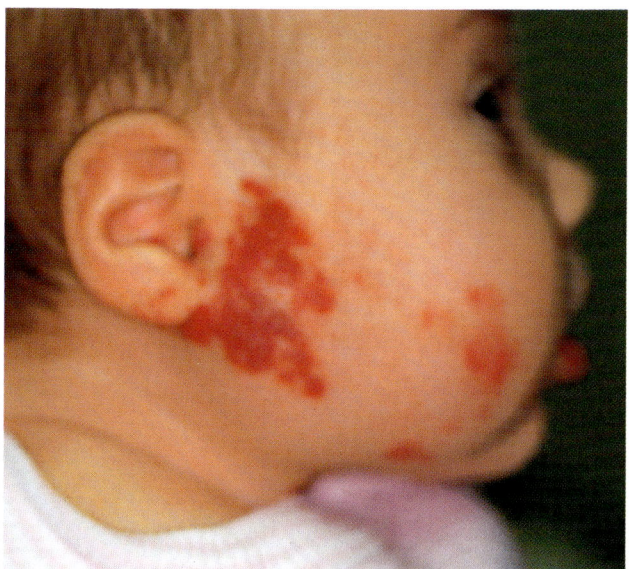
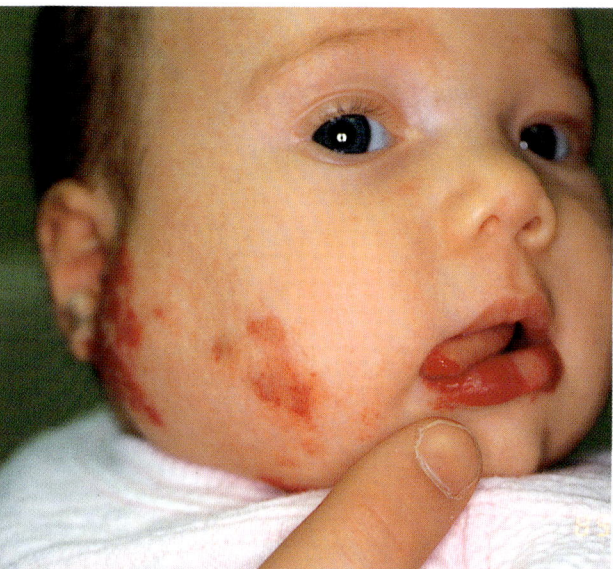

FIG. 7.1-A, B. Pre-operative enlarging vascular tumor of the right preauricular area, cheek, chin, and lower lip. The large bluish nodule in the preauricular area is a deeper cavernous hemangioma. The infant is 7 weeks old.

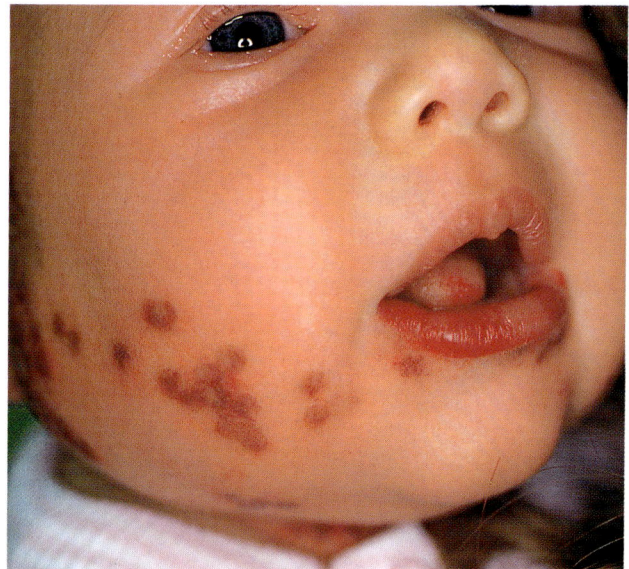

FIG. 7.1-C. The entire area, except the lip is treated at 6.0 J/cm^2, 585 nm, 400 μsec, 5 mm spot size. The pulses should be placed adjacent to each other, but should not overlap. With each pulse the tissue immediately turns a blue-gray which will darken to a deep purple black in a few minutes. The residual hemangioma is a much lighter pink when compared to the original lesion.

Case continues on following page.

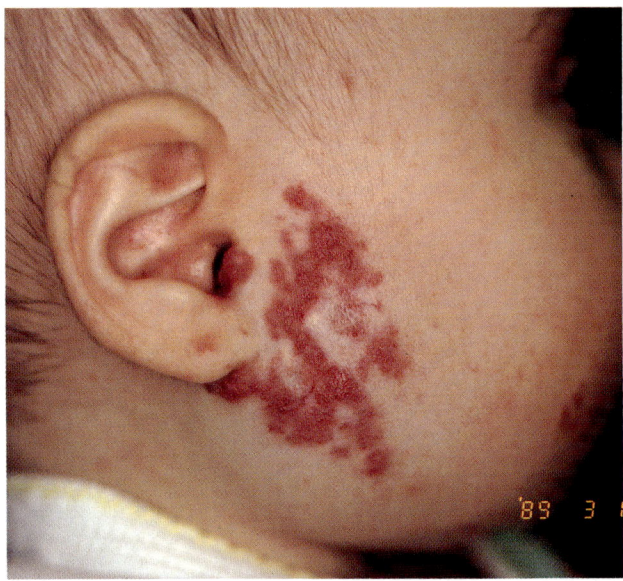

FIG. 7.1-D. The capillary hemangioma after treatments at 4 week intervals. The lesion had stopped growing and in areas is completely gone. The decision is made to continue treatment, attempting to completely ablate the hemangioma.

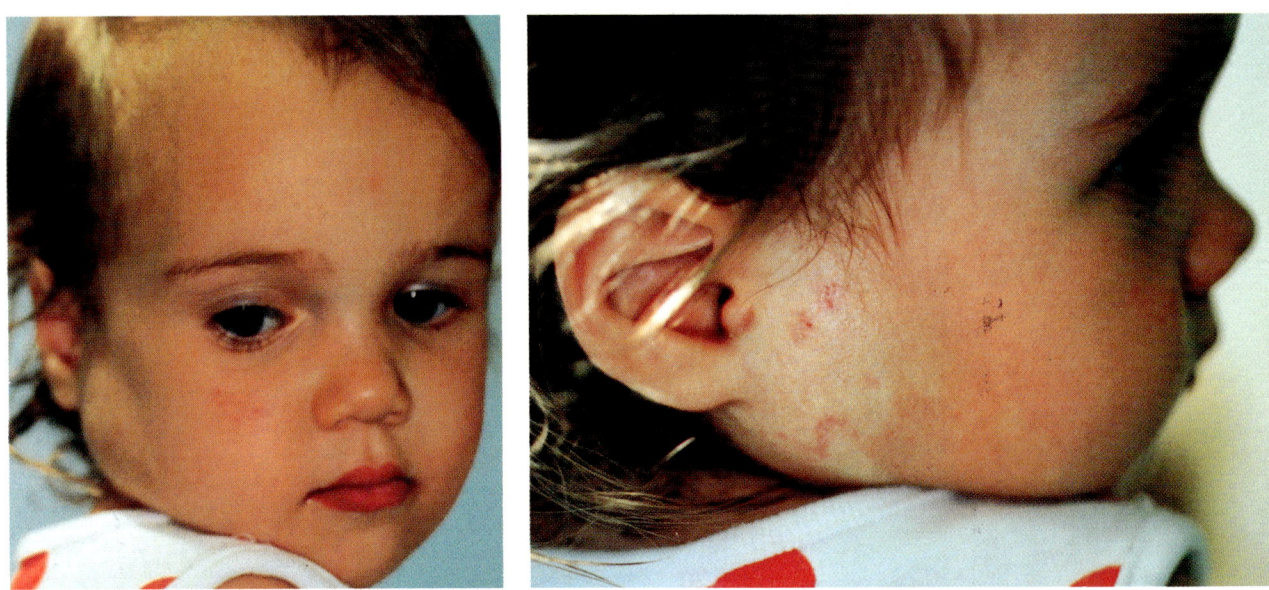

FIG. 7.1-E, F. After 12 treatments over 18 months, the capillary hemangioma is ablated. There are some small residual telangiectatic mats. The preauricular bluish cavernous hemangioma has not significantly changed. Note that the untreated capillary hemangioma on the lip is still present and that a spider angioma has developed on the right cheek.

Case courtesy of *Karen A. Sherwood*, M.D.

CASE 7.2
Diffuse Angiokeratoma

REVIEW OF CASE. This 15-year-old male had the onset of small angiokeratotic papules since childhood. Several biopsies and complete work-up by neurology and nephrology showed no evidence of Fabry's disease. In addition, there was no evidence of alpha-galactosidase deficiency. Enzyme levels of fucosidase enzyme were normal. It was felt that the patient had a benign form of angiokeratoma corporis diffusum. He requested treatment for cosmetic reasons. The angiokeratomas consisted of small, keratotic papules across the upper chest, neck, arms, and breast. The treatment area depicted in the figures is around the right breast area after one treatment. Treatment was given at 6.0 J/cm^2 fluence, each pulse 5.0 mm in size, and 158 pulses to treat the right breast area.

ADDITIONAL INFORMATION. Diffuse angiokeratomas of a variety of etiologies can be treated with the Candela laser. When the lesions are elevated and keratotic they often require several pulses. If they are flat and diffuse, single pulses minimally touching and not overlapping can be used to treat the involved areas. Blister formation, crust formation, or any sign of a significant amount of edema can be covered with systemic antibiotics to prevent secondary infection. This patient's major social embarrassment of having red areas around his breast was improved after one treatment.

POST-TREATMENT CARE. The patient was instructed to use topical antibiotics, normal soap and water and to cover the wounds with simple Telfa dressings for 48 hours.

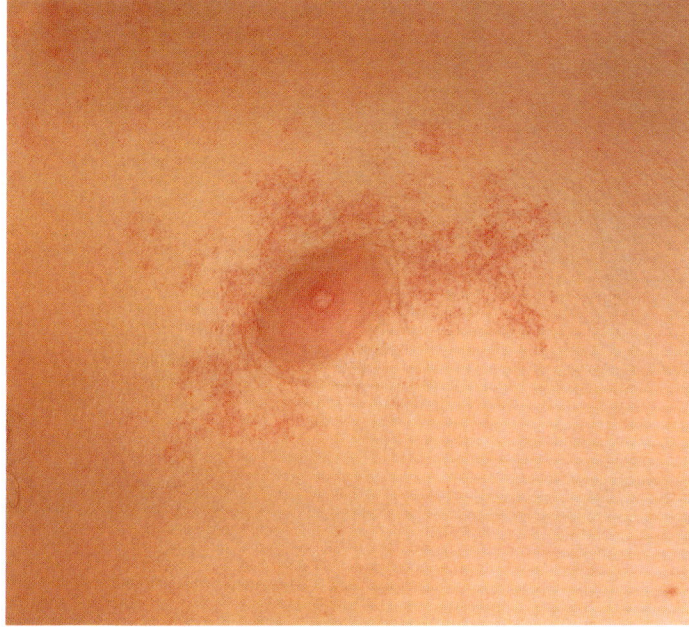

FIG. 7.2-A. Pre-operative plaques and papules of diffuse angiokeratomas around the right areola.

Case continues on following page.

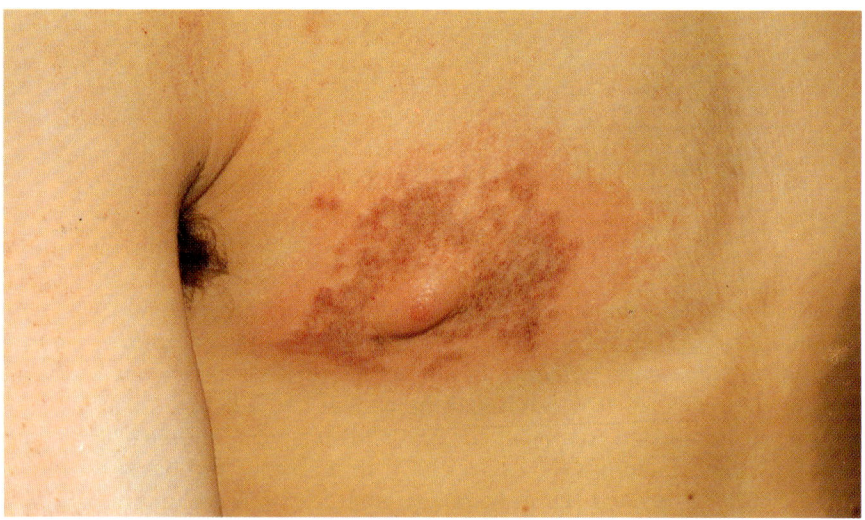

7.2-B. Immediate post-operative purpura from the Candela laser.

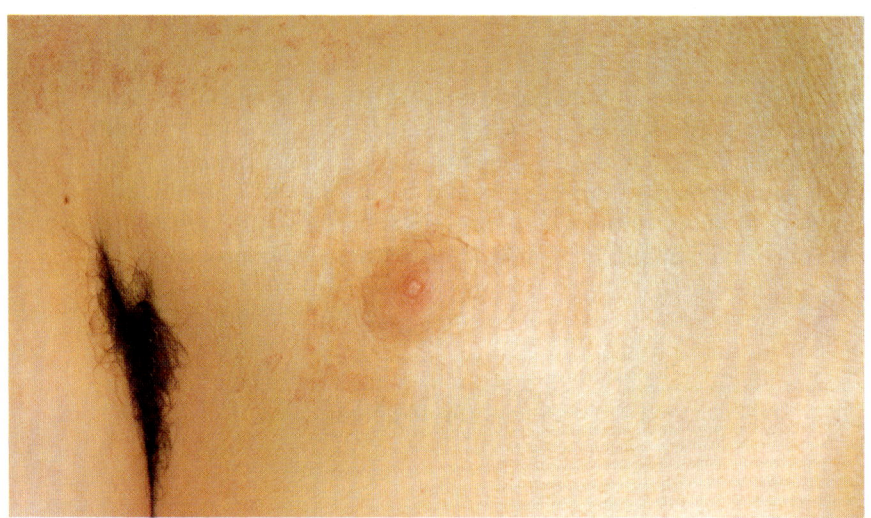

FIG. 7.2-C. One month follow-up, note residual hyperpigmentation from prior treatment.

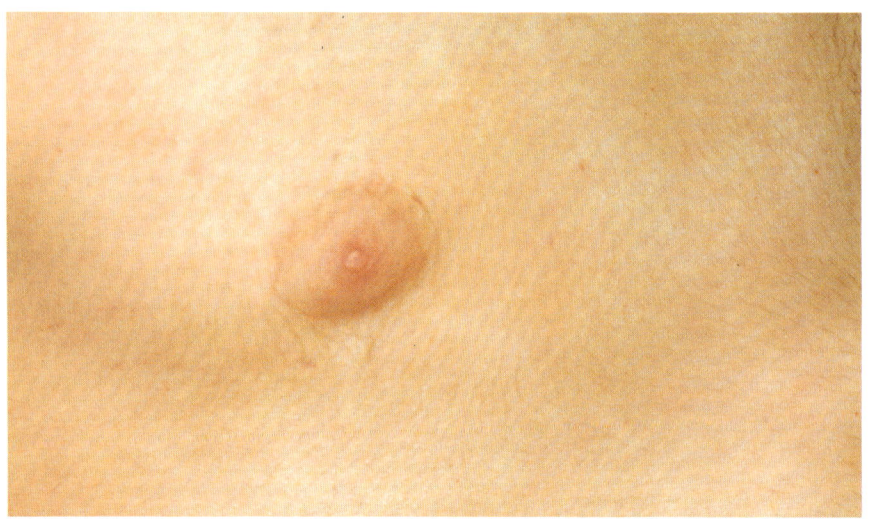

FIG. 7.2-D. Resolution of angiokeratoma and hyperpigmentation.

Case courtesy of ***Thomas O. McMeekin, M.D.***

CASE 7.3
Cherry Angioma

REVIEW OF CASE. This 48-year-old female presented with asymptomatic red papules across the forehead increasing in size and number without symptoms. She wished these to be removed for cosmetic reasons.

CHOICE OF LASER: TUNABLE DYE. The Candela flashed-pump tunable dye laser was chosen for its specificity for vascular lesions, its lack of scarring potential, and the ease of doing this procedure without anesthesia. The lesions were treated at two separate intervals approximately one month apart. The two lesions were treated initially with a pulse size of 5 mm, a dose of 6.0 J/cm^2 fluence, and each lesion received two pulses. Both lesions were again retreated at 6.25 J/cm^2 fluence, 5.0 mm lens, and three pulses each.

ADDITIONAL INFORMATION. Small cherry angioma and other benign telangiectatic vessels can be treated with multiple pulses if they are elevated. If a lesion is treated with more than three pulses however, the chance of blister formation or scar formation is increased. Elevated lesions usually take more than one treatment as opposed to flat, telangiectatic vessels which often respond to one treatment.

POST-TREATMENT CARE. For temporary pain or discomfort cool, wet compresses are applied in the first 24 hours. Otherwise, topical antibiotic such as Polysporin ointment is applied and the wounds left open to air.

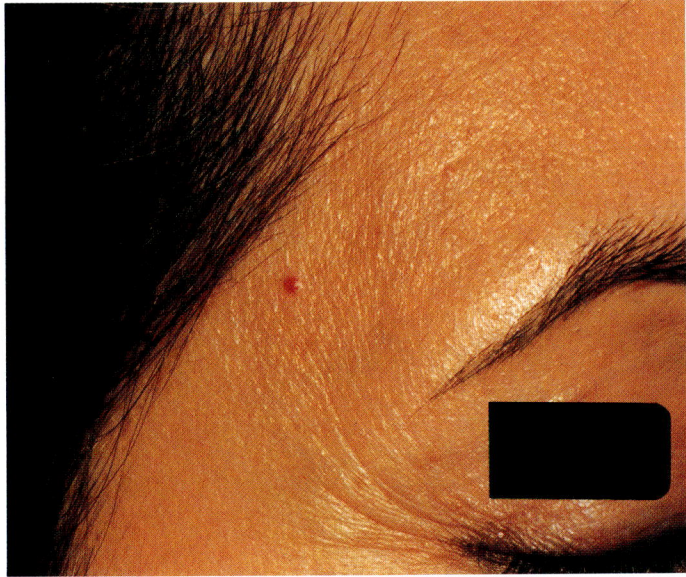

FIG. 7.3-A. Two pre-operative lesions on right forehead.

Case continues on following page.

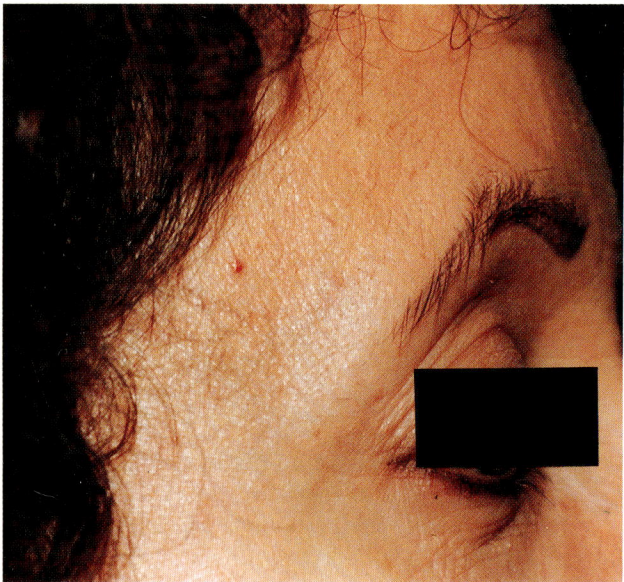

FIG. 7.3-B. 2½ weeks after one treatment.

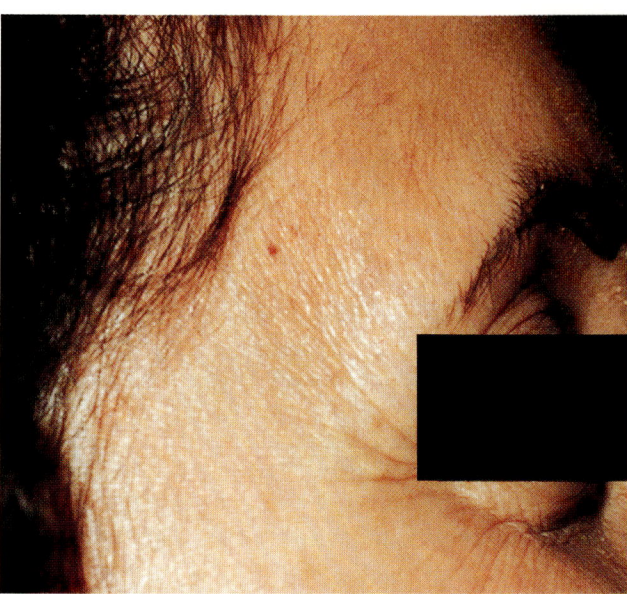

FIG. 7.3-C. Pre-operatively before the last or second treatment with one lesion almost completely cleared and the second lesion reduced to a small dot.

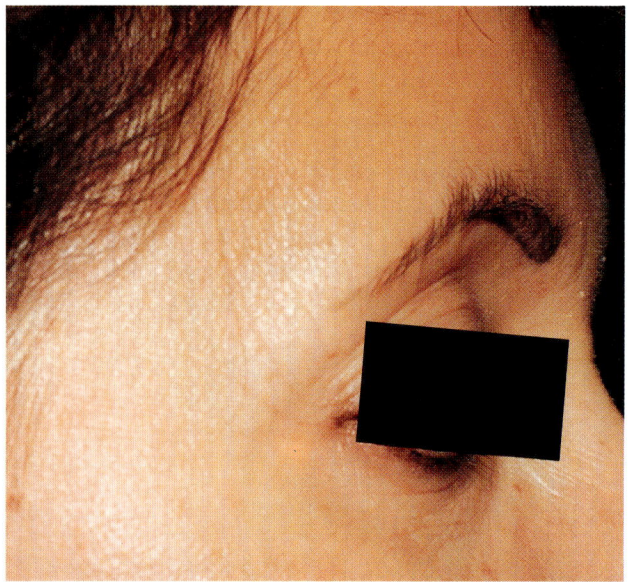

FIG. 7.3-D. Complete resolution of both cherry angiomas at the two-month interval. There is no sign of hyperpigmentation or texture change of the skin.

Case courtesy of *Thomas O. McMeekin*, M.D.

CASE 7.4
Cherry Hemangioma

REVIEW OF CASE. This 39-year-old woman presented with cherry angiomas on the left medial calf of several years duration.

CHOICE OF LASER: TUNABLE DYE. The tunable dye laser was selected to take advantage of the relatively selective absorption of yellow laser light by oxyhemoglobin. (argon or carbon dioxide lasers can also successfully be used on small lesions, but they are less selective and produce more nonspecific thermal damage and discomfort during treatment.) The 577 nm yellow wavelength was selected, however, 585 nm may provide slightly deeper penetration on thicker lesions.

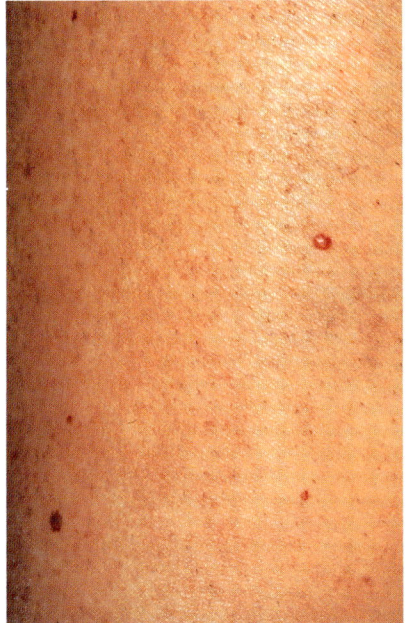 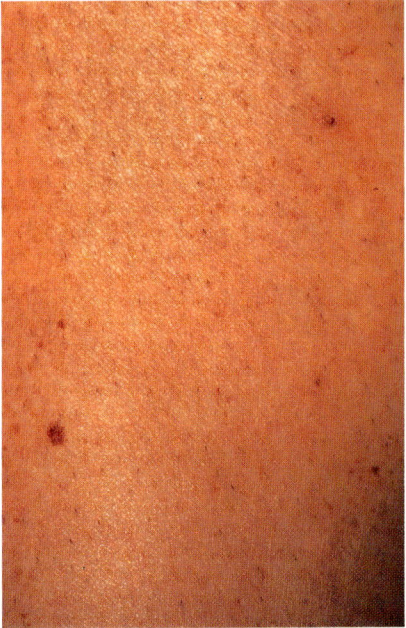 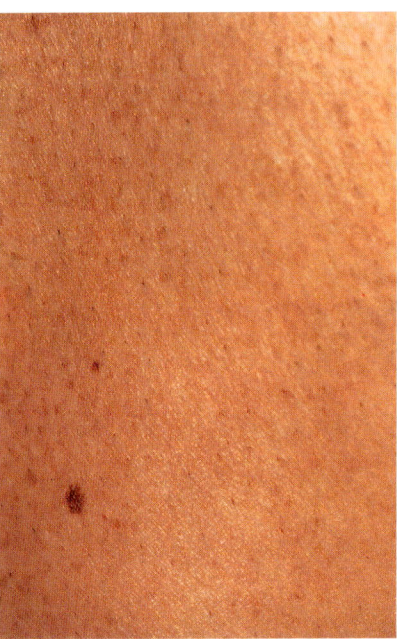

FIG. 7.4-A. Cherry hemangiomas prior to treatment.

FIG. 7.4-B. The angiomas were treated using a 577 nm yellow tunable dye laser with 1.0 mm spot diameter and 0.30 watts continuous mode focused power. The technique utilized was a "painting" technique where the beam is moved back and forth in a slightly overlapping "paint roller" type pattern using vessel disappearance and or slight color change from red to light grey as the treatment endpoint. Generally no anesthesia is required. If an endpoint of blanching is obtained, then the area has been overtreated and nonspecific thermal damage is being observed. The slight erythema immediately post-treatment is normal.

FIG. 7.4-C. Five weeks after treatment with the lesion sites being virtually unrecognizable.

Case courtesy of *David H. McDaniel, M.D.*

CASE 7.5

Hemangioma: Superficial/Capillary

REVIEW OF CASE. This 2-month-old female infant presented with a proliferating hemangioma over the dorsum of the right hand.

CHOICE OF LASER: TUNABLE DYE. Although these lesions will spontaneously involute with time, the therapeutic intervention with this laser may halt proliferation and eliminate the lesion much more rapidly than would occur naturally. The selective vascular damage using a 360 μsec pulse duration in the 580 nm range at 6.00 to 6.25 J/cm^2 allows for minimizing any adverse skin texture effects.

ADDITIONAL INFORMATION. Lesions which are raised off the surface of the skin higher than 3 mm become more difficult to eliminate. However, even with the thicker superficial lesions there is a good chance of halting the proliferative phase. The cavernous component of these lesions usually does not respond to this laser.

POST-TREATMENT CARE. A topical antibiotic ointment is used in all cases.

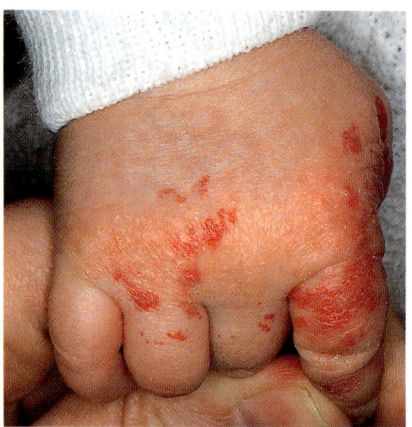

Fig. 7.5-A. Two-month-old female infant with hemangioma over dorsum of the right hand. The lesion is raised 1 to 2 mm from the skin surface.

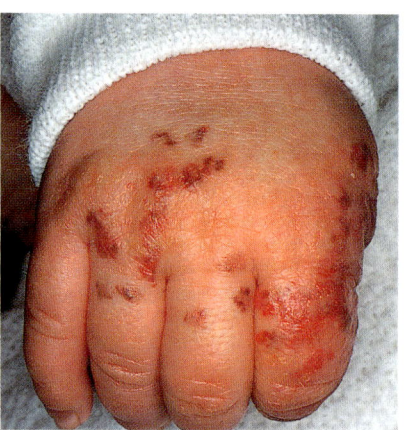

FIG. 7.5-B. Immediately post-treatment. The lesional darkening will resolve in 7 to 14 days.

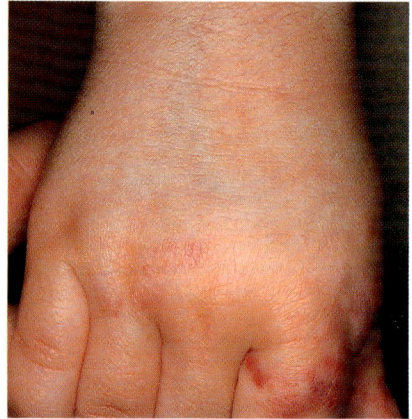

FIG. 7.5-C. Lesional area after three treatments performed at monthly intervals.

Case courtesy of *Jerome M. Garden*, M.D.

CASE 7.6
Large Telangiectasias

REVIEW OF CASE   This 72-year-old male presented with a history of many years of mild rosacea and large telangiectasias resulting in "drinker's nose." Previous treatment was unsuccessful with electrodessication. The patient complained of social embarrassment and rare episodes of bleeding with minor trauma.

CHOICE OF LASER: TUNABLE DYE.   The tunable dye (continuous wave (CW)) laser was chosen to accomplish selective vascular destruction of relatively large telangiectasias. Tunable dye and copper vapor CW lasers offer medium length pulse durations (0.02 seconds to continuous) sufficient to coagulate medium diameter and larger telangiectasias with concomitant long thermal relaxation times. It may be argued that such medium length pulses lack the thermal spatial confinement of the flashlamp excited dye laser (FEDL). However experience with these CW yellow lasers has shown complete clearance of telangiectasias with usually no clinically evident scar or texture change. Two key benefits of these CW yellow lasers besides their immediate efficacy is less discomfort than the FEDL (minimal pin-prick sensation) and the lack of purpura. The latter is a significant advantage for business people and others in the public eye. As our port wine stain and facial surgery patients have taught us for years, the purpuric color is difficult to cover with makeup.

ADDITIONAL INFORMATION.   Place the patient in a relaxed supine position. Sublingual Halcion may be used in anxious or sensitive patients. I begin with 1 watt (or maximum), pulse duration 0.04 second, and spot size 0.05 mm (or minimum) using a wave length between 577–588 nm. The laser is set in repeat pulse mode to deliver laser pulses to the target vessel one to two mm apart. Judge the efficacy of the first few pulses in photocoagulating the vessel. Small vessels may seal off without perceptible change in the overlying epidermis. Larger vessels may exhibit a whitening of the epidermis which is usually gone by the following day. Large vessels, particularly resistant ones retreated at longer pulse durations may show slight crusting within a few days of the treatment. If necessary increase the pulse duration to the next higher setting, e.g., 0.04 to 0.1 seconds. Try to avoid superimposing impulses unless encountering a resistant vessel. I usually proceed from the larger caliber portion of vessels toward their smaller aspect.

Occasionally the vessel will leak briskly. I then apply pressure with a cotton applicator to tamponade the source, defocus slightly, and lightly coagulate the site with a circular painting motion.

Patients overly concerned about vessels in the floor of the naris and coursing onto the mucosal aspect of the columnella should be advised of the especially high rate of recurrence (and sensitivity) in this location. One will generally need slightly longer pulse durations to proceed successfully.

POST-TREATMENT CARE.   No treatment is usually necessary. If crusting is observed apply antibiotic ointment ad libitum to keep the area soft and to aid re-epithelization.

Case continues on following page.

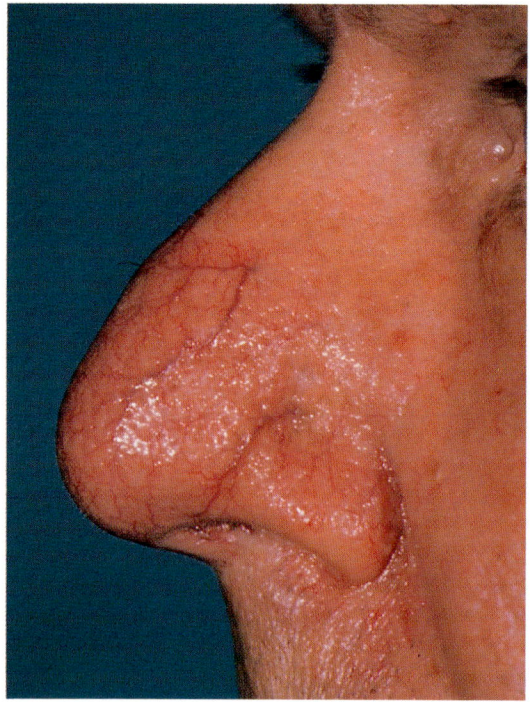

FIG. 7.6-A. Large facial telangiectasias before treatment, left profile.

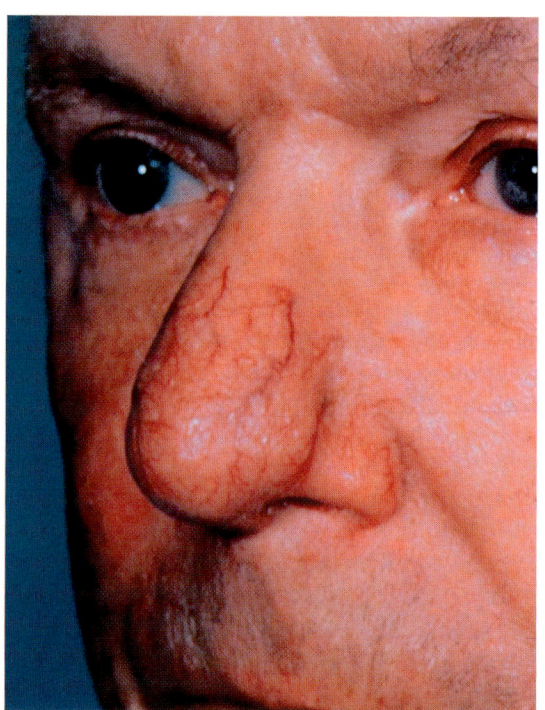

FIG. 7.6-B. Large facial telangiectasias before treatment, left three-quarters view.

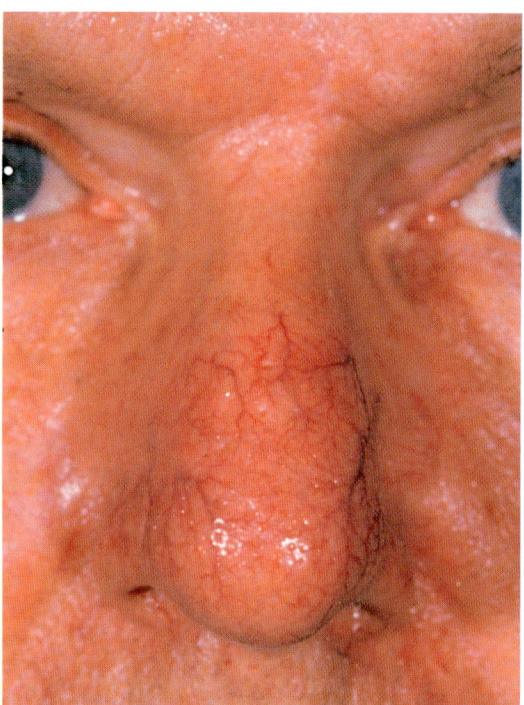

FIG. 7.6-C. Large facial telangiectasias before treatment, full facial view.

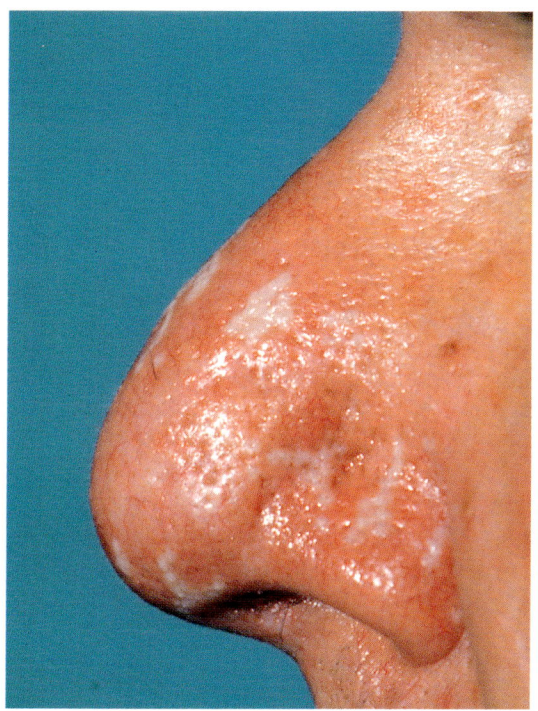

FIG. 7.6-D. Photocoagulated vessels with epidermal change, left profile.

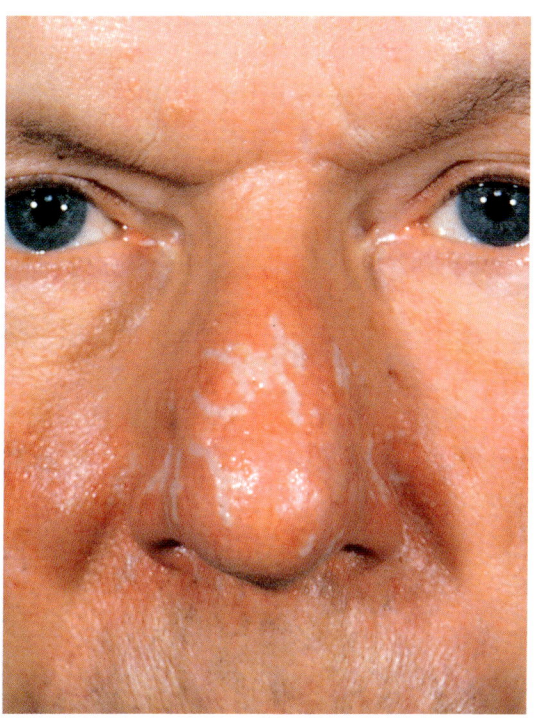

FIG. 7.6-E. Photocoagulated vessels with epidermal change, full facial view.

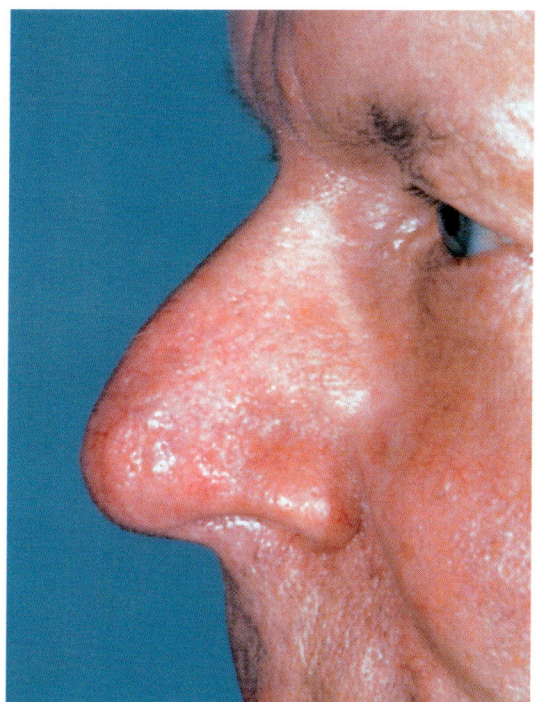

FIG. 7.6-F. Three weeks after CW tunable dye treatment, left profile.

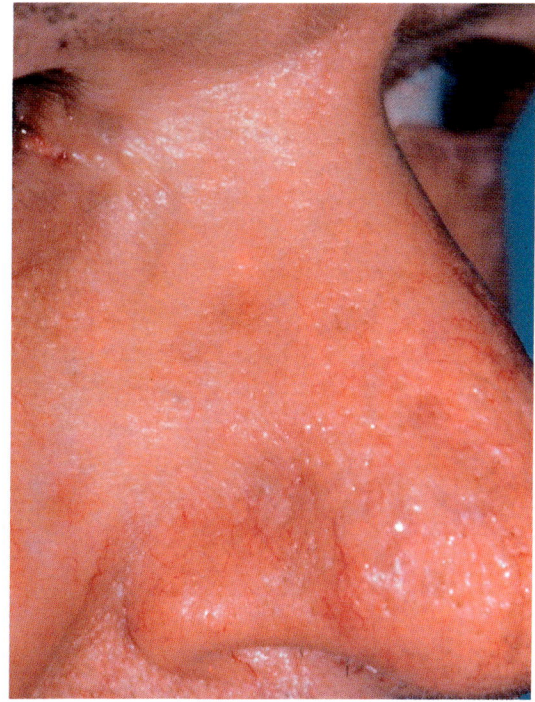

FIG. 7.6-G. Three weeks after CW tunable dye treatment, right three-quarter view.

Case courtesy of *Timothy J. Rosio*, M.D.

CASE 7.7

Mat Telangiectasias

Secondary to CRST Syndrome

REVIEW OF CASE. This 39-year-old male with a long-standing history of CRST syndrome had numerous telangiectatic vessels and mats of vessels across the cheeks and nose of several years duration. He requested treatment for cosmetic reasons.

CHOICE OF LASER: TUNABLE DYE. The Candela laser was chosen for its ease of application, low risk of scar formation, and its proven track record in treatment selective photothermolysis of dilated telangiectatic vessels. The area on the left cheek was treated three times over a 5-month period with initially 5.25 J/cm^2 fluence, and 23 pulses. On January 5, 1989 with 16 pulses at 5.5 J/cm^2 and on April 19, 1989, 7 pulses at 6.0 J/cm^2. Each pulse was 5.0 mm in size, greater than 50 μsec in duration and with the laser in the focused mode with the handpiece held at the preset in focus standard distance from the skin.

ADDITIONAL INFORMATION. Matted telangiectatic vessels can either take single or double pulses depending on whether they are flat or elevated. They respond easily to repeated treatments with the Candela flashed-pump tunable dye laser, but do take more than one treatment to show clearing or improvement. Treatment intervals can be as short as four weeks. There is minimum risk of infection and the purpura that is produced from the treatment persists for only 7–10 days. Because these areas are small, patients can be instructed in the use of cosmetic coverup makeups if the discoloration following the treatment is a problem. Patients have to be advised in the use of proper photo protection to prevent increased melanin formation and blockage of the absorption of the light by ectatic vessels.

POST-TREATMENT CARE. The wounds are left open and the patient is instructed to apply topical antibiotics for the first several days until the purpura had cleared. The patient is also instructed in the use of long wavelength sunblocks.

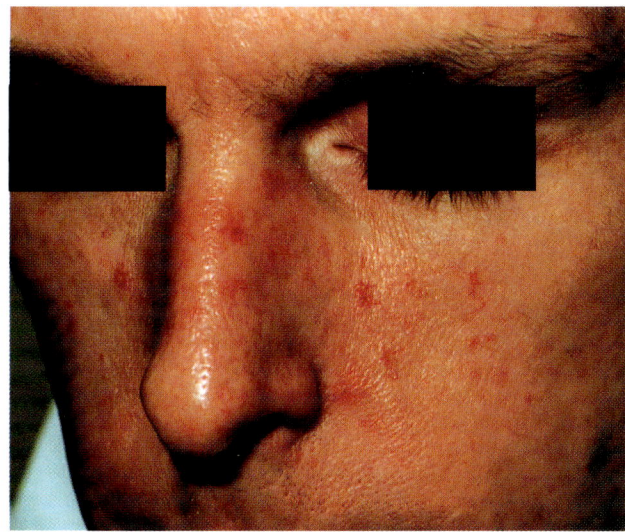

FIG. 7.7-A. Pre-operative mats of telangiectatic vessels. Note the presence of both elevated and flat vessels across the left cheek and nose.

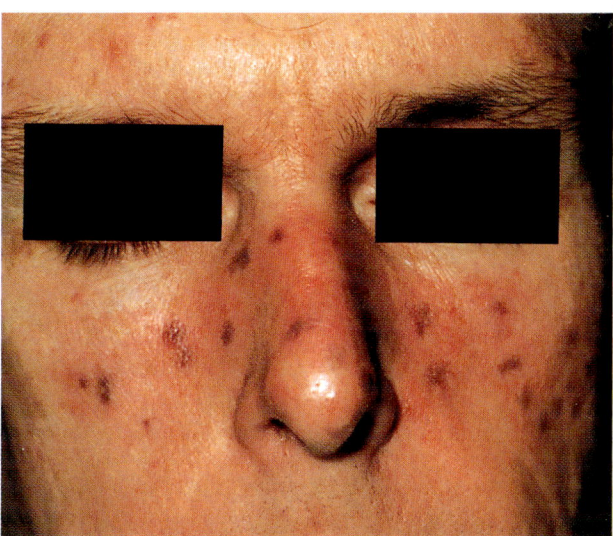

FIG. 7.7-B. Immediate post-operative purpura produced by the Candela laser.

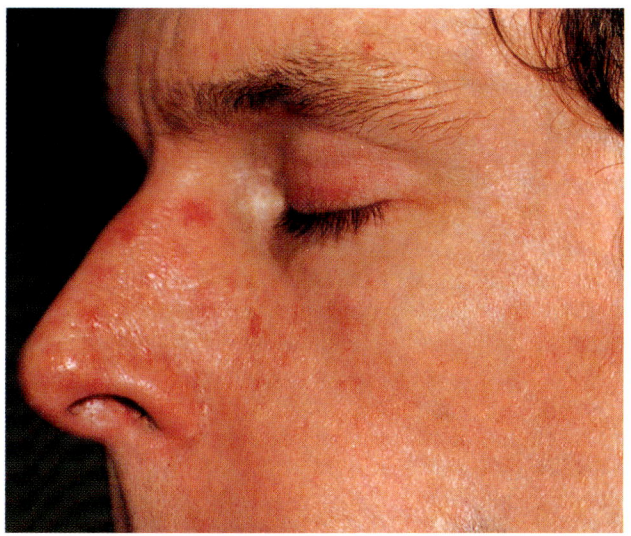

FIG. 7.7-C. One month following the first treatment.

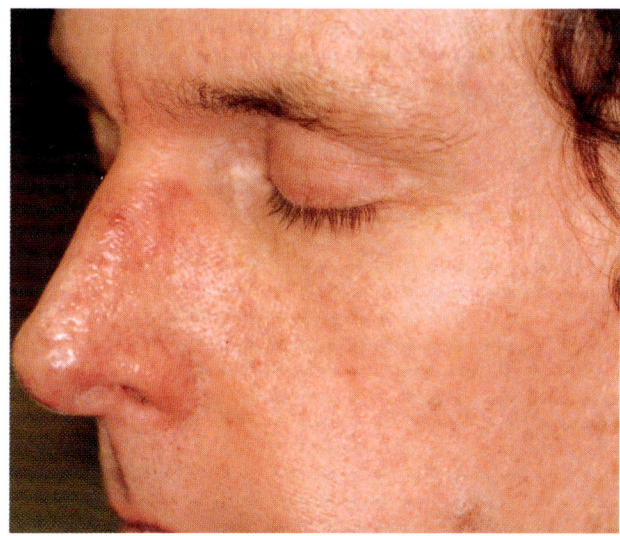

FIG. 7.7-D. Eight months following the last or third treatment of the ectatic vessels on the nose and left cheek. Note complete clearing of several matted telangiectatic vessels and partial clearing of those on the nose. Further treatments can be expected to clear this patient's face entirely.

Case courtesy of **Thomas O. McMeekin,** M.D.

CASE 7.8
Mat Telangiectasias

REVIEW OF CASE. This 59-year-old male with Rosacea had a 20 year history of numerous blanchable, bright red vascular macules and patches scattered over the lower two-thirds of the face, with occasional inflammatory papules or pustules. Previous treatment of topical agents and tetracycline eliminated only the papulopustular component. The patient complained of occasional itching or burning sensations and the spotted appearance of his face.

CHOICE OF LASER: FLASHLAMP EXCITED DYE (FEDL). Mat-like telangiectasias can occur sporadically, from actinic or physical trauma, and in association with a host of systemic problems including collagen-vascular disorders. The FED laser was chosen to eliminate the invisible to fine caliber, confluent telangiectatic vessels without inducing textural (scarring) or pigmentary irregularities (hypo/hyperpigmentation). Other yellow light lasers may be better suited for the large linear and arborizing vessels frequently seen in rosacea. Treatment physiology and mechanisms are summarized by the term "selective photothermolysis" which depends on four parameters: wavelength, pulse duration, peak power, and spot size.

Wavelength is optimized for peak absorption by the target chromophore and transmissive penetration to it. Experience has shown that a yellow light wavelength of between 577 nm to 585 nm is most efficiently absorbed by oxyhemoglobin. Penetration by 585 nm yellow light is demonstrably better than the blue-green argon wavelengths 488 and 514 nm. In small ectatic vessels (10–100 μm), short pulses of between 360–450 μseconds allow rapid delivery of the laser energy dose in a peak sufficient to damage the entire vessel diameter, and brief enough to dissipate without coagulating adjacent tissue. The thermal relaxation time describes influence of vessel diameter on rate of heat loss to adjacent tissue. Larger vessels with a longer thermal relaxation time may not be treated adequately with the very short fixed pulse duration of the FEDL, and require longer pulses from a continuous wave (CW) laser. A sufficiently high power peak may be distributed over a spot size greater than two mm which increases beam penetration depth. A wider beam diameter allows superimposition of refracted laser rays centrally and therefore deeper penetration of the therapeutic effect.

Power settings are generally 5 to 8 joules (derived by preliminary test spots of cosmetic units of sufficiently different skin thickness or texture); pulse duration is fixed at 450 μ seconds; spot size is generally 5 mm, but a 3 mm spot size is available for small individual vessels.

ADDITIONAL INFORMATION. Short-pulsed yellow light laser treatments may often be performed without anesthesia. However I administer local mental nerve blocks when feasible such as in the intra-oral and infra-orbital approach.

Eye protection is of utmost importance when using vascular target lasers. Opaque "suntanning" goggles are usually adequate when working on most areas of the face. For working over the eyelids or margins colored, opaque corneal shields should be used after topical anesthesia of the eye.

The margin of safety when treating macular vascular lesions has been greatly improved with the advent of the FEDL. Still, scarring can occur with injudicious power selection (including use of the same power settings in different cosmetic units), excessive overlap of treatment pulses, retreatment at too short intervals, or from skin injury soon after treatment.

Representative cosmetic units may be tested with as few as three to four pulses that overlap by 10–15%. This yields a club or cloverleaf-shaped laser purpura design (affectionately referred to by our patients as "laser hickeys.")

Extremely young or thin skin areas, or those prone to scarring may be tested at power settings just over the purpura threshold, and with barely contiguous laser spots. The rule-of-thumb "start low and work your way up" applies to power settings. An immediate prominent purpura response with marked gray color centrally argues for prompt consideration of reducing the power by 0.25 to 0.5 joules. If improvement is marginal and no crusting is reported by the patient a similar adjustment upwards may be warranted.

Overlapping impulses just sufficient to avoid or minimize significant nontreated areas (approximately 15%) may be facilitated by staggering or offsetting each row of pulses. Angling the handpiece slightly will produce an oval spot which may fit into corners better. The handpiece may be raised slightly from the skin to produce a more defocused beam and decreased tissue response for small adjacent areas judged to be thinner or more sensitive.

Re-treatment should be generally at six weeks or longer intervals, but never less than five weeks. I prefer even longer intervals in patients who develop a bronze hyperpigmentation. This is more frequently seen in older patients or those with thicker lesions and skin hypertrophy. One may mistake this fading pigment for residual vascular lesion.

Dressing treated areas with an ointment and nonstick bandage avoids shearing or scratching skin injury and provides reassurance and camouflage for the patient leaving the office. The frequent concern, "...but doctor, what happens if I accidentally scratch it in my sleep?", is eliminated for anxious patients and parents alike.

POST-TREATMENT CARE. Patients are given the same instructions as discussed above and a drawing of the respective body area after each test or treatment. The drawing is a copy of our record without the details of power settings and pulses. Patients are asked to grade response with the three grades: I, zero to mild flaking, II, crusting, and III, scabbing.

For the test areas and after the first treatment session, maintain the ointment and nonstick dressing intact overnight at least, and preferably until it is evident there will be no crusting. Dressings may be changed daily or dispensed with for older children and adults after treatment reaction is known. Only gentle tap water blotting or cleansing is suggested. If crusting or scabbing occurs note the location(s) and degree, the day of onset, and the day of resolution. Bring your map to each treatment session. A cool pack gently applied intermittently will alleviate areas of swelling (periorbit) or excess warmth. Scabbing or very prominent crusting should prompt a call to the doctor.

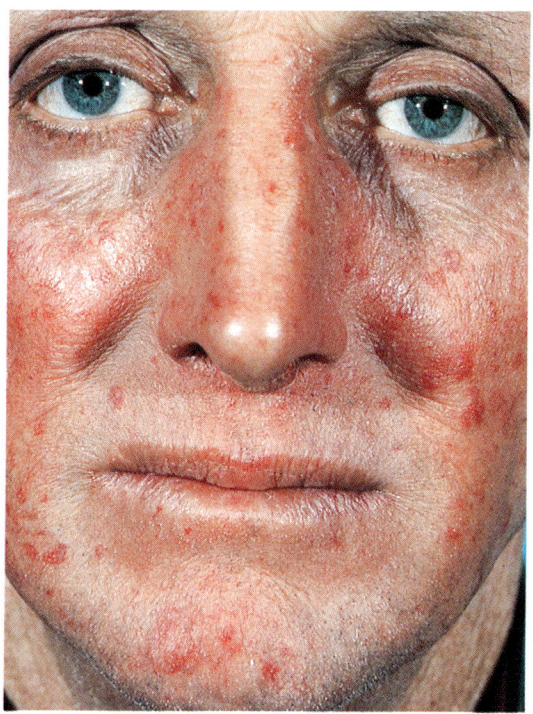

FIG. 7.8-A. Mat telangiectasias before FEDL treatment, front view.

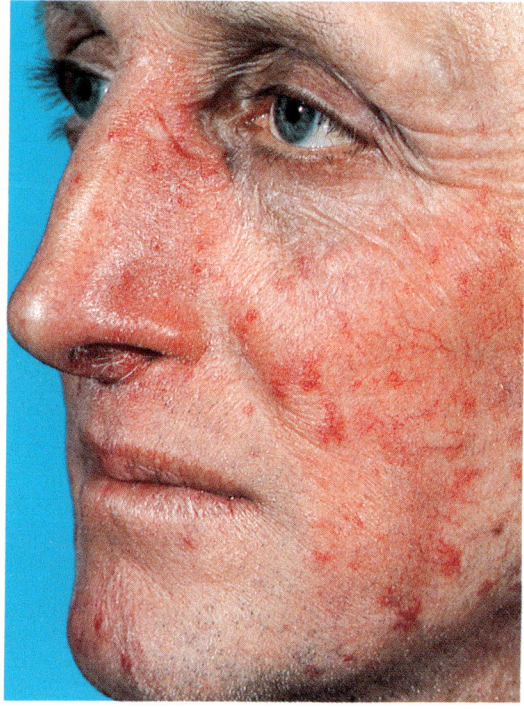

FIG. 7.8-B. Mat telangiectasias before FEDL treatment, side view.

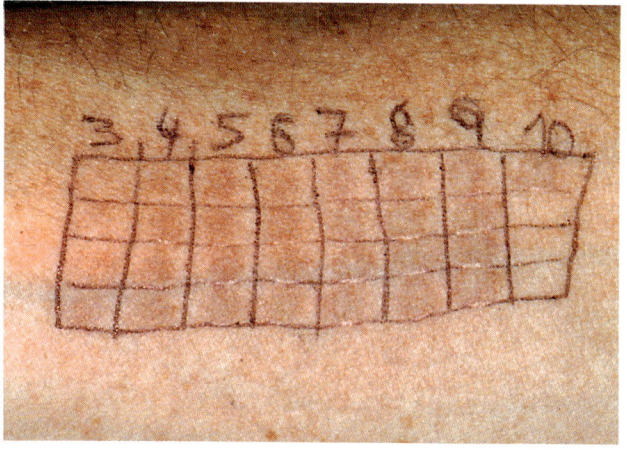

FIGS. 7.8-C. Close-up of laser purpura threshold; 3–10 joules in normal skin at 0 hours.

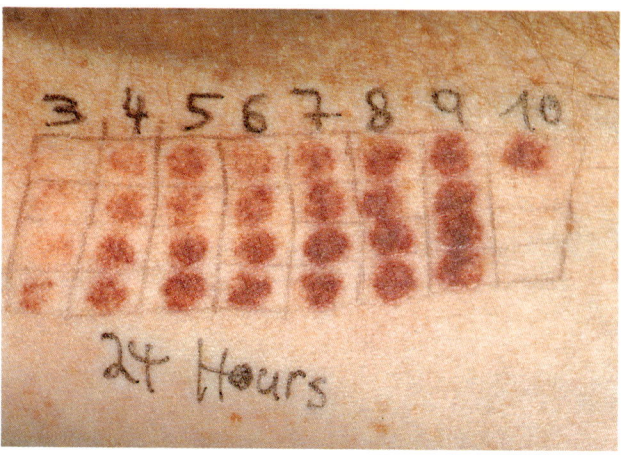

FIG. 7.8-D. Close-up of laser purpura threshold; 3–10 joules in normal skin at 24 hours.

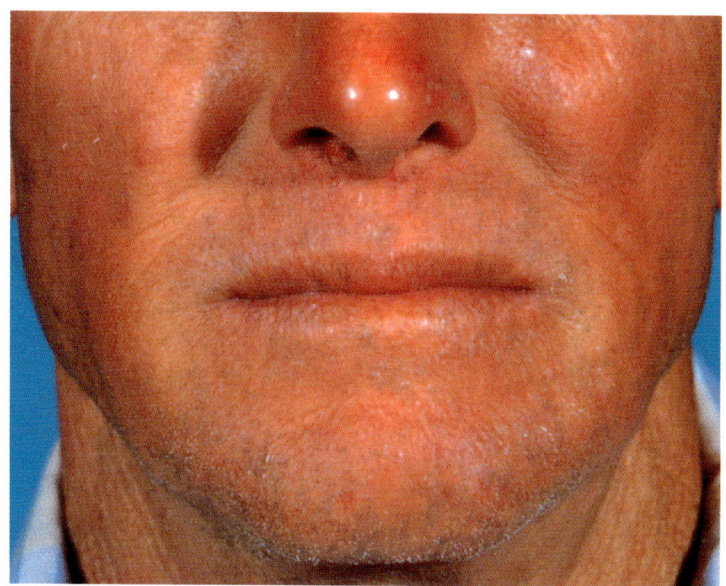

FIG. 7.8-E. Mat telangiectasias eight weeks after second FEDL treatment, front view.

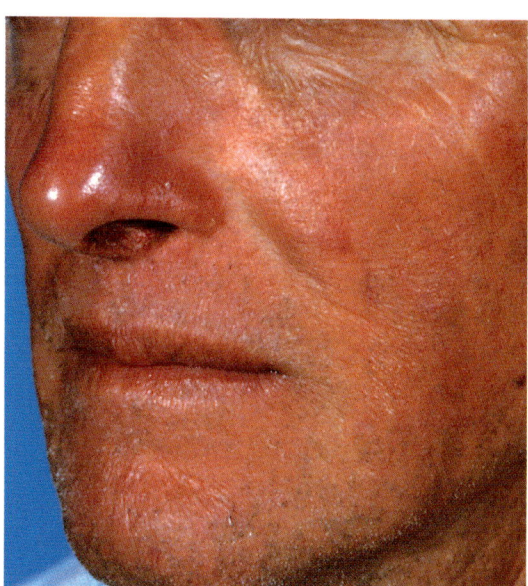

FIG. 7.8-F. Mat telangiectasias eight weeks after second FEDL treatment, side view.

Case courtesy of *Timothy J. Rosio*, M.D.

CASE 7.9

Nevus Araneus

REVIEW OF CASE. This 8-year-old Asian child presented with an asymptomatic lesion in the left cheek area of several months duration. There were no symptoms and the lesion had never bled.

CHOICE OF LASER: TUNABLE DYE. The Candela laser was chosen for its specificity for vascular structures, its relatively low risk of post-inflammatory hyperpigmentation, and because no anesthesia is required for a young child. The nevus araneus was treated initially with 5.25 J/cm^2 fluence with 5.0 mm pulse size, 2 pulses in the center and 5 pulses around the periphery. On the second treatment the dose was increased to 5.50 J/cm^2 fluence with the 5.0 mm lens and the center treated with 3 pulses and the surrounding skin with 4. At this dose slight bleeding occurred in the center. For the third treatment the dose was increased to 5.75 joules and 5 pulses were used overlapping the entire lesion at 5.75 joules using the 5.0 mm lens. For the fourth and final treatment 5.75 joules were used, 1 pulse in the center followed by 3 overlapping pulses around the central pulse.

ADDITIONAL INFORMATION. With type IV and V skin types lower doses have to be used to prevent hypopigmentation or marked blister formation with scar and resultant cicatrix formation. One can treat these lesions with multiple treatments at lower doses and minimize the potential for hyper- or hypopigmentation or scar formation. With multiple pulses at the center of a lesion one can, occasionally, get perforation of the vessel and local bleeding. Overlapping pulses are commonly used to treat elevated lesions, but one has to remember that multiple pulses increase the risk of blister formation. One has to use photo protection even in type IV to V skin to prevent excessive melanin protection with long wavelength photo blocks.

POST-TREATMENT CARE. The patient was treated with a topical antibiotic and a coverlet dressing for the first 48 hours. She was also advised to avoid contact sports while at school to minimize accidental injury to a healing wound. After 48 hours, the patient was allowed to leave the wound open to the air with just daily soap and water cleansing and topical antibiotics applied twice daily.

Case continues on following page.

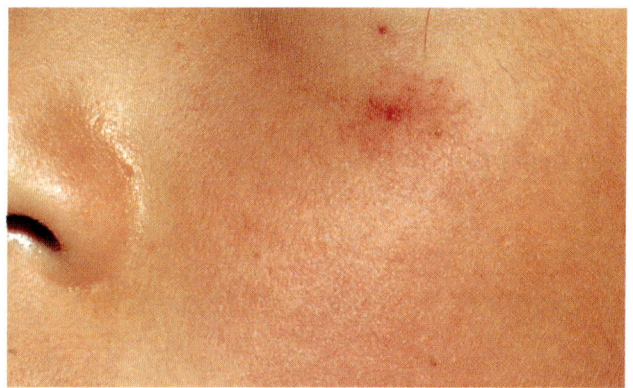

FIG. 7.9-A. Pre-treatment.

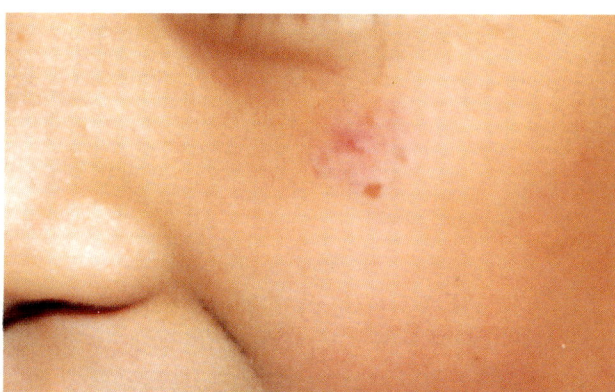

FIG. 7.9-B. One week after first treatment.

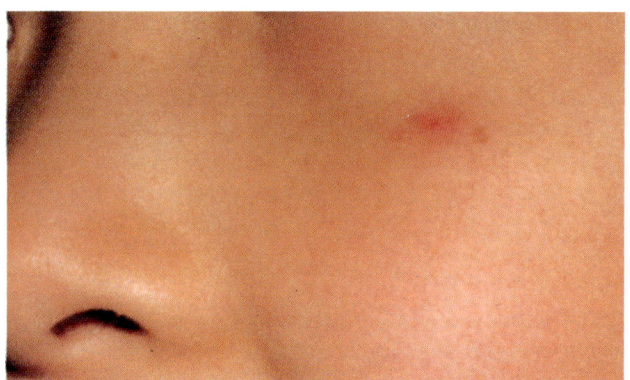

FIG. 7.9-C. Prior to third treatment.

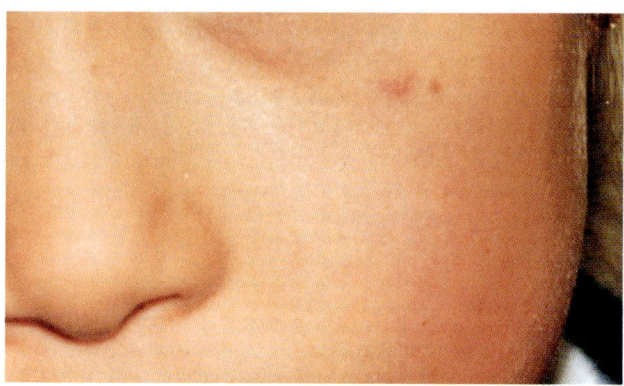

FIG. 7.9-D. Prior to fourth and final treatment.

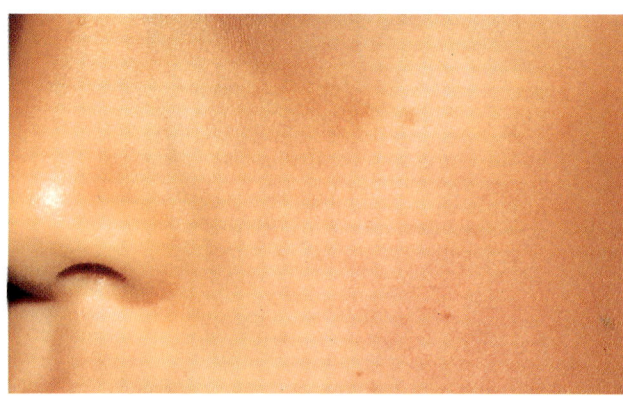

FIG. 7.9-E. Final result after four treatments in 7 months.

Case courtesy of *Thomas O. McMeekin,* M.D.

CASE 7.10
Port Wine Stain

REVIEW OF CASE. This 35-year-old white female presented with a splotchy, red, port wine stain of the right face, measuring 6 × 6 cm. She had recently noticed some red nodules developing within the birthmark which had revitalized her interest in seeking treatment. As a child, consultation regarding her birthmark resulted in discussion of treatment with liquid nitrogen and skin grafting, but no treatment was performed.

CHOICE OF LASER: TUNABLE DYE. A pulsed dye laser (585 nm) was chosen for treatment of this port wine stain. Numerous investigators have shown the pulsed dye laser to be very effective in lightening red, facial birthmarks. The incidence of scarring is rare. Because this port wine stain extends to the upper lip, it is particularly important to minimize the risk of scarring as the upper lip is known to be particularly prone to scarring. The nodules present in this birthmark would be expected to respond well to argon laser therapy. We chose the pulsed dye laser first, leaving the option of treating the nodules with the argon laser at a later time.

ADDITIONAL INFORMATION. When treating a large port wine stain with the argon laser, it is common practice to treat blocks while leaving adjacent untreated blocks. This facilitates rapid healing and minimizes the risk of scarring. This technique is unnecessary with the pulsed dye laser. It is safe and appropriate to expose even a very large birthmark to the laser light in only one treatment session. It is common to retreat the same area multiple times to achieve the desirable degree of fading. Some birthmarks may require as many as 5–7 treatments of the same area.

POST-TREATMENT CARE. Wash the area gently with tepid water. Avoid any creams, lotions, or makeup. Removal of makeup may disrupt re-epithelialization. Once the black color has faded, use of makeup may be resumed. Apply bacitracin ointment twice daily for 5–7 days following treatment. Avoid sun exposure for a full year following treatment. Routine use of sunscreen is strongly recommended.

Case continues on following page.

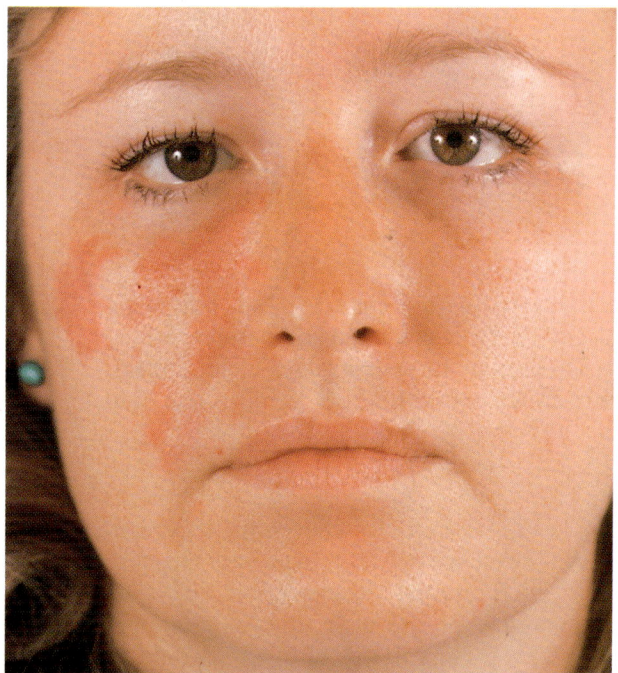

FIG. 7.10-A. At initial consultation, a red port wine stain involving the right cheek and upper lip is documented. Some nodules can be seen throughout this splotchy birthmark.

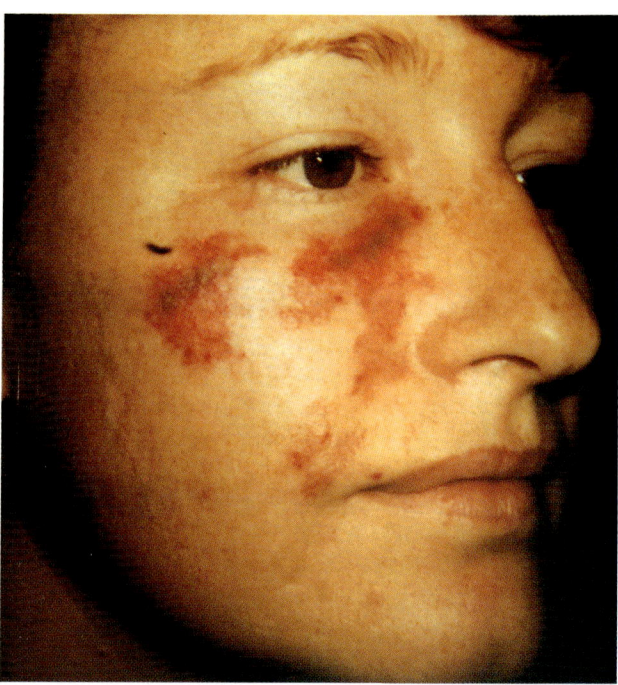

FIG. 7.10-B. Test spots of the right malar area and nasal area. In each anatomical area, 7.5, 8.0, 8.5, and 9.0 J/cm^2 were placed adjacent to one another. Note the eight pearl gray areas located centrally in these two areas.

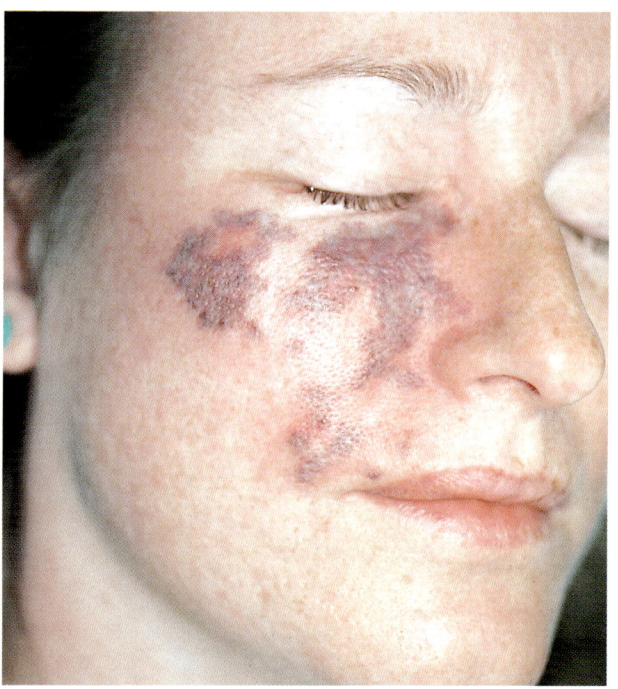

FIG. 7.10-C. At the conclusion of treatment, (with 9.0 J/cm^2) the typical pearl gray appearance of the skin and erythema are evident. The entire birthmark was exposed to the laser in this first treatment. Individual pulses were placed to overlap by approximately $\frac{1}{3}$ of the 5 mm spot size. A subsequent treatment was done five months later, again exposing the entire birth mark to the laser.

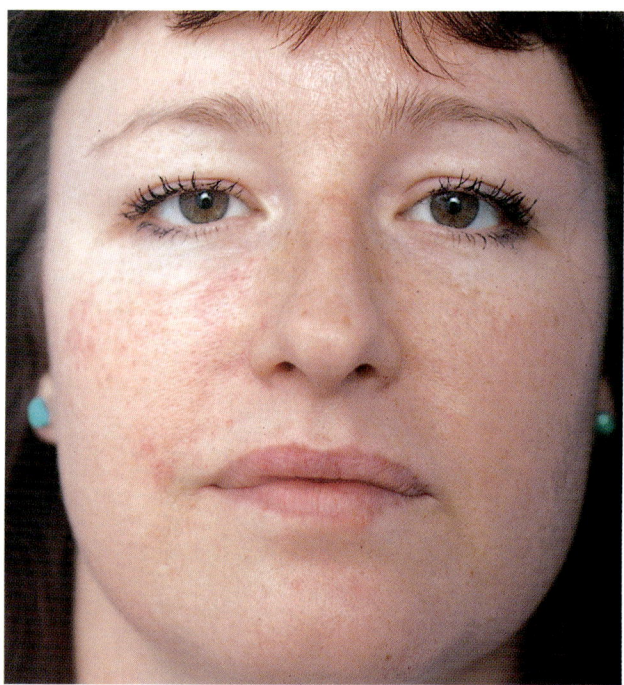

FIG. 7.10-D. Final result seven months after the second treatment.

Case courtesy of *Bruce M. Achauer*, M.D., and *Victoria M. Vander Kam*, R.N.

CASE 7.11

Vascular Malformation

Port Wine Stain

REVIEW OF CASE. This 4-month-old child presented for evaluation of a port wine stain. Examination revealed a purple facial birthmark involving the left forehead, left upper lid, and left glabella area. Pediatric consultation to rule out Sturge-Weber syndrome was recommended.

CHOICE OF LASER: TUNABLE DYE. Until the recent development of the pulsed dye laser (585 nm) we believed that infants and children with port wine stains were unsuitable candidates for laser treatment. Historically, children have responded poorly to argon laser therapy (488 nm, 514 nm). Argon laser treatment has been associated with a high incidence of scarring. Because the 585 nm wavelength is extremely specific to vascular tissue the incidence of scarring is exceptionally rare.

Using a 5 mm handpiece, ten test pulses were administered beginning at 8.0 J/cm^2 and increasing in 0.5 J/cm^2 increments to 10.0 J/cm^2. The pulse duration was 450 μsec. Two subsequent treatments were accomplished using 9.0 J/cm^2 (forehead), 8.5 J/cm^2 (eyelid), and 8.0 J/cm^2 (entire lesion), respectively.

ADDITIONAL INFORMATION. During treatment, individual spots are placed adjacent to one another with some overlap. Overlapping of the spots allows for a better aesthetic result with fewer treatment sessions. We have not experienced any complications from using this technique.

Two months following treatment there had been dramatic fading. Our recommendation at that time was to wait and allow the result to mature. Additional fading can be expected with the passage of time, even at 6–9 months.

We have successfully performed a test dose (8–12 pulses) on many infants and children without the aid of anesthesia. Although the application is not painless, discomfort is considered minimal. We have found it necessary to use general anesthesia for major treatments on infants and small children. Older children and adults can tolerate treatments without general or local anesthesia.

POST-TREATMENT CARE. Immediately following treatment, aloe vera gel was applied to cool and soothe the skin. The child's parents were instructed to apply bacitracin ointment twice daily for the first few days following treatment. Eschar is not expected, although it occasionally occurs. The following information regarding expected healing was given: The treated areas are expected to turn black within 24–48 hours. Over the next 7–10 days these black areas will fade. Fading of the birthmark may not be noticeable until several months after the treatment. Sun exposure should be avoided for a full year. Routine use of sunscreen is strongly recommended. Return at two months for evaluation after test and each treatment.

Case continues on following page.

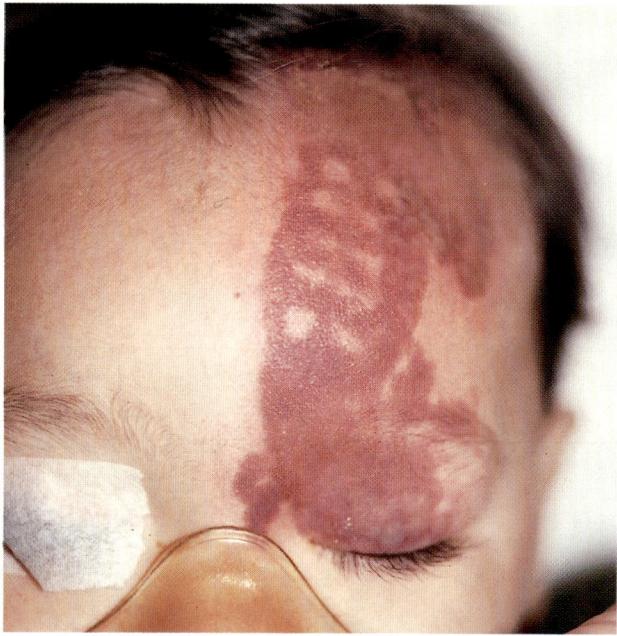

FIG. 7.11-A. The infant just prior to his first major treatment under general anesthesia. The ten, 5 mm test spots done three months prior can be seen as the light areas in the central portion of the forehead. The power chosen for treatment is the lowest power that produces the desired response of fading without scarring or skin texture changes.

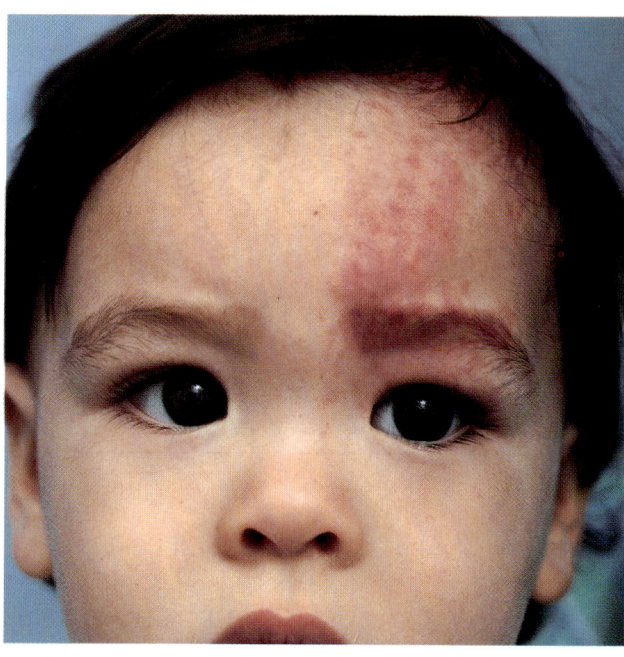

FIG. 7.11-B. Four months after treatment, there has been excellent fading. Additional fading can be expected from a second treatment.

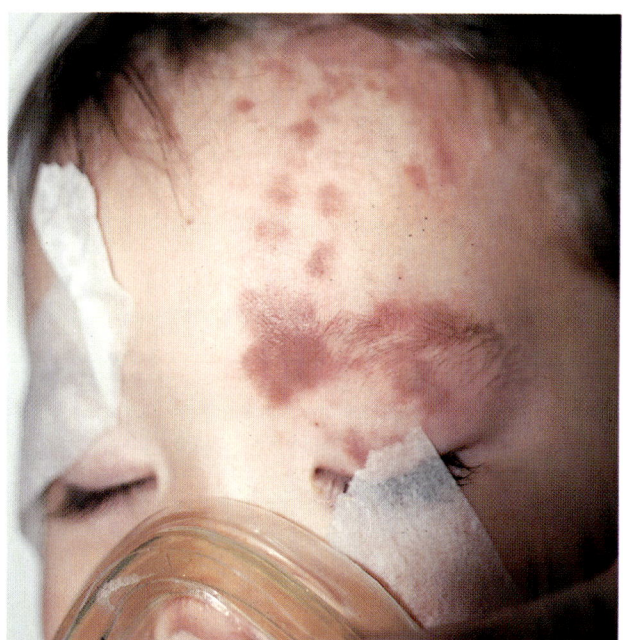

FIG. 7.11-C. At the conclusion of a second treatment using a lower power of 8.0 J/cm^2. The pearly gray color with moderate erythema is the typical tissue response immediately after exposure to the 585 nm wavelength. Note: Protective eye cover has been partially removed.

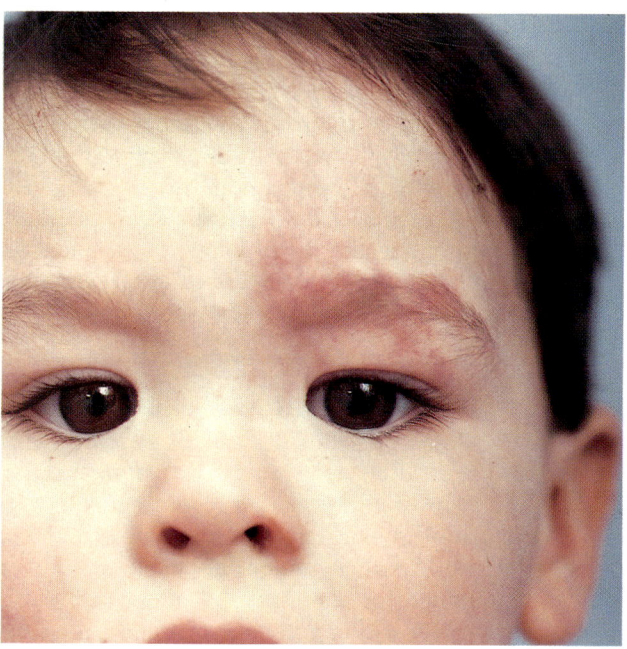

FIG. 7.11-D. Final result, two months after the second treatment.

Case courtesy of *Bruce M. Achauer, M.D.*, and *Victoria M. Vander Kam, R.N.*

CASE 7.12

Port Wine Stain Hemangioma of the Right Face

REVIEW OF CASE. This is a 48-year-old gentleman with a congenital port wine stain hemangioma of the right face and right lower orbit area. His previous treatment consisted of dry ice pencil treatment many years ago with some improvement, but in recent years the area had become more purplish. He desired removal primarily for cosmetic reasons. There was no history of glaucoma.

CHOICE OF LASER: TUNABLE DYE. The argon pumped continuous tunable dye laser was selected rather than the flashlamp pulsed dye laser because on examination of the vascular lesion with 5× loupes. A substantial component of individual vessels over 100 μm diameter were observed. Also the lesion was somewhat thickened and it was felt that the microspot tracing technique would be the preferred method, as it is for most adults.

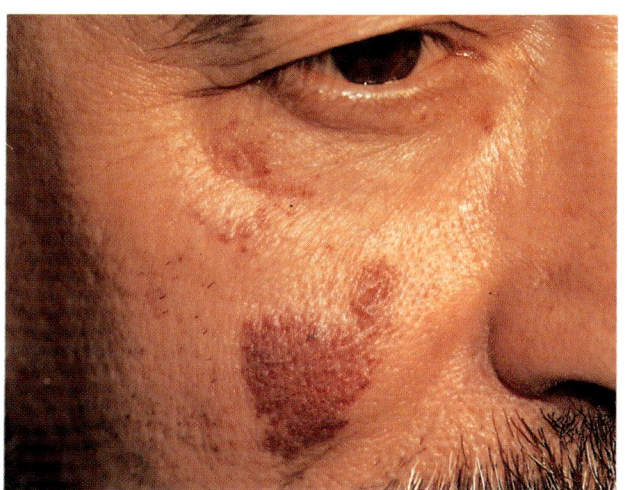

FIG. 7.12-A. Port wine stain prior to treatment. Note the two components of the angioma, the lower orbital area and the malar area. The malar portion was much thicker than the orbital portion.

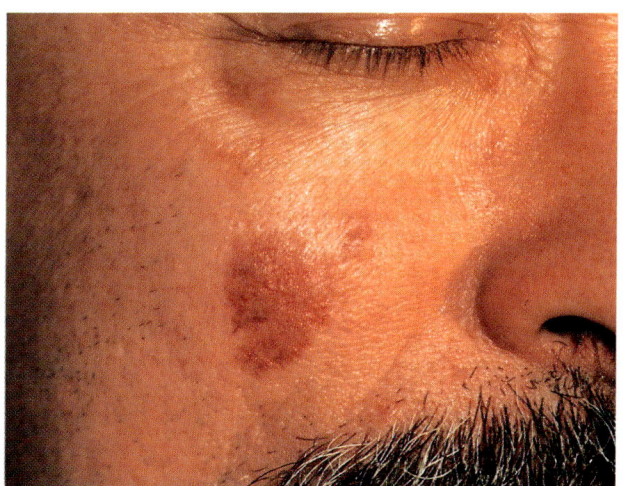

FIG. 7.12-B. Immediately post-treatment using the microspot tracing method, 0.130 mm spot, and 0.30 watts focused continuous wave with 5× telescopes and 577 nm light. This is a typical erythematous reaction obtained when vessel disappearance is used as endpoint (and not the white blanching typical of argon techniques.)

Case continues on following page.

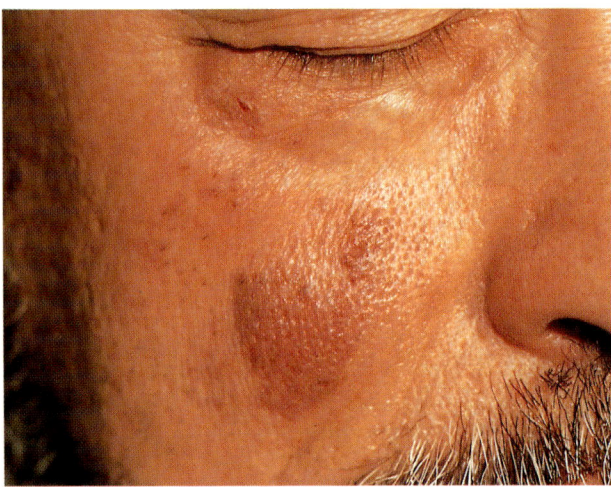

FIG. 7.12-C. Fifteen months after the first treatment and three months after the second treatment. Note the brown post-inflammatory hyperpigmentation in the orbital area which was produced by the second treatment. This is common with a pulsed dye laser but quite rare with the argon dye continuous laser techniques. Note also that there is more dramatic lightening of the upper (thinner) component of the port wine stain than the thicker malar component.

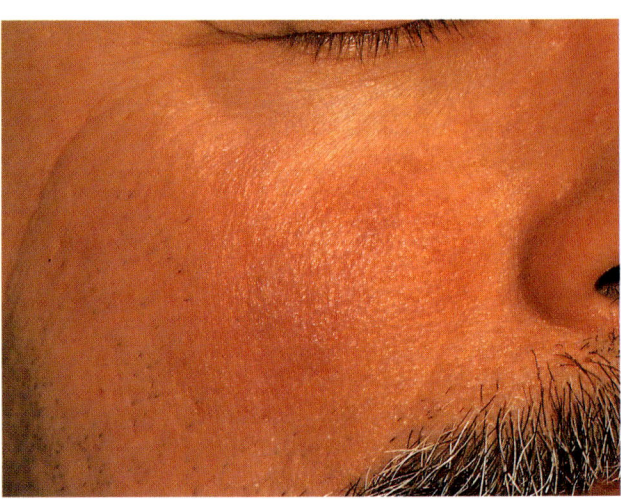

FIG. 7.12-D. Immediately post-treatment, approximately one year later than Fig. C. Note that the upper orbital area is essentially resolved and the hyperpigmentation is gone. Note again the typical reaction using the microspot tracing endpoint.

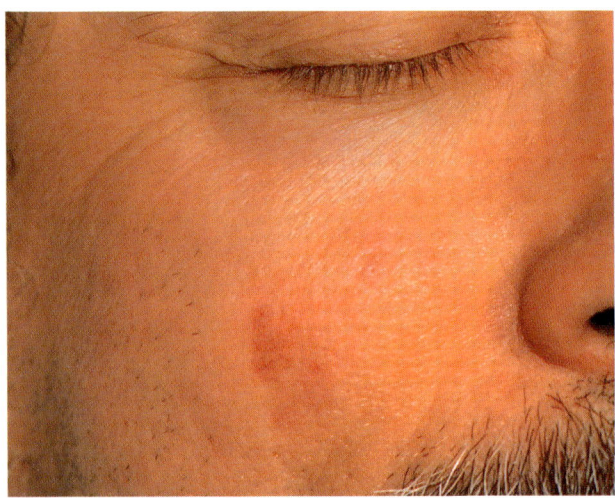

FIG. 7.12-E. Final photograph. Note the great improvement over the original treatment. Despite using both 577 nm and 585 nm wavelengths and multiple treatments, it was not possible to totally resolve this hemangioma. It is noteworthy that the majority of improvement in this case occurred with the first three treatment sessions but some slow, noticeable improvement did occur with treatments four through six. Many port wine stain hemangiomas cannot be *completely* removed with current tunable dye laser equipment and techniques.

Case courtesy of *David H. McDaniel*, M.D.

CASE 7.13
Port Wine Stain Hemangioma

CHOICE OF LASER: TUNABLE DYE.   The 577 nm wavelength was chosen as this is the wavelength best absorbed by oxyhemoglobin and with the least melanin absorption.

ADDITIONAL INFORMATION.   No anesthesia was used. The patient was treated using the following parameters: 0.1 mm spot size, 0.1 sec pulse duration, 0.7 watts of power. The individual capillaries were isolated using a 3× magnifying lens, and each of the vessels was followed along its course, one treatment field adjacent to the next. The patient underwent one treatment. Using these parameters and technique (tiny spot size, very short exposure time, and the appropriate wavelength), the damage to the surrounding tissue can be reduced to its minimum.

PRE-TREATMENT CARE.   The patient was advised to use a number 30 sunscreen daily for one month prior to treatment and to continue its use throughout the entire course of therapy. The patient was also given a topical antibiotic ointment to be applied twice a day until complete healing occurred (usually one week). The purpose of the sunscreen was twofold: (a) to reduce the absorption of light energy by melanin and thereby increase the light energy absorbed by hemoglobin and (b) to decrease the amount of damage to the epidermis.

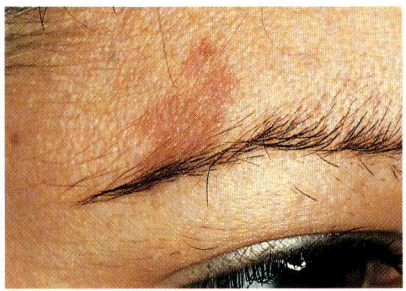

FIG. 7.13-A. Pre-treatment port wine stain hemangioma. Each blood vessel can be detected.

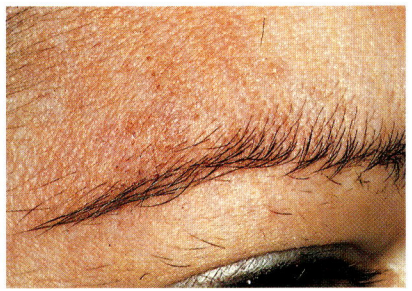

FIG. 7.13-B. Immediately post-treatment.

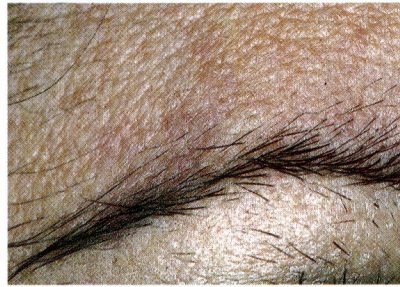

FIG. 7.13-C. Six months after one treatment.

Case courtesy of *Arie Orenstein*, M.D., and *J. Stuart Nelson*, M.D., Ph.D.

TUNABLE DYE LASER

CASE 7.14

Port Wine Stain

Macular Vascular Malformation

REVIEW OF CASE. This is an 11-year-old male with a history of a red, blanching macular vascular malformation of the right cheek since birth. The lesion has grown commensurately with the child and has never been treated.

CHOICE OF LASER: TUNABLE DYE. The Candela flashlamp-pulsed tunable dye laser has been shown to safely irradicate port wine stains in children. By employing the process of selective photothermolysis, whereby damage is limited to the target chromophore, in this instance hemoglobin; blood vessels are selectively ablated without thermal injury to surrounding tissues. It is because of this that the risk of scarring in children is extremely low (5%) when compared to the argon laser (50%).

Treatment of port wine stains should be started as soon as possible as it has been shown the number of treatment sessions required to irradicate a port wine stain increases with age. The average number of treatments for 0–6 year-olds is 6, while 7 to 14 year-olds average 8. This is in part due to the increasing thickness of skin, size of the vessels, and size of the lesion. Also, treatment at an early age can avoid significant psychological trauma to the child from the birthmark.

The laser parameters for the Candela flashlamp-pulsed tunable dye laser are wavelength 585 nm, pulse duration 400 μsec, and a 3 or 5 mm spot size.

ADDITIONAL INFORMATION. For treating lesions on the face, I generally recommend a test patch of 6.0 J/cm^2. For infants, I will decrease this by 0.5 J/cm^2 to 5.5 J/cm^2. I hardly ever employ energy densities above 6.5 J/cm^2 as I have found this may result in permanent hypopigmentation. For lesions on the neck and upper chest I recommend starting with an energy density of 5.5 J/cm^2.

POST-TREATMENT CARE. Warn the patient that the blue-gray will become a dark purple-black in the first twenty four hours. This will gradually lighten and disappear over two weeks. It will then appear as if no treatment has occurred. Reassure the patient that lightening of the port wine usually does not appear until 4 to 6 weeks after surgery. During the healing process bacitracin or a lubricant 2 or 3 times daily should be applied. A telfa dressing can be applied, but is not mandatory. Swimming and the application of makeup are forbidden during the healing process. Sunscreens should be used at all times to prevent tanning.

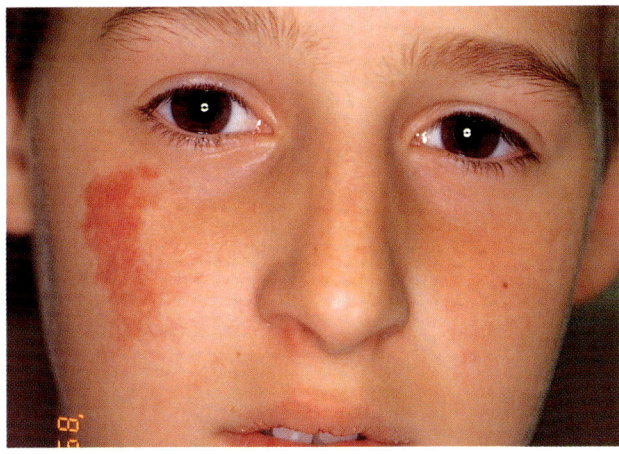

FIG. 7.14-A. Red macular vascular malformation of the right cheek consistent with a port wine stain.

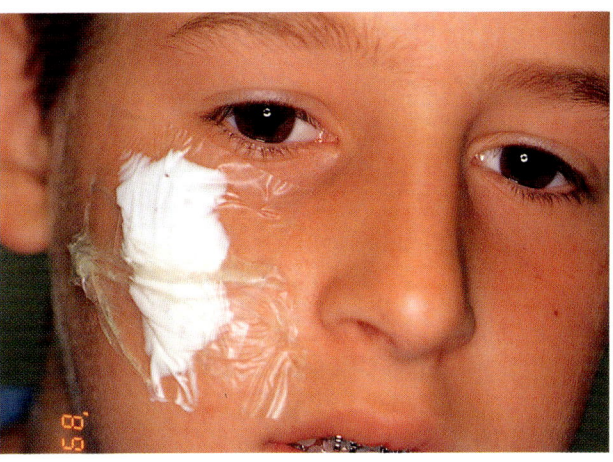

FIG. 7.14-B. The pain felt during the procedure can be compared to a "hot rubber band snap" on the skin. While one or two may be tolerated, a larger number can be overwhelming to a child. Intralesional Xylocaine is as uncomfortable as the actual laser treatment. It is for this reason that I use EMLA cream, a mixture of lidocaine and prilocaine, topically to numb the dermis. EMLA is applied generously and covered with a Tegaderm dressing. This is left on for at least two to three hours.

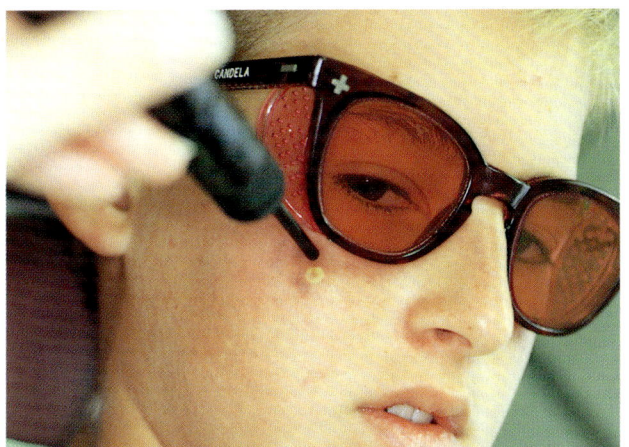

FIG. 7.14-C. Prior to starting the procedure, the patient's eyes must be shielded by appropriate goggles. When placing the handpiece on the patient, be sure that it is gently resting on the skin as shown here. If too much pressure is applied and the handpiece is pushed into the skin, the spot size will decrease thus increasing the energy density delivered. Increasing the energy density in this manner will increase the possibility of scarring. The placement of the green helium neon guiding beam is shown here.

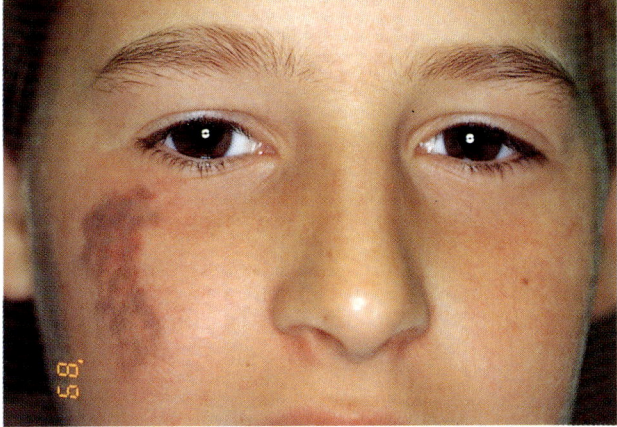

FIG. 7.14-D. This lesion was treated at 6.0 J/cm^2, 585 nm, 5 mm 400 μsec. To treat the entire area, outline it first, placing the individual pulses next to each other. Then fill in the center. One may overlap pulses slightly, but do not do so by more than one third of a pulse. As each pulse is placed the area immediately turns blue-gray. This is known as the purpuric response.

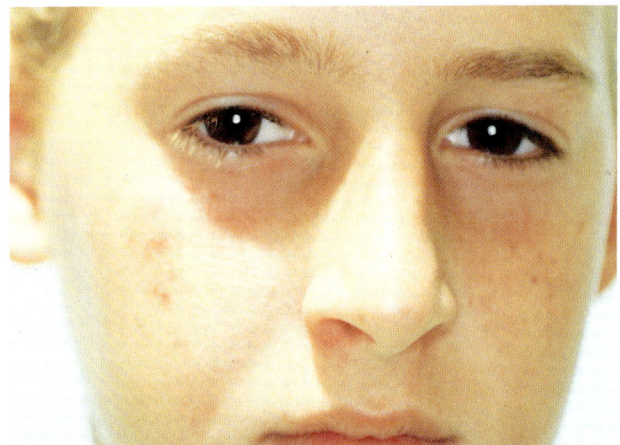

FIG. 7.14-E. The lesion completely healed after 6 treatments over 18 months. Note that there is normal skin texture without hypo- or hyperpigmentation.

Case courtesy of **Karen A. Sherwood**, M.D.

TUNABLE DYE LASER

CASE 7.15

Port Wine Stain Hemangioma

REVIEW OF CASE. This is a 51-year-old female with a history of port wine stain on the anterior chest since birth with no prior treatment. There is moderate chronic sun damage surrounding the lesion. This disturbed her since it was visible with most of her clothing.

CHOICE OF LASER: TUNABLE DYE. The tunable dye laser was selected because of the specificity of yellow light for cutaneous vascular disorders. In this situation, argon or CO_2 laser wavelengths could have been selected, however, the probability of hypopigmentation or hypertrophic scarring is much higher than using the tunable dye. The hypopigmented areas would be particularly noticeable in this case because of the surrounding chronic sun damage. Furthermore, this portion of the anterior chest is probably more likely to develop a scar. Thus, the tunable dye laser is the treatment of choice for this patient.

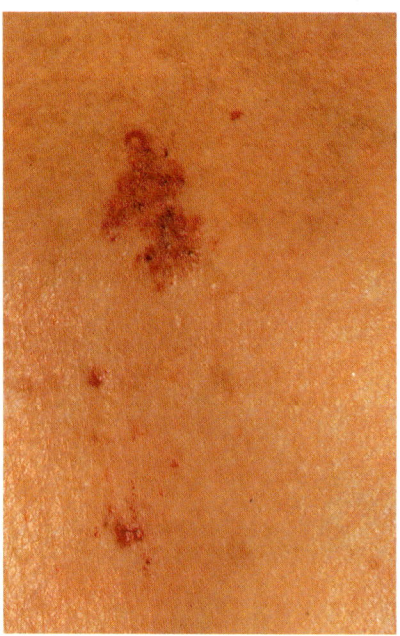

FIG. 7.15-A. Port wine stain prior to treatment.

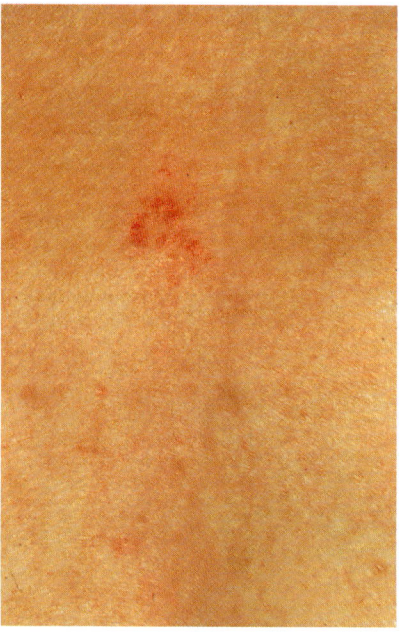

FIG. 7.15-B. After two treatments using the tunable dye laser at 577 nm yellow light, 0.130 mm spot, and 0.30 watts continuous wave. The technique utilized here is the "microspot tracing" technique (or Scheibner method) which utilizes 5× or 8× loupes and traces individual vessels to a vessel disappearance endpoint rather than the traditional argon blanching endpoint.

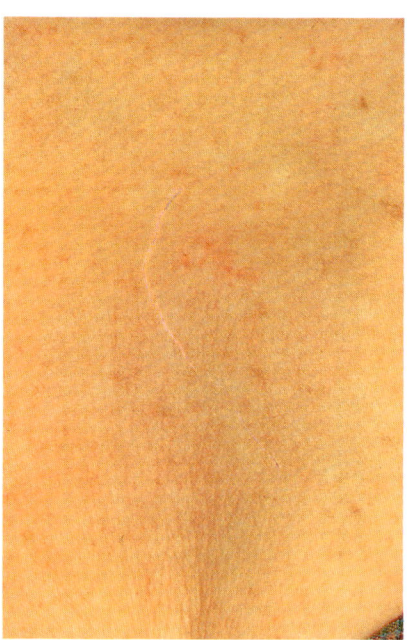

FIG. 7.15-C. After four treatment sessions. Treatment sessions are generally spaced at 2 to 3 month intervals to allow for the gradual vessel disappearance produced by this technique. Note the excellent match of color and texture.

Case courtesy of *David H. McDaniel*, M.D.

CASE 7.16

Port Wine Stain with Hypertrophy

REVIEW OF CASE. This 53-year-old female presented with a facial port wine stain which has become increasingly hypertrophic.

CHOICE OF LASER: TUNABLE DYE. The flashlamp-pumped tunable pulsed dye laser allows for the selective damage of vascular lesions, even with mild hypertrophy. A pulse duration of 360 μsec using a 580 nm range wavelength provides for thermal containment, after photothermal conversion within the blood vessel. This spares potential perivascular damage through thermal diffusion which can result in undesired skin texture changes or fibrosis and scarring.

ADDITIONAL INFORMATION. Each lesion is first evaluated using test sites of different energies to ascertain the best lightening with the least amount of energy. A 5 mm spot size is used with minimal overlap of the exposure sites. The lesion is retreated in 3-month intervals.

POST-TREATMENT CARE. In adult patients, no special care is necessary unless there are skin texture changes. Many patients apply makeup cover immediately after therapy. However, if any skin texture changes develop, a topical antibiotic ointment should be used. Pediatric patients must apply antibiotic ointment after treatment regardless of skin texture.

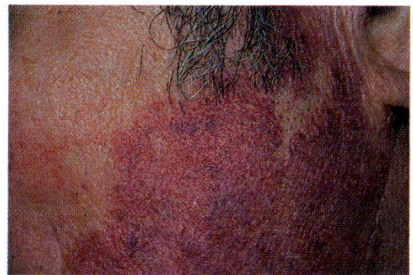

FIG. 7.16-A. Port wine stain over the left lateral face.

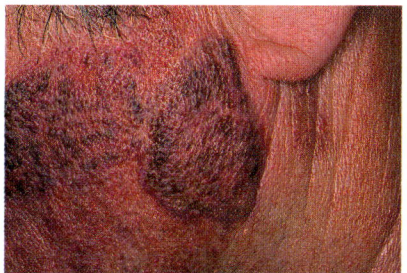

FIG. 7.16-B. Immediate post-laser exposure of 7.25 J/cm² at a pulse duration of 360 μsec and at the 580 nm range. The lesional darkening reflects an intravascular coagulum. The color remains dark for one to two weeks and the lesional lightening develops over the next three months.

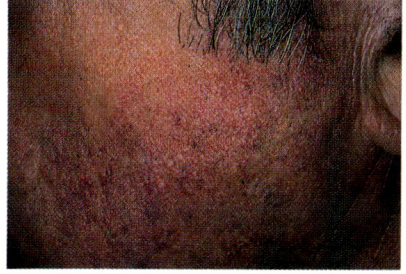

FIG. 7.16-C. Lesional area after four treatment sessions to the same area.

Case courtesy of *Jerome M. Garden*, M.D.

CASE 7.17

Port Wine Stain of the Left Cheek

REVIEW OF CASE. This 61-year-old female desired removal of a congenital hypertrophic hemangioma of the left cheek for cosmetic purposes.

CHOICE OF LASER: TUNABLE DYE. Indications for using the continuous wave tunable dye laser in the treatment of port wine stains are as follows: (a) patients under the age of 12, particularly infants and children; (b) areas of the trunk and extremities in patients of any age; (c) scar prone areas of the face such as the perioral, nasolabial, and nasal skin; (d) any deeply pigmented patients where hypopigmentation may be likely; and (e) patients who have previously been successfully but incompletely treated with the argon laser. In all of these instances, the tunable dye laser may produce satisfactory fading without scarring. Between 4 and 9 individual treatments separated by 3 to 6 months may be necessary for fading, which is never total. Some residual hemangioma may remain. Power settings vary from 10 to 40 joules depending on the color and hypertrophy of the lesion (power 0.4–0.8 watts, spot size 0.2–1 mm). The endpoint of the treatment is a "graying or disappearance" of the vessel but not a white blanching. Post-treatment skin changes should be minimal. Local anesthesia or sedation is required for treatments. Wavelengths of 577–595 nm may be easily tuned.

ADDITIONAL INFORMATION. The continuous wave tunable dye laser wavelength of 577–595 nm is selectively attracted by the hemoglobin in blood vessels. Overlying skin and melanocytes are relatively impervious to laser light at this wavelength. Therefore, selective injury to the blood vessels but not adjacent tissue occurs. The continuous wave tunable dye laser may be used with a hexascan device, an automated scanner that separates and diverges the 1 mm laser beams, or handpiece. Spot size for tracing individual vessels varies. It may be as small as 50 μm or as large as 300 μm. Tracing larger areas can be done with 1–5 mm spot sizes. Pulse duration may be as fast as 0.02 seconds. Joules vary between 10–45 and are determined by the endpoint of purpura or graying or disappearance of the vessel but not outright blanching. Between 2 to 7 treatments of the same area may be required for final clearing of the *hexascan* which is never total obliteration. Post-treatment crust and scab should be eliminated totally or very minimal.

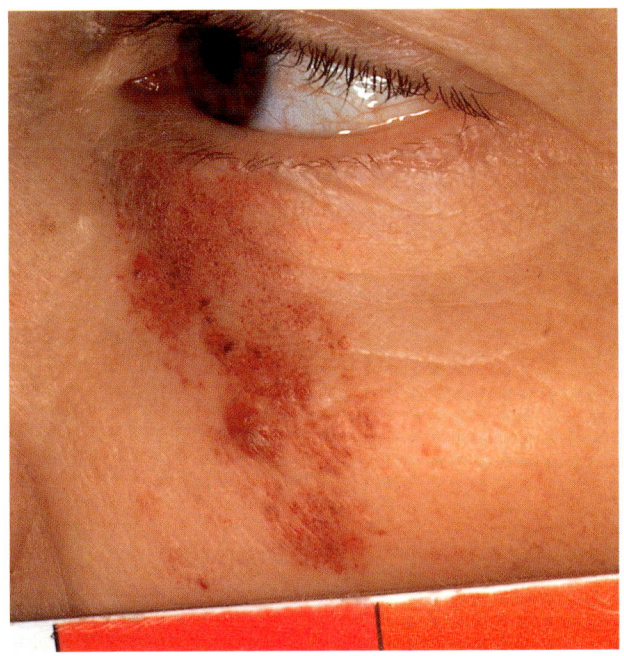

FIG. 7.17-A. Port wine stain of the left cheek and lower eyelid prior to treatment.

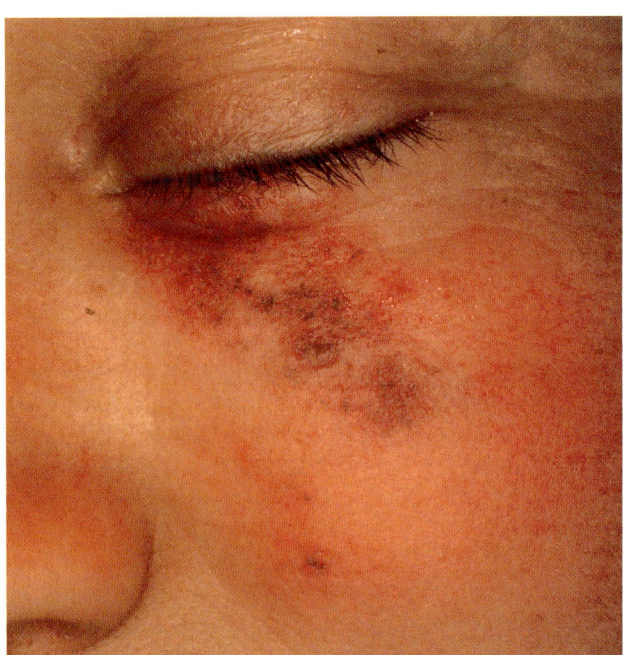

FIG. 7.11-B. Immediately following continuous wave tunable dye laser treatment with the handpiece.

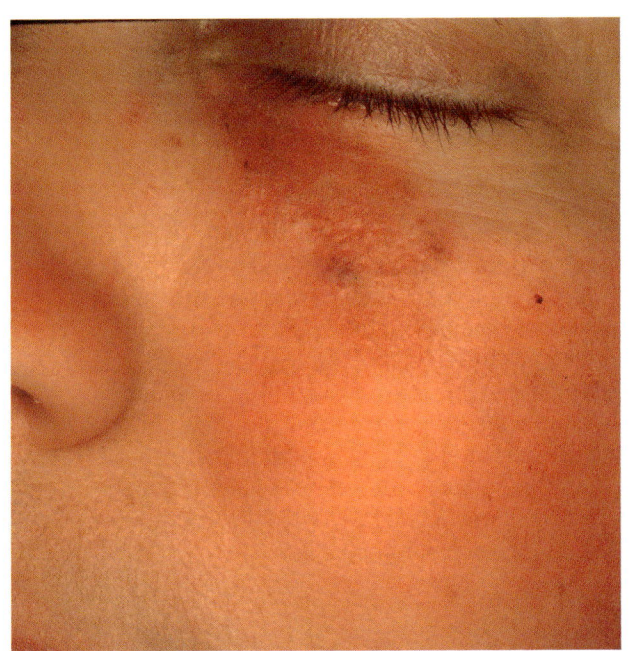

FIG. 7.17-C. Fading achieved after 12 weeks.

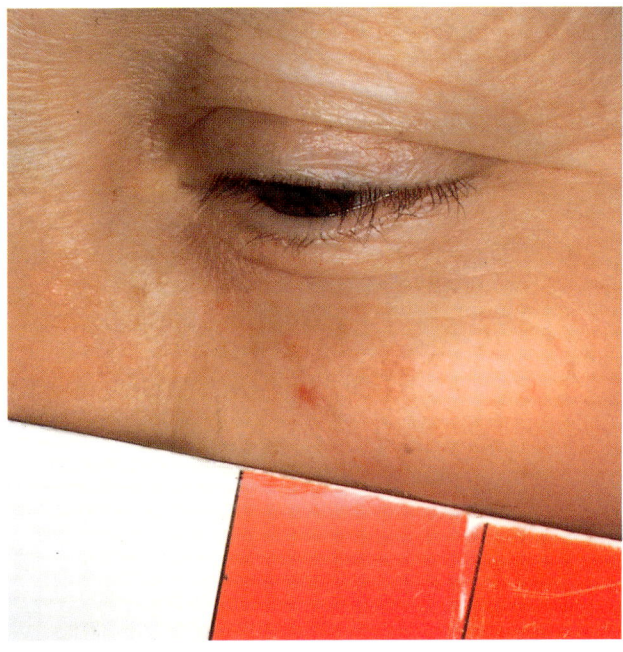

FIG. 7.17-D. Final fading without scar.

Case courtesy of *David B. Apfelberg*, M.D., and *Patricia Z. Spector*, R.N., MHS, P.A.-C.

CASE 7.18

Port Wine Stain of the Upper Lip

REVIEW OF CASE. This 26-year-old female desired removal of a congenital port wine stain for cosmetic reasons. The tunable dye laser was chosen to safely produce further blanching without scarring in the upper lip which had been previously treated with the argon laser. This area frequently scars after traditional argon laser treatment.

CHOICE OF LASER: TUNABLE DYE. Indications for using the continuous wave tunable dye laser in the treatment of port wine stains are as follows: (a) patients under the age of 12, particularly infants and children; (b) areas of the trunk and extremities in patients of any age; (c) scar prone areas of the face such as the perioral, nasolabial, and nasal skin; (d) any deeply pigmented patients where hypopigmentation may be likely; and (e) patients who have previously been successfully but incompletely treated with the argon laser. In all of these instances, the tunable dye laser may produce satisfactory fading without scarring. Between 4 and 9 individual treatments separated by 3 to 6 months may be necessary for fading, which is never total. Some residual hemangioma may remain. Power settings vary from 10 to 40 joules depending on the color and hypertrophy of the lesion (power 0.4–0.8 watts, spot size 0.2–1 mm). The endpoint of the treatment is a "graying or disappearance" of the vessel but not a white blanching. Post-treatment skin changes should be minimal. Local anesthesia or sedation is required for treatments. Wavelengths of 577–595 nm may be easily tuned.

ADDITIONAL INFORMATION. The continuous wave tunable dye laser wavelength of 577–595 nm is selectively attracted by the hemoglobin in blood vessels. Overlying skin and melanocytes are relatively impervious to laser light at this wavelength. Therefore, selective injury to the blood vessels but not adjacent tissue occurs. The continuous wave tunable dye laser may be used with a hexascan device, an automated scanner that separates and diverges the 1 mm laser beams, or handpiece. Spot size for tracing individual vessels varies. It may be as small as 50 μm or as large as 300 μm. Tracing larger areas can be done with 1–5 mm spot sizes. Pulse duration may be as fast as 0.02 seconds. Joules vary between 10 and 45 and are determined by the endpoint of purpura or graying or disappearance of the vessel but not outright blanching. Between 2 to 7 treatments of the same area may be required for final clearing of the *hexascan* which is never total obliteration. Post-treatment crust and scab should be eliminated totally or very minimal.

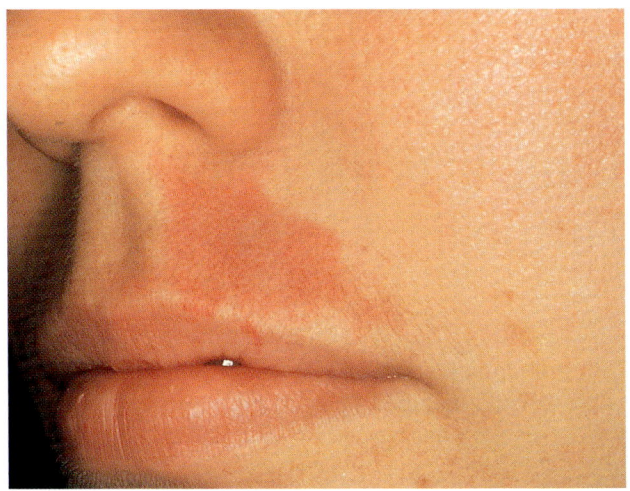

FIG. 7.18-A. Port wine stain upper lip prior to treatment.

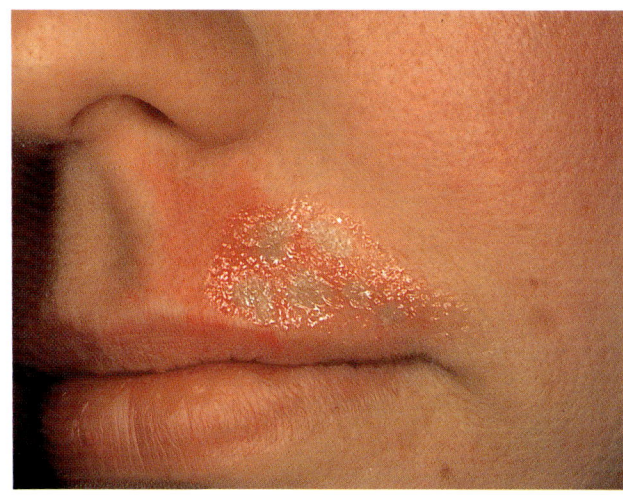

FIG. 7.18-B. "Polkadot" treatment with the argon laser.

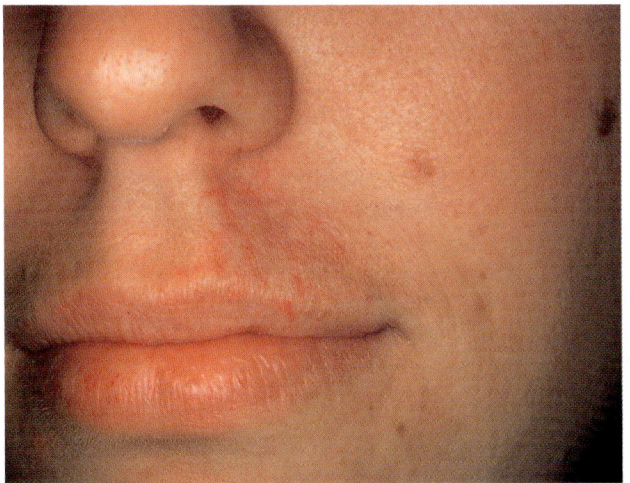

FIG. 7.18-C. Result of "polkadot" treatment.

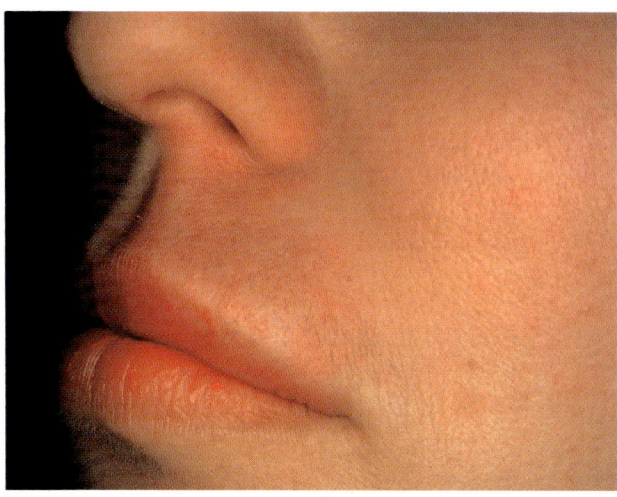

FIG. 7.18-D. Treatment with continuous wave tunable dye laser (577 nm) handpiece.

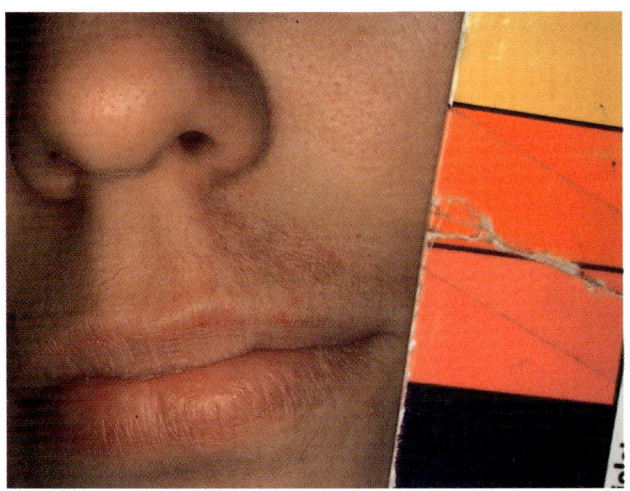

FIG. 7.18-E. Final fading without scarring.

Case courtesy of *David B. Apfelberg*, M.D., and *Teruko Smith*, R.N.

TUNABLE DYE LASER   375

CASE 7.19

Port Wine Stain Birthmark With Prior Dermal Tattoo

REVIEW OF CASE. This is a 65-year-old female with a lifelong history of port wine stain birthmark on the right hemiface V2 distribution. Previous treatments included flesh colored tattooing, argon laser treatments, x-ray, and surgical excision with results unacceptable to the patient.

CHOICE OF LASER: FLASHLAMP EXCITED DYE (FED). The FED laser was chosen to maximize therapeutic response without scarring or texture change in the skin. Higher joules were used than average patient usually requires due to laser scatter by dermal tattoo pigment, thicker skin, and scar tissue. A power setting of 7.5–8.5 joules, pulse duration 450 μsec, and spot size 5 mm was used.

ADDITIONAL INFORMATION. Power settings are arrived at with conventional testing. Gradual increases are determined by the patient's tolerance and the increases required to obtain therapeutic gains.

POST-TREATMENT CARE. Antibiotic ointment and nonadherent dressing is applied for 24 hours, then only as necessary.

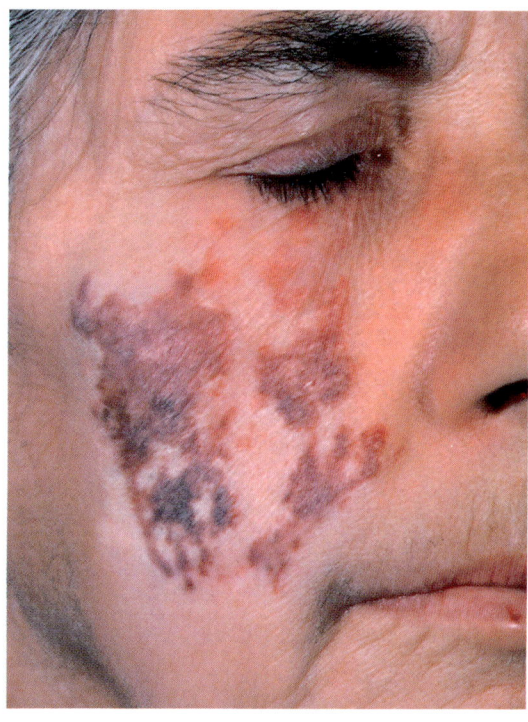

FIG. 7.19-A. Port wine stain birthmark with tattooing and scar tissue before treatment.

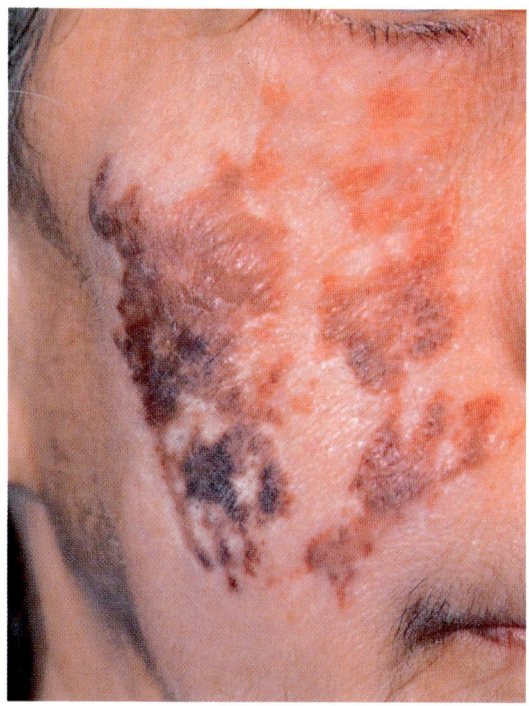

FIG. 7.19-B. Port wine stain birthmark with tattooing and scar tissue.

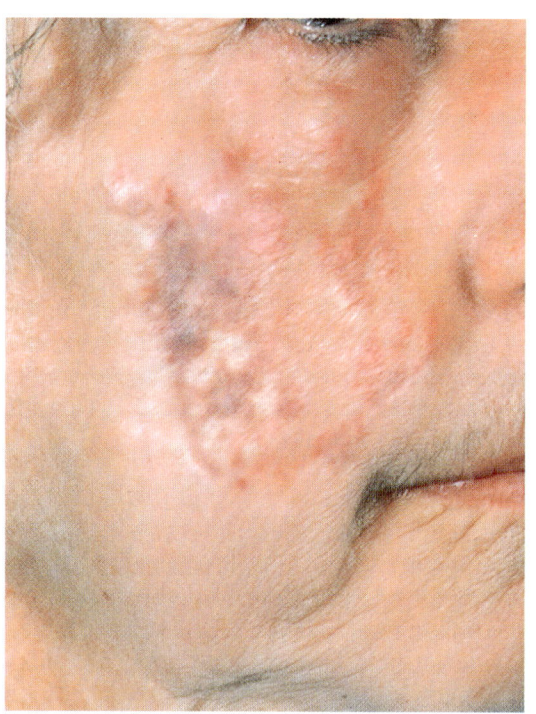

FIG. 7.19-C. Port wine stain birthmark with tattooing after four treatments (75% complete).

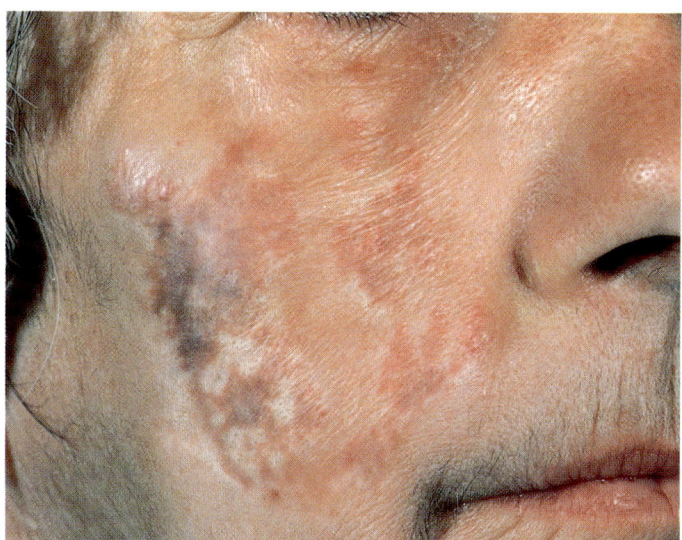

FIG. 7.19-D. Port wine stain birthmark with tattooing after four treatments (75% complete).

Case courtesy of *Timothy J. Rosio*, M.D.

FLASHLAMP EXCITED DYE LASER

CASE 7.20
Spider Angioma

REVIEW OF CASE. This is a 11-year-old male with a 5 year history of a 1½ cm spider-shaped vascular lesion in the right infraorbital area. In the last two years a central 1 mm papule had appeared and continued to enlarge. No previous treatment had been attempted. The patient complained of an intermittent burning sensation to the area.

CHOICE OF LASER: TUNABLE DYE. A continuous wave (CW) tunable dye laser was chosen to accomplish selective photocoagulation of the central feeding vessel of the angioma and its radiating arms in a single treatment. For a discussion of physiology and mechanisms, see Case 7.6. Small or early lesions often respond equally well to either FEDL, CW tunable dye/copper vapor lasers, or epilating needle electrodessication. In my experience with medium to large spider angiomas the diameter, depth, and pressure of the feeding vessel frequently causes failure of treatment, or requires multiple treatments due to recurrence. A power setting of 1 watt, pulse duration 0.04–0.2 second, and spot size 0.05 mm was used.

ADDITIONAL INFORMATION. Adults as well as children benefit from prior deep intradermal local anesthesia with 2% Xylocaine without epinephrine, or a nerve block. Smaller angioma feeding vessels may be treated directly with one to several pulses (0.04–0.1 second). Larger or resistant central vessels may be more readily treated by first marking it with dark ink from a fine point pen. Several laser pulses of 0.1–0.2 second result in drilling into the central vessel with the very small spot size beam. Deeper photocoagulation with minimal injury to adjacent tissue is accomplished. Small radiating arms of the spider may be treated at the shortest possible pulse duration.

POST-TREATMENT CARE. A band-aid dressing is used only for very young children.

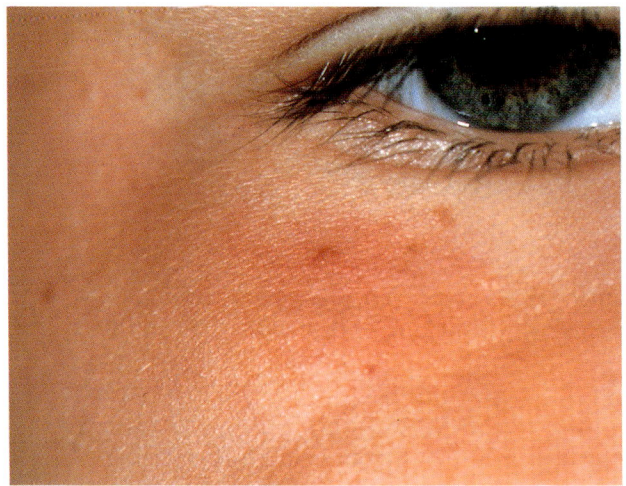

FIG. 7.20-A. Spider angioma before treatment.

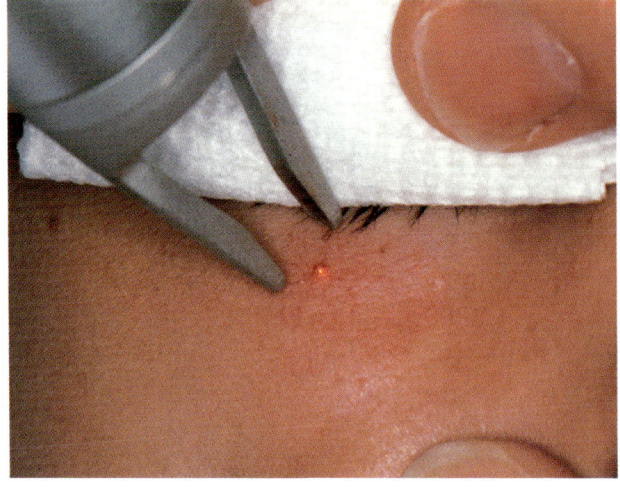

FIG. 7.20-B. Direct treatment of central vessel.

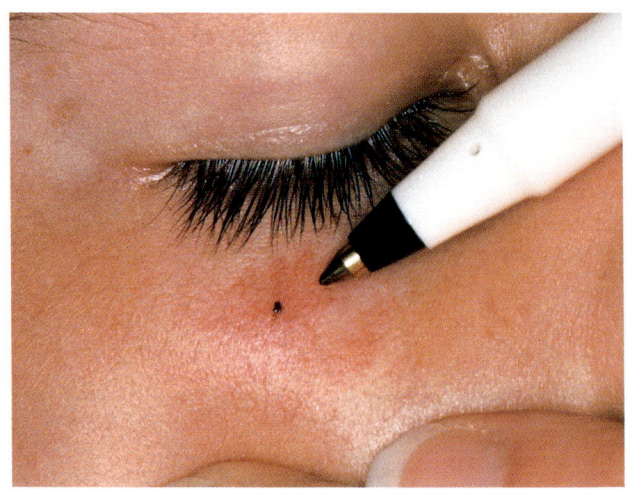

FIG. 7.20-C. Preliminary ink marking of central vessel.

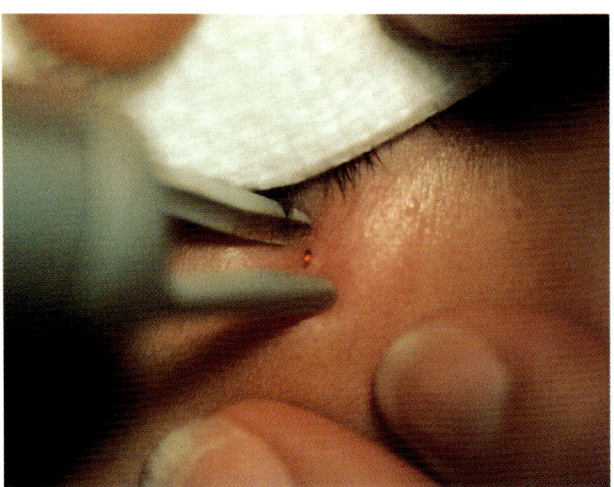

FIG. 7.20-D. Pulsed drilling of marked central vessel.

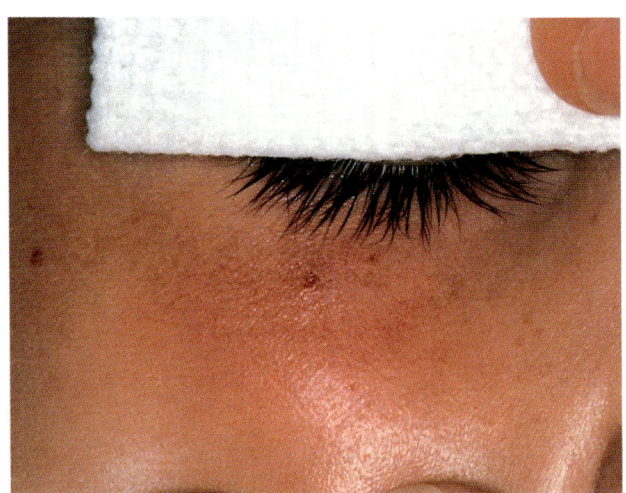

FIG. 7.20-E. Immediately post-laser treatment.

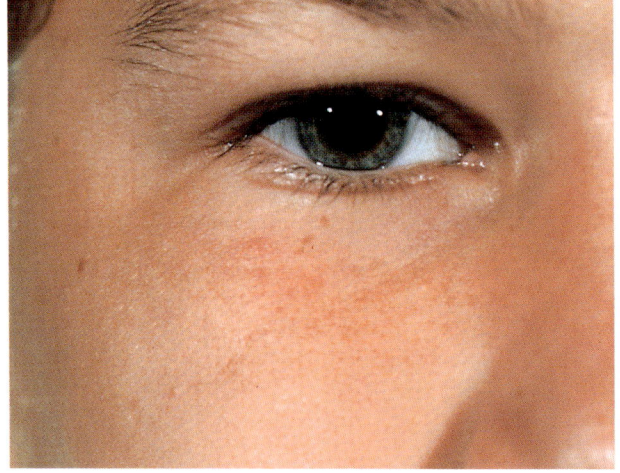

FIG. 7.20-F. Eight weeks after tunable dye laser treatment.

Case courtesy of *Timothy J. Rosio*, M.D.

CASE 7.21

Spider Hemangioma

REVIEW OF CASE. This 15-year-old female presented with a spider hemangioma of her upper nose which had been present for over a year and was slowly enlarging in diameter, the central punctum increasing in size and elevation.

CHOICE OF LASER: TUNABLE DYE. The tunable dye laser was chosen to utilize this selective absorption of the yellow light by hemoglobin and also because of the minimal risks of complications for this procedure. Additionally, the microspot tracing technique was selected wherein a small spot size matched approximately to the vessel diameter is used and tracing occurs with a 5× or 8× loupe, beginning peripherally and working centrally using vessel disappearance as an endpoint. The central punctum was then treated in a slightly defocused manner with a painting technique to vessel disappearance or slight graying. Caution in overtreating this area is required with these lesions since there is a risk of a minimally depressed scar. This risk seems to be enhanced if too much energy is used in this location. This author prefers multiple treatments to reduce the risk of this complication (which if it occurs usually resolves in 3 to 4 months). Although these often resolve in a single treatment this case was selected to illustrate that even small spider angiomas may require multiple treatments. In this situation, four treatments were performed at 4 to 6 week intervals using a 0.130 mm spot and 0.25 watts continuous wave focused microspot tracing technique and 5× loupes.

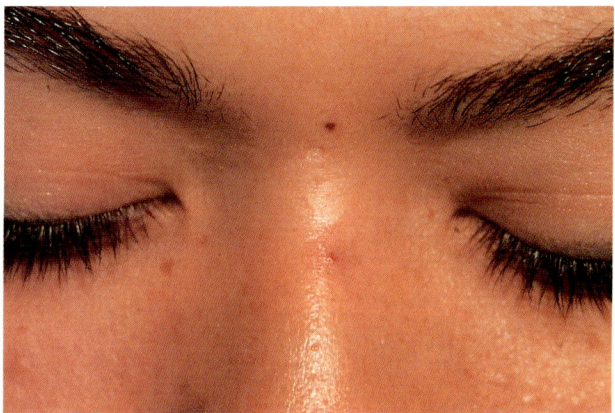

FIG. 7.21-A. Baseline pre-treatment of spider hemangioma prior to first treatment.

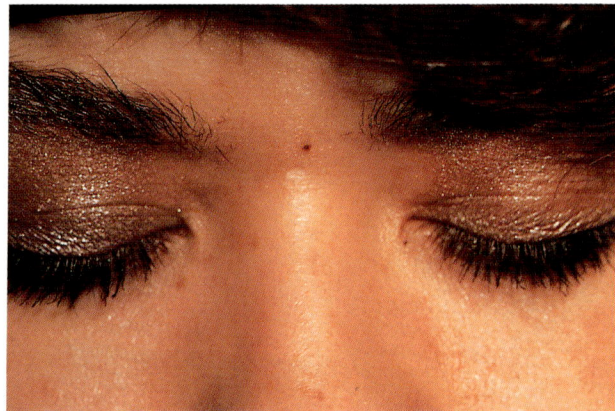

FIG. 7.21-B. Two months after last treatment. Note the lack of pigmentary texture or atrophic changes.

Case courtesy of *David H. McDaniel*, M.D.

CASE 7.22
Adult Onset Telangiectasia

REVIEW OF CASE. This 67-year-old female had progressive development of unsightly adult onset multiple telangiectasia of both cheeks. She desired removal for cosmetic reasons.

CHOICE OF LASER: TUNABLE DYE. Indications for the continuous wave tunable dye laser in the treatment of port wine stains are as follows: (a) patients under the age of 12, particularly infants and children; (b) areas of the trunk and extremities in any age patients; (c) scar prone areas of the face such as the perioral, nasolabial, and nasal skin; (d) any deeply pigmented patient where hypopigmentation may be likely; and (e) patients who have previously been successfully but incompletely treated with the argon laser. In all of these instances, the tunable dye laser may produce satisfactory fading without scarring. Between 4 and 9 individual treatments separated by 3 to 6 months may be necessary for fading, which is never total. Some residual hemangioma may remain. Power settings vary from 10 to 40 joules depending on the color and hypertrophy of the lesion (power 0.4–0.8 watts, spot size 0.2–1 mm). The endpoint of the treatment is a "graying or disappearance" of the vessel but not a white blanching. Post-treatment skin changes should be minimal. Local anesthesia or sedation is required for treatments. Wavelengths of 577–595 nm may be easily tuned.

ADDITIONAL INFORMATION. The continuous wave tunable dye laser wavelength of 577–595 nm is selectively attracted by the hemoglobin in blood vessels. Overlying skin and melanocytes are relatively impervious to laser light at this wavelength. Therefore, selective injury to the blood vessels but not adjacent tissue occurs. The continuous wave tunable dye laser may be used with a hexascan device, an automated scanner that separates and diverges the 1 mm laser beams, or a handpiece. Spot size for tracing individual vessels varies. It may be as small as 50 μm or as large as 300 μm. Tracing larger areas can be done with 1–5 mm spot sizes. Pulse duration may be as fast as 0.02 seconds. Joules vary between 10 and 45 and are determined by the endpoint of purpura or graying or disappearance of the vessel but not outright blanching. Between 2 to 7 treatments of the same area may be required for final clearing of the *hexascan* which is never total obliteration. Post-treatment crust and scab should be eliminated totally or very minimal.

Case continues on following page.

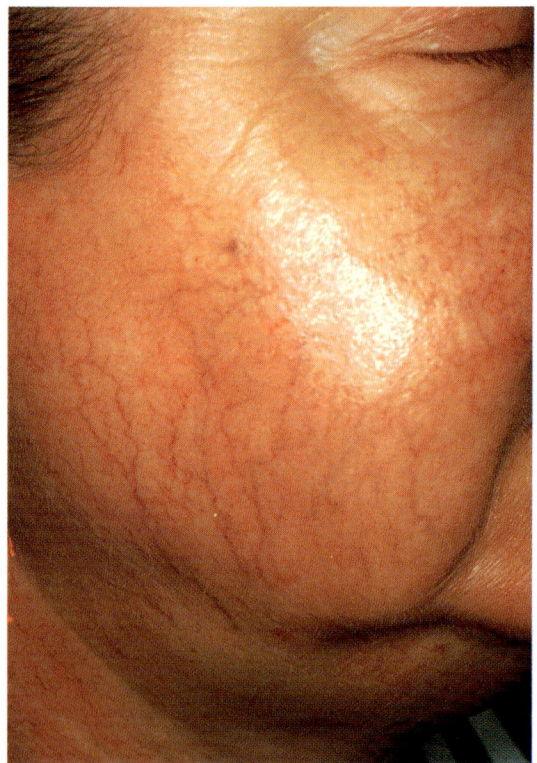

FIG. 7.22-A. Multiple telangiectasia of the right cheek prior to treatment.

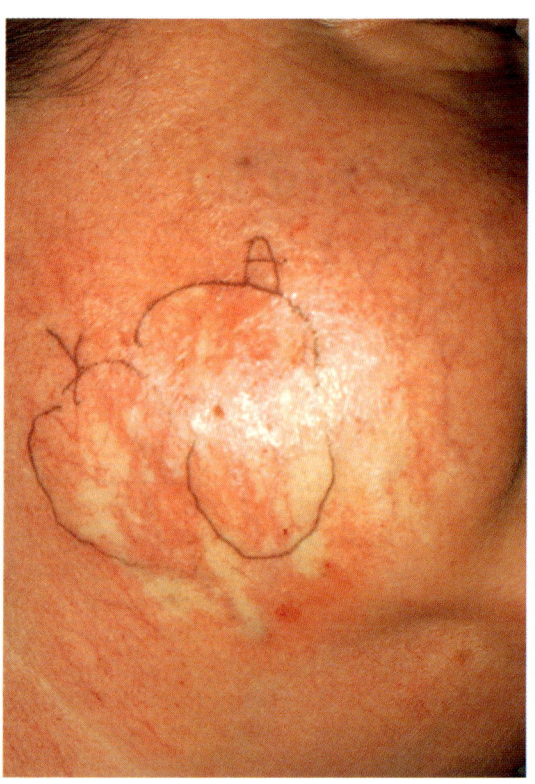

FIG. 7.22-B. Test patch with the argon laser (A) and the tunable dye laser (Y).

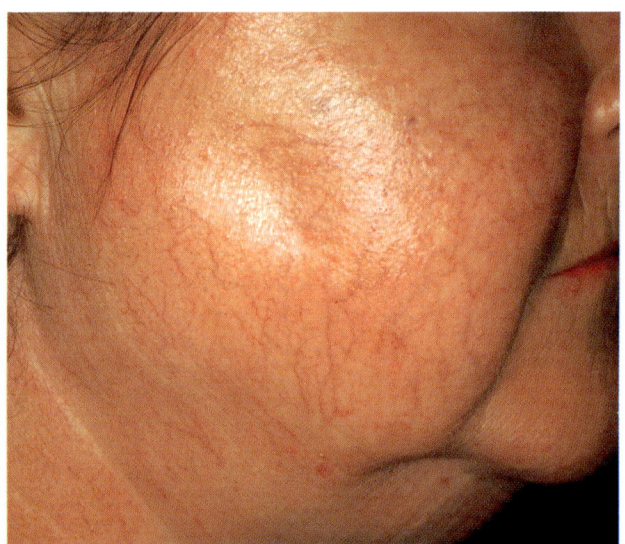

FIG. 7.22-C. Satisfactory result with fading of the test areas.

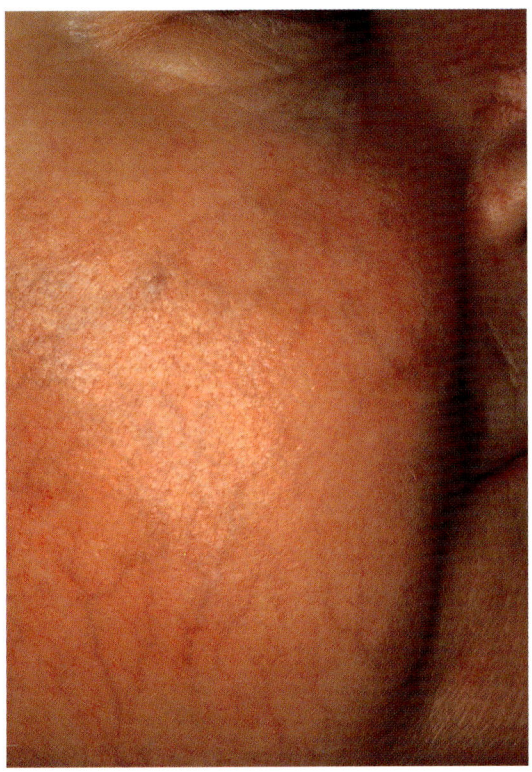

FIG. 7.22-D. Tracing of the telangiectasia with the tunable dye laser.

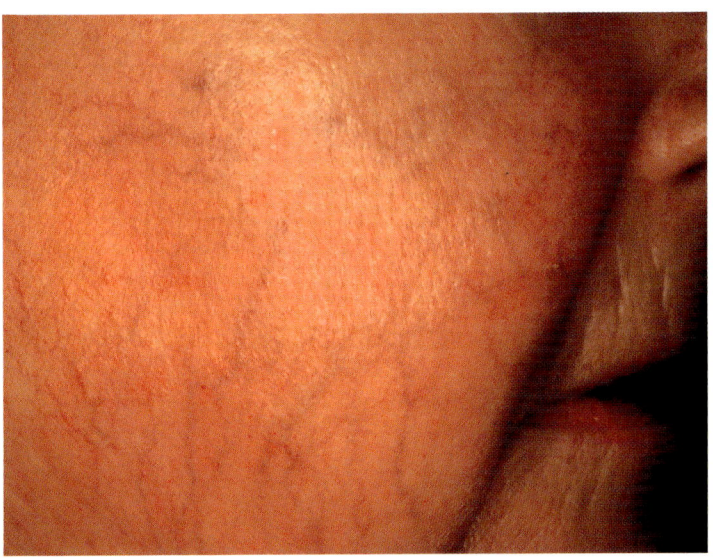

FIG. 7.22-E. Clearing of the telangiectasia 3 months following treatment.

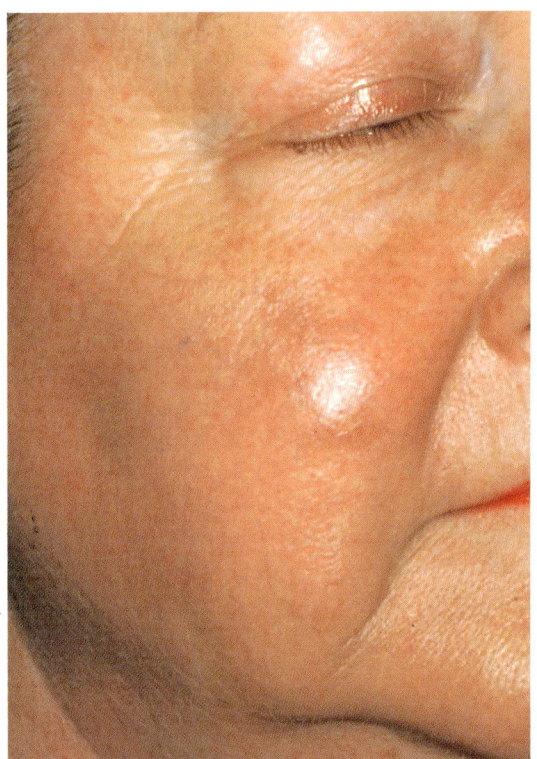

FIG. 7.22-F. Further clearing of the telangiectasia.

Case courtesy of *David B. Apfelberg*, M.D., and *Patricia Z. Spector*, R.N., MHS, P.A.-C.

TUNABLE DYE LASER

CASE 7.23
Essential Telangiectasia

REVIEW OF CASE. This 42-year-old male presented with a lifelong history of dilated blood vessels on both cheeks. He has a fair complexion and a moderate amount of sun damage or actinically damaged skin from prior exposure. His occupation as an electrician working outside for a power company has led to continual exposure to ultraviolet radiation. He requested treatment for the cosmetic benefit of decreasing the amount of red areas on his face especially when he flushes.

CHOICE OF LASER: TUNABLE DYE. The ability of the Candela laser to remove dilated vessels without scarring was the major reason for the choice in this patient. The concept of photothermolysis which is used in port wine stains is the same mechanism used to treat these dilated venules on the surface of the skin. The cheek was treated over a period of 7 months with treatment doses starting at 4.75 joules with 11 pulses used with the 5.0 mm lens on October 21, 1988. 5.0 J/cm^2 fluence with 62 pulses used to treat the right cheek on January 20, 1989 and an additional 121 pulses at 5.25 J/cm^2 were used and on 5/12/89 with 5.5 J/cm^2 191 pulses were used to treat the right cheek. All the treatments were given with individual pulses of 5.0 mm each pulse. The laser was in the focused mode with the handpiece held at the focal length of the lens.

ADDITIONAL INFORMATION. Fair, Celtic skin often requires 3–4 treatments to clear an area of telangiectatic vessels. One has to use broad spectrum photo-protective sunscreens and to almost cover an area with pulses that are minimally touching or slightly overlapping. The treatment can be repeated as short as four weeks from the initial treatment as long as there is no remaining purpura or hyperpigmentation from the last treatment. When an entire cheek is treated the purpura and wound reaction often persist longer than 7–10 days. Patients have to be forewarned about the purpura so they can plan their work schedule or activities accordingly. Patients can use makeups as long as they avoid trauma to the skin and the administration or removal of the makeups. The dose on subsequent treatments can be increased from .25 to .5 joules as long as there is no blister formation, crust formation or any marked edema or weeping from the prior treatment. Fair Celtic skin that burns easily and tans rarely can be treated with lower doses such as around 5.0 to 5.75 joules/sq. cm. Darker types III and IV skin can be treated with doses from 6.0 to 7.0 joules/sq. cm.

POST-TREATMENT CARE. The patient was told to use topical antibiotics and a telfa non-adherent dressing for 48 hours. After the 48 hours, the wound was cleansed daily with soap and water with thin amounts of a topical antibiotic and the major part of the wound being allowed to remain open to the air. If there is any sign of crust formation or severe blister reaction patients are normally treated with oral antibiotics as a preventative or prophylactic measure. This patient experienced no secondary infection in four treatments.

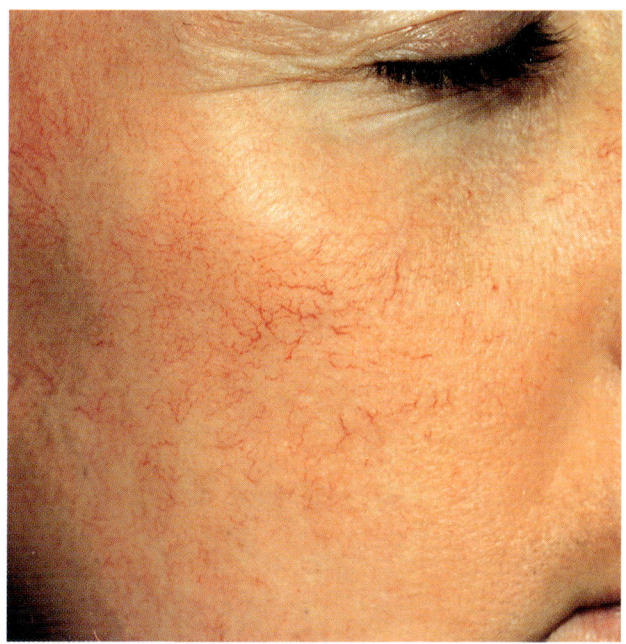

FIG. 7.23-A. Pre-operative dilated telangiectatic vessels on the right cheek.

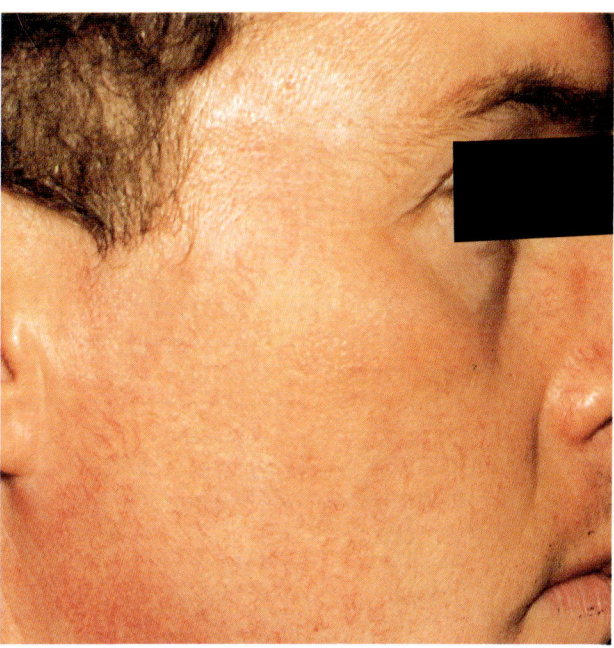

FIG. 7.23-B. Pre-operative clearing of the telangiectatic vessels on the right cheek.

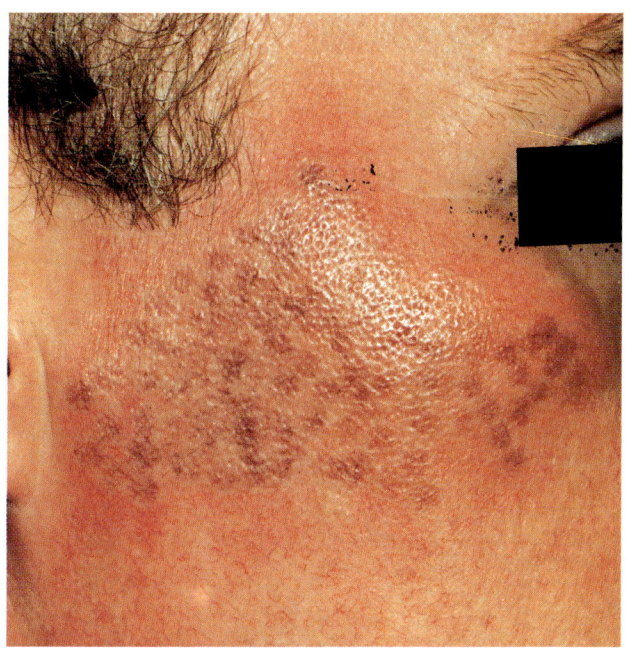

FIG. 7.23-C. Immediately post-operative wound with purpura and surrounding erythema from the treatment.

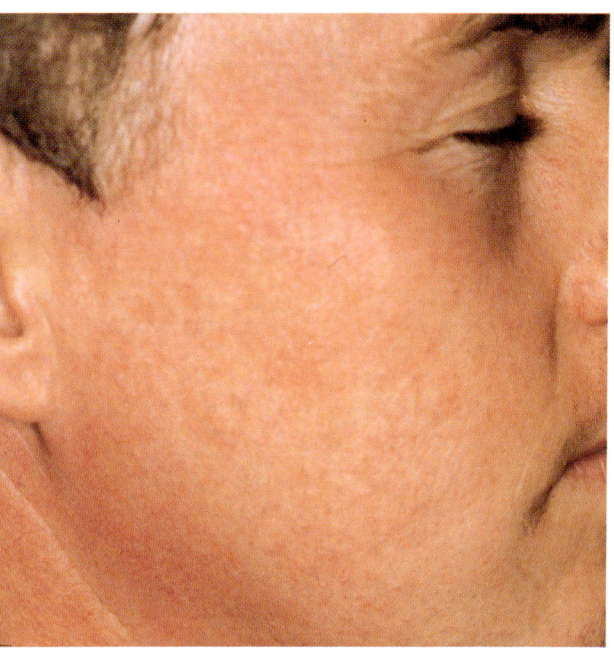

FIG. 7.23-D. Three months post-operation. Note there is no evidence of the large telangiectatic vessels and no dilated ectatic vessels in most of the central parts of the right cheek.

Case courtesy of *Thomas O. McMeekin,* M.D.

TUNABLE DYE LASER   385

CASE 7.24

Essential Facial Telangiectasia

REVIEW OF CASE. This is a 61-year-old gentleman with progressive essential facial telangiectasia present since childhood without history of acne rosacea. He had previously received electrosurgical treatment in the distant past and also, more recently, some treatment with the CO_2 laser resulting in some slight hypopigmentation.

CHOICE OF LASER: TUNABLE DYE. The tunable dye laser was selected in order to utilize the microspot tracing technique and the yellow wavelengths for selective destruction of the ectatic vessels.

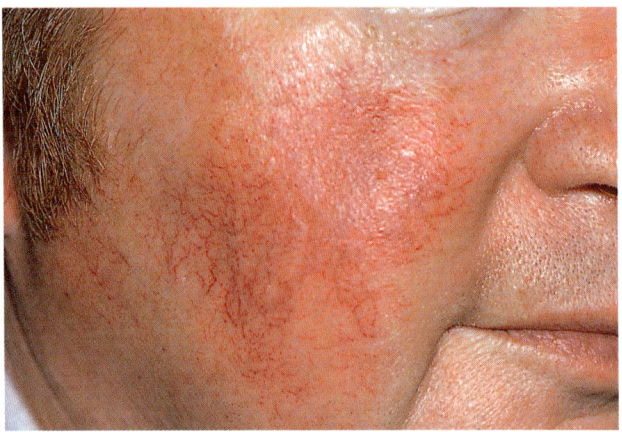

FIG. 7.24-A. Baseline photograph prior to dye laser treatment. He received 4 treatments at approximately 6 week intervals using 577 nm with 100 to 130 μm spot size and 0.20 to 0.30 watts continuous wave microspot tracing technique with 5× Zeiss loupes with vessel disappearance as the desired endpoint. No anesthesia was used.

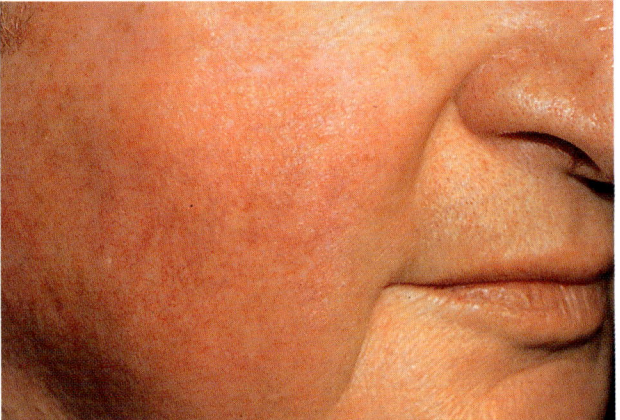

FIG. 7.24-B. This is about one year after the previously described treatments. The remaining telangiectatic areas were treatable but, more for economic reasons than technical reasons, some residual fine vessels are left untreated. It is possible to treat further with this technique or to overtreat the area rapidly for the finer vessels using the same wavelength with the hexascan robotic scanner or flash lamp pulsed dye laser. Intervals of up to 3 months are more commonly selected to allow maximum fading. However, retreatment at 6 week intervals is acceptable when travel or other constraints require more rapid treatment.

Case courtesy of *David H. McDaniel*, M.D.

CASE 7.25
Facial Telangiectasia

REVIEW OF CASE. This 40-year-old female presented with facial telangiectasia that are worsening with time.

CHOICE OF LASER: TUNABLE DYE. The tunable dye laser selectively damages vascular lesional component while allowing the perivascular area to remain intact. This occurs without the sequela of skin texture change.

ADDITIONAL INFORMATION. The whole vessel should be treated. Any retreatment sessions can occur after two months.

POST-TREATMENT CARE. There is no need of special care. If any skin texture changes occur, a topical antibiotic ointment should be used.

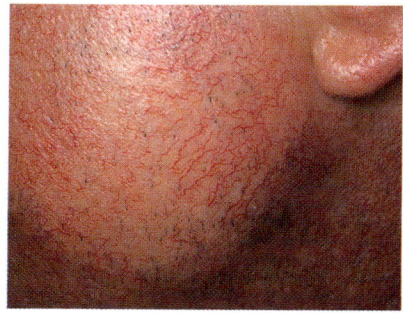

7.25-A. Telangiectases over the left lower face.

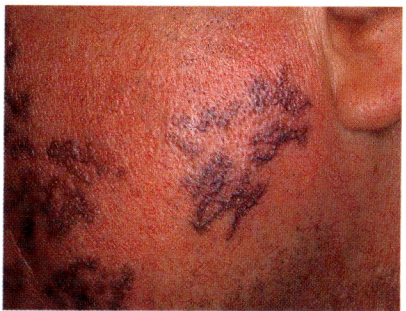

FIG. 7.25-B. Immediate post-operative appearance using a 3 mm spot size emitting in the 580 nm range at a 360 μsec pulse duration at 6.75 J/cm^2. The darkening remains from 5 to 10 days.

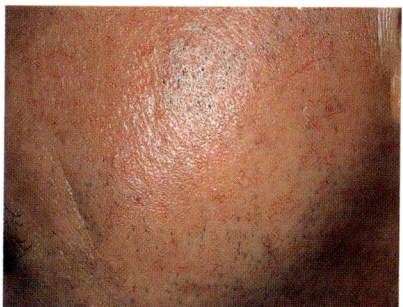

FIG. 7.25-C. Area after one treatment session to each location.

Case courtesy of *Jerome M. Garden, M.D.*

CASE 7.26

Facial Telangiectasia

REVIEW OF CASE.   A 39-year-old white female suffered from facial telangiectasia for 6 years. She had no prior treatment.

CHOICE OF LASER: TUNABLE DYE.   The yellow 577 nm wavelength was chosen as this is the wavelength best absorbed by oxyhemoglobin with least melanin absorption.

ADDITIONAL INFORMATION.   No anesthesia used. The patient was treated using the following parameters: 0.1 mm spot size, 0.1 sec pulse duration, and 0.7 watts of power. The individual capillaries were isolated using a 3× magnifying lens, and each of the vessels was followed along its course, one treatment field adjacent to the next. The patient underwent one treatment (Fig. B). Using these parameters and technique (tiny spot size, very short exposure time; and the appropriate wavelength), the damage to the surrounding tissue can be reduced to its minimum.

POST-TREATMENT CARE.   The patient was advised to use a #30 sunscreen daily for one month prior to treatment, and to continue use throughout the entire course of therapy. The patient was also given a topical antibiotic ointment to be applied twice a day until complete healing occurred (usually one week). The purpose of the sunscreen was twofold: a) to reduce the absorption of light energy by melanin, and thereby increase the light energy absorbed by hemoglobin; b) to decrease the amount of damage to the epidermis.

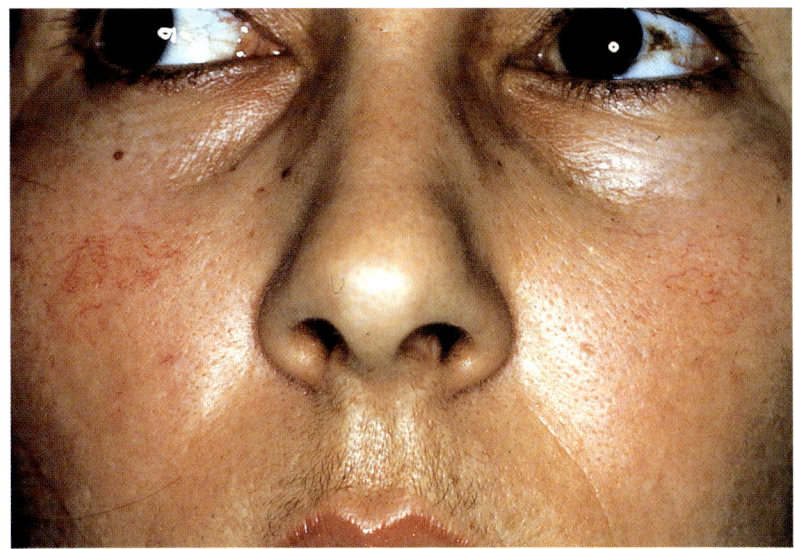

FIG. 7.26-A. Multiple facial telangiectasias of cheeks.

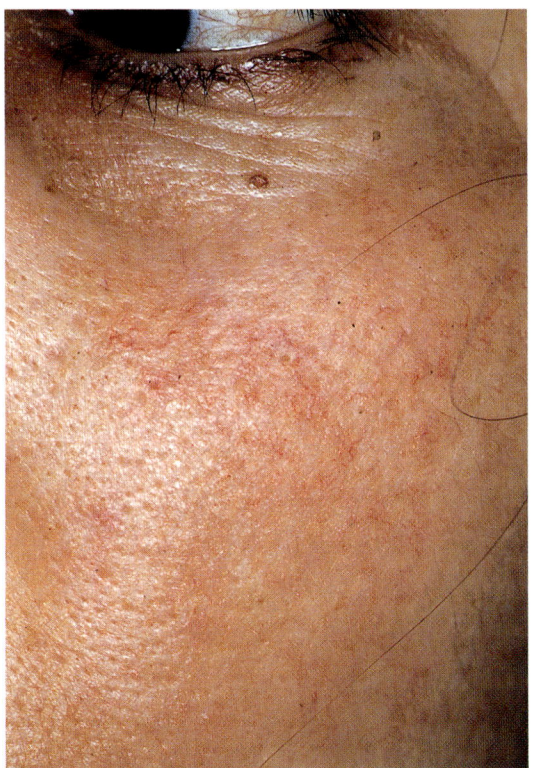

FIG. 7.26-B. Immediately post-treatment appearance of left check.

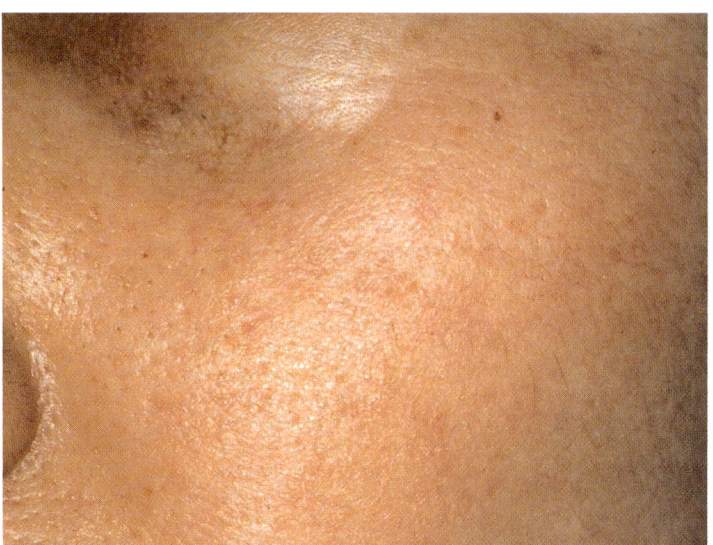

FIG. 7.26-C. Final result six months post-treatment.

Case courtesy of *Arie Orenstein, M.D.*

TUNABLE DYE LASER 389

CASE 7.27
Nasal Venous Telangiectasia

CHOICE OF LASER: TUNABLE DYE. The yellow 577 nm wavelength was chosen as this is the wavelength best absorbed by oxyhemoglobin with least melanin absorption.

ADDITIONAL INFORMATION. 0.1 mm spot size, 0.05–0.10 seconds pulse duration, and 0.8–1.0 watts were used. A 3× magnifying lens was used to view the vessel clearly and to precisely "hit" it with the laser beam (Fig. B). The patient was treated at two month intervals in two treatment sessions.

POST-TREATMENT CARE. The patient was advised to use a #30 sunscreen daily for one month prior to treatment, and to continue use throughout the entire course of therapy. The patient was also given a topical antibiotic ointment to be applied twice a day until complete healing occurred (usually one week). The purpose of the sunscreen was twofold: a) to reduce the absorption of light energy by melanin, and thereby increase the light energy absorbed by hemoglobin; b) to decrease the amount of damage to the epidermis.

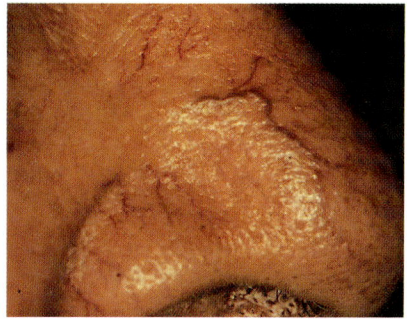

FIG. 7.27-A. Pre-treatment nasal venous telangiectasia.

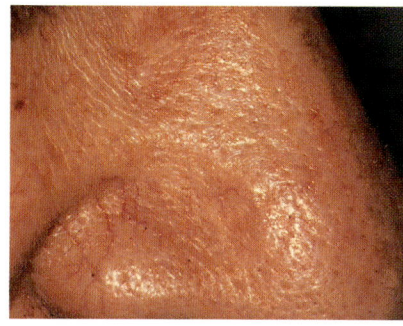

FIG. 7.27-B. Immediately post-treatment.

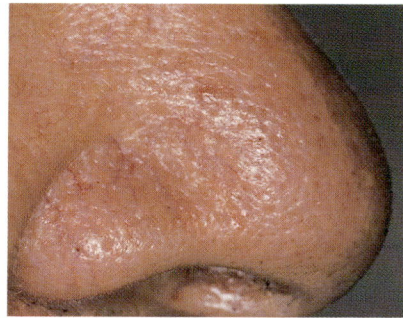

FIG. 7.27-C. Three months post-treatment.

Case courtesy of *Arie Orenstein*, M.D.

CASE 7.28
Telangiectatic Congenital Vascular Malformation

REVIEW OF CASE. This is a 15-year-old female with a history of a vascular anomaly on the left upper anterior thigh from birth which had progressed somewhat in recent years with the telangiectatic component becoming more pronounced and the angiomatous component becoming more elevated. She was concerned about this primarily for cosmetic reasons but also the elevated portion produced difficulty in shaving her legs.

CHOICE OF LASER: TUNABLE DYE. The tunable dye laser was selected because of the selective absorption of the visible yellow light wavelengths by oxyhemoglobin and to minimize the risk of adverse reaction such as color and texture changes or hypertrophic scarring.

This case was selected to illustrate the ability to treat *small* telangiectatic vessels with the tunable dye laser. However, in general, the essential telangiectatic vessels or "spider leg veins" commonly encountered are probably best treated at the present time using sclerotherapy rather than dye laser.

Please also note the small hypopigmented area in this case which represents a previous test area using older lasers. Note that the final photographs shows no such areas with the tunable dye laser.

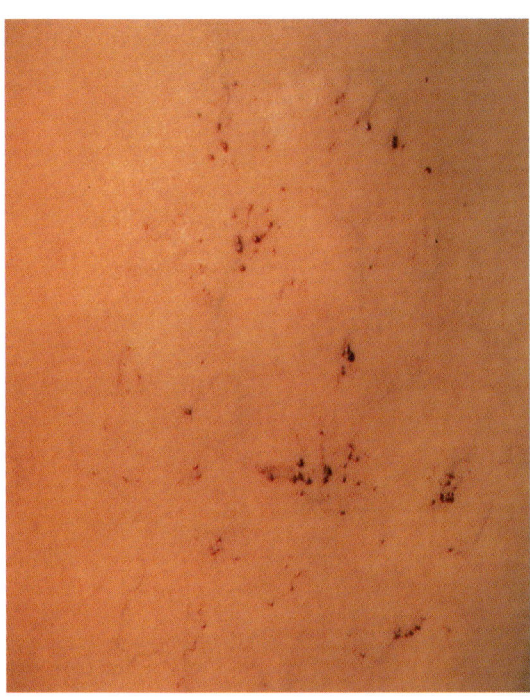

7.28-A. Telangiectatic vascular anomaly of the left upper anterior thigh prior to treatment.

Case continues on following page.

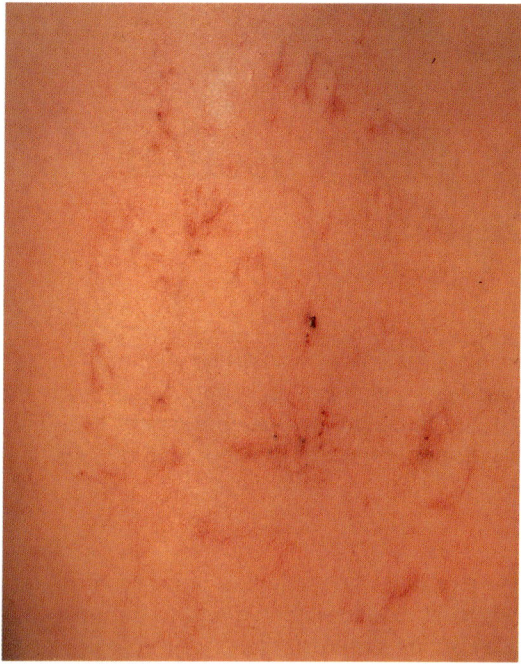
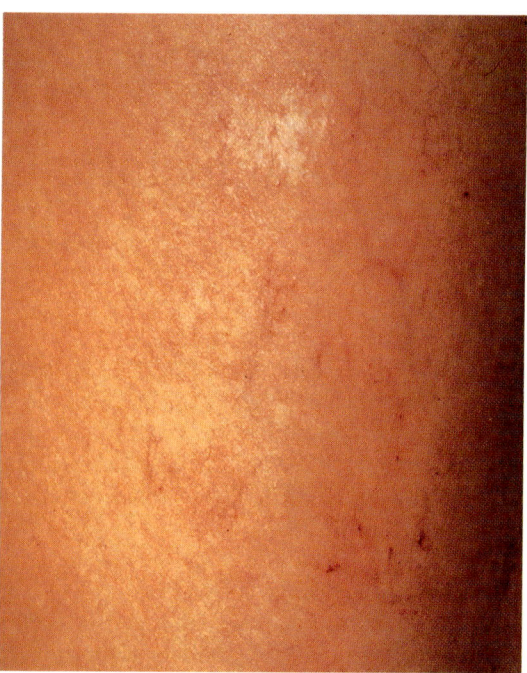

FIG. 7.28-B. Area immediately post-treatment with 577 nm yellow tunable dye laser treatment 0.130 mm spot and 0.30 watts using continuous wave mode focused beam 5× size loupes and microspot tracing technique with vessel disappearance as the endpoint. Note the typical wheal and erythema seen after treatment. Occasionally fine crusting vesiculation can develop.

FIG. 7.28-C. Area 3 months after the first treatment and prior to treatment number two.

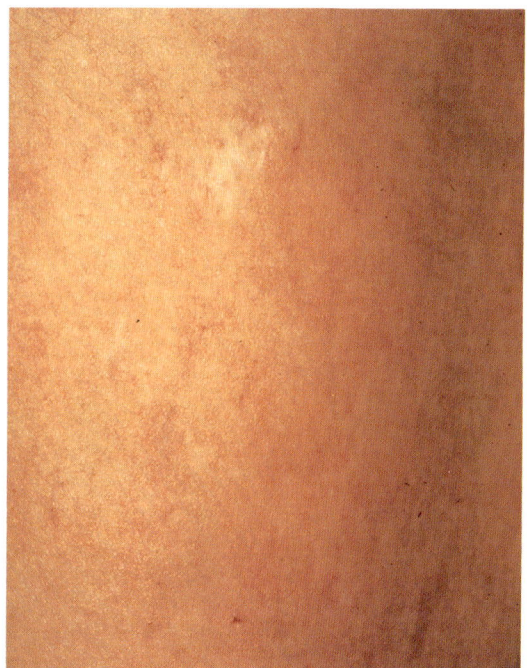

FIG. 7.28-D. Site one month after the second treatment and a total of 4 months after the first treatment showing nice resolution in the anomaly and no further hypopigmentation after using the dye laser.

Case courtesy of *David H. McDaniel*, M.D.

CASE 7.29
Telangiectatic Leg Vein/Telangiectatic Matting

REVIEW OF CASE. This 56-year-old female noted the progressive onset of telangiectatic leg veins over the past 10 years. She noted that her veins are getting larger and more numerous with time. In addition, she noted that her legs have a dull ache after prolonged standing. At the time of treatment she was not taking estrogen supplements. After the telangiectatic leg veins were treated with sclerotherapy by another physician, she developed a flare of "new" vessels (telangiectatic matting) at the treatment site. She was referred to our practice for laser treatment.

CHOICE OF LASER: TUNABLE DYE. Although sclerotherapy treatment was highly effective for eradicating both varicose, reticular and telangiectatic veins, as with any therapeutic modality, adverse sequelae may occur. Telangiectatic matting has been estimated to occur in approximately 15% of patients (30% if patients are on systemic estrogen therapy or oral contraceptives). The Candela SPTL-1 pulsed dye laser was developed to treat vascular abnormalities. The laser parameters of pulsed power output are primarily established for the treatment of blood vessels less than 0.1 mm in diameter. This is to keep the laser-generated thermal damage to within the thermal relaxation time of the targeted blood vessel. Therefore, sclerotherapy must be performed on *all* blood vessels over 0.1 mm in diameter in addition to all blood vessels which drain or feed into the telangiectatic area. Only after sclerotherapy is performed is the use of the Candela pulsed dye laser efficacious.

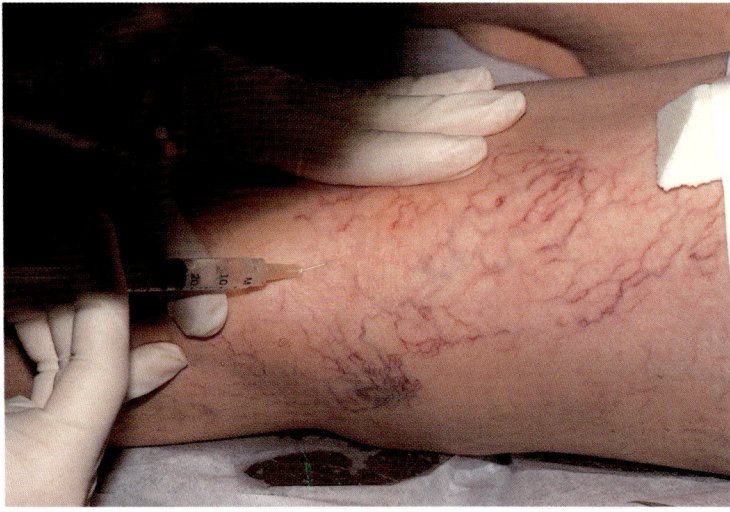

FIG. 7.29-A. These blood vessels are best treated by sclerotherapy. The red telangiectatic leg veins measure 0.2–0.4 mm in diameter. Note a blue reticular "feeding" vein 2 mm in diameter. (This photograph is not of the patient described above).

For literature pertaining to this case see References section.

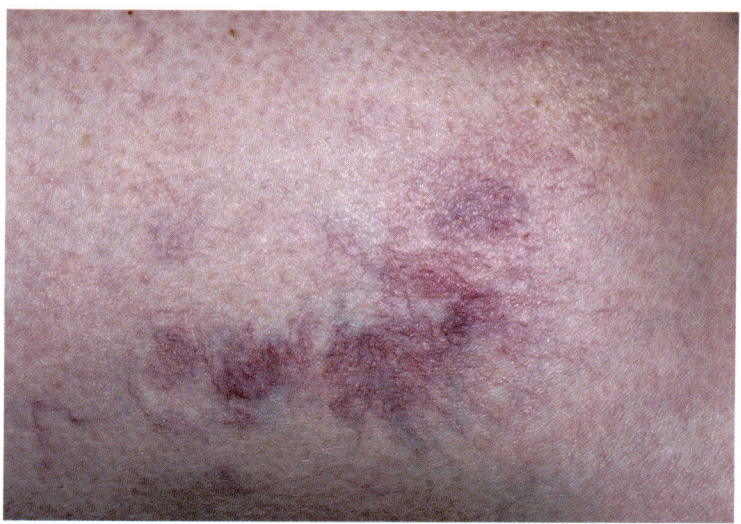

FIG. 7.29-B. Initial presentation of the patient. An extensive "mat" of red telangiectatic vessels <0.1 mm in diameter is present. This area was treated with three laser patch tests utilizing 10, 5 mm diameter pulses at 7.0, 7.25, and 7.5 J/cm^2.

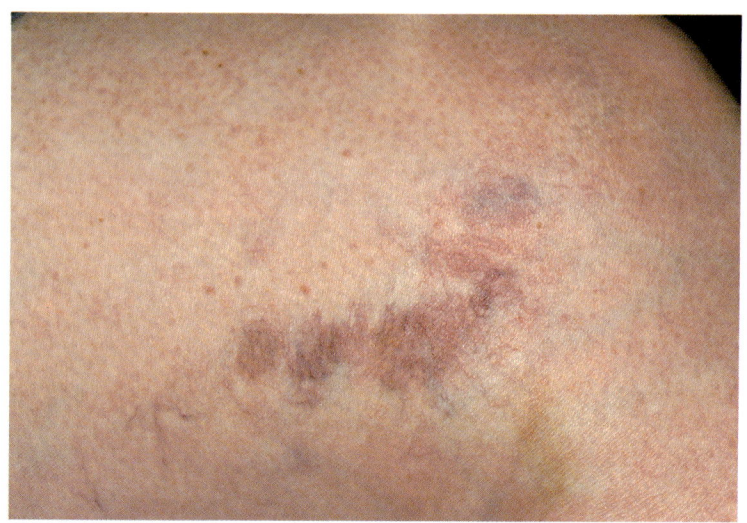

FIG. 7.29-C. One month after initial laser patch tests. There is no noticeable improvement, in fact associated reticular veins are more prominent (*arrows*).

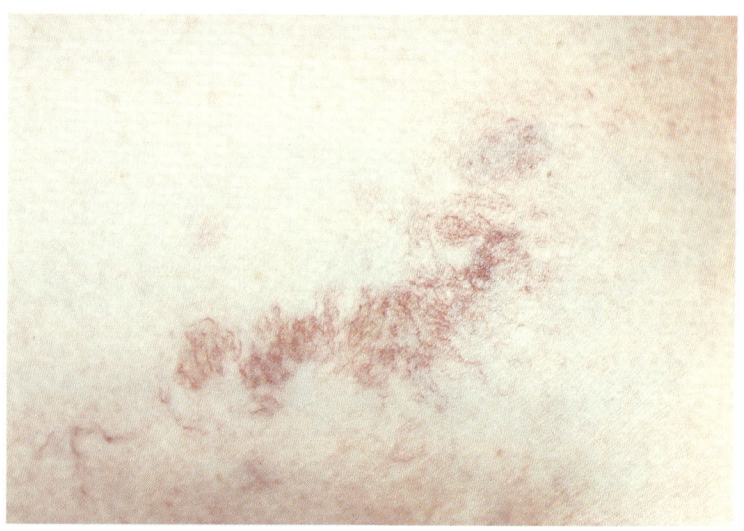

FIG. 7.29-D. Three weeks after treatment of reticular veins with 1 ml total of Polidocanol 0.75%. Note the resolution of reticular veins without change in the telangiectatic matting.

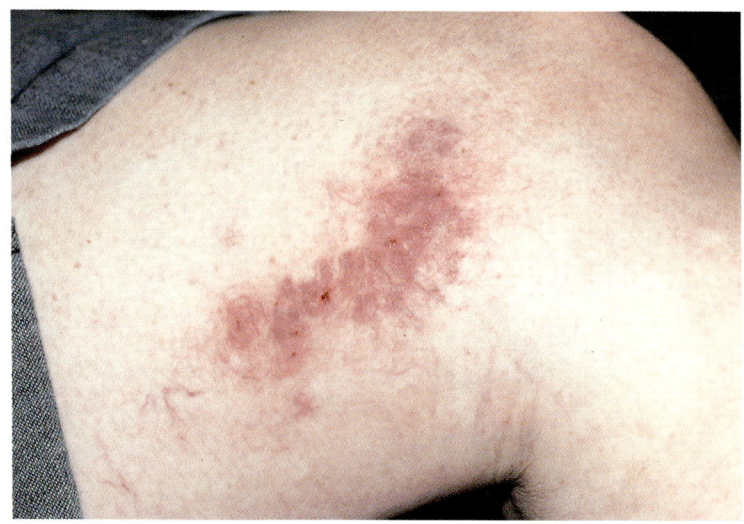

FIG. 7.29-E. Laser induced ecchymosis immediately following treatment of the telangiectatic matting utilizing 40, 5 mm diameter pulses at 7.25 J/cm^2. Polidocanol 0.5% was injected into a single feeding reticular vein (*arrow*).

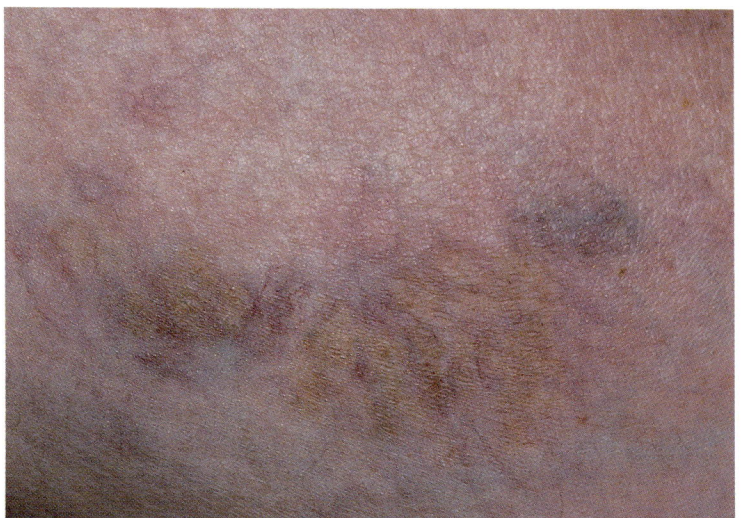

FIG. 7.29.F. Four weeks after treatment. Note some persistent hyperpigmentation.

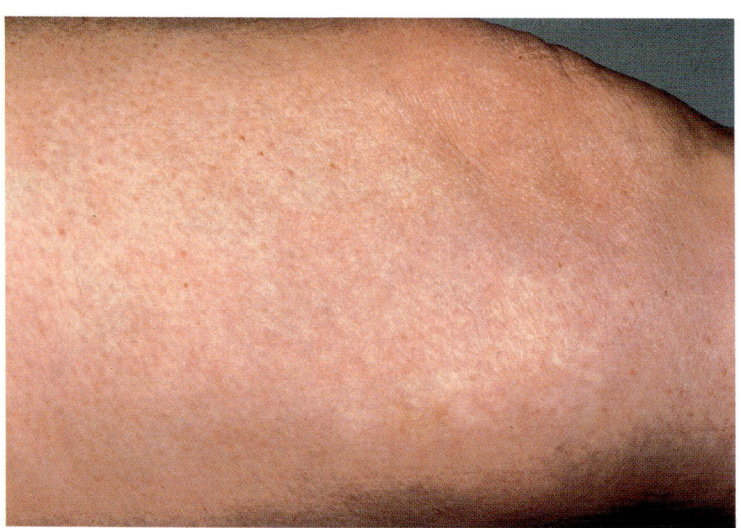

FIG. 7.29-G. Fourteen months after initial treatment. Note complete resolution of both reticular and telangiectatic veins.

Case courtesy of *Mitchel P. Goldman*, M.D., and *Richard E. Fitzpatrick*, M.D.

CASE 7.30

Telangiectasia on the Ala Nasi

REVIEW OF CASE. This 44-year-old female presented with a 1 year history of increasingly visible red lines around the nose which became more prominent with any flushing reaction. She denied any signs or symptoms of inflammatory rosacea including the appearance of pustules or papules. She requested treatment for cosmetic reasons.

CHOICE OF LASER: TUNABLE DYE. The Candela laser was chosen for its known effect on small blood vessels and the minimum risk of scar formation and the ability to do this without anesthesia. The vessels were treated over a period of five months with four individual treatments. The vessels were treated initially on November 8 with 5.50 J/cm^2 fluence with 10 pulses. On January 6, 7 additional pulses at 5.75 J/cm^2 were used. On March 7, an additional 11 pulses at 6.0 J/cm^2 were used and, finally, on April 18, 7 additional pulses at 6.50 J/cm^2 with a pulse size of 5.0 mm were used. All the pulses were administered at the focal length of the Candela handpiece with the laser in the focused mode.

ADDITIONAL INFORMATION. Large vessels about the ala nasi or columella of the nose often require more than one treatment. The four treatments that these vessels required is fairly standard for vessels of this size. Each treatment is given at approximately 3–4 week intervals with pulses that are immediately touching and usually not overlapping. The post-operative purpura and erythema normally persist for 5–7 days. Patients can use topical coverup makeups as long as they minimize wound irritation when they remove them. Patients also have to be instructed in the use of long wavelength photo blockers to prevent excessive tanning which competes for the absorption of the 585 nm pulse width of this laser.

POST-TREATMENT CARE. The patient was instructed to use topical antibiotics and normal soap and water to clean the wound. There was no wound dressing applied and the patient was allowed to use makeup after the first 48 hours.

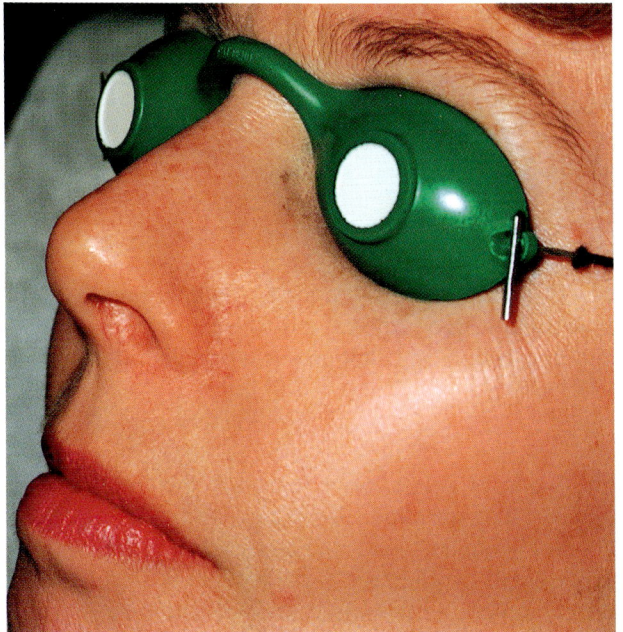

FIG. 7.30-A. Pre-treatment ala nasi.

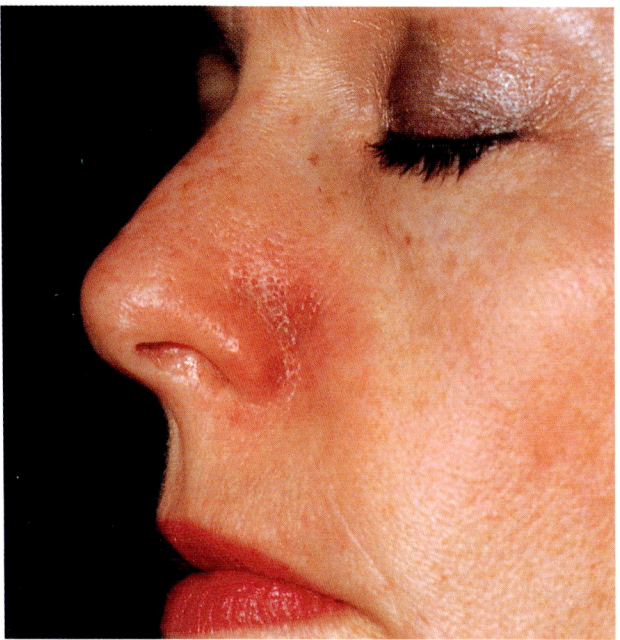

FIG. 7.30-B. Immediately post-operative erythema and purpura occurring with each treatment that lasts 5–7 days.

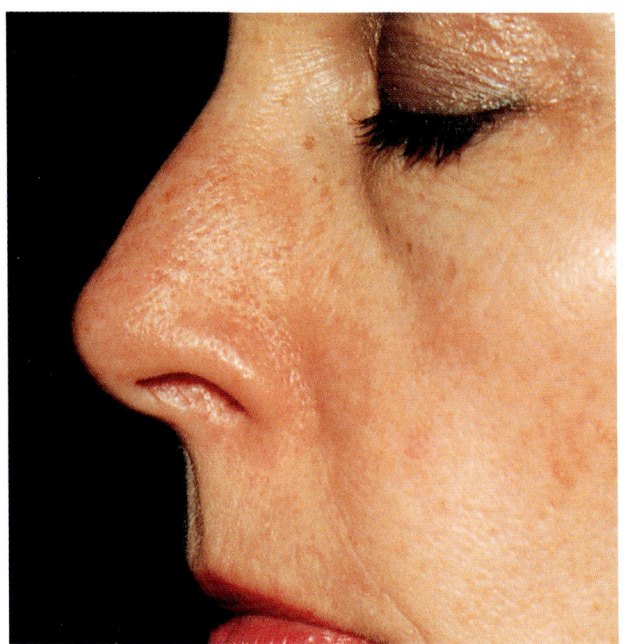

FIG. 7.30-C. One month post-laser treatment. Note complete resolution of dilated telangiectatic vessels around the ala nasi. There is no skin texture change, hyperpigmentation, or scar formation.

Case courtesy of *Thomas O. McMeekin*, M.D.

TUNABLE DYE LASER

CASE 7.31

Venous Lake

REVIEW OF CASE. This is a 65-year-old female with a 10 year history of a gradually enlarging blue-black compressible vascular papule on the lower vermilion. No previous treatment has been received. The patient complained of being able to feel the lesion and that strangers frequently attempted to point out that she had "ink on her lip."

CHOICE OF LASER: TUNABLE DYE. The tunable dye laser was chosen to match the long thermal relaxation time of the large vessel with a sufficient pulse duration. Physiology and mechanisms are reviewed in the case of FEDL treatment of mat telangiectasias and continuous wave tunable dye laser treatment of large telangiectasias. Experience with medium-to-larger ectatic skin vessels as seen in rosacea and also in venous lakes has demonstrated the importance of matching thermal relaxation time to the laser selection. A power setting of 1 watt, continuous wave, and spot size of 2 mm was used.

ADDITIONAL INFORMATION. Diascopy technique is used to compress the separated venous walls into contiguity. A slow circular painting motion is used to direct the beam through the transmissive glass until moderate whitening indicates sufficient photocoagulation is accomplished. Note: without diascopy or with smaller beam sizes or with inadequate movement of the beam, rupture of the venous lake wall is likely. If this occurs blot the area dry and use diascopy with a larger beam size.

POST-TREATMENT CARE. Antibiotic ointment should be applied frequently to prevent dryness or friction. Avoid irritation and trauma. The patient should be advised that the area may heal only to re-form a smaller second crust or scab at the end of a week to ten days.

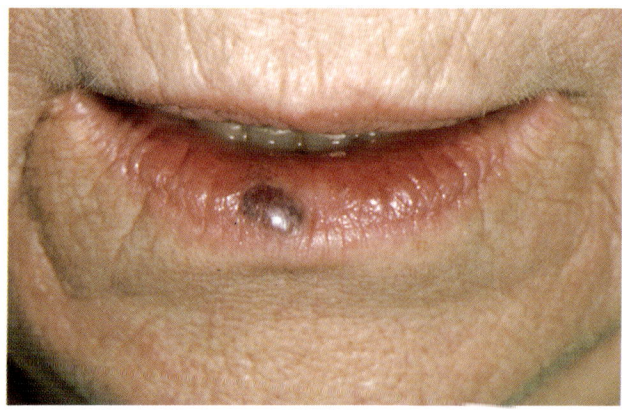

FIG. 7.31-A. Venous lake before treatment.

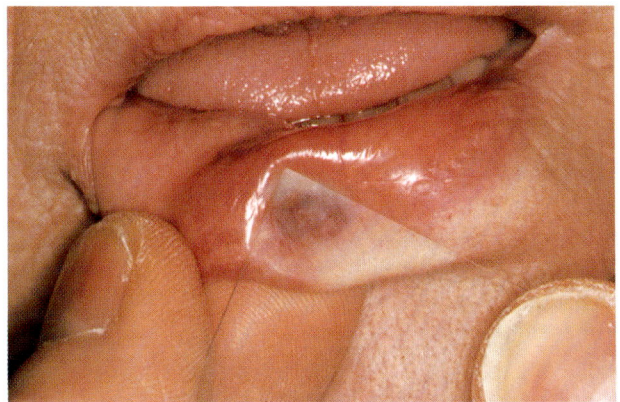

FIG. 7.31-B. Diascopy during laser treatment.

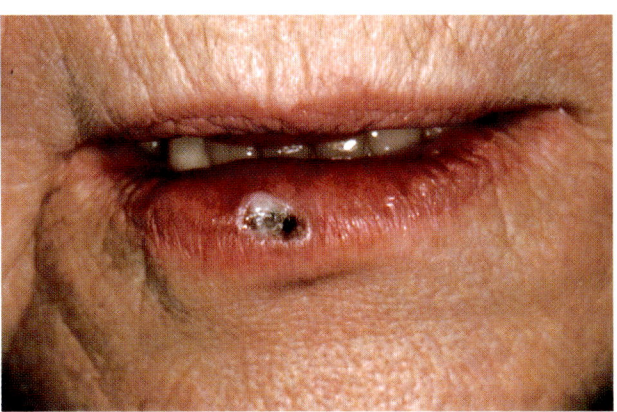

FIG. 7.31-C. Immediately post-laser photocoagulation.

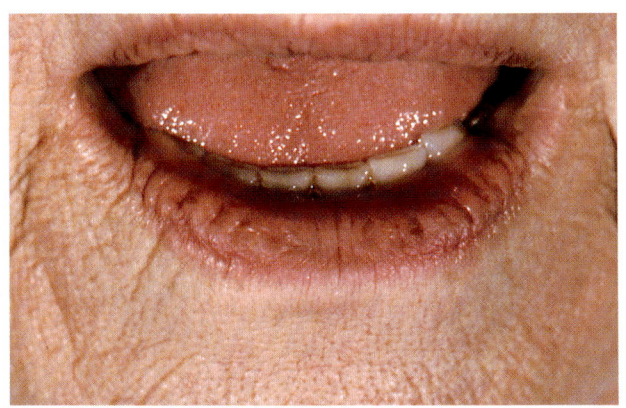

7.31-D. Close up of open mouth eight weeks after tunable dye laser treatment.

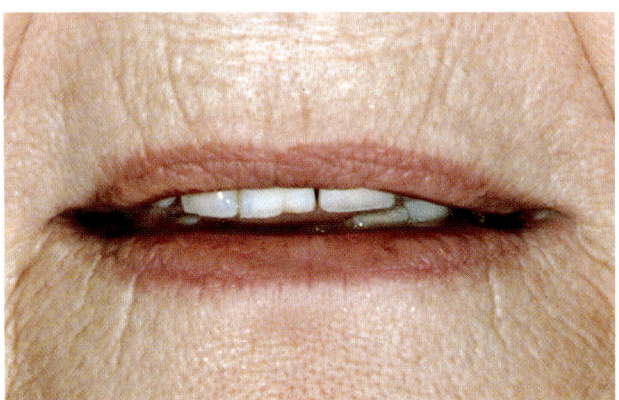

FIG. 7.31-E. Mouth in relaxed position eight weeks after tunable dye laser treatment.

Case courtesy of *Timothy J. Rosio*, M.D.

CASE 7.32
Venous Lake of the Lower Lip

REVIEW OF CASE. This 52-year-old healthy woman presented with a two year history of venous lake on her lower lip. It had been slowly increasing in size.

CHOICE OF LASER: TUNABLE DYE. The tunable dye laser was selected because of its specificity for the vascular lesion and also to minimize the risk of scarring or damage to the vermilion in this important cosmetic portion of the face.

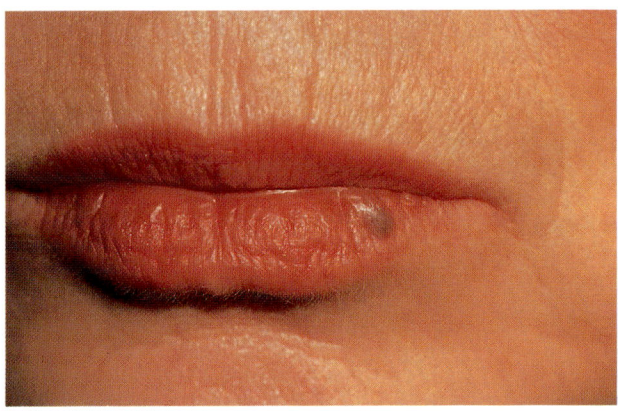

FIG. 7.32-A. Pre-treatment venous lake. The area was subsequently treated with yellow tunable dye laser 585 nm using 0.130 mm spot, 0.25 watts continuous mode, and microspot tracing technique. Vessel disappearance endpoint was utilized. Some graying of the overlying epidermis occurred. The area subsequently required a second treatment which was performed using 590 nm yellow light, 0.130 mm spot, and 0.45 watts continuous wave defocused power using a painting technique to attempt to seal off the deeper vessels. Also, in this circumstance slight greying but not a severe blanching was used as the endpoint.

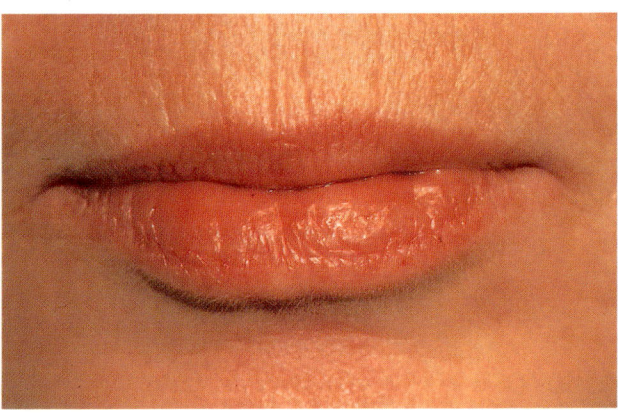

FIG. 7.32-B. Two weeks post-final treatment with excellent cosmetic result. Only topical anesthesia was used during this treatment.

Case courtesy of *David H. McDaniel*, M.D.

8

NEW TECHNOLOGIES

Copper Vapor Laser, Gold Vapor Laser, Hexascan Device, KTP, Photodynamic Therapy

VASCULAR AND RELATED LESIONS
8.1 Capillary hemangioma of the nose [KTP]
8.2 Congenital port wine stain of the face [copper vapor with hexascan]
8.3 Port wine stain of the face [CW tunable dye with hexascan]
8.4 Port wine stain of the face [CW tunable dye with hexascan]
8.5 Port wine stain of the face and neck [CW tunable dye with hexascan]
8.6 Port wine stain of the upper lip [CW tunable dye with hexascan]
8.7 Port wine stain of the leg [CW tunable dye with hexascan]
8.8 Port wine hemangioma of the extremity with angiokeratomas [CW tunable dye with hexascan]
8.9 Port wine stain of the face [gated argon/copper laser technique]
8.10 Port wine stain hemangioma of the lower leg [tunable dye with hexascan]
8.11 Port wine hemangioma of the face and neck [argon dye with hexascan]
8.12 Port wine hemangioma of the face and neck [KTP]
8.13 Telangiectasia of the face with persistent erythema [argon dye with hexascan]

MALIGNANT AND PRE-MALIGNANT LESIONS
8.14 Basal cell carcinoma of the nose [photodynamic therapy]
8.15 Basal cell carcinoma of the nose [photodynamic therapy]
8.16 Squamous cell carcinoma of the eyelid [photodynamic therapy]

TATTOO
8.17 Blue/black amateur tattoo [ruby]
8.18 Amateur decorative tattoo [ruby]
8.19 Amateur decorative tattoo [ruby]
8.20 Decorative tattoo [KTP]

MISCELLANEOUS
8.21 Cafe-au-lait lesion [argon dye with hexascan]
8.22 Divided nevus of the right eyelid [ruby]
8.23 Epidermal melanosis secondary to post-traumatic hyperpigmentation [ruby]
8.24 Epidermal melanosis secondary to cafe-au-lait spot [ruby]
8.25 Lentigo senilis of the left cheek [ruby]
8.26 Nevus cell nevus of the lower leg [ruby]
8.27 Nevus cell nevus of the left shoulder [ruby]
8.28 Nevus Ota of the left eyelid [ruby]
8.29 Nevus spilus of the left cheek [ruby]
8.30 Nevus spilus of the left knee [ruby]
8.31 Seborrheic keratosis of anterior part of the left ear [ruby]

CASE 8.1
Capillary Hemangioma of the Nose

REVIEW OF CASE. This is a 3-month-old female with a rapidly growing strawberry capillary hemangioma. The hemangioma covers the dorsum of the nose, more prominently on the right than on the left, and involves the columella, and the right nasal ala. A crust or eschar had previously appeared in the midportion of the right ala and on its removal a full-thickness defect of the right ala was present extending from the alar edge approximately 10 mm up the nose.

CHOICE OF LASER: KTP. The KTP laser was chosen because the green light at 532 nm is attracted to the hemoglobin in the vessels. Light is converted to heat and heat has the ability to coagulate the vessels. Adjacent skin appendages such as hair follicles and pilosebaceous glands are spared, aiding in the healing of the laser wound.

ADDITIONAL INFORMATION. The patient and all personnel in the room must have proper eye protection for the frequency doubled Nd:YAG laser.

POST-TREATMENT CARE. Iced compresses and antibiotic ointment are used.

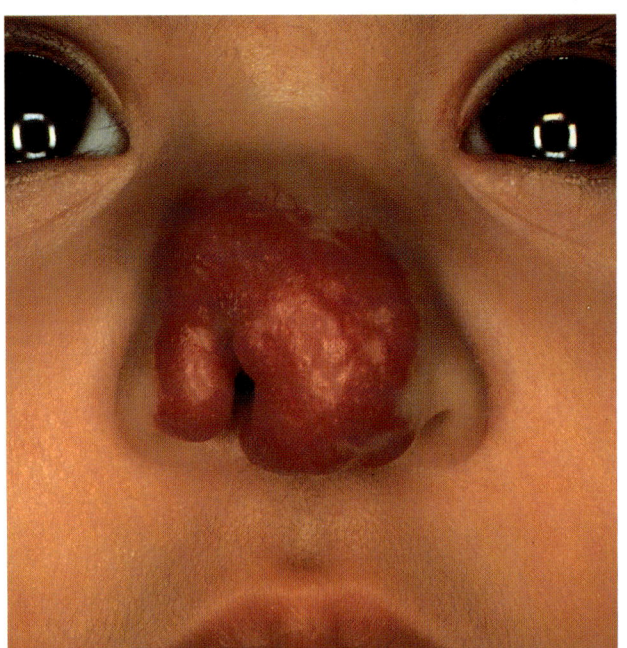

FIG. 8.1-A. Pre-operative capillary hemangioma of the nose. Note extensive lesion and full-thickness loss in the right ala.

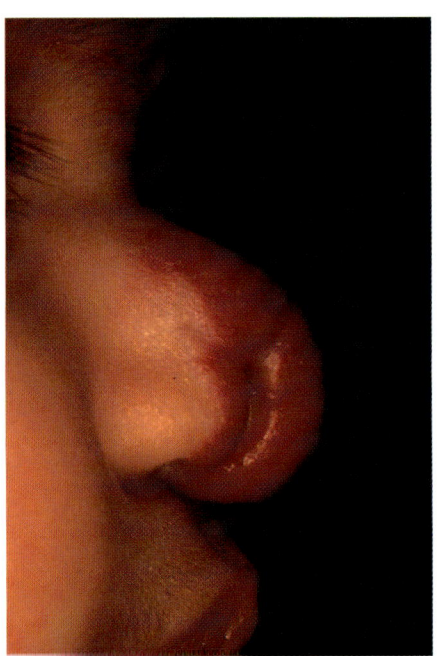

FIG. 8.1-B. Pre-operative capillary hemangioma of the nose. Note extensive lesion and full thickness in the right ala.

Reprinted with permission of Wiley-Liss, a division of John Wiley & Sons, Inc.
For literature pertaining to this case see References section.

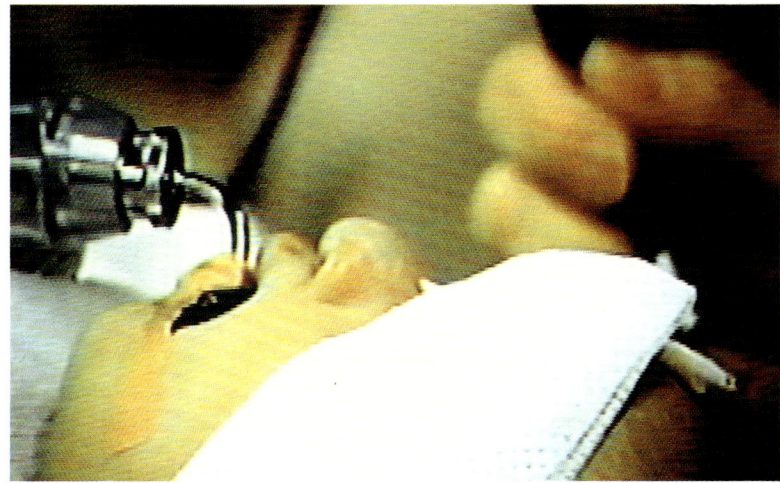

FIG. 8.1-C. Blanching produced by the KTP laser.

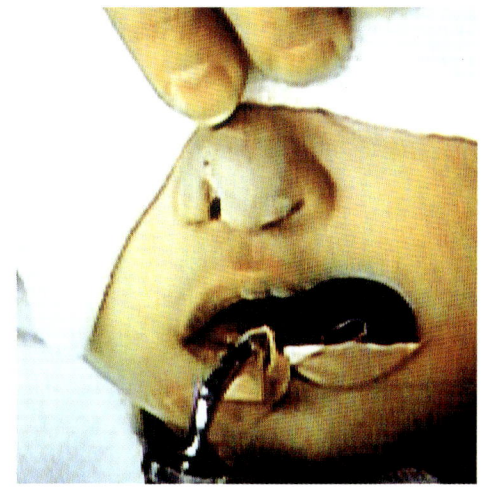

FIG. 8.1-D. Blanching produced by the KTP laser.

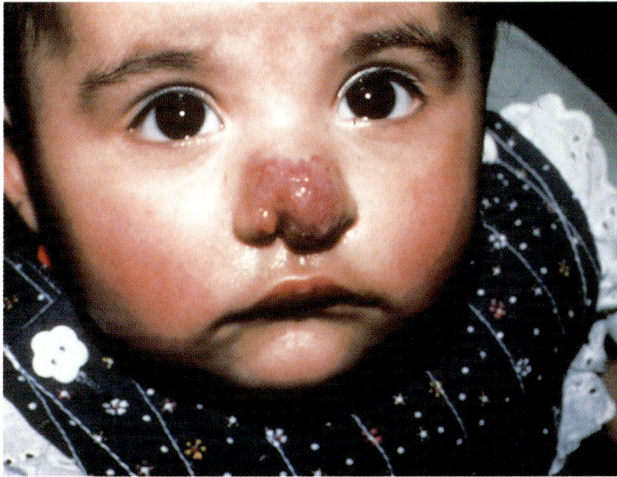

FIG. 8.1-E. Blanching 48 hours post-treatment with inflammatory reaction and superficial skin loss.

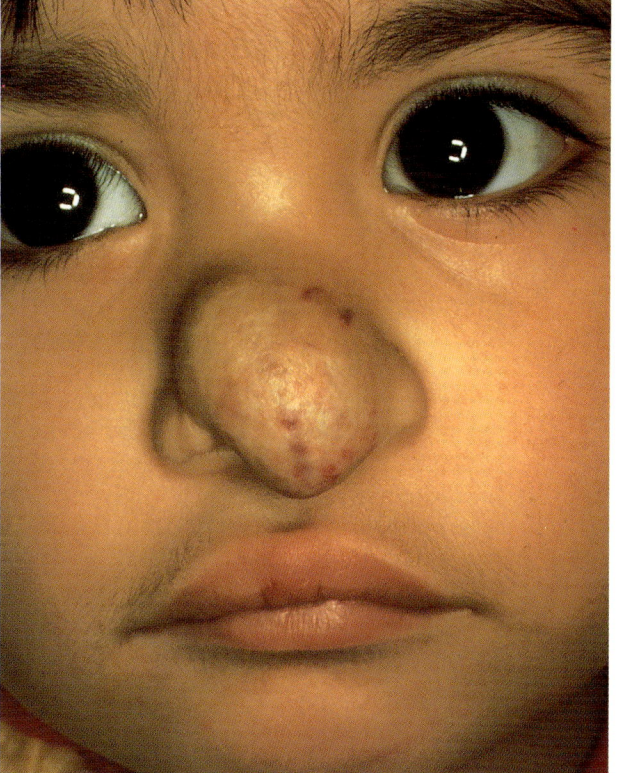

FIG. 8.1-G. Final result showing marked shrinkage and blanching of the hemangioma with restoration of the right alar deficit.

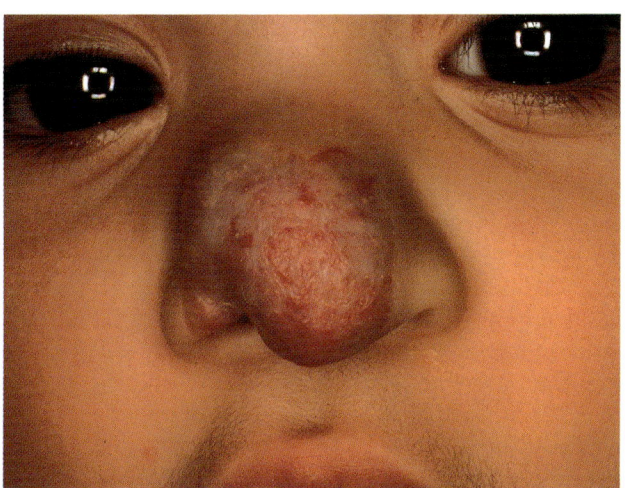

FIG. 8.1-F. Final result showing marked shrinkage and blanching of the hemangioma with restoration of the right alar deficit.

Case courtesy of ***David B. Apfelberg***, M.D.

CASE 8.2
Congenital Port Wine Stain of the Face

REVIEW OF CASE. This 32-year-old male presented first in 1979 at age 22 for testing with the argon laser. He at that time had a good response to the argon test but did not decide to proceed with definitive therapy. He appeared again in 1988 for re-evaluation at which time he was tested witih the argon laser again and simultaneously in other spots with the continuous wave tunable dye laser at 578 nm and copper vapor laser. At six months, he was approximately 40% cleared using the argon and continuous tunable dye lasers but approximately 50% clear using the copper laser. At that time treatment was begun using only the copper laser, for the most part performed with a hexascan scanner with a 13 mm grid pattern which provides 127 bursts per 13 mm grid. The spot size individual burst was 1 mm and the shutter (pulse) duration was 0.2 seconds. The power setting was at 350 to 380 milliwatts. No anesthesia was required.

CHOICE OF LASER: COPPER VAPOR WITH HEXASCAN. This patient would have had good results with any of the three lasers utilized. Copper vapor laser was chosen because its effects seemed to be somewhat better than the others and thus a more prompt improvement or degree of resolution could be anticipated with it. In potentially difficult cases of port wine stains, it is best to test simultaneously with several different lasers if they are available or to anticipate treating with first one and then later with another if the level of improvement seems to diminish drastically with repeated treatments. Copper vapor laser, then, seems to be effective when argon or pulsed dye laser have reached their limit of ability to improve the port wine stain. This may be because of the deeper penetration of yellow light in the copper vapor laser and the greater thermal damage which occurs in both the argon and pulsed dye lasers.

Telangiectases and small or irregular areas of port wine stain are best treated freehand using the copper vapor laser with a 200 μm spot size for the former and 1 mm spot size for the latter. For very large port wine stains the hexascan scanner provides the most convenient method of treatment and insures uniform dispersal of laser energy through the entire grid and in a very fast (faster than freehand) manner. Only intermittent bursts either freehand or (of necessity) in hexascan mode are suggested. Continuous air brush application of the copper vapor laser is not suggested as too much energy may be delivered and only an imprecise estimation of its amount can be given. Too much thermal damage increases the risk of poor healing with hypertrophic scarring or unnecessary opacification.

ADDITIONAL INFORMATION. As in argon laser surgery, port wine stains treated by copper vapor laser may continue to lighten for up to one year. The minimal dose technique of Cosman is used for either freehand or hexascan treatments with the copper vapor laser. Local anesthesia is not usually necessary in adults but will be in children and general anesthesia may be required for young children. It is useful to mark areas treated with gentian violet at the tips of the hexagon since with the minimal dose technique it is often times difficult to visualize the exact area treated. This will prevent unnecessary overlap and unnecessary skip intervals. Because the beam profile is not uniform and the individual 1 mm spots in the grid do not overlap, there also frequently will be a polka dot pattern appearing after use of the hexascan unless high enough doses are utilized which produce more diffuse thermal damage. The use of smaller hexagons than 13 mm may be difficult. It is sometimes more useful to continue to use the 13 mm grid but to obstruct the application of the laser by inserting a white gauze over normal skin underneath the grid pattern. This allows for increased speed of operation and accuracy of placement of the grids but obviously interferes with the ability to know precisely the number of bursts which have been applied to the port wine stain.

POST-TREATMENT CARE. Copper vapor laser produces a through-and-through second degree burn even when the minimal dose technique of Cosman is utilized. The area therefore must be scrupulously cared for post-operatively. A semi-permeable dressing should be utilized at all times and changed daily or twice daily. Gentle hydrogen peroxide cleansing without rubbing and then application of an antibacterial ointment (not cream) under this dressing is necessary. Edges of the dressing should be sealed well on all four edges particularly near the nose and the mouth so that bacteria from these orifices do not contaminate the wound. Such contamination can occur within hours of the laser treatment. Hypertrophic scarring can occur with the copper vapor laser. If the port wine stain extends to the hairline, a portion of the hairline should be shaved so that tape can be sealed beyond the edge of the treated area.

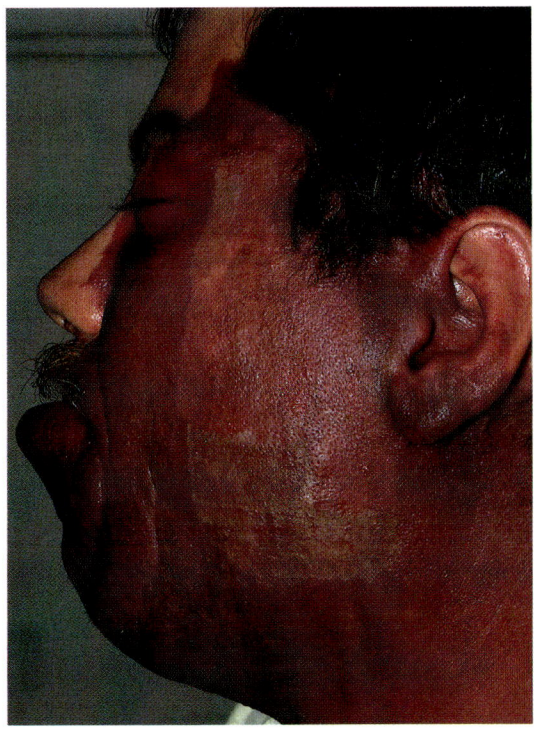

FIG. 8.2-A. Patient during treatment. The port wine stain was uniformly colored prior to treatment. The upper portion of the treated area shows clearly the dramatic improvement in the port wine stain though there is substantial residual in such a hypertrophic port wine stain. The lower portion exhibits the "milk scald" appearance of epidermal injury which is apparent immediately after application of the laser. The minimum dose technique of Cosman is utilized wherein the smallest power setting to produce such a light grey-white appearance is used.

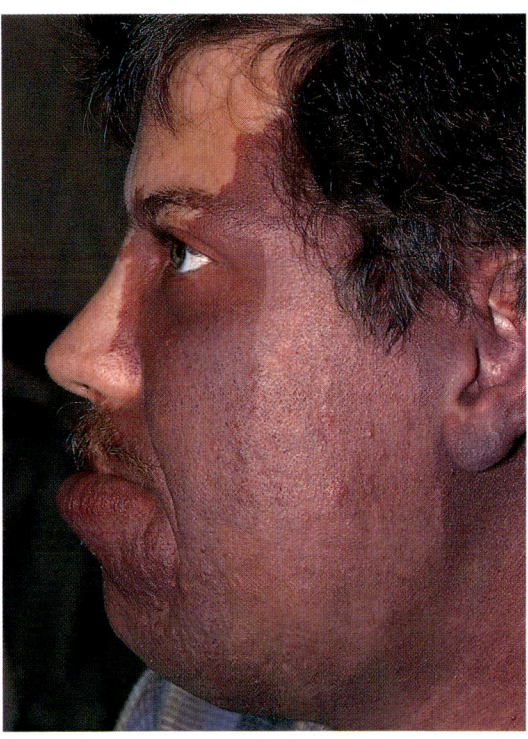

FIG. 8.2-B. Follow-up two months after subsequent treatments. Note degree of improvement of the treated area.

Case courtesy of *Gary J. Brauner*, M.D., and *Alan Schliftman*, M.D.

CASE 8.3
Port Wine Stain of the Face

REVIEW OF CASE. This 24-year-old male presented with a congenital port wine stain of the face. He desires removal for cosmetic purposes.

CHOICE OF LASER: TUNABLE DYE WITH HEXASCAN. Indications for the hexascan with either the argon laser or tunable dye lasers in the treatment of port wine stains are as follows: (a) in patients under the age of 12, particularly infants and children; (b) in areas of the trunk and extremities in any age patients; in scar prone areas of the face such as the perioral, nasolabial, and nasal skin; (c) in any deeply pigmented patient where hypopigmentation may be likely; and (d) in patients who have previously been successfully but incompletely treated with the argon laser. In all of these instances, either the argon laser or the tunable dye laser with hexascan may produce satisfactory fading without scarring. Between 4 and 9 individual treatments separated by 3 to 6 months may be necessary for fading, which is never total. Some residual hemangioma may remain. Power settings vary from 10 to 40 joules depending on the color and hypertrophy of the lesion. The endpoint of the treatment is a "graying or disappearance" of the vessel but not a white blanching. Post-treatment skin changes should be minimal. Local anesthesia or sedation is required for treatments. Wavelengths of 577–595 nm may be easily tuned.

ADDITIONAL INFORMATION. The hexascan is a computerized, automated scanning device that allows for the rapid and easily reproducible treatment of large areas of skin using either the argon or tunable dye lasers. The scanning pattern is designed to promote uniform energy fluence and minimize unwanted thermal damage to non-target tissue. The 1 mm spots are assembled into hexagons of 3, 5, 9, 11, or 13 mm diameter. The scanning pattern is designed to separate consecutive spots 2 mm apart at 1 μmsec intervals in a precise non-adjacent pattern. This allows dissipation of undesired thermal energy between pulses. Approximately 20 seconds are required to treat the largest hexascan of 13 mm which contains 127 separate spots. The hexascan device is indicated for any situation where traditional "tracing" by the argon laser technique is likely to produce scarring. It may also be used in conjuction with continuous wave tunable dye laser to break up the beam so that thermal damage is minimal. This results in a safer treatment which may be equivalent to the "selective photothermolysis" of the flashlamp pump dye laser but produced by a different physical parameter. Instead of supershort pulses of 350 μsecond which do not exceed the thermal relaxation time of adjacent tissue, the hexascan produces random short pulses which are widely divergent such that dissipation of unwanted thermal energy occurs between pulses.

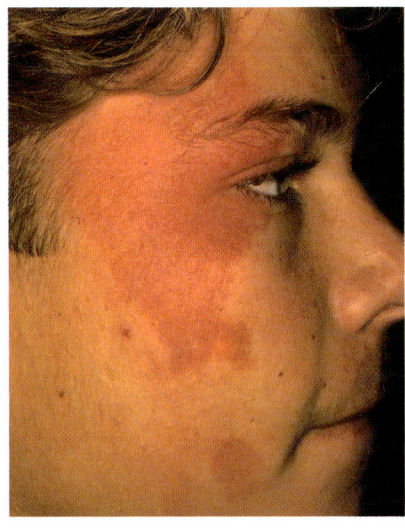

FIG. 8.3-A. Port wine stain of right temple, eyelid, and cheek prior to treatment.

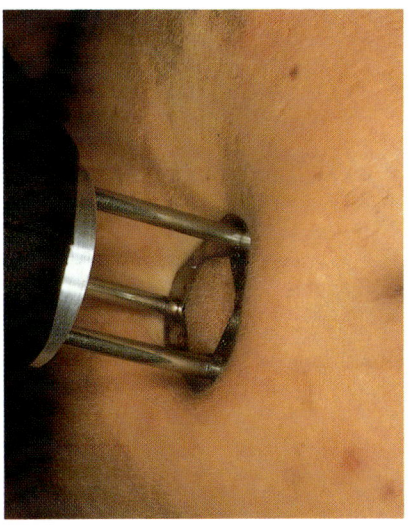

FIG. 8.3-B. Hexascan device.

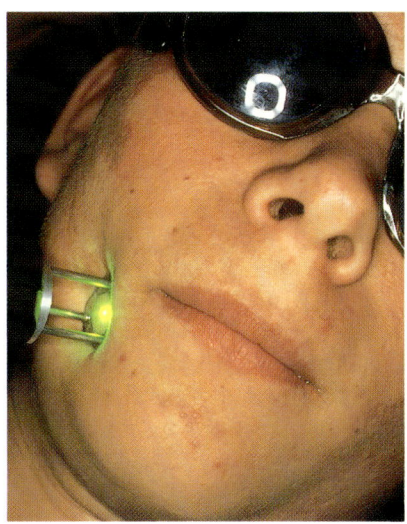

FIG. 8.3-C. Hexascan device.

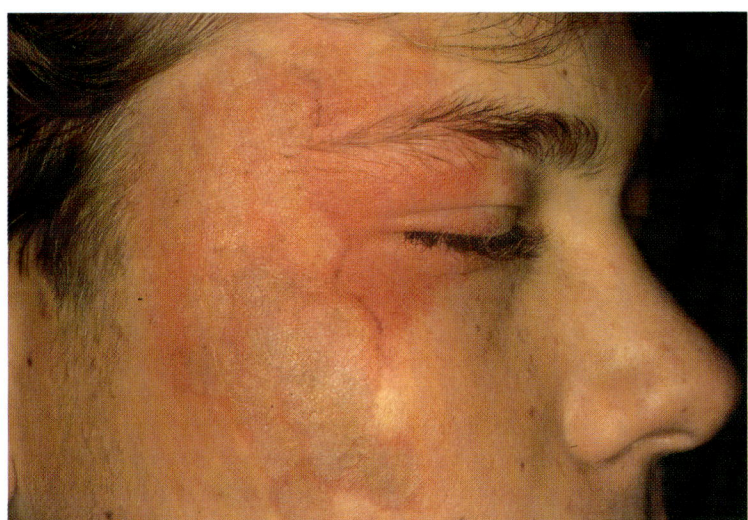

FIG. 8.3-D. Hexascan treatment areas immediately following treatment.

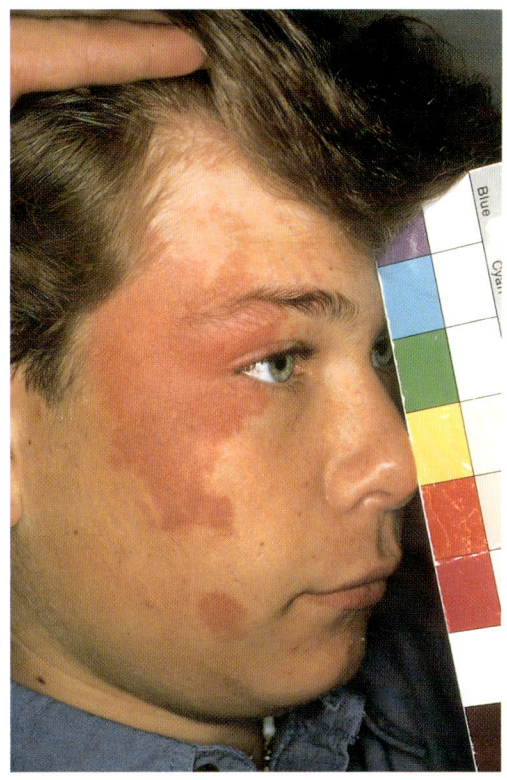

FIG. 8.3-E. Modest fading without scarring 5 months post-treatment.

Case courtesy of *David B. Apfelberg*, M.D., and *Teruko Smith*, R.N., P.A.-C.

TUNABLE DYE LASER WITH HEXASCAN   407

CASE 8.4

Port Wine Stain of the Face

REVIEW OF CASE. This 26-year-old male presented with a port wine stain of the cheek, lower eyelid, nose, and upper lip. Due to his dark complexion and possible interference of laser absorption by melanin particles in the dermis, the continuous wave tunable dye laser was chosen. In addition, the upper lip and side of the nose are areas in which treatment frequently results in hypertrophic scarring.

CHOICE OF LASER: TUNABLE DYE WITH HEXASCAN. Indications for the hexascan with either the argon laser or tunable dye lasers in the treatment of port wine stains are as follows: (a) in patients under the age of 12, particularly infants and children; (b) in areas of the trunk and extremities in any age patients; (c) in scar prone areas of the face such as the perioral, nasolabial, and nasal skin; (d) in any deeply pigmented patient where hypopigmentation may be likely; and (e) in patients who have previously been successfully but incompletely treated with the argon laser. In all of these instances, either the argon laser or the tunable dye laser with hexascan may produce satisfactory fading without scarring. Between 4 and 9 individual treatments separated by 3 to 6 months may be necessary for fading, which is never total. Some residual hemangioma may remain. Power settings vary from 10 to 40 joules depending on the color and hypertrophy of the lesion. The endpoint of the treatment is a "graying or disappearance" of the vessel but not a white blanching. Post-treatment skin changes should be minimal. Local anesthesia or sedation is required for treatments. Wavelengths of 577–595 nm may be easily tuned.

ADDITIONAL INFORMATION. The hexascan is a computerized, automated scanning device that allows for the rapid and easily reproducible treatment of large areas of skin using either the argon or tunable dye lasers. The scanning pattern is designed to promote uniform energy fluence and minimize unwanted thermal damage to non-target tissue. The 1 mm spots are assembled into hexagons of 3, 5, 9, 11, or 13 mm diameter. The scanning pattern is designed to separate consecutive spots 2 mm apart at 15 μsec intervals in a precise non-adjacent pattern. This allows dissipation of undesired thermal energy between pulses. Approximately 20 seconds are required to treat the largest hexascan of 13 mm which contains 127 separate spots.

The hexascan device is indicated for any situation where traditional "tracing" by the argon laser technique is likely to produce scarring. It may also be used in conjunction with the continuous wave tunable dye laser to break up the beam so that thermal damage is minimal. This results in a safer treatment which may be equivalent to the "selective photothermolysis" of the flashlamp pump dye laser but produced by a different physical parameter. Instead of supershort pulses of 350 μsecond which do not exceed the thermal relaxation time of adjacent tissue, the hexascan produces random short pulses which are widely divergent such that dissipation of unwanted thermal energy occurs between pulses.

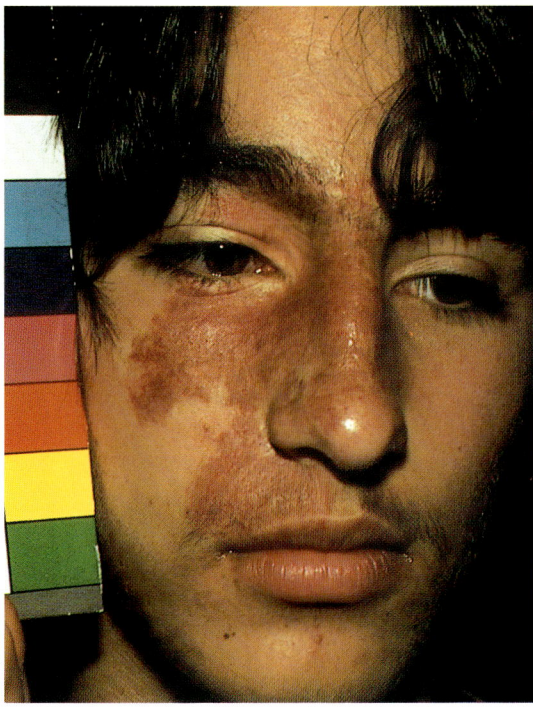

FIG. 8.4-A. Port wine stain of cheek, lower eyelid, nose and upper lip.

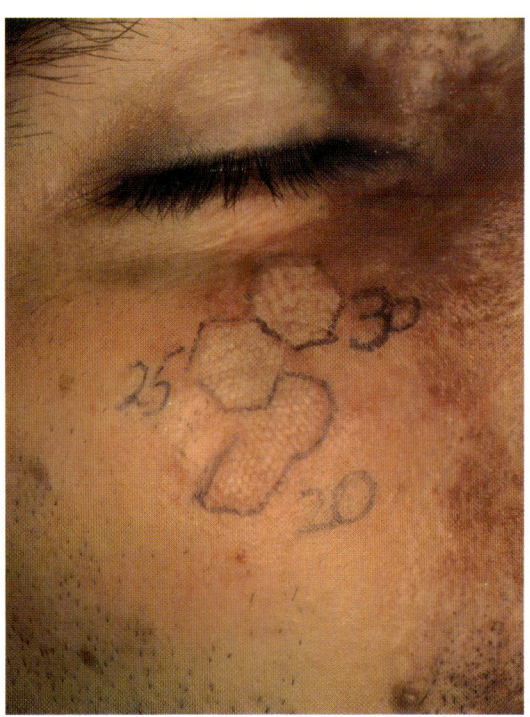

FIG. 8.4-B. Result of hexascan at varying power levels to the cheek.

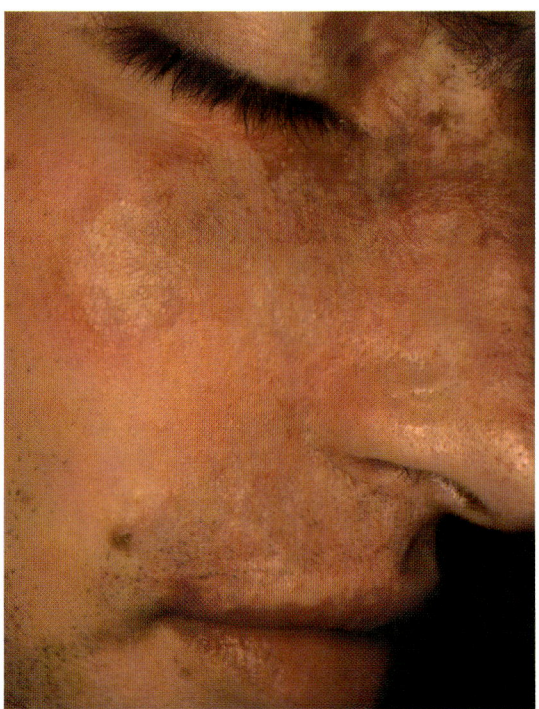

FIG. 8.4-C. Result of hexascan 3 months following the first treatment of the cheek and the upper lip.

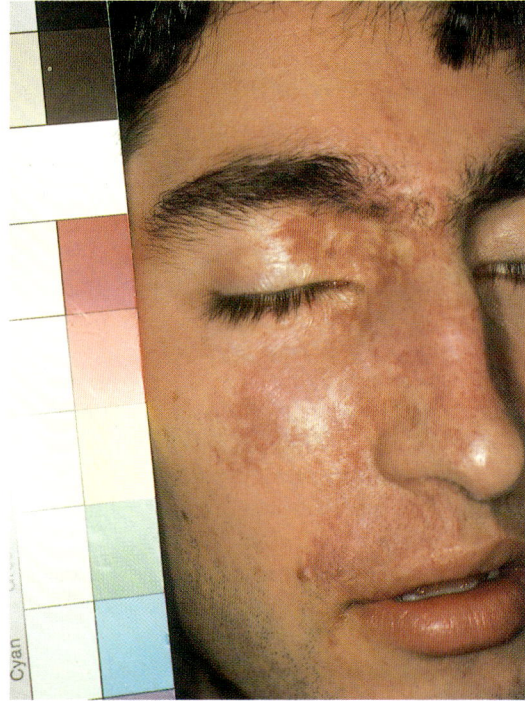

FIG. 8.4-D. Satisfactory fading without scarring 9 months following the first treatment and 6 months following the second treatment.

Case courtesy of *David B. Apfelberg*, M.D., and *Patricia Z. Spector*, R.N., MHS, P.A.-C.

TUNABLE DYE LASER WITH HEXASCAN   409

CASE 8.5

Port Wine Stain of the Face and Neck

REVIEW OF CASE. This 27-year-old female desired removal of a congenital port wine stain of the face and neck for cosmetic reasons. The tunable dye laser was chosen because more traditional argon laser treatment of the neck often results in hypopigmentation or scarring.

CHOICE OF LASER: TUNABLE DYE WITH HEXASCAN. Indications for the hexascan with either the argon laser or tunable dye lasers in the treatment of port wine stains are as follows: (a) in patients under the age of 12, particularly infants and children; (b) in areas of the trunk and extremities in any age patients; (c) in scar prone areas of the face such as the perioral, nasolabial, and nasal skin; (d) in any deeply pigmented patient where hypopigmentation may be likely; and (e) in patients who have previously been successfully but incompletely treated with the argon laser. In all of these instances, either the argon laser or the tunable dye laser with hexascan may produce satisfactory fading without scarring. Between 4 and 9 individual treatments separated by 3 to 6 months may be necessary for fading, which is never total. Some residual hemangioma may remain. Power settings vary from 10 to 40 joules depending on the color and hypertrophy of the lesion. The endpoint of the treatment is a "graying or disappearance" of the vessel but not a white blanching. Post-treatment skin changes should be minimal. Local anesthesia or sedation is required for treatments. Wavelengths of 577–595 nm may be easily tuned.

ADDITIONAL INFORMATION. The hexascan is a computerized, automated scanning device that allows for the rapid and easily reproducible treatment of large areas of skin using either the argon or tunable dye lasers. The scanning pattern is designed to promote uniform energy fluence and minimize unwanted thermal damage to non-target tissue. The 1 mm spots are assembled into hexagons of 3, 5, 9, 11, or 13 mm diameter. The scanning pattern is designed to separate consecutive spots 2 mm apart at 15 μsec intervals in a precise non-adjacent pattern. This allows dissipation of undesired thermal energy between pulses. Approximately 20 seconds are required to treat the largest hexascan of 13 mm which contains 127 separate spots.

The hexascan device is indicated for any situation where traditional "tracing" by the argon laser technique is likely to produce scarring. It may also be used in conjunction with the continuous wave tunable dye laser to break up the beam so that thermal damage is minimal. This results in a safer treatment which may be equivalent to the "selective photothermolysis" of the flashlamp pump dye laser but produced by a different physical parameter. Instead of supershort pulses of 350 μsecond which do not exceed the thermal relaxation of adjacent tissue, the hexascan produces random short pulses which are widely divergent such that dissipation of unwanted thermal energy occurs between pulses.

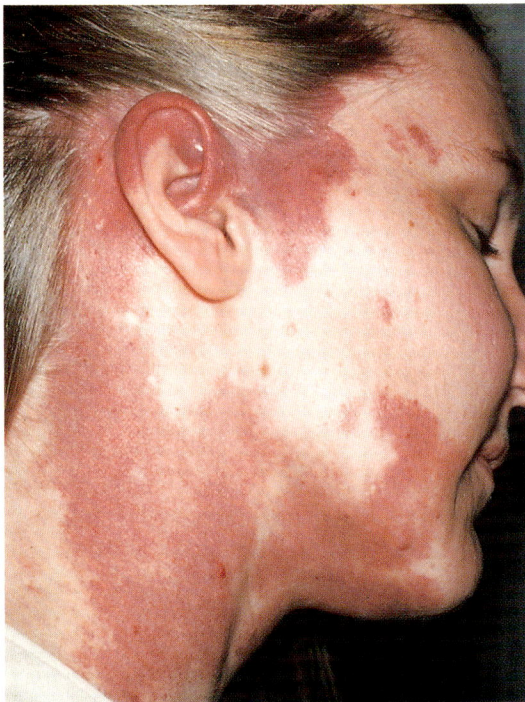

FIG. 8.5-A. Port wine stain of face and neck prior to treatment.

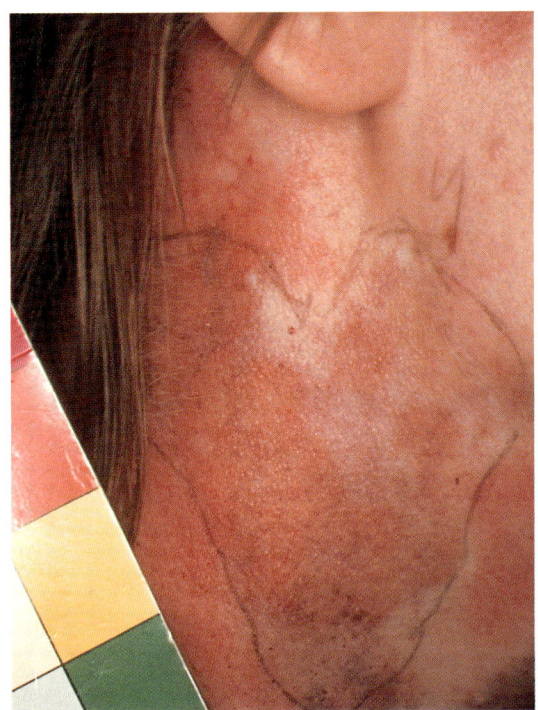

FIG. 8.5-B. Result of hexascan treatment of the neck.

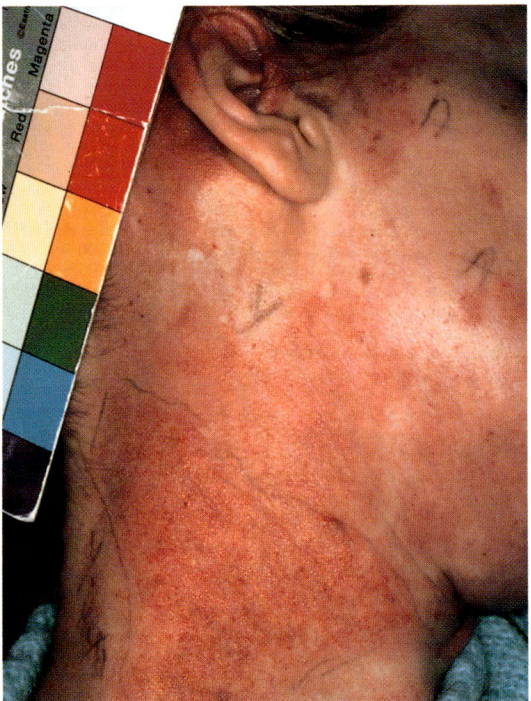

FIG. 8.5-C. Further result of hexascan treatment of the neck.

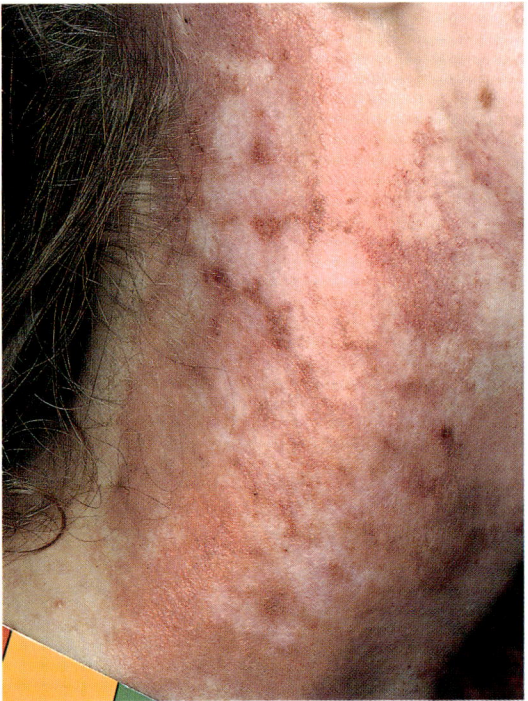

FIG. 8.5-D. Interim result showing marked blanching without scarring or hypopigmentation in hexascan areas of the neck—interspaces need to be traced with the handpiece.

Case courtesy of *David B. Apfelberg*, M.D., and *Teruko Smith*, R.N., P.A.-C.

CASE 8.6
Port Wine Stain of the Upper Lip

REVIEW OF CASE. This 9-year-old male sought treatment for a congenital port wine stain of the upper lip. The tunable laser was chosen because argon laser treatment frequently results in hypertrophic scarring in the upper lip, especially in children.

CHOICE OF LASER: TUNABLE DYE WITH HEXASCAN. Indications for the hexascan with either the argon laser or tunable dye lasers in the treatment of port wine stains are as follows: (a) in patients under the age of 12, particularly infants and children; (b) in areas of the trunk and extremities in any age patients; (c) in scar prone areas of the face such as the perioral, nasolabial, and nasal skin; (d) in any deeply pigmented patient where hypopigmentation may be likely; and (e) in patients who have previously been successfully but incompletely treated with the argon laser. In all of these instances, either the argon laser or the tunable dye laser with hexascan may produce satisfactory fading without scarring. Between 4 and 9 individual treatments separated by 3 to 6 months may be necessary for fading, which is never total. Some residual hemangioma may remain. Power settings vary from 10 to 40 joules depending on the color and hypertrophy of the lesion. The endpoint of the treatment is a "graying or disappearance" of the vessel but not a white blanching. Post-treatment skin changes should be minimal. Local anesthesia or sedation is required for treatments. Wavelengths of 577–595 nm may be easily tuned.

ADDITIONAL INFORMATION. The hexascan is a computerized, automated scanning device that allows for the rapid and easily reproducible treatment of large areas of skin using either the argon or tunable dye lasers. The scanning pattern is designed to promote uniform energy fluence and minimize unwanted thermal damage to non-target tissue. The 1 mm spots are assembled into hexagons of 3, 5, 9, 11, or 13 mm diameter. The scanning pattern is designed to separate consecutive spots 2 mm apart at 15 μsec intervals in a precise non-adjacent pattern. This allows dissipation of undesired thermal energy between pulses. Approximately 20 seconds are required to treat the largest hexascan of 13 mm which contains 127 separate spots.

The hexascan device is indicated for any situation where traditional "tracing" by the argon laser technique is likely to produce scarring. It may also be used in conjunction with continuous wave tunable dye laser to break up the beam so that thermal damage is minimal. This results in a safer treatment which may be equivalent to the "selective photothermolysis" of the flashlamp pump dye laser but produced by a different physical parameter. Instead of supershort pulses of 350 μsecond which do not exceed the thermal relaxation time of adjacent tissue, the hexascan produces random short pulses which are widely divergent such that dissipation of unwanted thermal energy occurs between pulses.

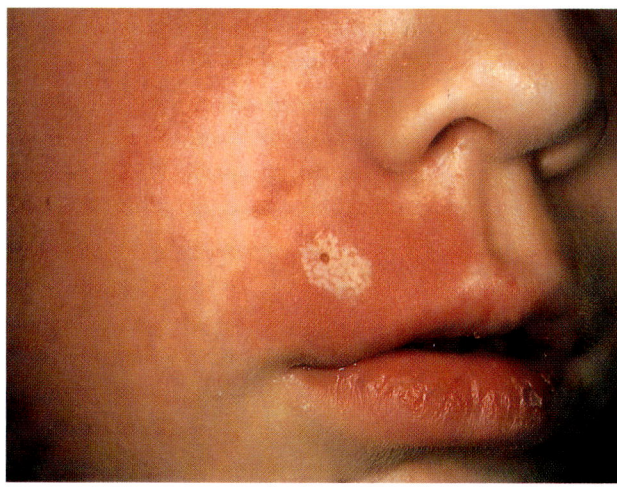

FIG. 8.6-A. Port wine stain of the upper lip prior to treatment with a visible test patch from the continuous wave tunable dye laser.

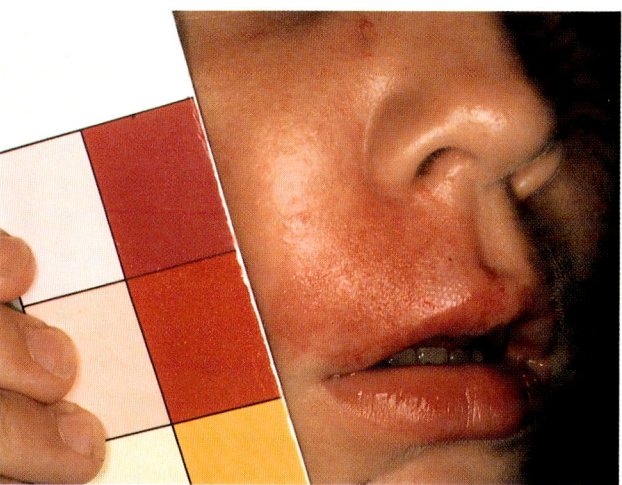

FIG. 8.6-B. Complete hexascan treatment of the upper lip area.

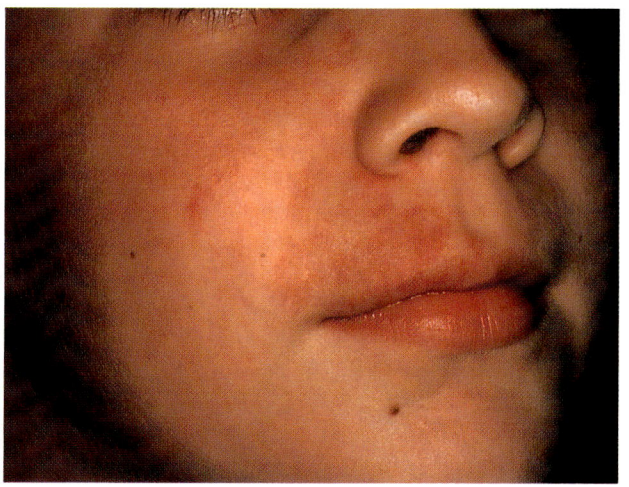

FIG. 8.6-C. Result after hexascan treatment with satisfactory fading.

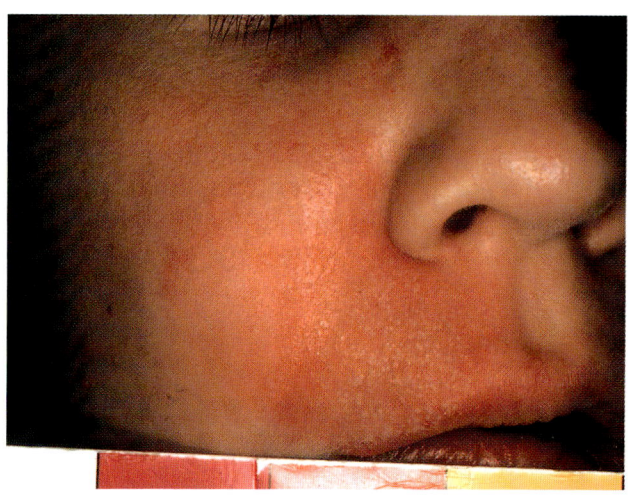

FIG. 8.6-D. Immediately following second hexascan treatment.

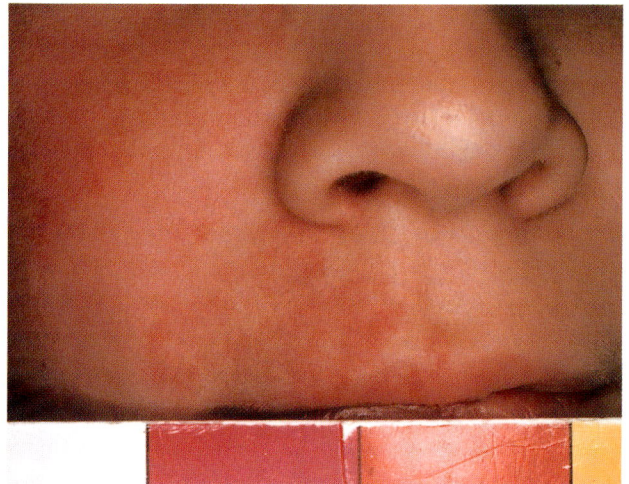

FIG. 8.6-E. Final result with satisfactory blanching and no scarring.

Case courtesy of *David B. Apfelberg*, M.D., and *Teruko Smith*, R.N., P.A.-C.

CASE 8.7

Port Wine Stain of the Leg

REVIEW OF CASE. This 4-year-old female presented with a diffuse port wine stain of the lower extremity. Previous test patches with the argon laser and CO_2 laser resulted in scarring. The tunable laser with hexascan was chosen to prevent further scarring.

CHOICE OF LASER: TUNABLE DYE WITH HEXASCAN. Indications for the hexascan with either the argon laser or tunable dye lasers in the treatment of port wine stains are as follows: (a) in patients under the age of 12, particularly infants and children; (b) in areas of the trunk and extremities in any age patients; (c) in scar prone areas of the face such as the perioral, nasolabial, and nasal skin; (d) in any deeply pigmented patient where hypopigmentation may be likely; and (e) in patients who have previously been successfully but incompletely treated with the argon laser. In all of these instances, either the argon laser or the tunable dye laser with hexascan may produce satisfactory fading without scarring. Between 4 and 9 individual treatments separated by 3 to 6 months may be necessary for fading, which is never total. Some residual hemangioma may remain. Power settings vary from 10 to 40 joules depending on the color and hypertrophy of the lesion. The endpoint of the treatment is a "graying or disappearance" of the vessel but not a white blanching. Post-treatment skin changes should be minimal. Local anesthesia or sedation is required for treatments. Wavelengths of 577–595 nm may be easily tuned.

ADDITIONAL INFORMATION. The hexascan is a computerized, automated scanning device that allows for the rapid and easily reproducible treatment of large areas of skin using either the argon or tunable dye lasers. The scanning pattern is designed to promote uniform energy fluence and minimize unwanted thermal damage to non-target tissue. The 1 mm spots are assembled into hexagons of 3, 5, 9, 11, or 13 mm diameter. The scanning pattern is designed to separate consecutive spots 2 mm apart at 15 μsec intervals in a precise non-adjacent pattern. This allows dissipation of undesired thermal energy between pulses. Approximately 20 seconds are required to treat the largest hexascan of 13 mm which contains 127 separate spots.

The hexascan device is indicated for any situation where traditional "tracing" by the argon laser technique is likely to produce scarring. It may also be used in conjunction with continuous wave tunable dye laser to break up the beam so that thermal damage is minimal. This results in a safer treatment which may be equivalent to the "selective photothermolysis" of the flashlamp pump dye laser but produced by a different physical parameter. Instead of supershort pulses of 350 μsecond which do not exceed the thermal relaxation time of adjacent tissue, the hexascan produces random short pulses which are widely divergent such that dissipation of unwanted thermal energy occurs between pulses.

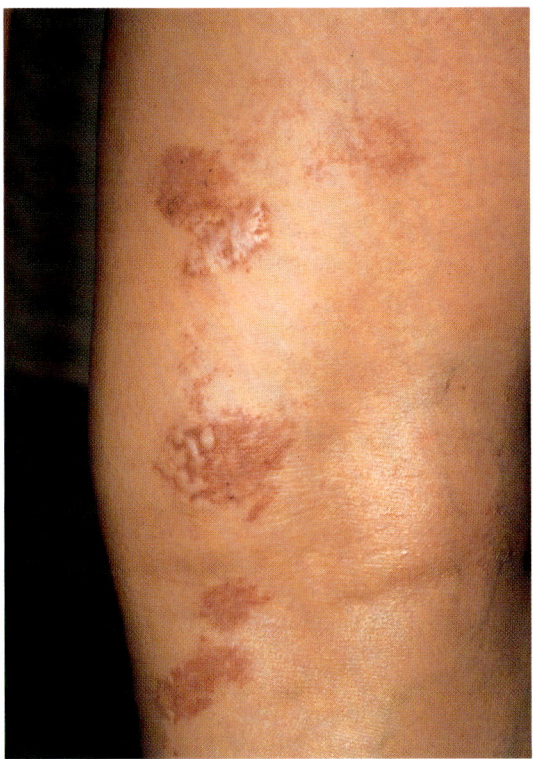

FIG. 8.7-A. Port wine stain of the leg in a 4-year-old child. Scars represent previous test patches with the argon laser and CO_2 laser.

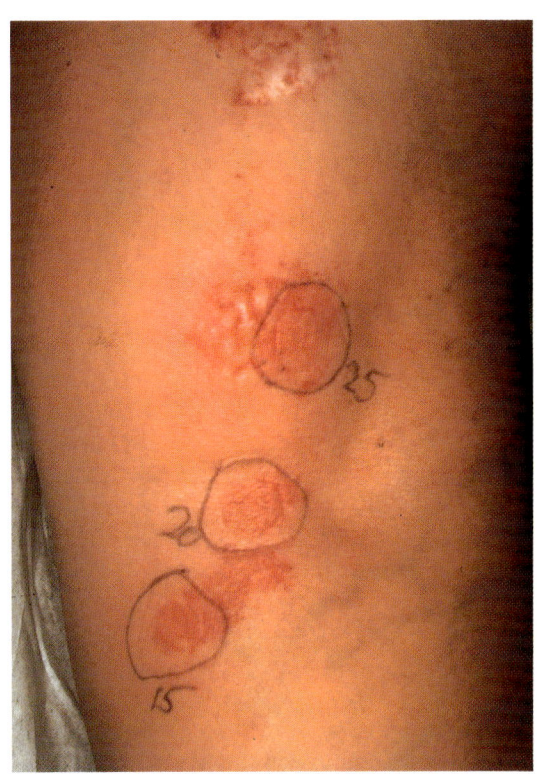

FIG. 8.7-B. Result after hexascan treatment of the areas.

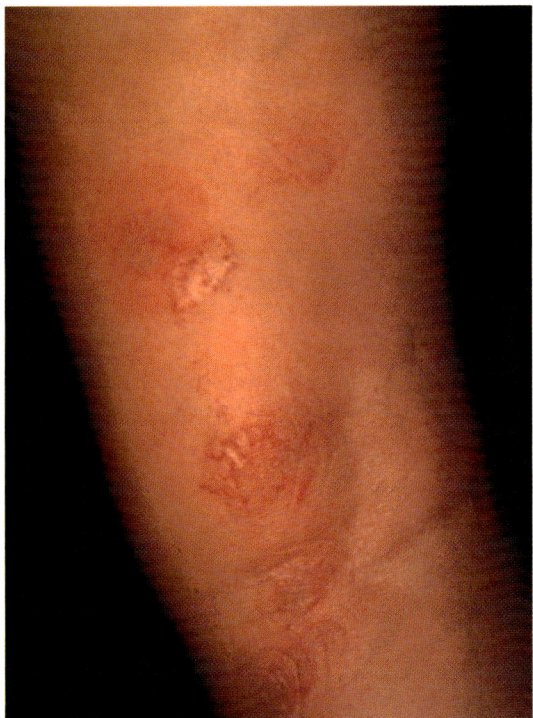

FIG. 8.7-C. Second hexascan treatment of the areas done eight months following the first treatment.

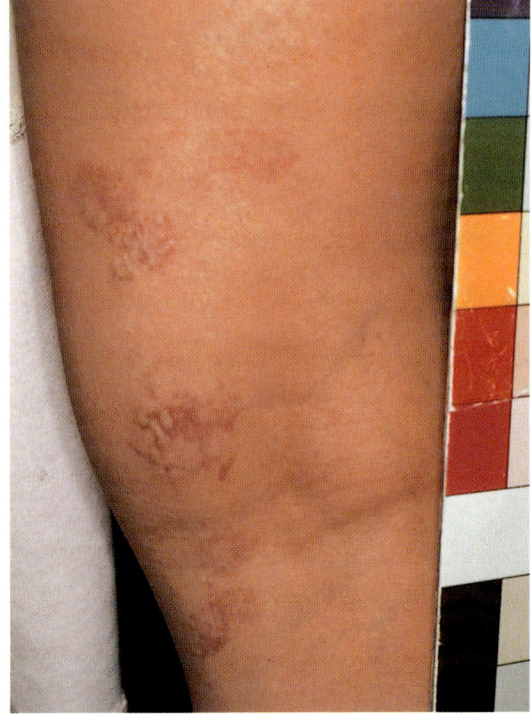

FIG. 8.7-D. Marked blanching and fading 12 months following the first treatment and 3 months following the second treatment.

Case courtesy of *David B. Apfelberg, M.D.*, and *Patricia Z. Spector, R.N., MHS, P.A.-C.*

CASE 8.8

Port Wine Hemangioma of the Extremity with Angiokeratomas

REVIEW OF CASE. This 72-year-old female with a congenital port wine stain of the lower extremity had experienced progressive growth, hypertrophy, and development of angiokeratomas. She had frequent episodes of bleeding with minor trauma.

CHOICE OF LASER: TUNABLE DYE WITH HEXASCAN. Indications for the hexascan with either the argon laser or tunable dye lasers in the treatment of port wine stains are as follows: (a) patients under the age of 12, particularly infants and children; (b) areas of the trunk and extremities in patients of any age; (c) scar prone areas of the face such as the perioral, nasolabial, and nasal skin; (d) any deeply pigmented patient where hypopigmentation may be likely; and (e) patients who have previously been successfully but incompletely treated with the argon laser. In all of these instances, either the argon laser or the tunable dye laser with hexascan may produce satisfactory fading without scarring. Between 4 and 9 individual treatments separated by 3 to 6 months may be necessary for fading, which is never total. Some residual hemangioma may remain. Power settings vary from 10 to 40 joules depending on the color and hypertrophy of the lesion. The endpoint of the treatment is a "graying or disappearance" of the vessel but not a white blanching. Post-treatment skin changes should be minimal. Local anesthesia or sedation is required for treatments. Wavelengths of 577–595 nm may be easily tuned.

ADDITIONAL INFORMATION. The hexascan is a computerized, automated scanning device that allows for the rapid and easily reproducible treatment of large areas of skin using either the argon or tunable dye lasers. The scanning pattern is designed to promote uniform energy fluence and minimize unwanted thermal damage to non-target tissue. The 1 mm spots are assembled into hexagons of 3, 5, 9, 11, or 13 mm diameter. The scanning pattern is designed to separate consecutive spots 2 mm apart at 15 μsec intervals in a precise non-adjacent pattern. This allows dissipation of undesired thermal energy between pulses. Approximately 20 seconds are required to treat the largest hexascan of 13 mm which contains 127 separate spots.

The hexascan device is indicated for any situation where traditional "tracing" by the argon laser technique is likely to produce scarring. It may also be used in conjunction with continuous wave tunable dye laser to break up the beam so that thermal damage is minimal. This results in a safer treatment which may be equivalent to the "selective photothermolysis" of the flashlamp pump dye laser but produced by a different physical parameter. Instead of supershort pulses of 350 μsecond which do not exceed the thermal relaxation time of adjacent tissue, the hexascan produces random short pulses which are widely divergent such that dissipation of unwanted thermal energy occurs between pulses.

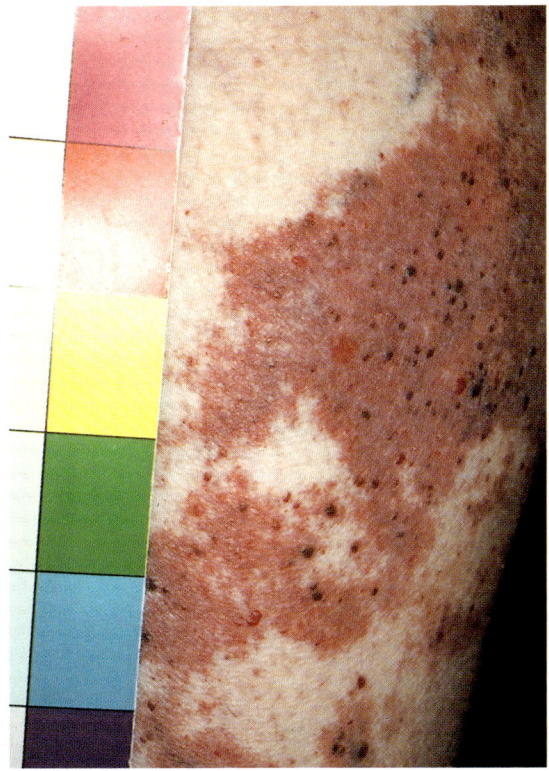

FIG. 8.8-A. Pre-treatment port wine stain of extremity with numerous angiokeratomas.

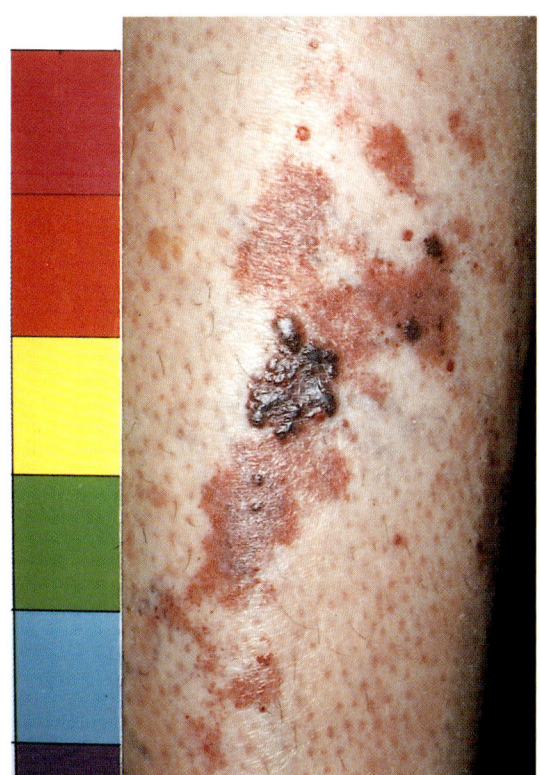

FIG. 8.8-B. Close-up of angiokeratoma area.

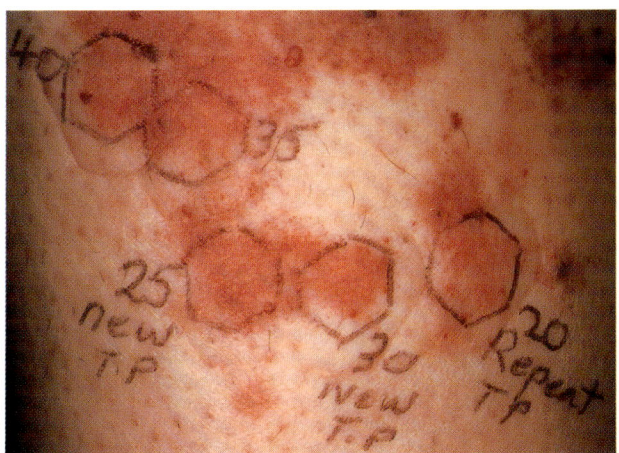

FIG. 8.8-C. Result of hexascan treatment with varying power levels.

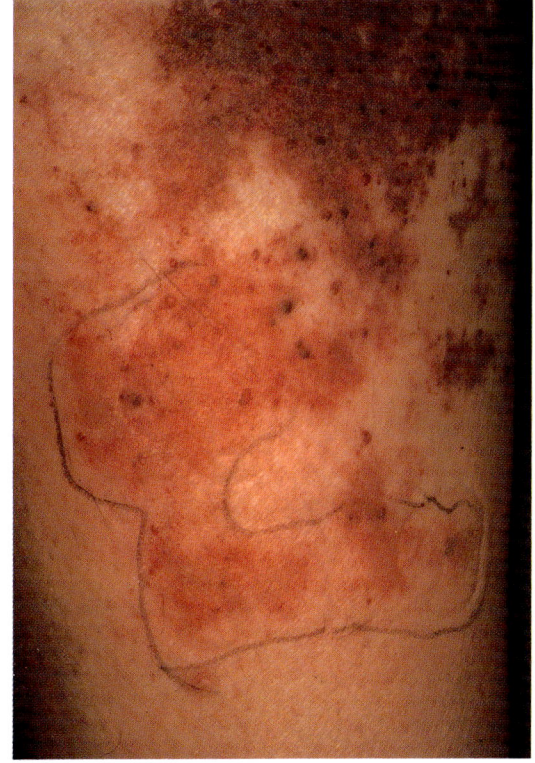

FIG. 8.8-D. Result of hexascan treatment with varying power levels.

TUNABLE DYE LASER WITH HEXASCAN   417

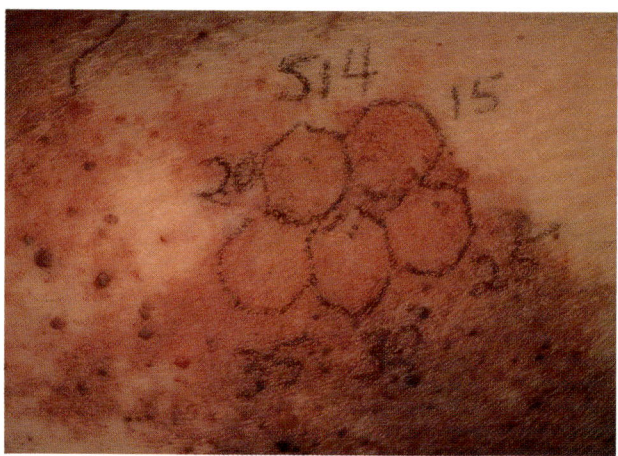

FIG. 8.8-E. Result of further hexascan treatment with varying power levels.

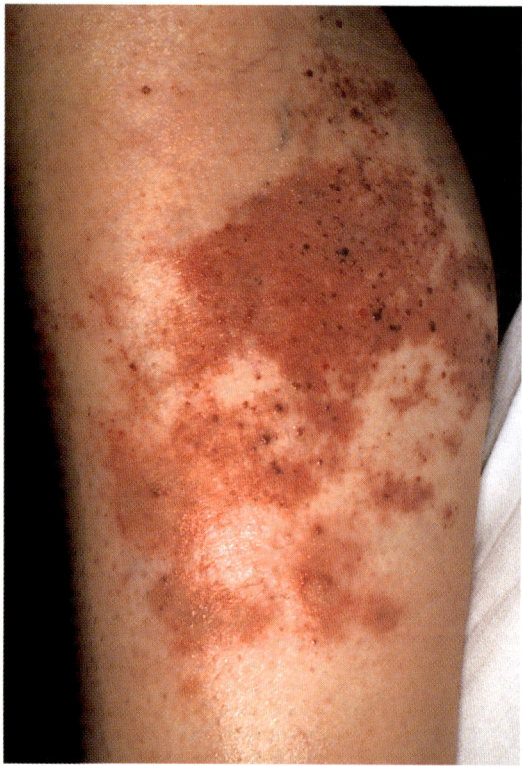

FIG. 8.8-F. Satisfactory fading of port wine stain and angiokeratomas.

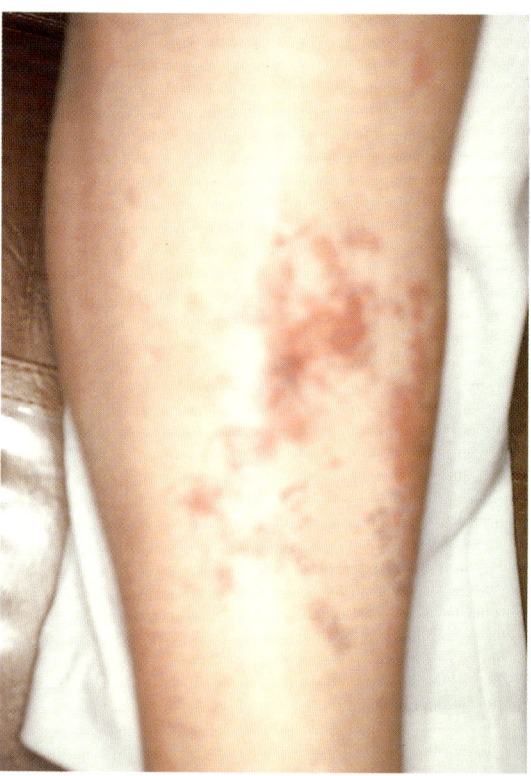

FIG. 8.8-G. Further fading of port wine stain and angiokeratomas.

Case courtesy of *David B. Apfelberg, M.D.*, and *Patricia Z. Spector, R.N., MHS, P.A.-C.*

CASE 8.9
Port Wine Stain of the Face

REVIEW OF CASE. This is a 37-year-old male with a red port wine stain of the left upper lip, nose, and nasolabial fold.

CHOICE OF LASER: GATED ARGON/COPPER LASER TECHNIQUE. The minimal gated laser dose technique is an attempt to reduce the risk of scarring in the treatment of vascular disorders by using various laser systems such as Cosman-argon, copper, and argon dye. The justification is that the maximum total laser dose needed to destroy the targeted vascular tissue can be determined for any given system. Uniform maintenance of this dose will ensure even tissue exposure. Thus a maximum effective dose can be delivered with reduction in overtreatment. Such overtreatment may result in an increased risk of scarring due to increased non-target tissue heating without a subsequent increase in vessel ablation.

ADDITIONAL INFORMATION. Several parameters need to be controlled to offer safe therapy. These include definable and repeatable power density and fluence levels from surgeon to surgeon. Thus gating the laser output ensures an exact pulse width and energy output to a corresponding uniform beam diameter. Patients are first tested with a 1 mm beam at either 0.1–0.2 second pulse widths. The energy output should be in the range of approximately 0.2 watts and increased by 0.05 watts until clinical blanching is achieved. It appears that this level will achieve maximum clinical response. This technique can be adapted for all beam sizes, desired pulsed widths, appropriate laser systems, and multiple clinical entities. It should be obvious that it is difficult to measure the actual fluence incidence upon tissue when a continuous beam is utilized in that even a slight change in speed of movement of the beam can dramatically alter these energy levels.

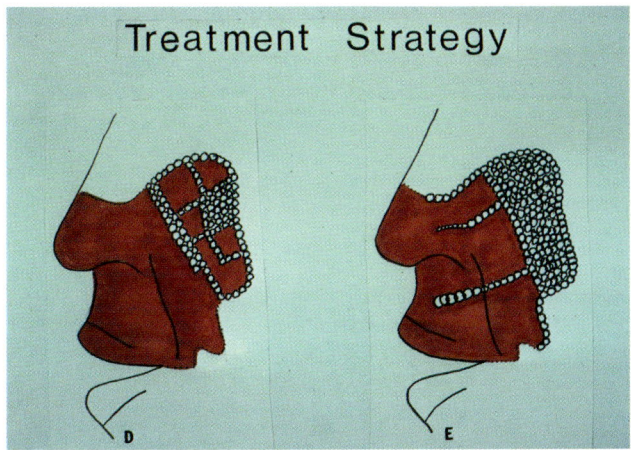

FIG. 8.9-A. Diagram of multiple gated 1 mm pulses placed side by side to accurately and uniformly treat a desired area.

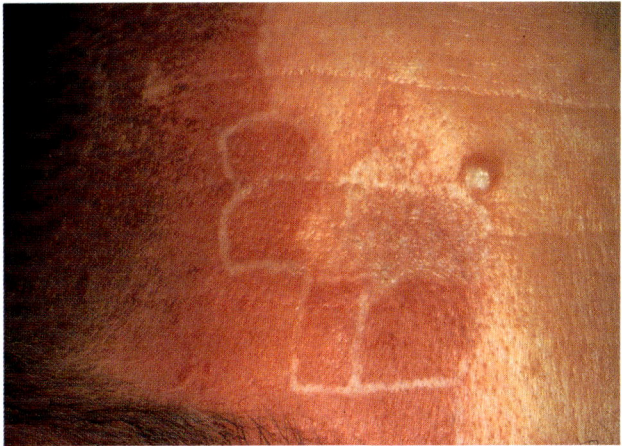

FIG. 8.9-B. Corresponding clinical effects on a port wine stain demonstrate this uniformity.

Case courtesy of *Alan Schliftman*, M.D., and *Gary Brauner*, M.D.

CASE 8.10
Port Wine Stain Hemangioma of the Lower Leg

REVIEW OF CASE. This is a 23-year-old female with a large port wine stain hemangioma involving the left lower leg.

CHOICE OF LASER: TUNABLE DYE WITH HEXASCAN. The hexascan robotic scanning handpiece was selected in this case because of its proven ability to perform well on extremity port wine stain and also because of the rapidity of treating large areas. This could also have been treated with the flashlamp pulsed dye laser or microspot tracing with the argon pumped dye laser but the hexascan was selected because of its ability to produce the best results with the fewest number of treatments.

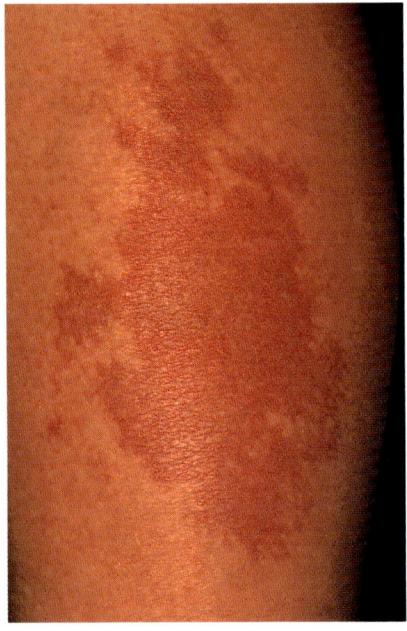 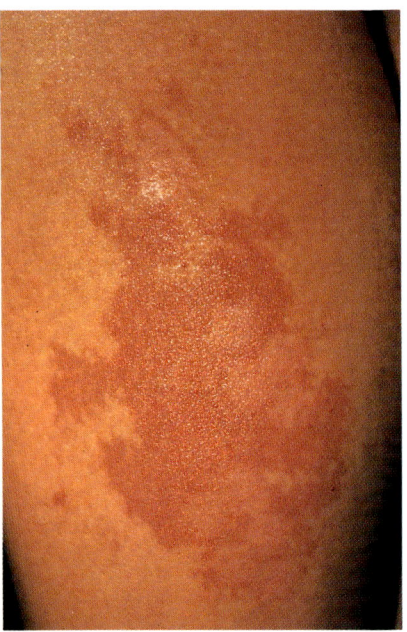 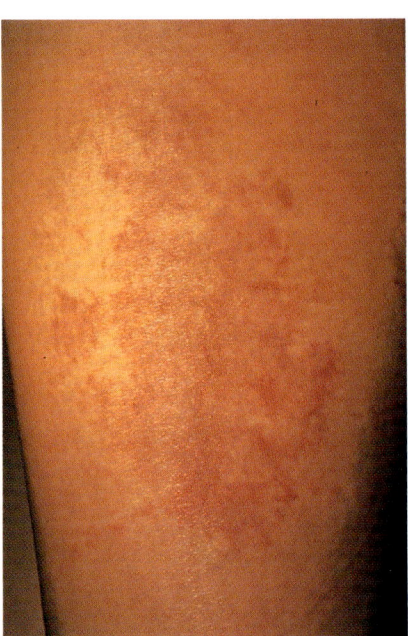

FIG. 8.10-A. Baseline photograph of port wine stain hemangioma. This area was treated using topical 30% Xylocaine cream applied 1 hour prior to treatment.

FIG. 8.10-B. Six weeks after two sets of test areas were performed using 13 mm hexagonal treated fields. Note the dramatic lightening after only a short time interval.

FIG. 8.10-C. Area 3 months after the entire area received one treatment using 585 nm light, 13 mm hexagonal field size, and 20 joules energy at 130 μsec pulse length.

Case courtesy of *David H. McDaniel*, M.D.

CASE 8.11
Port Wine Hemangioma of the Face and Neck

REVIEW OF CASE. This is a 20-year-old female with a large congenital port wine stain of the right hemiface and neck (about 150 cm^2). No previous treatment has been received.

CHOICE OF LASER: ARGON DYE WITH HEXASCAN. Argon laser was chosen to photocoagulate this port wine stain. During the last ten years, this laser was proved to be efficient for this indication. Because of high absorption at the green light, the treatment is achieved by thermal coagulation of abnormal vessels in the upper part of the dermis. The hexascan was chosen because it is the only device capable of performing laser sessions easily, rapidly, and with a great reproducibility with different physicians. This system includes a control of heat diffusion in the treated area, and it was proved to be efficient and safe, giving far less hypertrophic scar than a conventional handpiece.

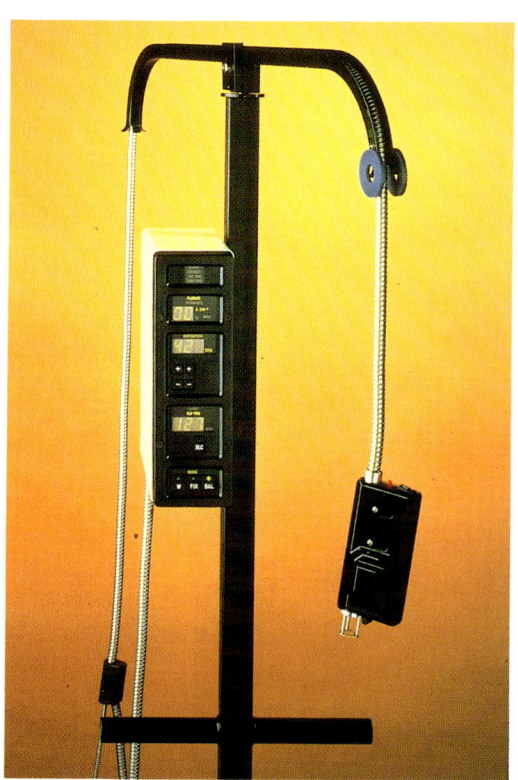

FIG. 8.11-A. The hexascan includes: (a) a control box with microprocessor, displaying the following parameters: power, fluence, pulse length, and size of hexagonal fields (3 to 13 mm); (b) a scanning handpiece which is put on the skin surface and provides a hexagonal irradiation pattern; and (c) an optic fiber easily adaptable to the laser source.

Case continues on following page.

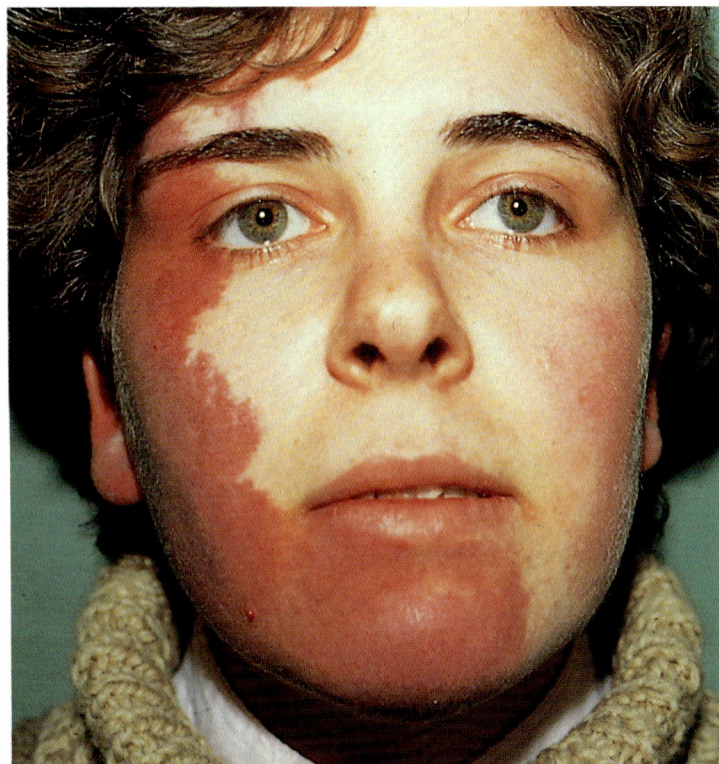

FIG. 8.11-B. Port wine stain prior to treatment. Note the large size and the purple color of the lesion. After several successful test patches, the treatment program was begun, including monthly outpatient sessions.

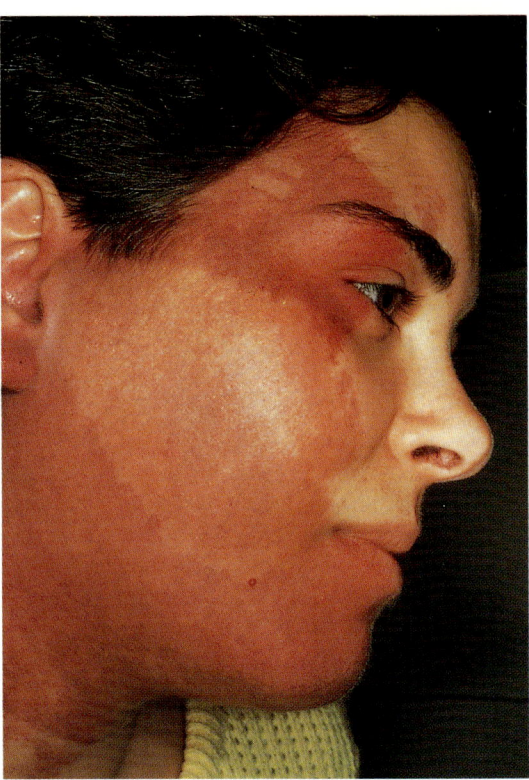

FIG. 8.11-C. Result one month after first laser session. The whole cheek was treated (about 40 cm^2). Note the homogeneity of blanching. The parameters were: fluence = 18 J/cm^2, pulse length = 40 μsec, spot diameter = 1 mm, and output power = 3–5 watts.

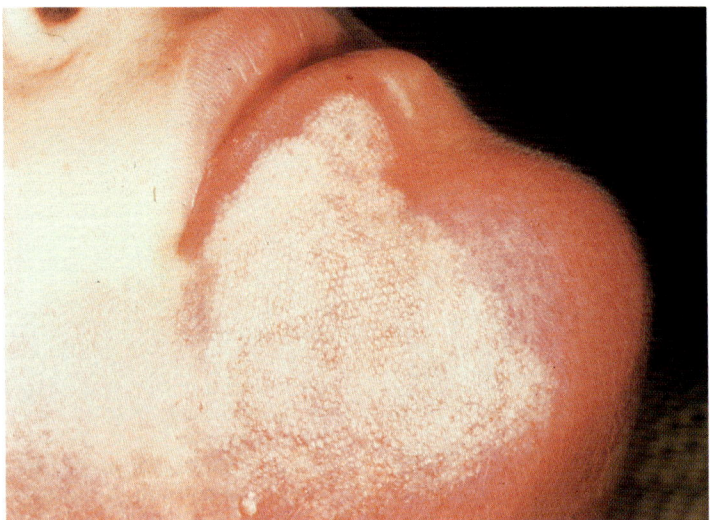

FIG. 8.11-D. Immediately after second session, 25 hexagonal fields of 13 mm were juxtaposed on the chin. Identical parameters were used. Note the white grayish appearance immediately after laser impacts.

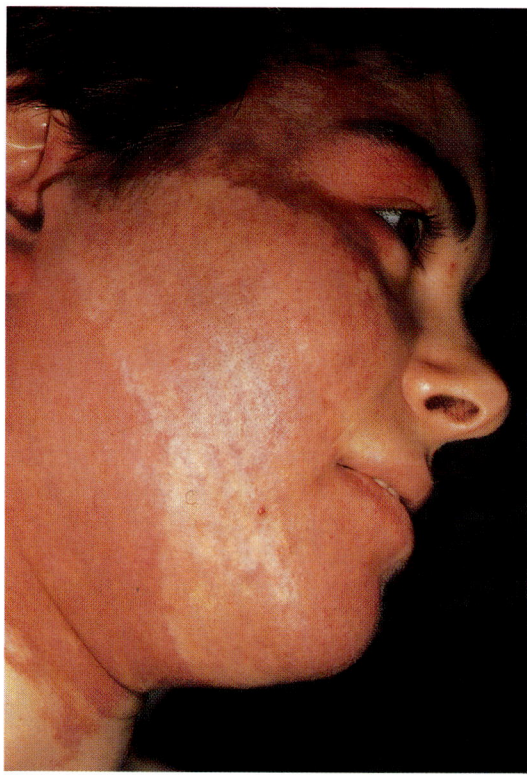

FIG. 8.11-E. Result one month after second session.

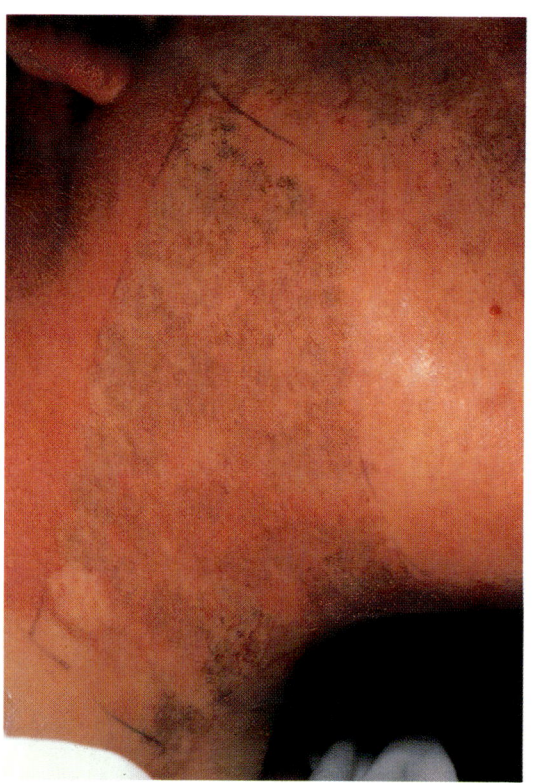

FIG. 8.11-F. Immediately after treatment of a large area of the neck. Such a scanning with the hexascan takes about 10 minutes. Note the test patch previously performed (at bottom of figure).

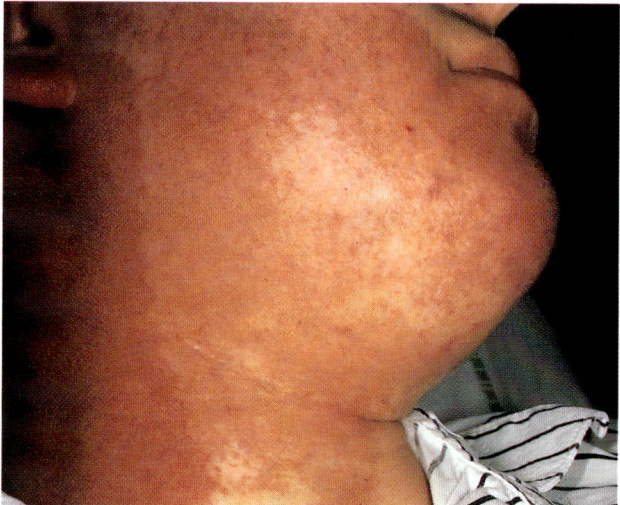

FIG. 8.11-G. One month later. Note the quality of blanching and the lack of pathologic scar.

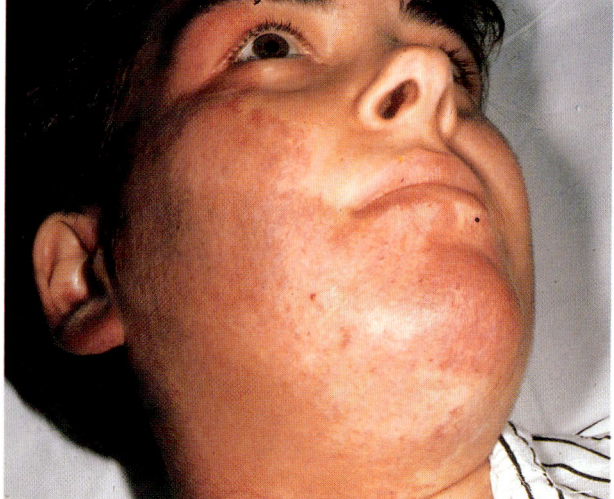

FIG. 8.11-H. Final appearance after six outpatient sessions. After every session, the patient was instructed to keep the wound dry during the crust stage (the first week) and to apply sunscreen for several months thereafter.

Case courtesy of *Guy Rotteleur,* M.D., *Serge Mordon,* Ph.D., and *J. M. Brunetaud,* M.D.

CASE 8.12

Port Wine Hemangioma of the Face and Neck

REVIEW OF CASE. This 27-year-old male presented with a deep purple, slightly hypertrophic port wine hemangioma of the face and neck.

CHOICE OF LASER: KTP. The KTP laser is a frequency doubled neodymium:YAG laser producing all its output at 532 nm. The green light is directed through a series of fiberoptics from the source to the end output. The green light is preferentially absorbed by hemoglobin in abnormal vasculature, converted to heat, and this heat coagulates vessels. Adjacent skin appendages are relatively spared by the laser light and aid in the healing of the laser wound. For this study, a power of 0.5 to 0.9 watts, spot size of 1 mm, and continuous setting according to skin blanching was used.

ADDITIONAL INFORMATION. In this study, the argon laser and the KTP 532 nm laser were evaluated in a side by comparison. Identical parameters of power, spot size, and pulse duration were utilized in each area. Clinical and histological results proved equivalent between the two lasers.

POST-TREATMENT CARE. Iced saline compresses and topical antibiotic ointment with open wound treatment were used.

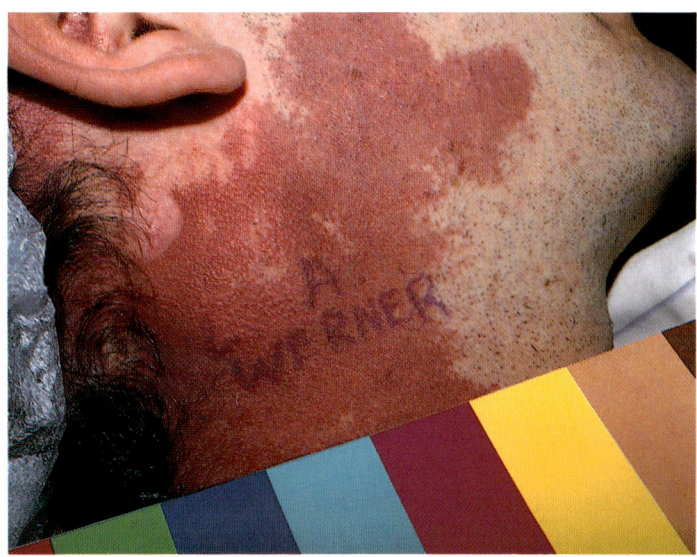

FIG. 8.12-A. Port wine hemangioma of face and neck prior to treatment.

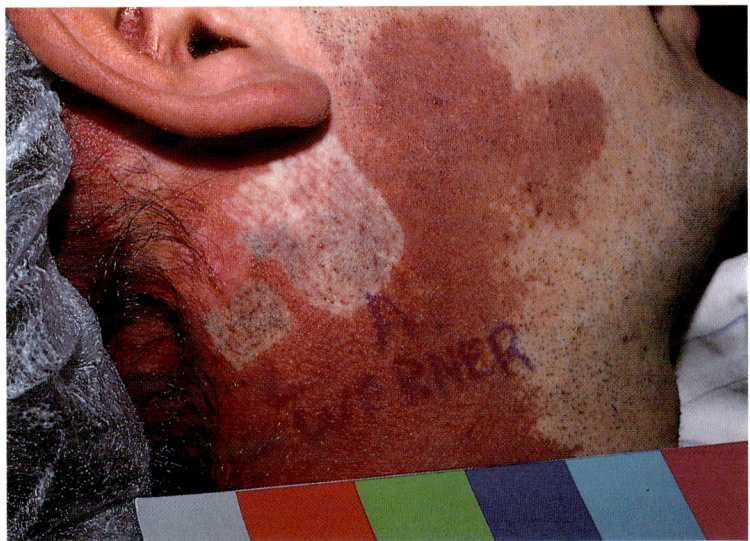

FIG. 8.12-B. Immediately after treatment, a dark gray photocoagulation effect is visible in both the argon (A) and the KTP 532 nm (Laserscope L) areas.

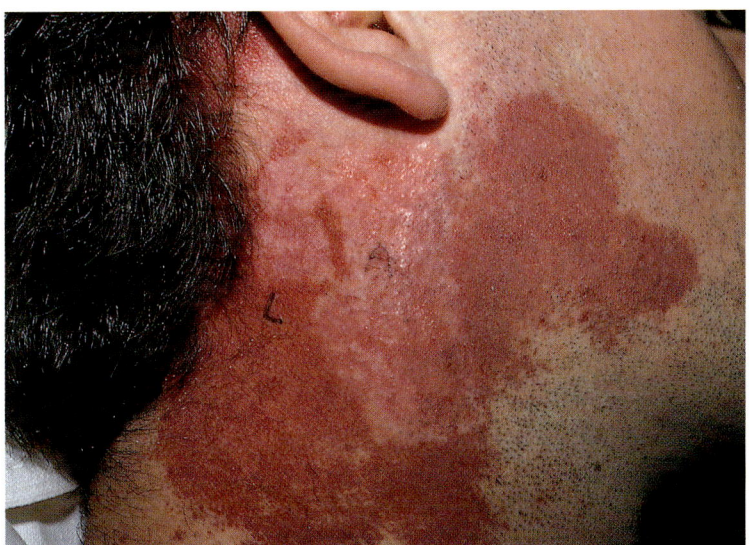

FIG. 8.12-C. Final clinical result demonstrating satisfactory blanching of hemangioma 4 months after treatment, with results equivalent between the argon and the KTP lasers.

Case courtesy of *David B. Apfelberg*, M.D.

Reprinted with permission of Wiley-Liss, a division of John Wiley and Sons, Inc, copyright © 1986.
For literature pertaining to this case see References section.

CASE 8.13

Telangiectasia of the Face with Persistent Erythema

REVIEW OF CASE. This is a 39-year-old female with a dense network of facial telangiectasia and persistent erythema. No topical corticosteroid has been previously applied. The telangiectasia appeared progressively and the persistent erythema was preceded by attacks of facial flushes for several years. There was no episode of papulopustular eruption.

CHOICE OF LASER: ARGON DYE WITH HEXASCAN. The argon laser was chosen to photocoagulate these telangiectasia because it is the most suitable laser for vascular abnormalities. Because of the important vessel network and the existence of a persistent erythema, classical electrocauterization was not appropriate. Dermabrasion and chemical peeling were not considered because of the risk of scarring. The use of a classical handpiece with the argon laser was not suitable for these widespread telangiectasias. On the other hand, a robotized scanning handpiece such as hexascan has indisputable advantages: (a) shorter treatment time (about 10 minutes in an outpatient session for coagulating 20 cm^2), (b) easy to use, (c) persistent control of energy dosage during the treatment, (d) more reproducibility with different physicians and from one session to another one, and (e) greater homogeneity in blanching. Moreover, the persistent erythema is treated at the same time. The whole area is treated just like a port wine stain.

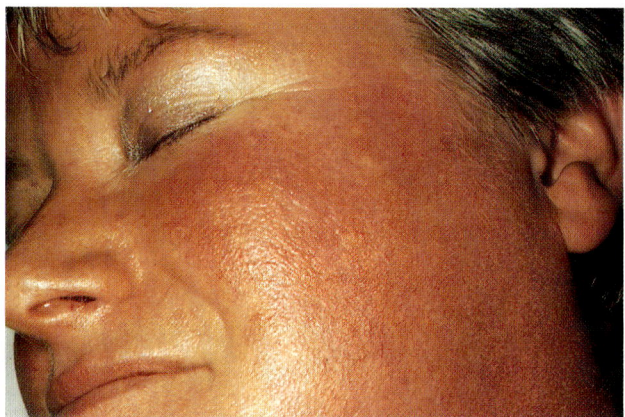

FIG. 8.13-A. Widespread telangiectasia of the face with persistent erythema just before the first session.

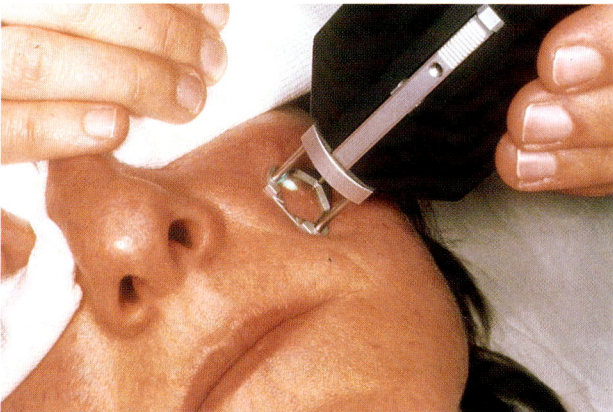

FIG. 8.13-B. Hexascan handpiece during the treatment. A 20 cm² area was photocoagulated in the middle of the cheek with the hexascan (13 mm hexagonal field, fluence 16 J/cm², spot diameter 1 mm, pulse length 40 μsec, and output power 3 watts).

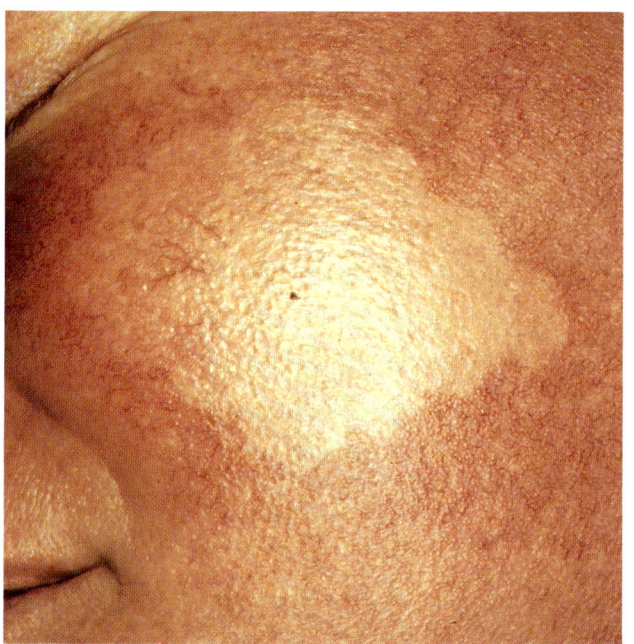

FIG. 8.13-C. One month after the first session. Note the quality and homogeneity of blanching and the absence of scar.

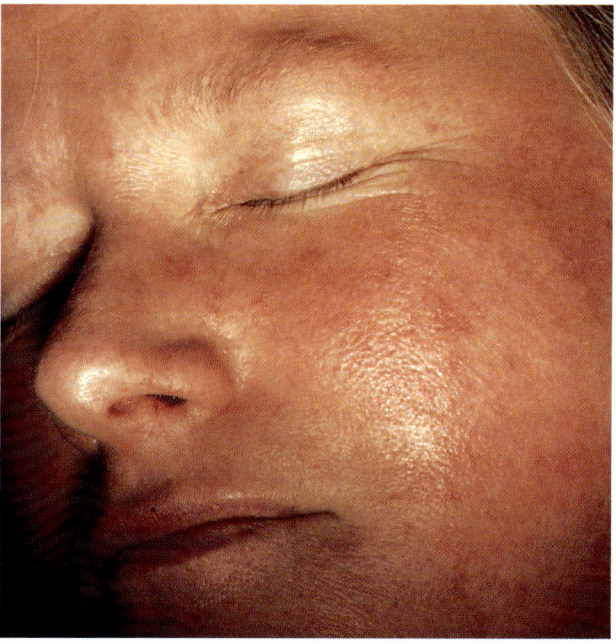

FIG. 8.13-D. Final appearance after 8 outpatient sessions. Every treatment session was carried out without anesthesia. The only post-operative care consisted of the application of sunscreen for several months.

Case courtesy of *Guy Rotteleur, M.D., Serge Mordon, Ph.D.,* and *J. M. Brunetaud, M.D.*

CASE 8.14
Basal Cell Carcinoma of the Nose

REVIEW OF CASE. This patient is an 80-year-old female with extensive basal cell (basosquamous variety) carcinoma of the nose. She has had a previous horizontally controlled serial excision auriculectomy for a similar lesion on the left ear. She is neither medically fit for a rhinectomy and reconstruction nor desirous of this procedure.

With our current treatment regimen, photofrin is infused intravenously 48 hours prior to treatment as an outpatient in a dose of 1 mg/kg. Areas of retention of photofrin in the tumors are detected by inciting fluorescence with a krypton laser operating in the 408 nm violet range (Figs. A and B). The entire nose and right nasolabial area are treated with a surface dose of 250 J/cm^2 using an argon dye laser at 630 nm (Fig. C). The tumor in the right nasolabial area is implanted with cylinder implants utilizing a dose of an additional 200 J/cm^2 of cylinder to cover all areas of possible spread (Fig. D). Balloon treatment inside the nares was not used in this instance.

Retreatment of selected areas that biopsied positive for tumor was necessary 6 weeks later in this instance. A complete response of the tumor was obtained. The patient died of other causes more than 4 years after photodynamic therapy (PDT), but had been free of tumor at her death (Figs. E and F). Cosmetically, the nose appeared normal without evidence of scar.

CHOICE OF LASER: ARGON DYE AND KRYPTON. PDT was chosen for this patient because of the amount of multifocal disease, the age and infirmity of the patient, and the mutilation and recovery that would be required to resect these tumors (a rhinectomy with forehead flap reconstruction).

ADDITIONAL INFORMATION. For PDT to be effective, all areas of potential tumor spread must be treated with 630 nm laser light in adequate dosage. Penetration of laser light through skin and tumor reaches a depth of approximately 0.5 cm. Areas deeper than this need to be either implanted with light-bearing probes or retreated after more superficial tumor has sloughed. Alternately the areas of superficial tumor can be debrided with a CO_2 laser and the deeper tumor treated with PDT.

The nasoalar area is one of the most difficult to treat as tumor can travel along embryologic fusion planes. This must be taken into account during the treatment process. Pre-surgical planning and treatment of all potential areas of tumor spread is essential.

In a large series, this regimen of PDT was shown to have an 88% complete response (CR) rate with one treatment. The CR rate increased to 100% with one retreatment. We have found that photodynamic therapy is particularly useful and effective for auricular tumors where mutilation of the auricle is necessary. This application is of interest because of the poor control rates with other therapeutic modalities.

POST-TREATMENT CARE. After injection with 1 mg/kg of Photofrin, patients experience a transient photosensitivity and must avoid direct sunlight for 3–6 weeks. Patients may travel to work, but should keep exposed skin covered.

An eschar will form in treated areas where tumor is present. Healing will take place over 3–5 weeks in heavily involved areas of tumor. During this time patients should shower frequently to keep the area clean and apply ointments such as Silvadene to the area.

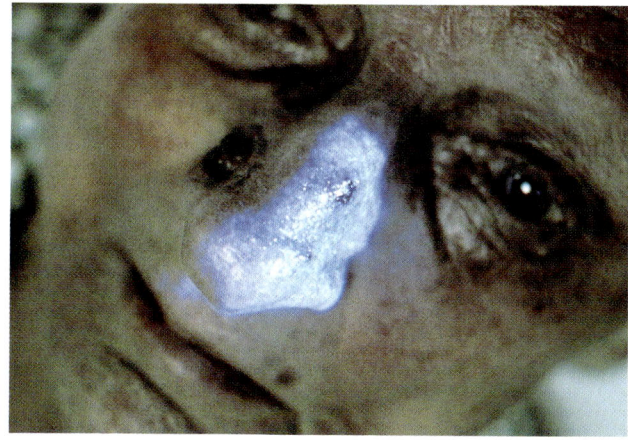

FIG. 8.14-A. Violet light from a krypton laser illuminates the left nose.

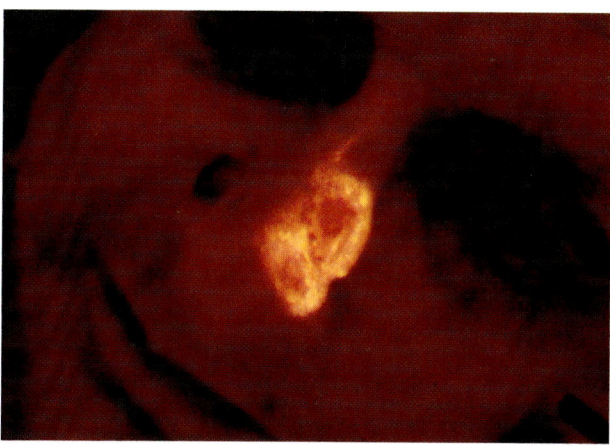

FIG. 8.14-B. Area viewed through an argon safety glass to filter out the violet. Salmon pink fluorescence (630–650 nm) of tumor areas can now be visualized.

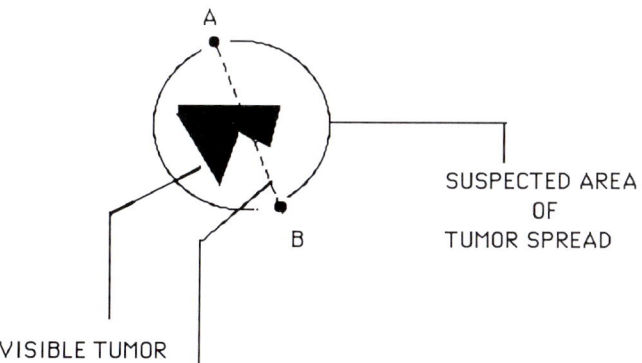

1. Place dots (A&B) to delineate the diameter of the proposed treatment area circle. The treatment area circle encompasses all suspected areas of tumor spread.
2. Use a micrometer to measure the diameter (D) in cm. D = AB.
3. Calculate area of treatment circle in cm^2. Area = $\pi \times$ (1/2 D)^2.
4. Establish delivery rate (>0.2 W/cm^2) to minimize hyperthermia.
5. Calculate laser power settings in watts. W/cm^2 = 0.2 W = 0.2 × Area.
6. Establish treatment dosage: 200 – 250 J/cm^2 based on experience for basal cell carcinoma with an injected dose of 1.0 mg/kg of Photofrin II.
7. Calculate treatment time (t). J/cm^2 = W/cm^2 × t. t = J/cm^2/W/cm^2.
8. Focus laser circle from microlens fiber so that it falls between the two dots. Set laser to desired power using global power meter. Treat for calculated period of time.

FIG. 8.14-C. Forward surface treatment for PDT. Most tumors can be treated with this method alone.

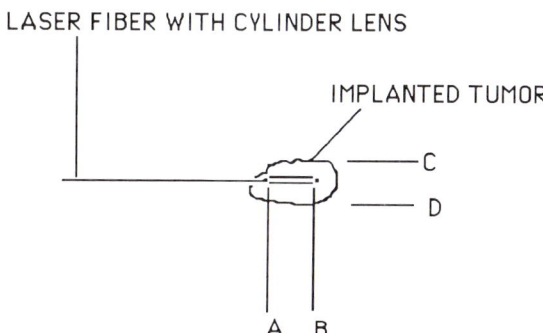

1. AB = length of cylinder diffusing lens implanted into tumor.
2. Premise: since tumor is inserted into tissue, an exact area distribution of light cannot be made. Therefore, all energy distribution is calculated on the basis of energy (J)/fiber length (cm).
3. Establish the delivery rate: since the cylinder is inserted into tissue that acts as a heat sink, we increase our dose delivery rate to 0.4 W/cm.
4. Calculate laser power settings in watts: W = 0.4 × AB.
5. Establish treatment dosage: 200 J/cm in this case based on our experience.
6. Calculate laser time setting: time (t) = total dose/dose rate. t = 200 J/cm/0.4 W/cm.
7. Place cylinder into global power meter and set to calculated power (W). Implant cylinder into tumor. Treat for calculated period of time. If three dimensional tumor is greater than 0.8 cm (CD), parallel insertions will need to be made.

FIG. 8.14-D. Cylinder implantation for PDT.

Case continues on following page.

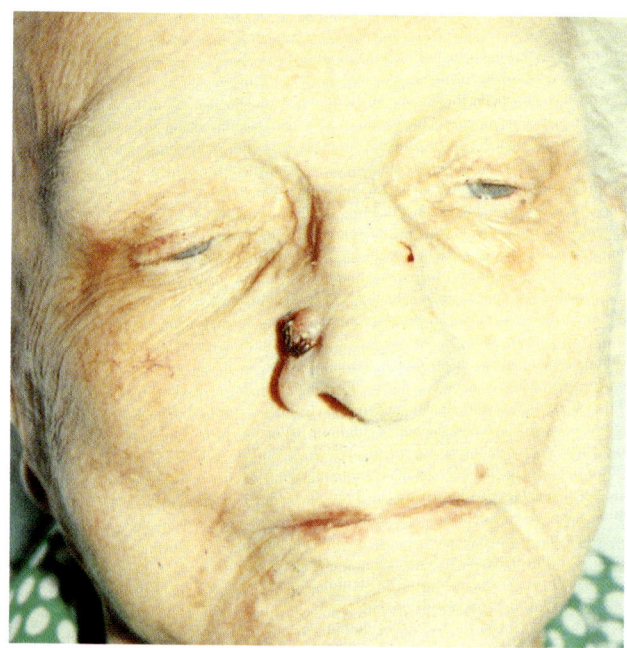

FIG. 8.14-E. Pre-operative patient with multifocal basal cell carcinoma of the nose.

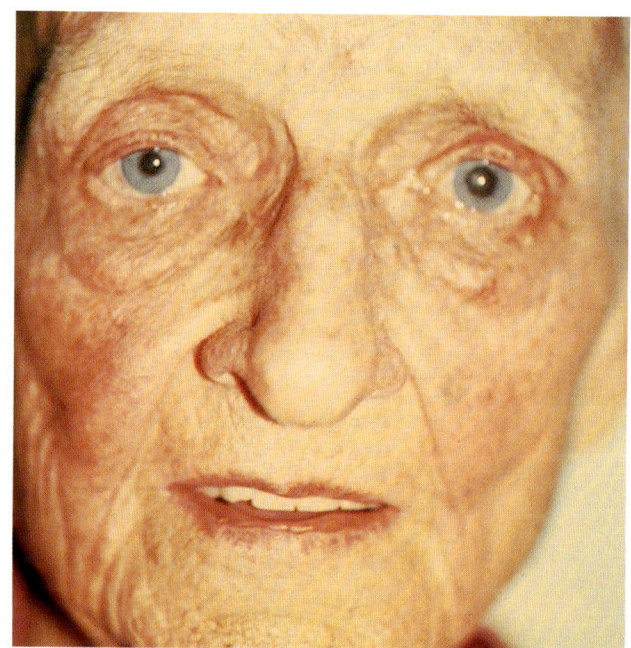

FIG. 8.14-F. Patient 1 year post-operation. Note absence of scar. Patient was tumor-free 4 years post-operation before her death of other causes.

Case courtesy of *Gregory S. Keller, M.D.*

CASE 8.15
Basal Cell Carcinoma of the Nose

REVIEW OF CASE. This 75-year-old male presented at the dermatology clinic with a history of basal cell carcinoma. Seven biopsy-proven basal cell carcinoma sites were found. One lesion on the nose was of particular importance, measuring 3–3.5 cm diameter on the surface. The other sites ranged from 0.5–1.0 cm diameter. The lesion on the nose was open, ulcerated, painful, and had chronic drainage.

CHOICE OF LASER: ARGON DYE. Photodynamic therapy (PDT) utilizing the argon dye laser was chosen to treat the lesions. This investigational procedure involves the i.v. injection of the photosensitizing drug Photofrin, which is selectively retained by tumor cells at a higher concentration than most normal tissues. Upon activation with 630 nm light from the dye laser via a fiberoptic, the drug in an excited state may transfer the absorbed energy to endogenous molecular oxygen. The excited state of oxygen which results, singlet oxygen, is a powerful oxidizing agent which may then proceed to kill the cell, if enough has been produced. The overall result is a selective cytotoxic effect on tumor cells, while only sublethally affecting the surrounding normal skin. The only side effect of this therapy is prolonged cutaneous photosensitivity which may last 4–6 weeks. With the proper choice of drug and light combinations a significant depth effect may be attained, thereby making it possible to treat large tumors at various depths and sparing normal tissues. It has been shown that using a 1 mg/kg injected dose of the photosensitizer Photofrin II doses of upwards of 225 J/cm^2 may be effectively given to achieve necrosis of ~2 cm in the tumor yet sparing the surrounding normal tissues. Healing of the treated area may be complete within 4 weeks post-treatment for smaller tumors 1.0 cm, or may take 6–8 weeks for larger tumors >1.0 cm. The primary option for this patient consisted of surgical removal, which would have resulted in the loss of a substantial section of his nose necessitating surgical reconstruction.

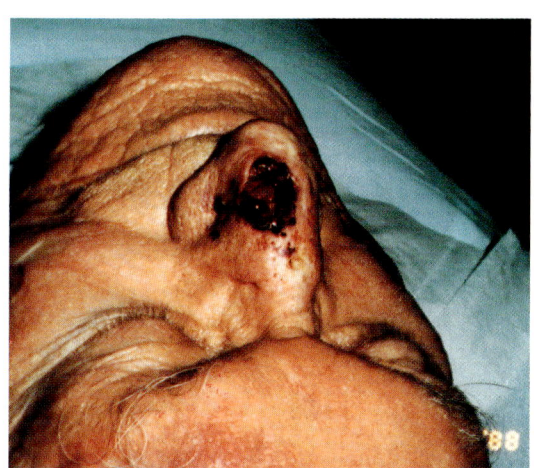

FIG. 8.15-A. Large ulcerative basal cell carcinoma that is draining and mildly painful. The lesion measured 2.5 cm in diameter. This lesion had been treated unsuccessfully with surgery in the past. PDT was given as an option due to the extent of the lesion. The patient's only other option was extensive surgery, which would result in a considerable defect with resultant reconstructive surgery. It was determined, due to the size of this lesion, that two treatment sessions with two injections of Photofrin would be required to eradicate this tumor.

Case continues on following page.

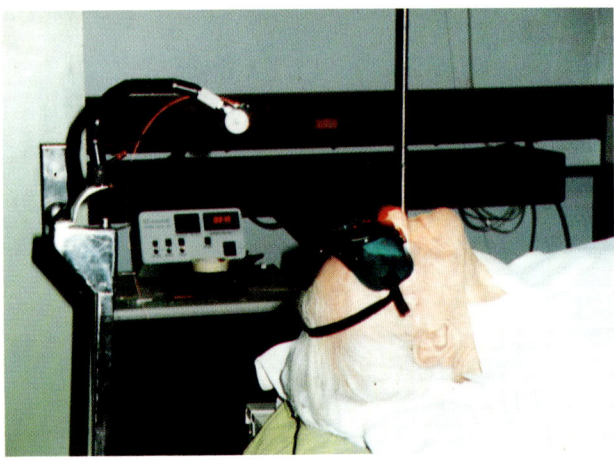

FIG. 8.15-B. PDT was administered 48 hours post-injection of 1 mg/kg of Photofrin i.v. Using an argon dye laser, 630 nm (red) light was delivered via fiberoptic with a diverging lens tip. The light was focused on a 3 cm spot, thus giving a 5 mm margin around the tumor diameter. The light was delivered at a power density of 150 mW/cm^2 for a total dose of 250 J/cm^2.

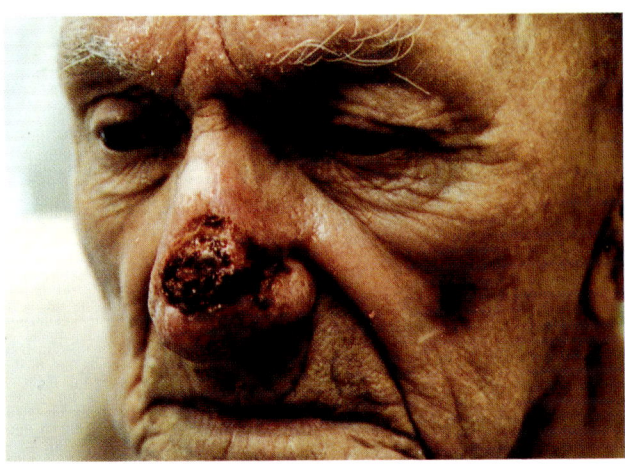

FIG. 8.15-C. Ten days post-treatment the mass of the tumor is necrotic. Normal tissue damage surrounding the tumor is absent. Some necrotic tissue was debrided, and the patient received a second injection of Photofrin (1 mg/kg) on the 21st day post-number 1 injection. The nose was retreated using 150 mW/cm^2, for a total dose of 225 J/cm^2 in the same manner as previously described.

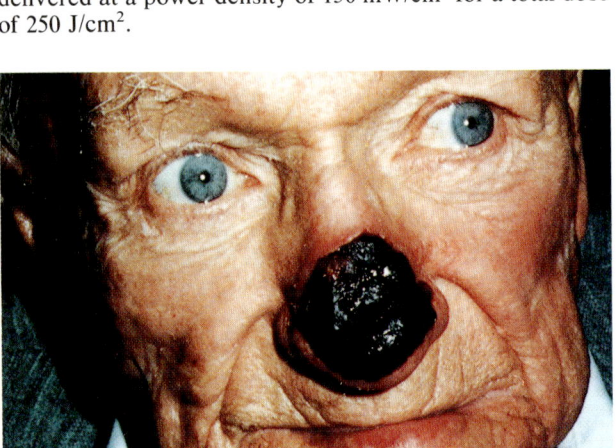

FIG. 8.15-D. Two weeks post-second PDT administration. A large scab formed over the necrotic debris of the full tumor dimension. Normal tissue which had been included in the treatment volume was not irreversibly damaged.

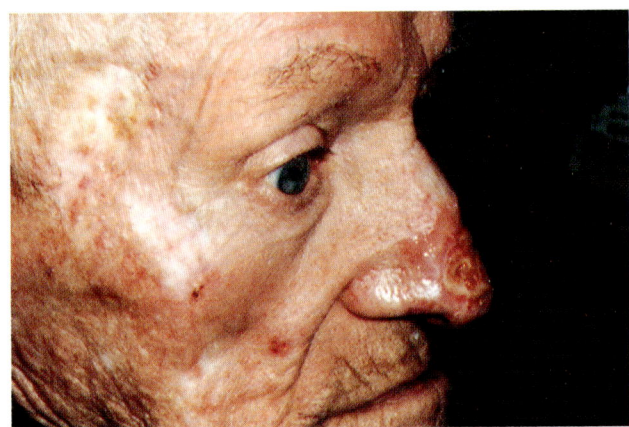

FIG. 8.15-E. Six weeks post-treatment. Scab has been removed non-surgically. Re-epithelialization is apparent. No residual tumor is clinically evident.

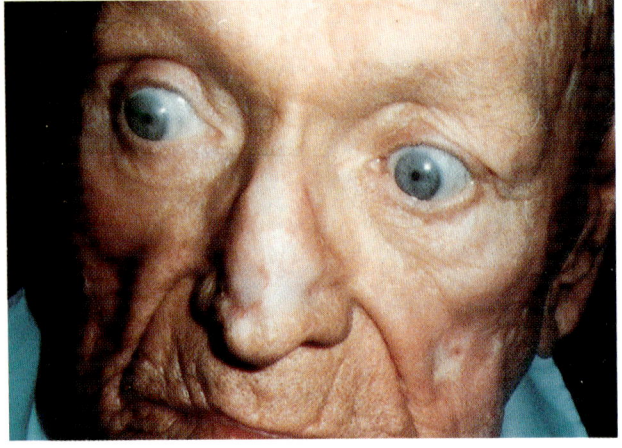

FIG. 8.15-F. Approximately 8 months post-second treatment. Area is completely healed with no further evidence of tumor. Last follow-up at 18 months post-treatment showed treatment area was free of tumor with excellent cosmetic results.

Case courtesy of **Brummitte D. Wilson**, M.D., **Thomas S. Mang**, Ph.D., and **Thomas J. Dougherty**, Ph.D.

CASE 8.16

Squamous Cell Carcinoma of the Eyelid

REVIEW OF CASE. A squamous cell cancer was present on the eyelid of an 83-year-old man with severe Parkinson's disease and severe cardiac disease. Accordingly, he was considered a high risk for general anesthesia. Local anesthesia appeared to be unsuitable for the extent of the resection that would be required and the location of the cancer made the radiotherapist reluctant to use ionizing irradiation. Therefore he received three surface irradiations of 8 minutes each, three and five months apart following presensitization with i.v. DHE or HPD before each photodynamic therapy treatment (PDT).

CHOICE OF LASER: ARGON DYE. Since the photosensitizer absorbs 630 nm wavelength light (red) and this has the deepest penetration of tissue (0.5 to 1.0 cm), the light energy for the activation of the sensitizer is generated by a tunable argon dye laser system. This permits couling of the red light beam to quartz fibers which can then be used with modifications to treat external surface tumors, inserted interstitially directly into large tumors, passed through any endoscope to treat intraluminal tumors, or inserted behind the retina to treat tumors of the retina.

ADDITIONAL INFORMATION. PDT is a new form of treatment of malignant tumors by high intensity light which selectively destroys cancers previously sensitized by a photosensitizer. Following the i.v. injection of the photosensitizer dihematoporphyrin either (DHE, Lederle, Quadralogic) the sensitizer goes to all the cells. However, it clears from normal tissue more rapidly than from cancerous tissue so in two or three days there is a higher concentration in the cancer cells relative to the adjacent normal tissue. When the cancer is exposed to light of the proper wavelength the sensitizer absorbs the light energy and produces singlet oxygen radical which then destroys the cancer cell. Since there is less sensitizer in the adjacent normal tissue it reacts less or not at all. A simplistic analogy is the formation of oxygen by green plants when they absorb sunlight.

In the last ten years over 4000 patients have been treated world-wide in phase two studies. Currently world-wide phase three investigational studies of the treatment of esophageal, endobronchial, and urinary bladder tumors are being performed to obtain FDA approval to remove this from investigational status and make it available for general use.

One month after 72 photodynamic therapy sessions to 27 different patients for cutaneous and subcutaneous malignant tumors 67% of the areas treated showed no clinical evidence of viable tumor. 26% had more than a 50% reduction in tumor size or number. Of 31 treatment sessions that resulted in a complete response, 48% retained this status one year after PDT.

For literature pertaining to this case see References section.

Case continues on following page.

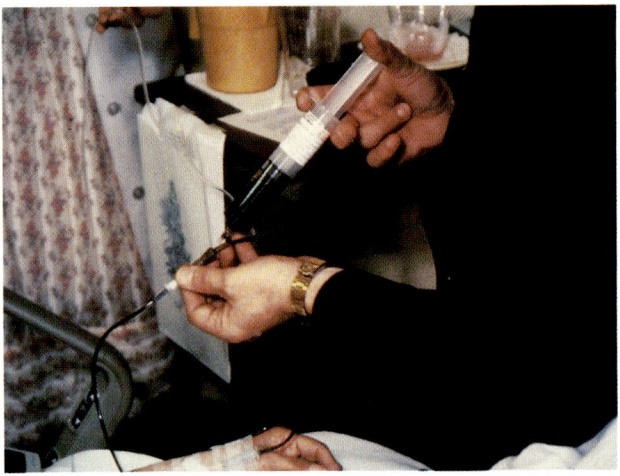

FIG. 8.16-A. DHE (2 mg/kg body weight) is injected intravenously two or three days prior to the PDT treatment.

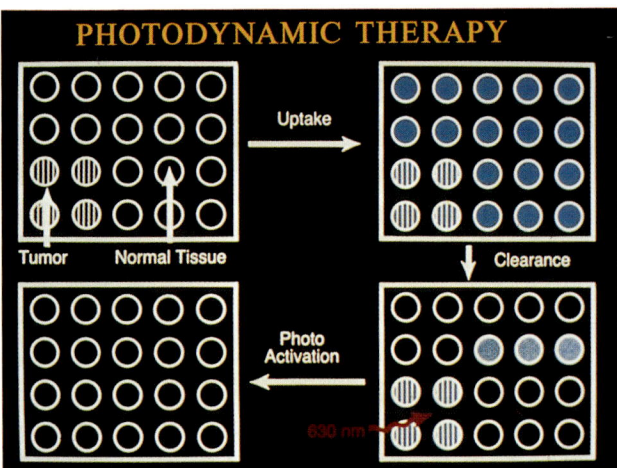

FIG. 8.16-B. Tumor and normal cells taking up the DHE and then clearing the DHE from the normal cells. When the sensitizer is activated by the red (630 nm) light the tumor cells are destroyed and the normal tissue has little or no reaction.

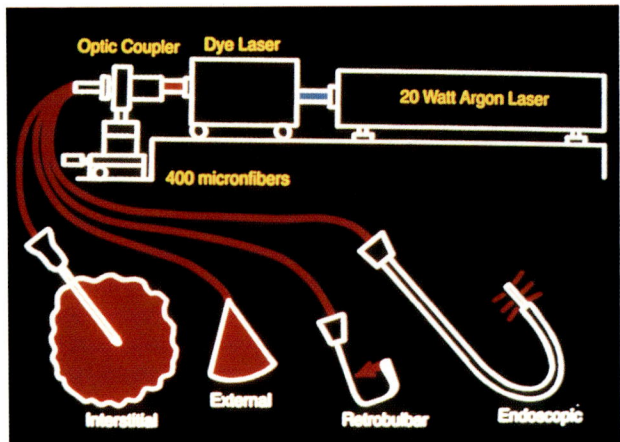

FIG. 8.16-C. Generation of energy by 20 watt argon laser causing the red dye circulating in the dye laser to produce a red laser beam. It is this red beam that is used for PDT.

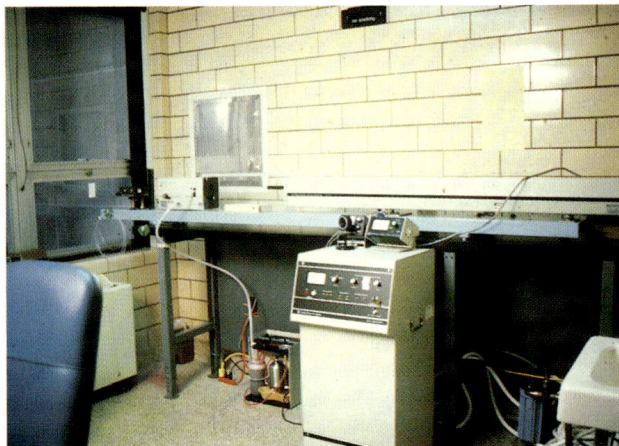

FIG. 8.16-D. The long argon laser and smaller dye laser are located adjacent to an operating room permitting the passage of the light carrying fibers through the wall into the operating room for use during operative procedures.

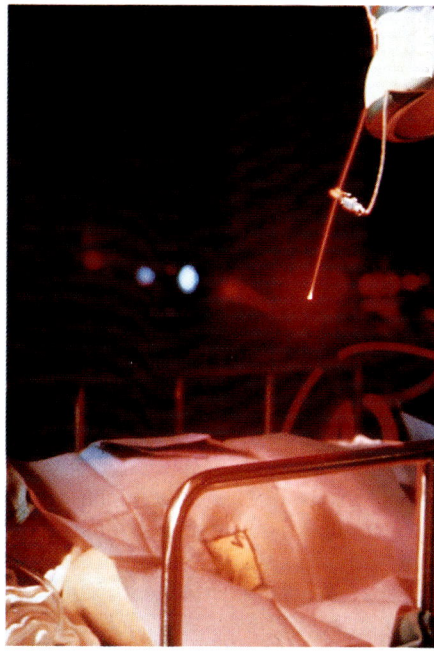

FIG. 8.16-E. Technique of surface PDT. Area to be treated is masked off and external red light is applied to tumor bearing area.

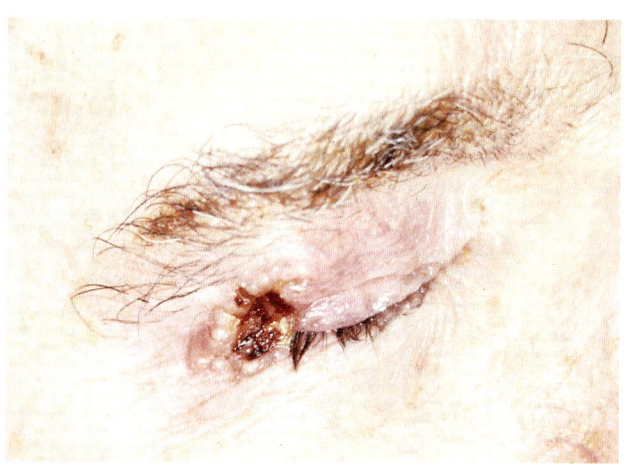

FIG. 8.16-F. Pre-treatment squamous cell carcinoma of right upper eyelid.

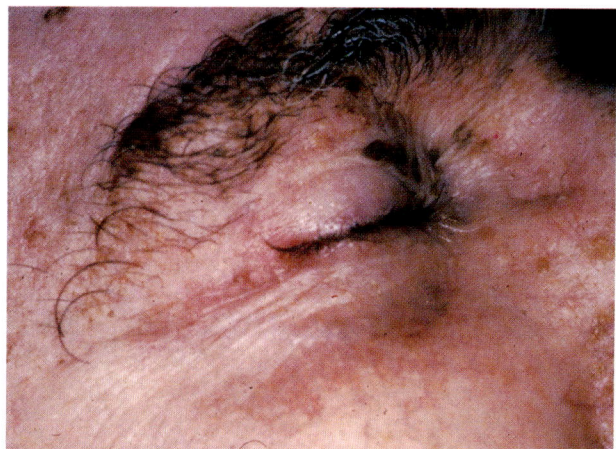

FIG. 8.16-G. Two years after third treatment with PDT. There was no recurrence. The patient is now 6.5 years post-treatment with no recurrence.

Case courtesy of *James S. McCaughan*, Jr., M.D.

CASE 8.17

Blue/Black Amateur Tattoo

REVIEW OF CASE. This 23-year-old male patient inflicted this "amateur" tattoo by stabbing his left hand with a sewing needle through a layer of india ink. This procedure results in a tattoo composed of a large range of pigment aggregate sizes at various depths in the dermis. Treatment was requested due to the negative social reaction the tattoo provoked.

CHOICE OF LASER: RUBY. The Q-switched pulsed ruby laser treatment of blue/black tattoos has proven very successful in that pigment can be broken down through a photo-mechanical shock wave process. The short pulse duration, typically 40 nanoseconds, ensures virtually no thermal damage to the tissues while the ruby wavelength of 694 nm is preferentially absorbed by the dark pigment. The smaller fragments of pigment are then believed to be removed via phagocytosis. Using a 3 mm spot diameter, the working energy density (fluence) range of 4–8.5 J/cm^2 provides efficacious treatment of superficial and deep tattoos.

ADDITIONAL INFORMATION. Some hypopigmentation may occur due to the destruction of the overlying melanin leaving the appearance of a light border around the tattoo. This will persist through the course of treatments and for some months post-treatment. Generally, the melanocytes will then migrate into the treated area resulting in a normal pigmented appearance.

A minimum of 4 weeks is left between treatments of a given area. This allows the body sufficient time to remove as much pigment as possible while repair of localized tissue damage can occur. By allowing such time between treatments the incidence of scarring is virtually nonexistent.

A test area may be irradiated at the lower end of the fluence range to assess the required treatment parameters. This is found by increasing the energy until the white steam vacuoles appear.

The number of treatments required to treat a tattoo by this technique is variable due to the variable nature of tattoos. Small, superficial tattoos may only require 2 or 3 treatments while the larger or deeper ones could require up to 10 or 12 repeat treatments. Typically the fading process will not appear uniform over a tattoo which results in some areas fading after a few treatments leaving adjacent areas requiring further treatments. This is primarily due to the variable depth and density of the pigment which cannot be accurately assessed by visual inspection alone.

The white appearance immediately following irradiation becomes less pronounced as further treatments occur, until it is almost unnoticeable by about the fourth or fifth treatment.

Occasionally hemhorraging may occur at the treatment sites. This is thought to be due to superficial pigment shattering close to nearby vessels. The blood does not absorb the laser light directly but local mechanical disturbance can rupture the vessel wall. Decreasing the fluence either by lowering the energy or increasing the spot diameter will usually remedy this effect.

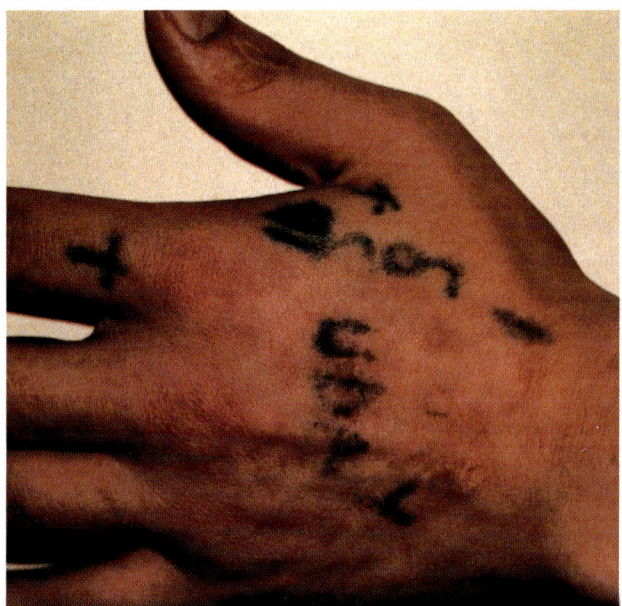

FIG. 8.17-A. Blue/black amateur tattoo on hand with no previous treatment history.

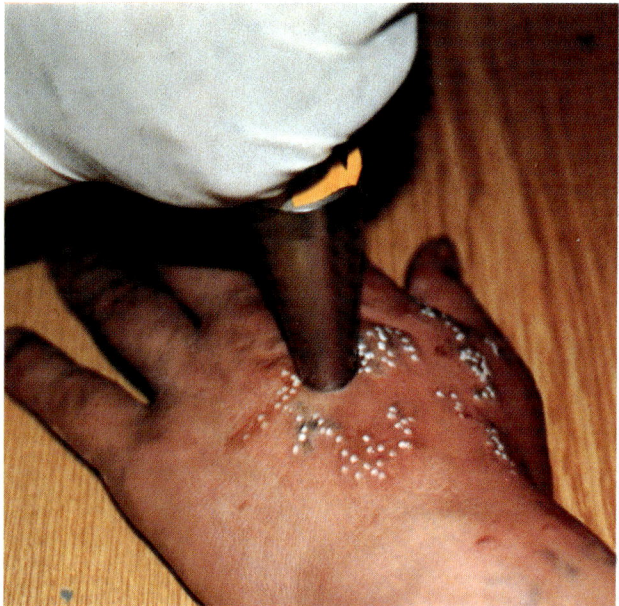

FIG. 8.17-B. The site is first shaved to reduce competition for the laser energy by hair and then cleaned to remove dirt and grease. Local anesthetic (1% lignocaine without epinephrine) is injected intradermally using dental needles to minimize discomfort. The laser handpiece is then placed in contact with the skin to prevent leakage of laser light. The very high power beam is such that even a low percentage of reflected light entering the unprotected eye may cause damage. For this reason all personnel in the treatment room must wear goggles throughout the procedure. Removal or coverage of all jewelry near the treatment area is advised to further reduce the risk of reflected light.

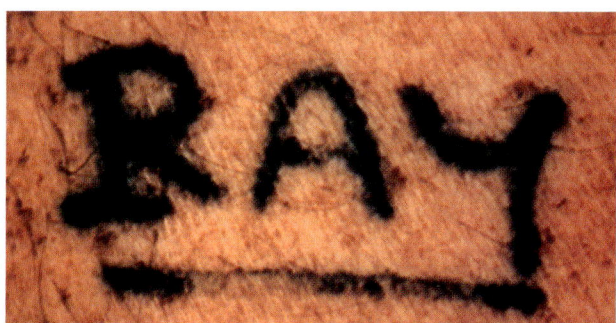

FIG. 8.17-D. This 27-year-old male patient possessed a typical self-inflicted "amateur" tattoo on the dorsal surface of his forearm.

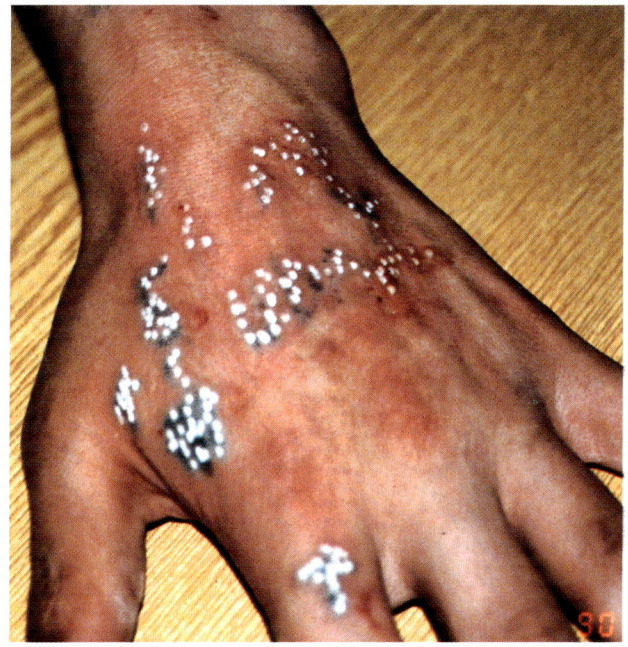

FIG. 8.17-C. Using a 3 mm spot diameter with 0.5 joules of energy (fluence = 7 J/cm^2) the tattoo is traced by the operator firing one pulse at each location. Immediately following irradiation the treated area appears white due to steam vacuoles forming around the pigment particles. Re-treatment over these sites is futile as the beam will be almost totally reflected. This white appearance lasts for between 10 and 60 minutes after which the tattoo reappears. This treatment is currently under progress and so a completed similar case history is shown in figs. D and E.

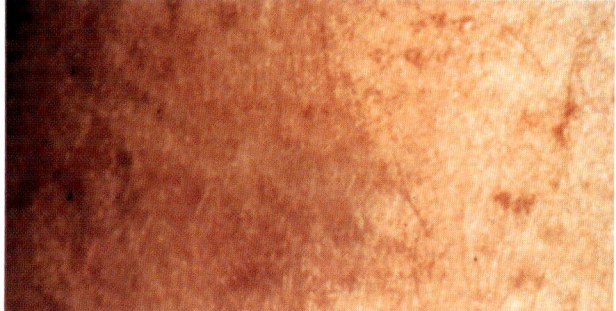

FIG. 8.17-E. After only 3 treatments the tattoo has almost completely faded with no evidence of tissue damage.

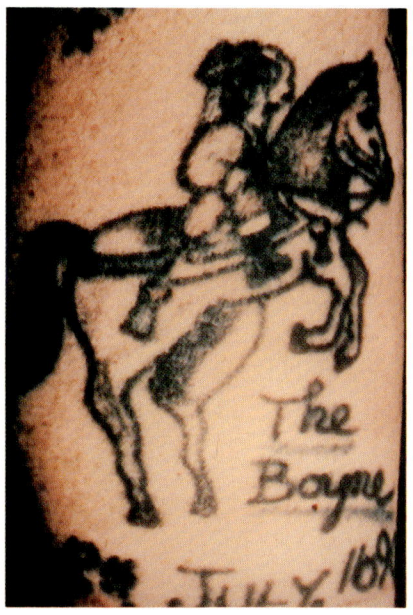

FIG. 8.17-F. This patient had a typical professionally applied tattoo on his forearm. Originally it had contained some colored pigment (horseman's jacket, horse's head, neck, and body) but this had faded over the 12 year period since the tattoo had been applied.

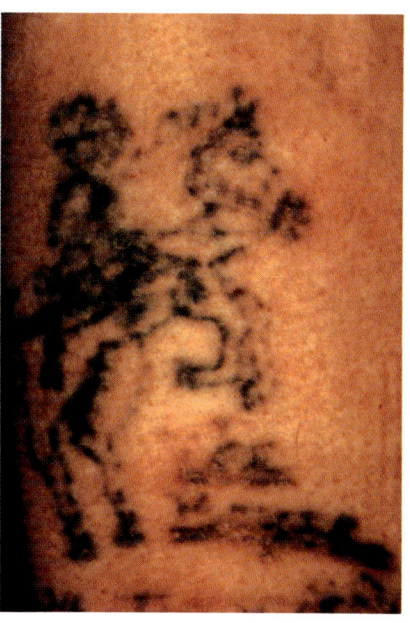

FIG. 8.17-G. After 4 treatments the writing above the horseman had completely faded while the rest of the tattoo was breaking up.

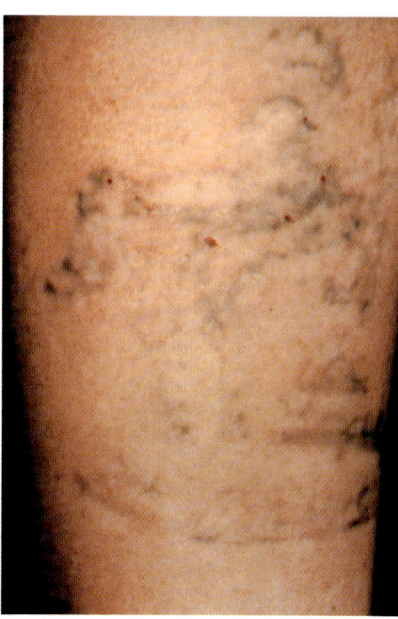

FIG. 8.17-H. Two further treatments and the tattoo is now indistinguishable with only a small amount of pigment remaining.

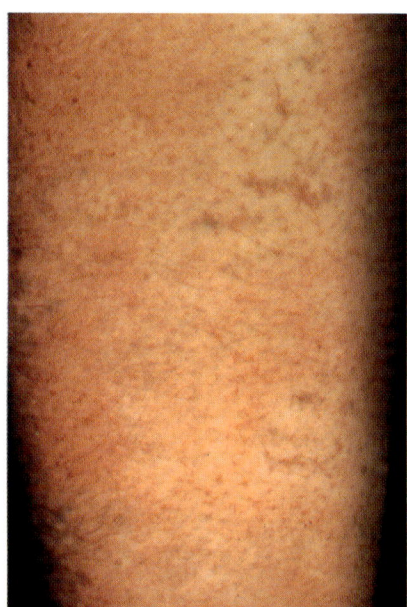

FIG. 8.17-I. After a course of 9 treatments over the whole tattoo there is virtually no pigment left. Some slight hypopigmentation is evident although there is no evidence of hypertropic scarring at all.

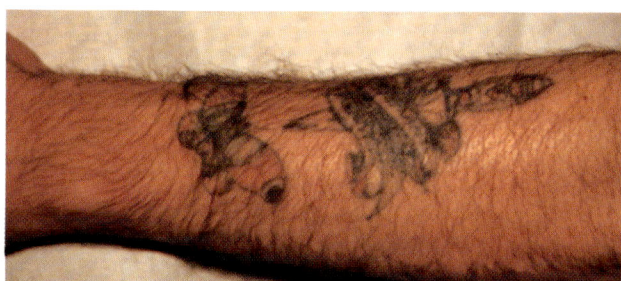

FIG. 8.17-J. This patient possessed two professionally applied tattoos which contained some red and green pigment. The ruby laser emits a red beam so it is pointless treating the red part directly as the laser light will be mostly reflected. However, evidence shows that by treating the dark borders around red pigment the subsequent phagocytotic reaction can also remove the red ink.

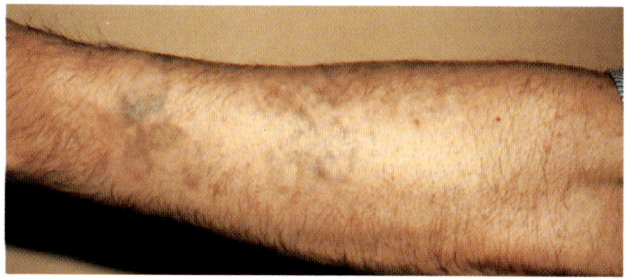

FIG. 8.17-K. After 6 treatments most of the blue/black pigment has faded, as has the red pigment. However, some patches of the green pigment remains. Once again, there is no evidence of scarring at this site or any of this patient's other treated areas.

Case courtesy of **William H. Reid,** M.D., **Michael J. Murphy,** Ph.D., and **Iain D. Miller,** M.D.

CASE 8.18
Amateur Decorative Tattoo

REVIEW OF CASE. The patient is a 23-year-old Hispanic male with amateur tattoos on the fingers of his left hand present for 7 years.

CHOICE OF LASER: RUBY. The Q-switched ruby laser emits nanosecond pulses with extremely high peak powers (megawatts). The red 694 nm wavelength of the laser penetrates several millimeters into the dermis and is well absorbed by carbon, india ink, and other organometallic dyes typically found in dark blue-black amateur and professional tattoos, relative to other optically absorbing structures. Furthermore, the nanosecond pulse duration produced by this laser closely matches the thermal relaxation time for tattoo pigment thereby confining the laser energy to the targeted pigment before much heat is lost by thermal diffusion.

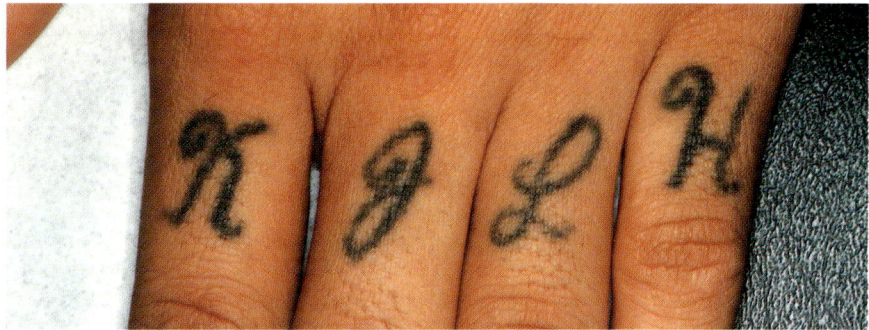

FIG. 8.18-A. Amateur decorative tattoos on fingers of the left hand prior to laser treatment.

Case continues on following page.

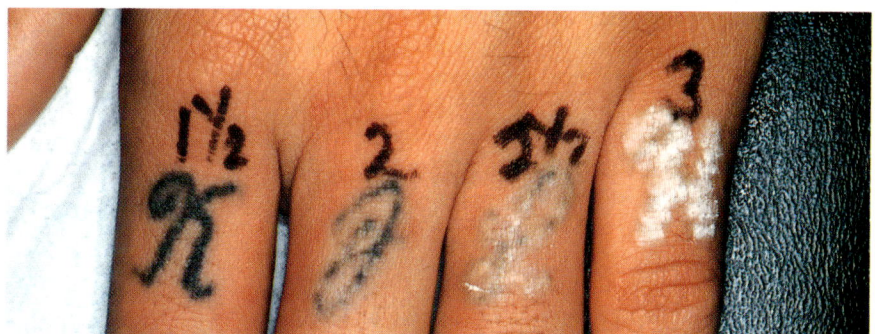

FIG. 8.18-B. Immediately post Q-switched ruby laser treatment using energy densities of 1.5–3.0 J/cm^2. Laser energy is transmitted through an articulating arm which terminates in a microlens that focuses laser radiation on a 5 mm circular spot of uniform light intensity. The treatment, which is described as feeling like a hot elastic band snapped against the skin, is well tolerated. Immediately after treatment, a white-ash discoloration is seen. This opaque white appearance in the skin is caused by the formation of vacuoles in the dermis probably due to the production of steam.

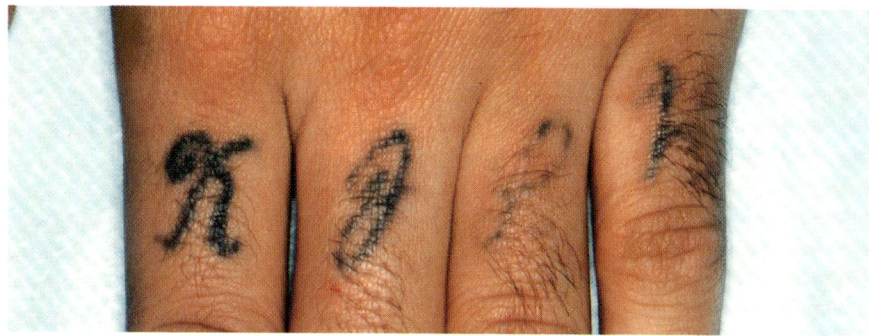

FIG. 8.18-C. Examination 4 weeks after first laser treatment reveals moderate fading, particularly of the tattoos treated with 2.5–3.0 J/cm^2.

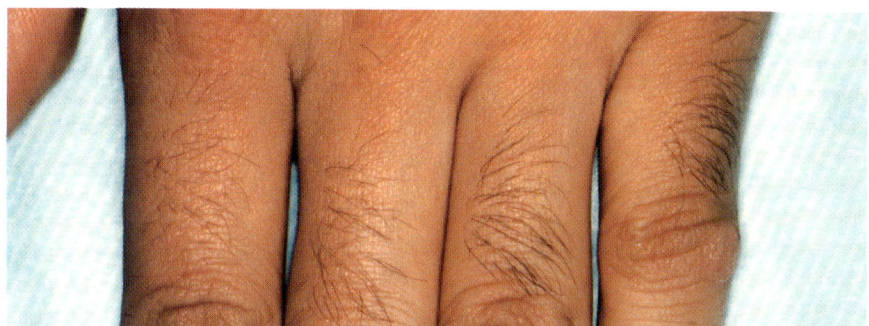

FIG. 8.18-D. Examination 4 weeks after third laser treatment. Both second and third laser treatments were performed using an energy density of 3 J/cm^2. The tattoos have been completely removed with no skin textural changes or scarring. The fading and removal of ink is brought about by two mechanisms. First, the dye absorbs light energy and converts it to heat causing the production of steam with probable chemical alteration of the ink into colorless compounds. Second, there is an increase in macrophage activity in subsequent weeks and months post-operatively. The large deposits of ink are broken up into smaller particles which are then removed by phagocytosis.

Case courtesy of *J. Stuart Nelson*, M.D., Ph.D.

CASE 8.19
Amateur Decorative Tattoo

REVIEW OF CASE. The patient is a 31-year-old white male with an amateur tattoo on the left hand present for 10 years.

CHOICE OF LASER: RUBY. The Q-switched ruby laser emits nanosecond pulses with extremely high peak powers (megawatts). The red 694 nm wavelength of the laser penetrates several millimeters into the dermis and is well absorbed by carbon, india ink, and other organometallic dyes typically found in dark blue-black amateur and professional tattoos, relative to other optically absorbing structures. Furthermore, the nanosecond pulse duration produced by this laser closely matches the thermal relaxation time for tattoo pigment thereby confining the laser energy to the targeted pigment before much heat is lost by thermal diffusion.

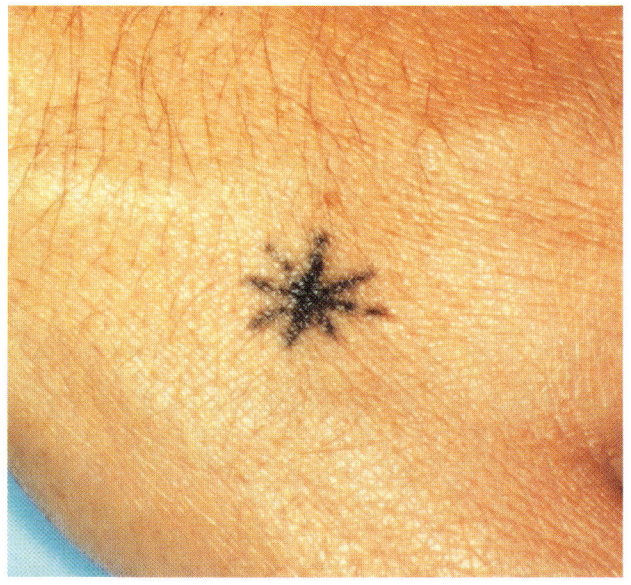

FIG. 8.19-A. Amateur decorative tattoo on the left hand prior to laser treatment.

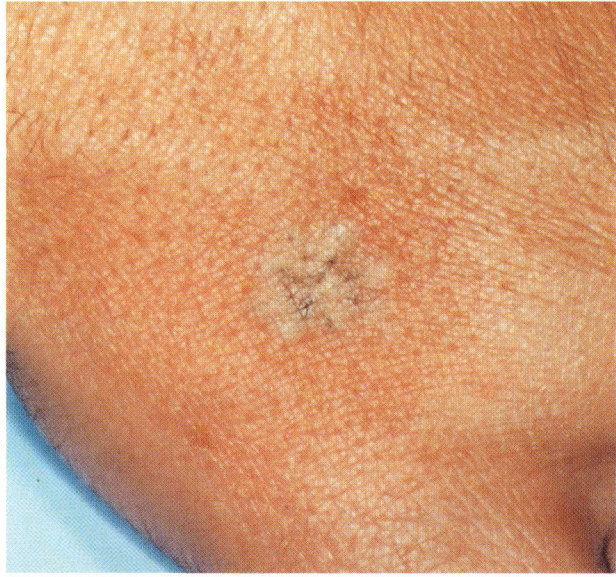

FIG. 8.19-B. Immediately post Q-switched ruby laser treatment using 4 J/cm^2. Laser energy is transmitted through an articulating arm which terminates in a microlens that focuses laser radiation on a 5 mm circular spot of uniform light intensity. The treatment, which is described as feeling like a hot elastic band snapped against the skin, is well tolerated. Immediately after treatment, a white-ash discoloration is seen. This opaque white appearance in the skin is caused by the formation of vacuoles in the dermis probably due to the production of steam.

Case continues on following page.

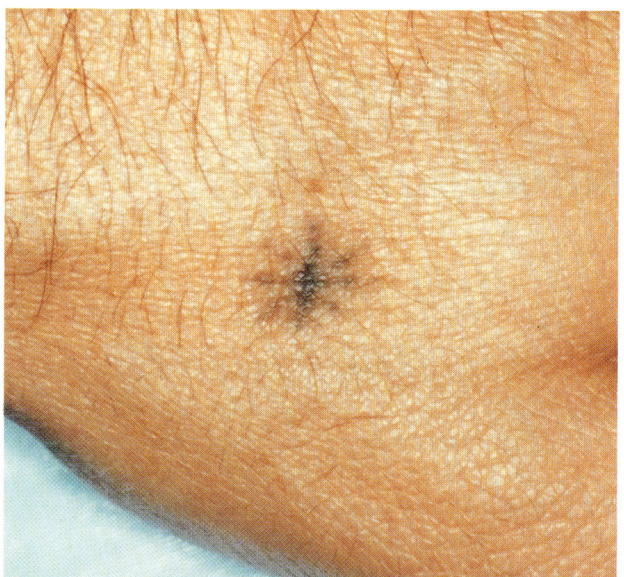

FIG. 8.19-C. Examination 4 weeks after first laser treatment reveals moderate fading.

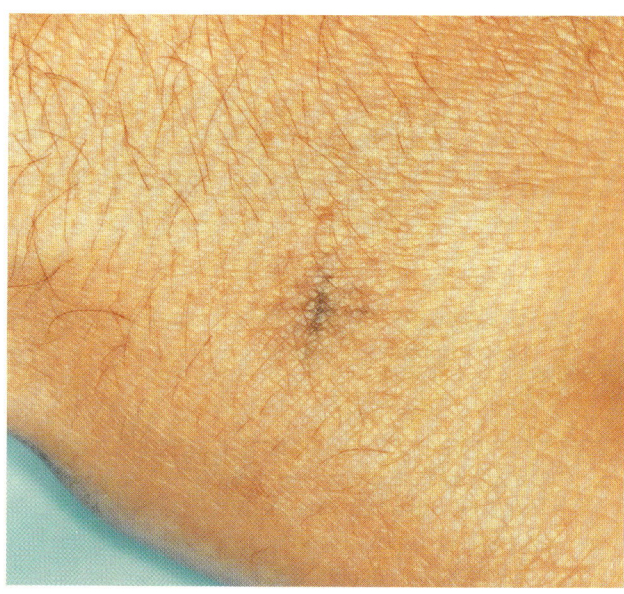

FIG. 8.19-D. Examination 4 weeks after second laser treatment using 4 J/cm^2 reveals significant fading.

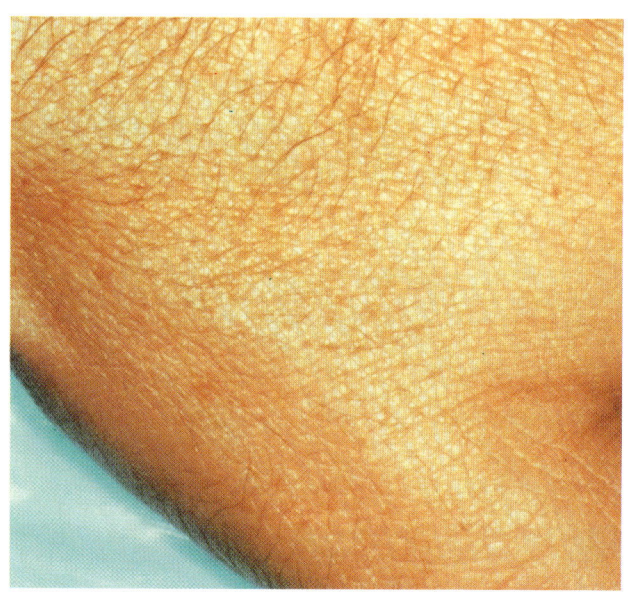

FIG. 8.19-E. Examination 4 weeks after fourth laser treatment using 4 J/cm^2. The tattoo has been completely removed with no skin textural changes or scarring. The fading and removal of ink is brought about by two mechanisms. First, the dye absorbs light energy and converts it to heat causing the production of steam with probable chemical alteration of the ink into colorless compounds. Second, there is an increase in macrophage activity in subsequent weeks and months postoperatively. The large deposits of ink are broken up into smaller particles which are then removed by phagocytosis.

Case courtesy of *J. Stuart Nelson,* M.D., Ph.D.

CASE 8.20

Decorative Tattoo

REVIEW OF CASE.   This is a 32-year-old male with a nonprofessional decorative tattoo of the left upper arm, desiring removal for cosmetic purposes.

CHOICE OF LASER: KTP.   The KTP laser is a frequency doubled neodymium:YAG laser producing all its output at 532 nm. The green light is directed through a series of fiberoptics from the source to the end output. The green light is absorbed by tattoo pigment partially suspended in the upper dermis. The absorbed light is converted to heat and the dye particles, regardless of color in a gaseous form, are expelled during the localized vaporization of the surrounding cells as part of the laser "plume." There follows an inflammatory wound phase with secondary washout of remaining dye particles in the accompanying exudate and subsequent eschar. The result is usually the obliteration of the tattoo pigment, replaced by a shiny superficial scar or texture change. The laser is used with a continuous power setting, 1 watt of power, and a 1 mm spot size.

ADDITIONAL INFORMATION.   In this study, the argon and KTP 532 lasers were evaluated in a side by side comparison. Identical parameters of power, spot size, and pulse duration were utilized in each area. Clinical and histological results proved equal between the two lasers.

POST-TREATMENT CARE.   Iced saline compresses and topical antibiotic ointment and closed wound dressings are used.

Reprinted with permission of Wiley-Liss, a division of John Wiley & Sons, Inc.
For literature pertaining to this case see References section.

Case continues on following page.

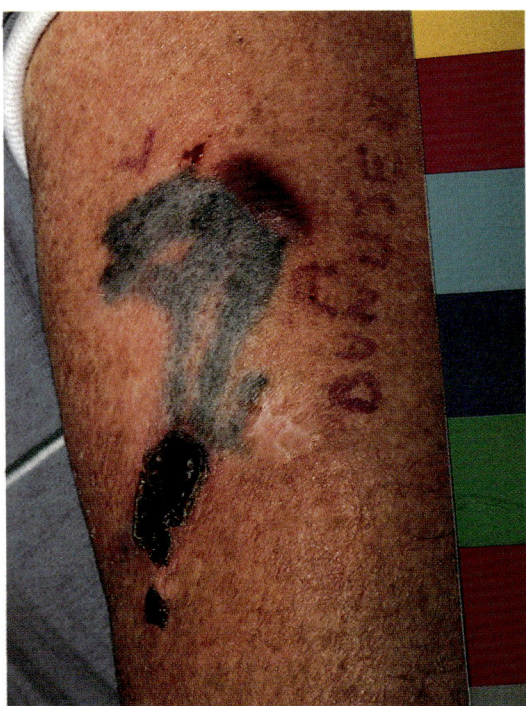

FIG. 8.20-A. Decorative tattoo prior to treatment.

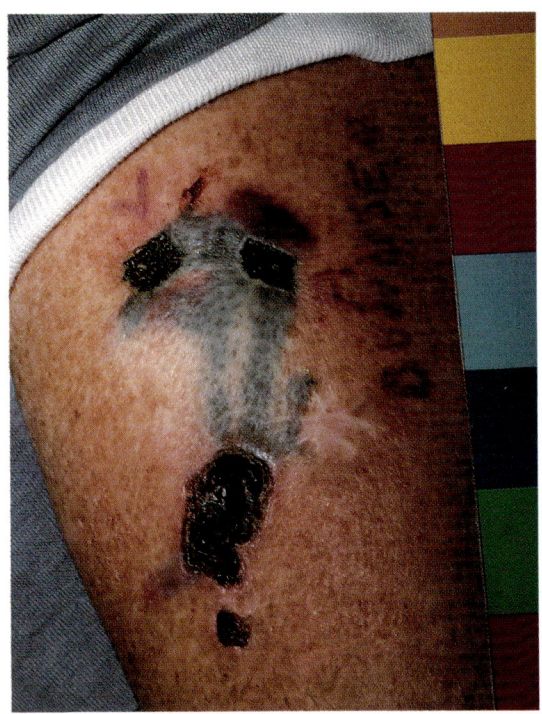

FIG. 8.20-B. Immediately post-treatment result with the argon laser (A) and KTP 532 laser (Laserscope, L) demonstrating vaporization of the tattoo pigment.

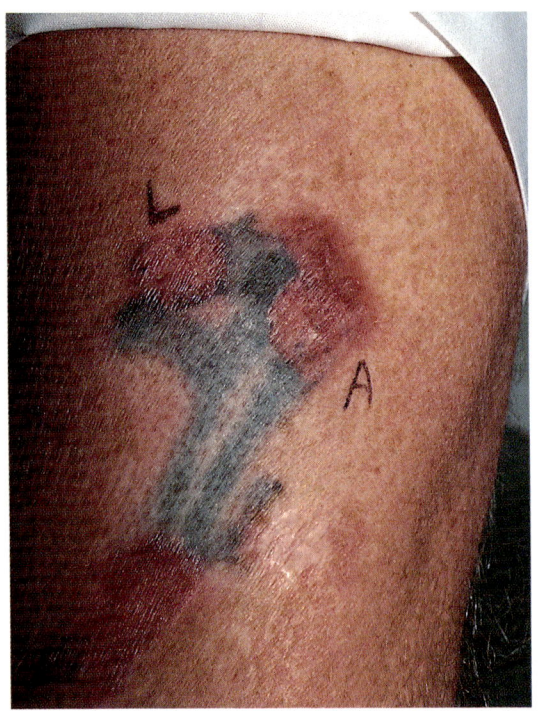

FIG. 8.20-C. Final result with total clearing of the tattoo pigment in both areas with residual texture change of the skin.

Case courtesy of *David B. Apfelberg*, M.D.

CASE 8.21
Cafe-Au-Lait Lesion

REVIEW OF CASE. This is a 34-year-old woman with a lifetime history of this cafe-au-lait lesion on the right anterior upper right leg. The lesion produced some self-consciousness and she desired treatment.

CHOICE OF LASER: ARGON DYE WITH HEXASCAN. The green only wavelength from the tunable dye laser was selected because of its increased absorption at melanin wavelengths. The robotic scanning device, hexascan, was chosen because of its ability to precisely deliver, in a reproducible fashion, a carefully measured energy fluence. The ability to treat large areas rapidly and uniformly with minimal discomfort and concern about hypopigmentation or hypertrophic scarring from nonuniform treatment were also a factor.

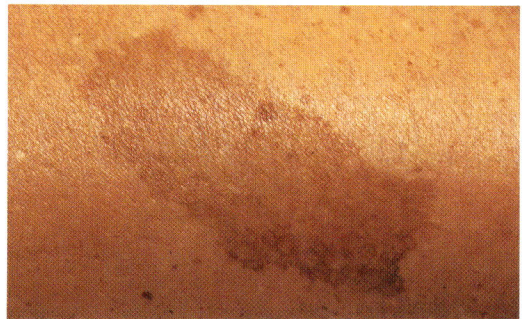

FIG. 8.21-A. Cafe-au-lait lesion prior to treatment.

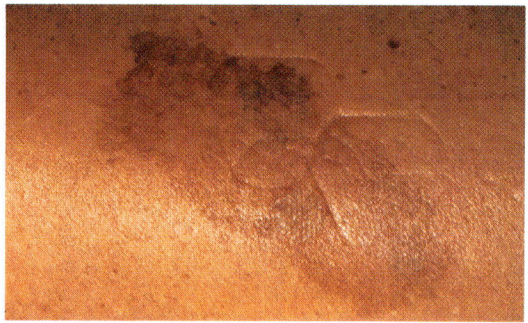

FIG. 8.21-B. A 13 mm hexagonal "test" treatment field has been performed. Note the slightly hyperpigmented appearance in the mid-portion of the figure. This increased pigmentation begins almost immediately as well as mild erythema which rapidly fades. The hyperpigmentation persists for two to four weeks and then lightening rapidly occurs.

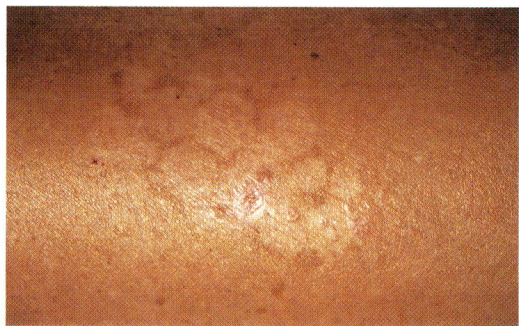

FIG. 8.21-C. Area 4 weeks post-treatment with 10 joules 514 nm green only argon light delivered using a 13 mm field size with the hexascan robotic scanning device. Note the small skip areas where the 13 mm hexagonal fields were not perfectly assembled. These areas required touchup using 1 mm single pulsed mode or small 3 mm or 5 mm hexagons.

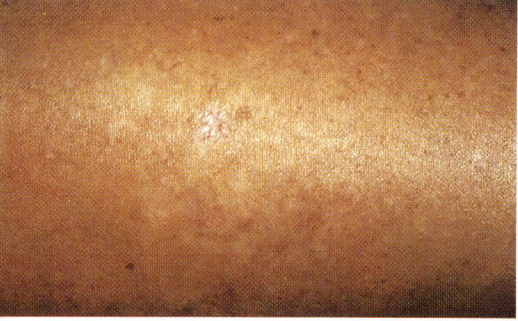

FIG. 8.21-D. Area 8 weeks after the original treatment and 4 weeks after the touchup.

Case courtesy of *David H. McDaniel,* M.D.

CASE 8.22
Divided Nevus of the Right Eyelid

REVIEW OF CASE. This is a 16-year-old male patient who had a divided nevus since birth.

CHOICE OF LASER: RUBY. The ruby laser is absorbed selectively by melanin granules, causing very little effect on melanin pigmentation. It does not readily cause scarring. Compared with the dye laser, argon laser, and CO_2 laser, the ruby laser has better selectivity and far-reaching capabilities. Treatment can be conducted on an outpatient basis, and the method is quite simple. In many cases, local anesthetics are not required, and pain is minimal after treatment. Epithelialization is completed in 7 to 10 days. Pigmentation disappears completely, without scarring.

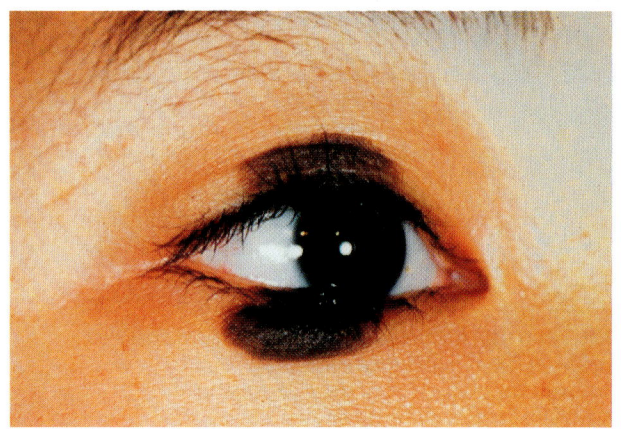

FIG. 8.22-A. Blackish divided nevus on the right eyelid.

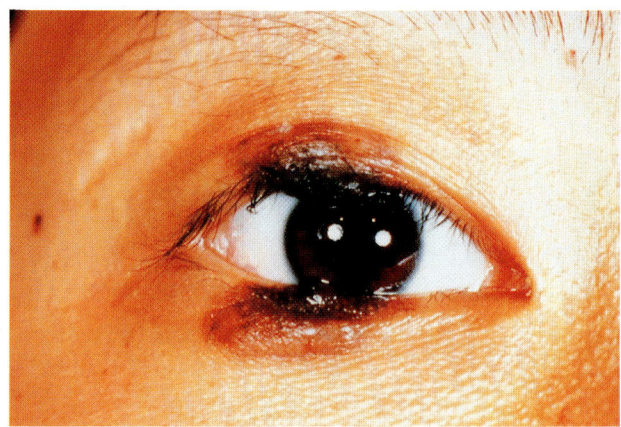

FIG. 8.22-B. One month after a single ruby laser treatment of 20 J/cm^2. The pigmentations on both upper and lower eyelids are lighter.

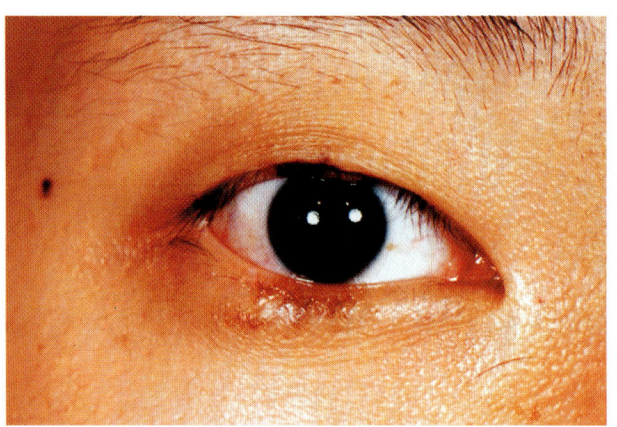

FIG. 8.22-C. One year after undergoing five 20 J/cm^2 ruby laser treatments. Although pigmentation remains in one area, no signs of recurrence or scarring could be found.

Case courtesy of *Muneo Miyasaka,* M.D., *Ryuzaburo Tanino,* M.D., *Taichin Morita,* M.D., *Hiroto Yamada,* M.D., and *Mitsuhiro Osada,* M.D.

CASE 8.23
Epidermal Melanosis
Secondary to Post-Traumatic Hyperpigmentation

REVIEW OF CASE. This patient is a 40-year-old Oriental female with a history of receiving a hot water burn to her right cheek 20 years ago. The patient reports the burned area has gotten progressively darker over the past 10 years.

CHOICE OF LASER: RUBY. The Q-switched ruby laser emits nanosecond pulses with extremely high peak powers (megawatts). The red 694 nm wavelength of the laser penetrates several millimeters into the dermis and is well absorbed by epidermal melanin, relative to other optically absorbing structures. Furthermore, the nanosecond pulse duration produced by this laser closely matches the thermal relaxation time for intracellular melanosomes thereby causing highly specific damage to melanin-containing cells.

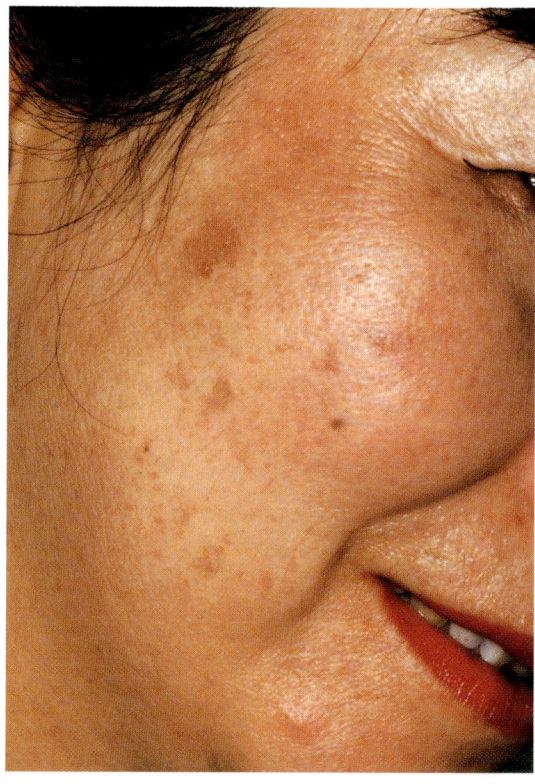

FIG. 8.23-A. Epidermal melanosis secondary to post-traumatic hyperpigmentation on right cheek prior to Q-switched laser treatment.

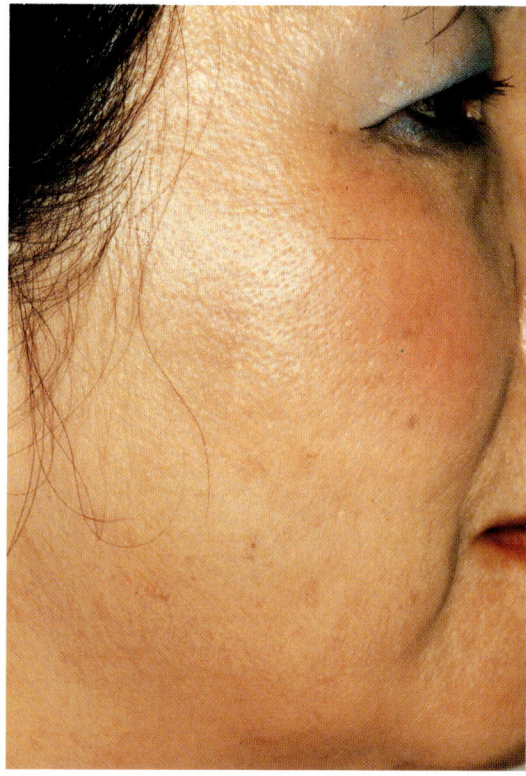

FIG. 8.23-B. Examination 6 months after one laser treatment using 3 J/cm^2. Pigmentation has been completely removed with no skin textural changes or scarring.

Case courtesy of *J. Stuart Nelson*, M.D., Ph.D.

CASE 8.24

Epidermal Melanosis

Secondary to Cafe-Au-Lait Spot

REVIEW OF CASE.   This patient is a 17-year-old white female with a cafe-au-lait spot of the left upper lip.

CHOICE OF LASER: RUBY.   The Q-switched ruby laser emits nanosecond pulses with extremely high peak powers (megawatts). The red 694 nm wavelength of the laser penetrates several millimeters into the dermis and is well absorbed by epidermal melanin, relative to other optically absorbing structures. Furthermore, the nanosecond pulse duration produced by this laser closely matches the thermal relaxation time for intracellular melanosomes thereby causing highly specific damage to melanin-containing cells.

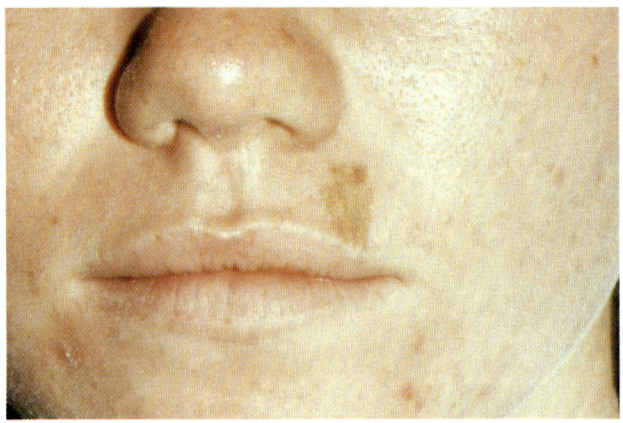

FIG. 8.24-A. Cafe-au-lait spot on left upper lip prior to Q-switched laser treatment.

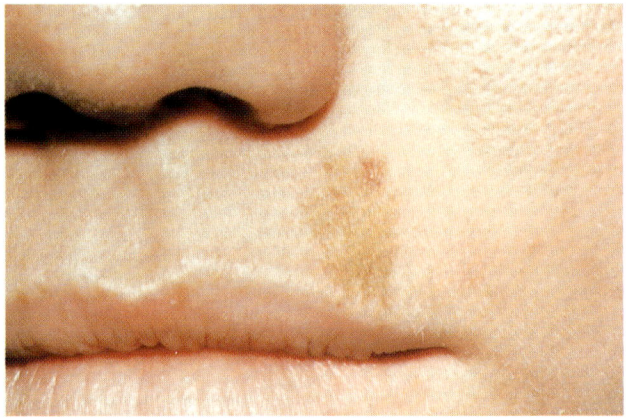

FIG. 8.24-B. Same patient as in Fig. A, higher magnification.

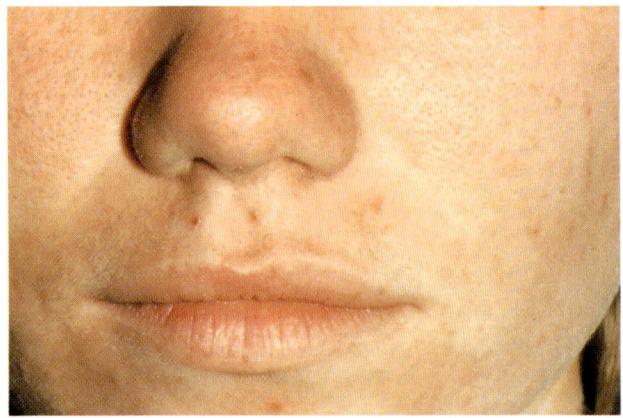

FIG. 8.24-C. Examination 6 weeks after one laser treatment using 3 J/cm^2. Pigmentation has been completely removed with no skin textural changes or scarring.

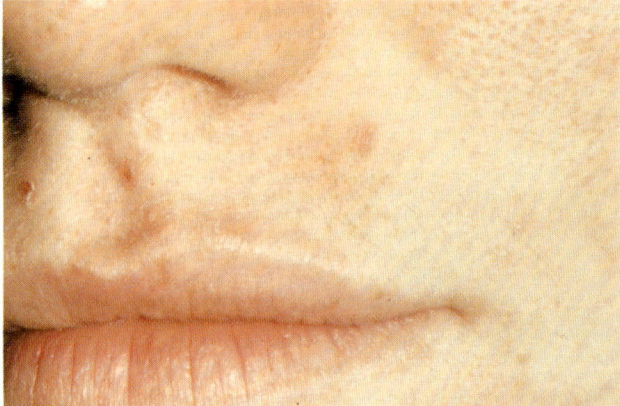

FIG. 8.24-D. Same patient as in Fig. C, higher magnification.

Case courtesy of *J. Stuart Nelson*, M.D., Ph.D.

CASE 8.25
Lentigo Senilis of the Left Cheek

REVIEW OF CASE. A 45-year-old female with pigmentation which first appeared on the left cheek two years ago and gradually became more conspicuous. The use of various cosmetics did not improve the situation. A great deal of the patient's time was spent on makeup to conceal the pigmentation.

CHOICE OF LASER: RUBY. The ruby laser is absorbed selectively by melanin granules, causing very little effect on the melanin pigmentation. It does not readily cause scarring. Compared with the dye laser, argon laser, and CO_2 laser, the ruby laser has better selectivity and far-reaching capabilities. Treatment can be conducted on an outpatient basis, and the method is quite simple. In many cases, local anesthetics are not required, and pain is minimal after treatment. Epithelialization is completed in 7 to 10 days. Pigmentation disappears completely, without scarring.

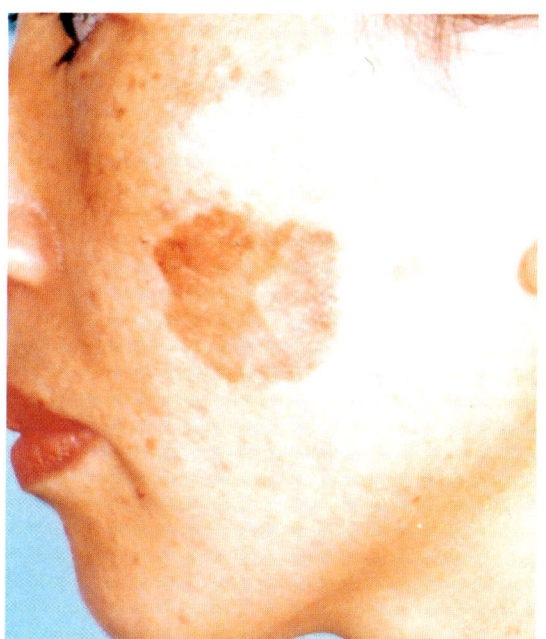

FIG. 8.25-A. Brownish lentigo senilis, 5 × 4 cm, on the left cheek.

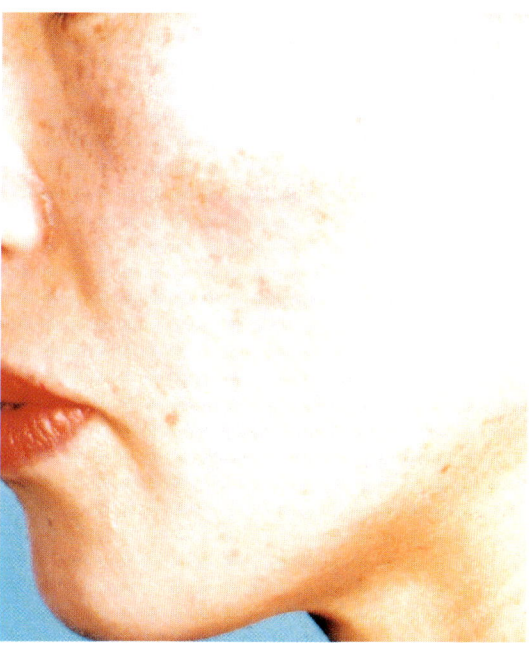

FIG. 8.25-B. One year after being treated twice with the ruby laser (30 J/cm^2). Some redness still remains, but there are no scars or signs of recurrence.

Case courtesy of *Muneo Miyasaka*, M.D., *Ryuzaburo Tanino*, M.D., *Taichin Morita*, M.D., *Hiroto Yamada*, M.D., and *Mitsuhiro Osada*, M.D.

CASE 8.26

Nevus Cell Nevus of the Lower Leg

REVIEW OF CASE. This is a 3-year-old male patient who has had nevus cell nevus on his left lower leg since birth.

CHOICE OF LASER: RUBY. The ruby laser is absorbed selectively by melanin granules, causing very little effect on melanin pigmentation. It does not readily cause scarring. Compared with the dye laser, argon laser, and CO_2 laser, the ruby laser has better selectivity and far-reaching capabilities. Treatment can be conducted on an outpatient basis, and the method is quite simple. In many cases, local anesthetics are not required, and pain is minimal after treatment. Epithelialization is completed in 7 to 10 days. Pigmentation disappears completely, without scarring.

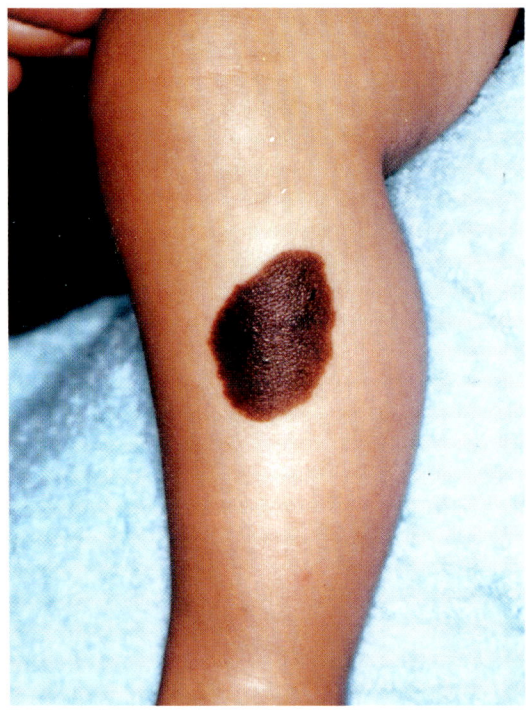

FIG. 8.26-A. Blackish nevus cell nevus, 7 × 5 cm in size, on his left lower leg.

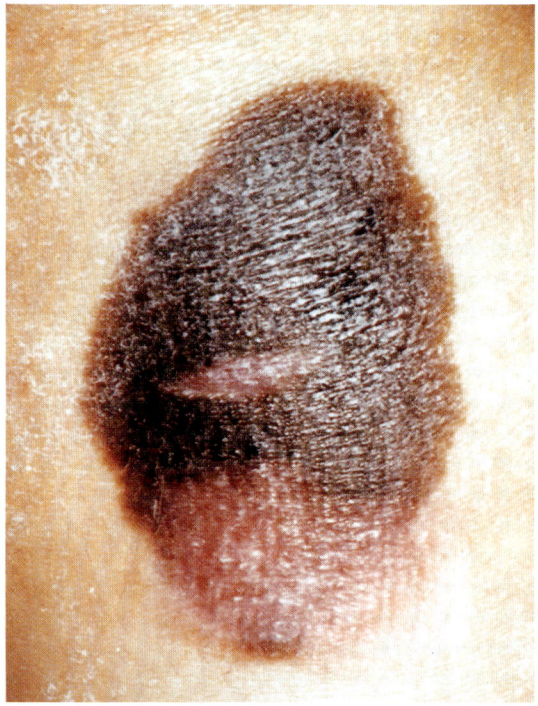

FIG. 8.26-B. Two weeks after undergoing biopsy and trial irradiation. The pigmentation where irradiated on a trial basis is paler.

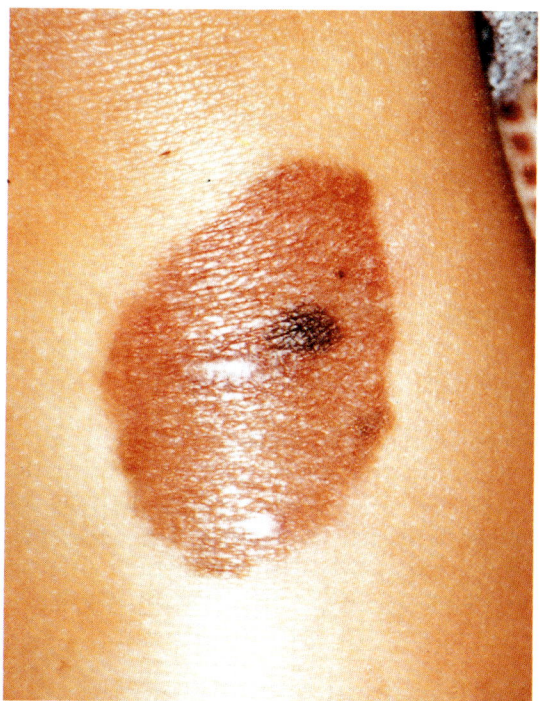

FIG. 8.26-C. Two weeks after undergoing one ruby laser treatment. Pigmentation still remains.

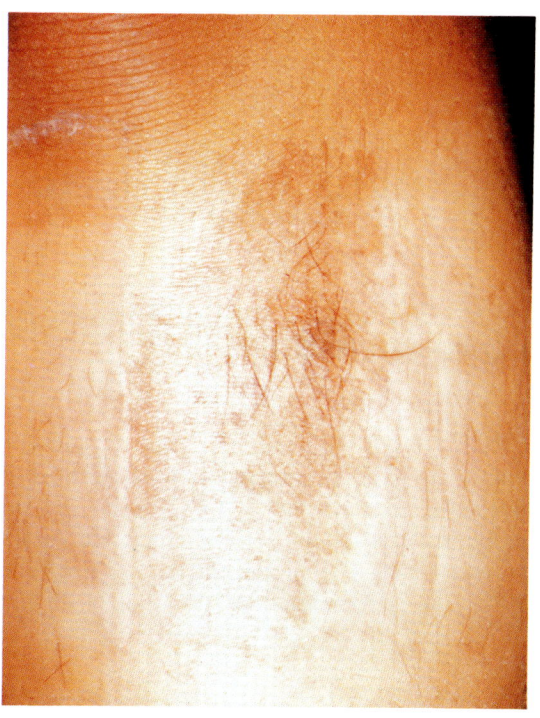

FIG. 8.26-D. One year after 5 treatments of 40 J/cm² ruby laser. No scar formation or recurrence observed.

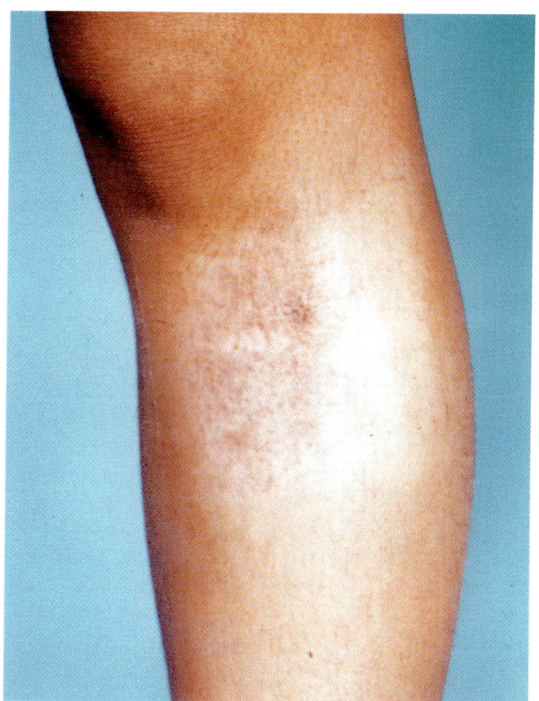

FIG. 8.26-E. Five years after receiving ruby laser treatment. Absolutely no recurrence is present.

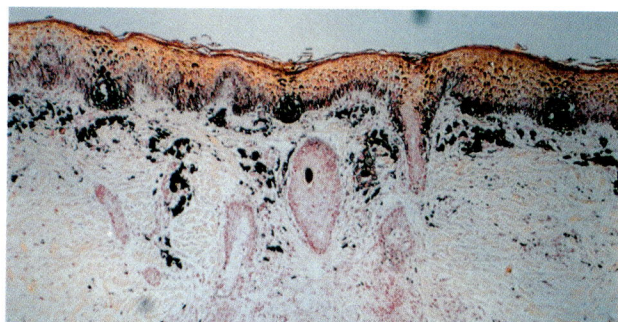

FIG. 8.26-F. Tissue specimen prior to ruby laser treatment using Masson-Fontana stain: A melanin deposit can be seen in the upper dermis layer.

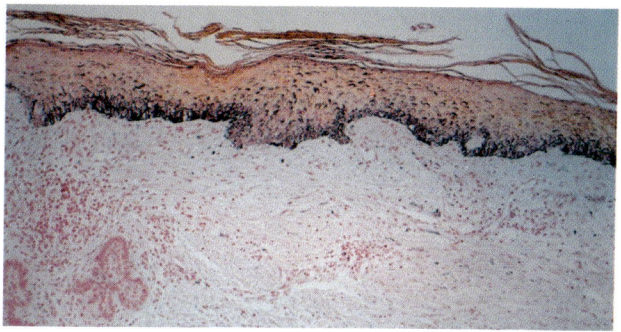

FIG. 8.26-G. Tissue specimen after ruby laser treatment: Melanin deposit has disappeared.

Case courtesy of *Muneo Miyasaka*, M.D., *Ryuzaburo Tanino*, M.D., *Taichin Morita*, M.D., *Hiroto Yamada*, M.D., and *Mitsuhiro Osada*, M.D.

CASE 8.27
Nevus Cell Nevus of the Left Shoulder

REVIEW OF CASE. This is a 25-year-old male patient who has had nevus cell nevus on the left shoulder since birth.

CHOICE OF LASER: RUBY. The ruby laser is absorbed selectively by melanin granules, causing very little effect on melanin pigmentation. It does not readily cause scarring. Compared with the dye laser, argon laser, and CO_2 laser, the ruby laser has better selectivity and far-reaching capabilities. Treatment can be conducted on an outpatient basis, and the method is quite simple. In many cases, local anesthetics are not required, and pain is minimal after treatment. Epithelialization is completed in 7 to 10 days. Pigmentation disappears completely, without scarring.

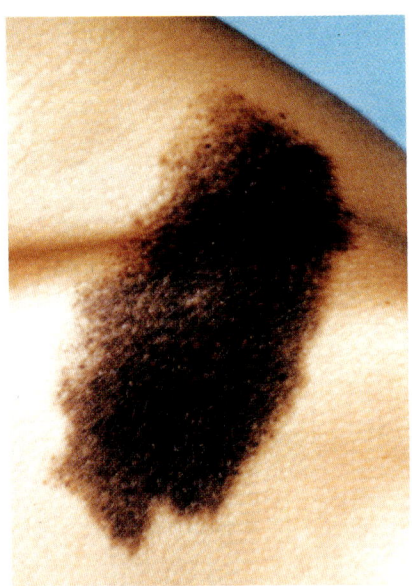

FIG. 8.27-A. Pilous nevus cell nevus, 7 × 14 cm on the left shoulder.

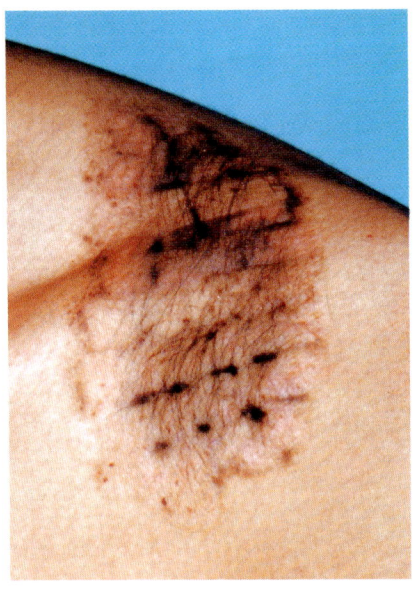

FIG. 8.27-B. Two months after undergoing two 35 J/cm^2 ruby laser treatments. Pigmentation still remains where irradiation was uneven.

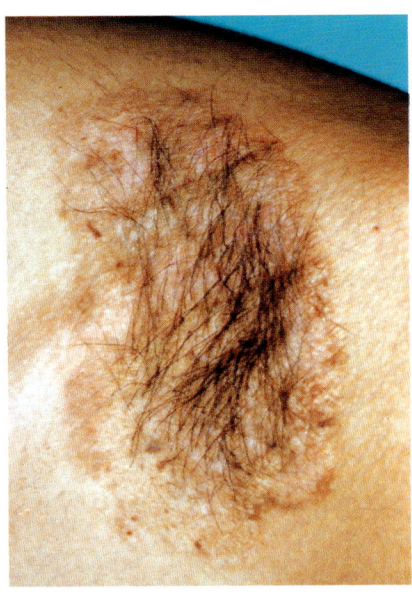

FIG. 8.27-C. One year after three 35 J/cm^2 ruby laser treatments. No recurrence is seen and the scar is hardly noticeable. The patient is currently undergoing depilatory treatment.

Case courtesy of *Muneo Miyasaka*, M.D., *Ryuzaburo Tanino*, M.D., *Taichin Morita*, M.D., *Hiroto Yamada*, M.D., and *Mitsuhiro Osada*, M.D.

CASE 8.28

Nevus Ota of the Left Eyelid

REVIEW OF CASE. This 50-year-old female patient had pigmentation around the left eyelid since birth. The spot began growing larger and darker from approximately 8 years of age. The patient had given up hope that nevus Ota could be treated.

CHOICE OF LASER: RUBY. The ruby laser is absorbed selectively by melanin granules, causing very little effect on melanin pigmentation. It does not readily cause scarring. Compared with the dye laser, argon laser, and CO_2 laser, the ruby laser has better selectivity and far-reaching capabilities. Treatment can be conducted on an outpatient basis, and the method is quite simple. In many cases, local anesthetics are not required, and pain is minimal after treatment. Epithelialization is completed in 7 to 10 days. Pigmentation disappears completely, without scarring.

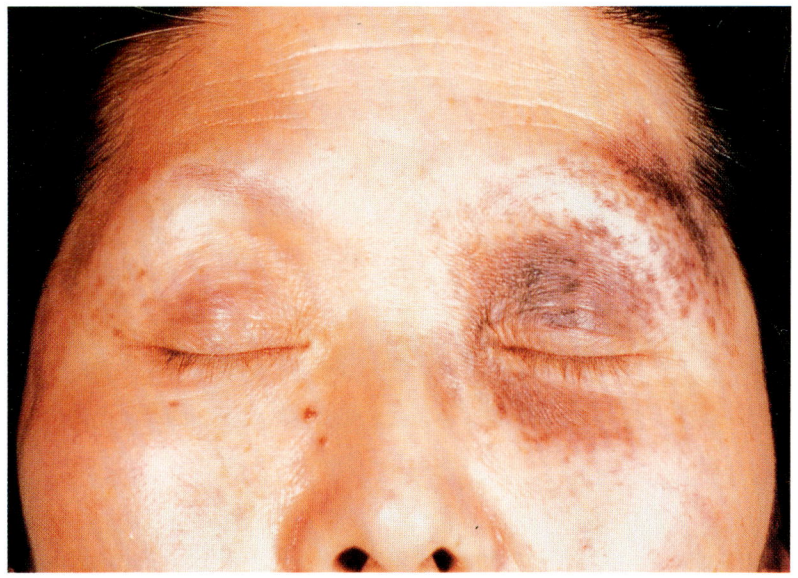

FIG. 8.28-A. Blackish-brown pigmentation from the area around the left eyelid to the forehead.

Case continues on following page.

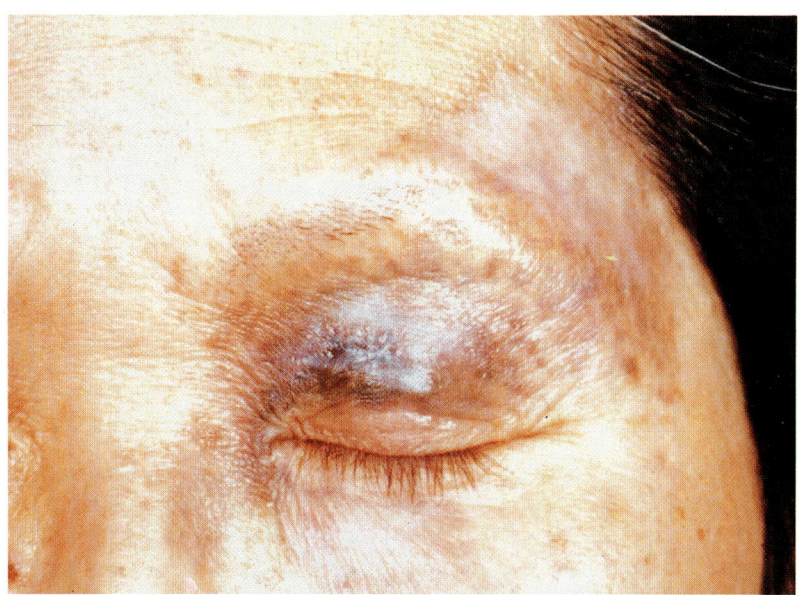

FIG. 8.28-B. Two months after three 10 J/cm² ruby laser treatments. Pigmentation on lower eyelid has completely disappeared with no scarring present.

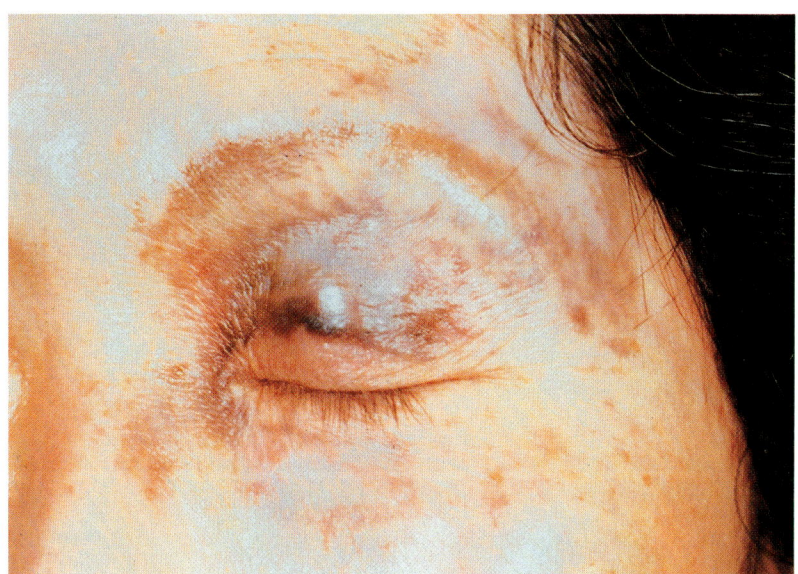

FIG. 8.28-C. Five months after five 10 J/cm² ruby laser treatments. Although some pigmentation still remains on the upper eyelid, the lesion is completely healed, without any scars.

Case courtesy of *Muneo Miyasaka,* M.D., *Ryuzaburo Tanino,* M.D., *Taichin Morita,* M.D., *Hiroto Yamada,* M.D., and *Mitsuhiro Osada,* M.D.

CASE 8.29
Nevus Spilus of the Left Cheek

REVIEW OF CASE. This 22 year-old male presented with innate nevus spilus of the left cheek.

CHOICE OF LASER: RUBY. The ruby laser is absorbed selectively by melanin granules, causing very little effect on melanin pigmentation. It does not readily cause scarring. Compared with the dye laser, argon laser, and CO_2 laser, the ruby laser has better selectivity and far-reaching capabilities. Treatment can be conducted on an outpatient basis, and the method is quite simple. In many cases, local anesthetics are not required, and pain is minimal after treatment. Epithelialization is completed in 7 to 10 days. Pigmentation disappears completely, without scarring.

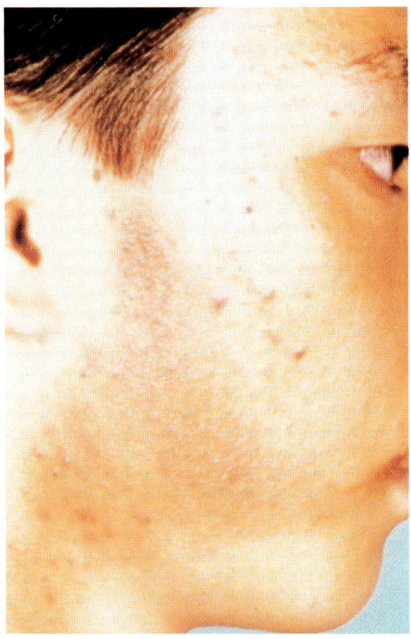

FIG. 8.29-A. The lesion is dark brownish in color and extends from the left cheek to the corners of the mouth.

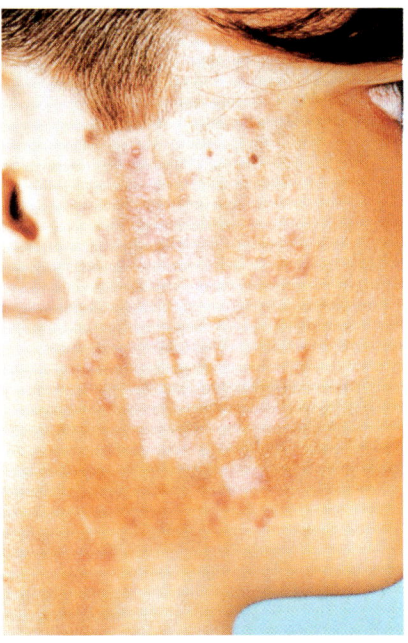

FIG. 8.29-B. One month after initial ruby laser treatment (35 J/cm^2), pigmentation where the laser was irradiated had disappeared completely.

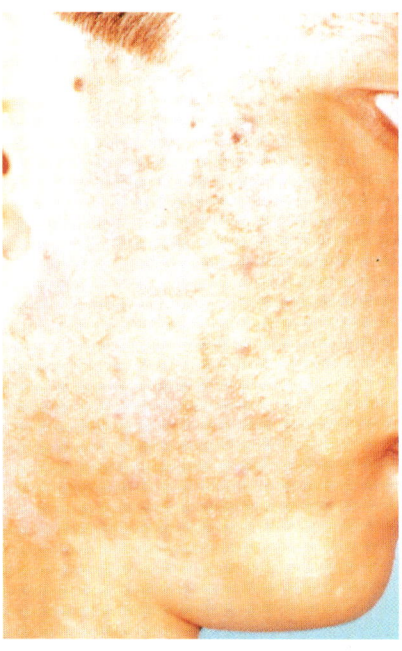

FIG. 8.29-C. One year after undergoing four ruby laser treatments (35 J/cm^2). No recurrence or scarring is present.

Case courtesy of *Muneo Miyasaka*, M.D., *Ryuzaburo Tanino*, M.D., *Taichin Morita*, M.D., *Hiroto Yamada*, M.D., and *Mitsuhiro Osada*, M.D.

CASE 8.30
Nevus Spilus of the Left Knee

REVIEW OF CASE. This patient is a 22-year-old female who had a nevus spilus since birth. The lesion had been treated in the past with dry ice without success.

CHOICE OF LASER: RUBY. The ruby laser is absorbed selectively by melanin granules, causing very little effect on melanin pigmentation. It does not readily cause scarring. Compared with the dye laser, argon laser, and CO_2 laser, the ruby laser has better selectivity and far-reaching capabilities. Treatment can be conducted on an outpatient basis, and the method is quite simple. In many cases, local anesthetics are not required, and pain is minimal after treatment. Epithelialization is completed in 7 to 10 days. Pigmentation disappears completely, with no scarring.

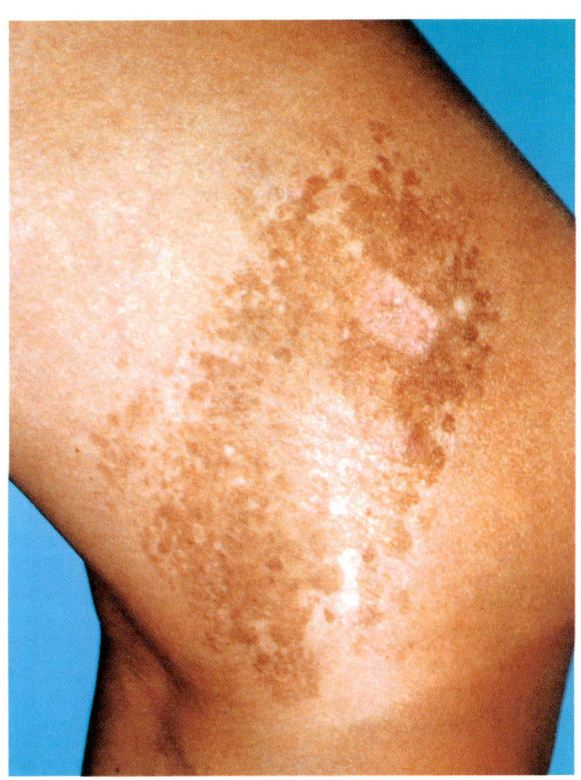

FIG. 8.30-A. The lesion is dark brownish in color and about 12 × 5 cm in size. One month after initial ruby laser test irradiation (25 J/cm^2), pigmentation where the laser was irradiated has disappeared completely.

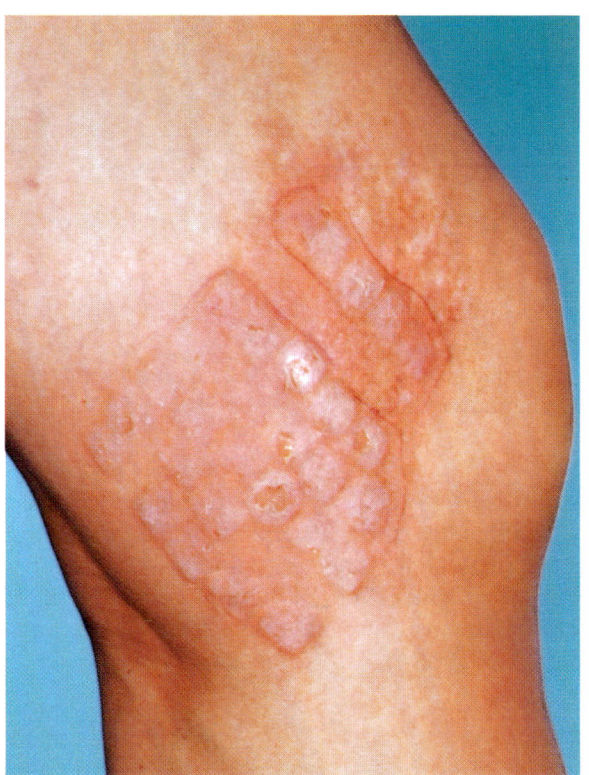

FIG. 8.30-B. Immediately after ruby laser treatment.

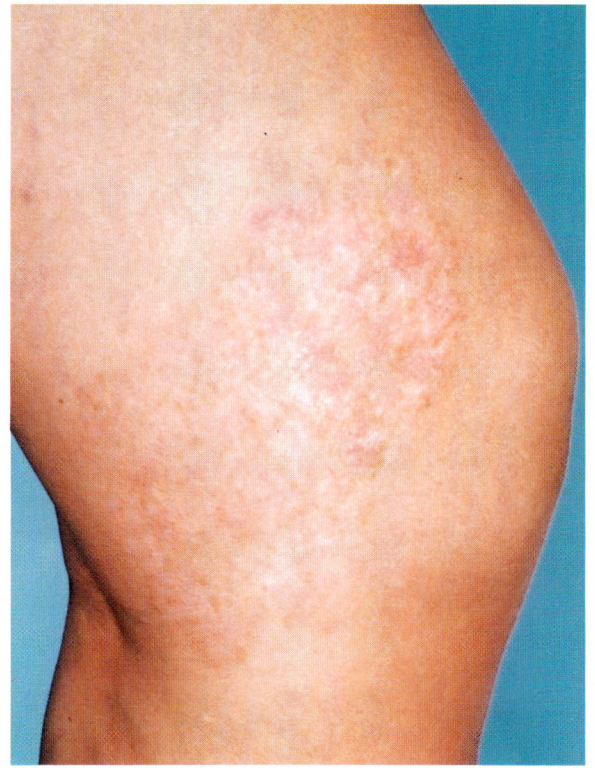

FIG. 8.30-C. One year after undergoing four 30 J/cm² ruby laser treatments. Some redness still remains, but there are no signs of recurrence or scarring.

Case courtesy of *Muneo Miyasaka*, M.D., *Ryuzaburo Tanino*, M.D., *Taichin Morita*, M.D., *Hiroto Yamada*, M.D., and *Mitsuhiro Osada*, M.D.

CASE 8.31

Seborrheic Keratosis of Anterior Part of the Left Ear

REVIEW OF CASE. This patient is a 61-year-old male who had a mole appear on the anterior part of the left ear 10 years ago. The lesion has gradually enlarged.

CHOICE OF LASER: RUBY. The ruby laser is absorbed selectively by melanin granules, causing very little effect on melanin pigmentation. It does not readily cause scarring. Compared with the dye laser, argon laser, and CO_2 laser, the ruby laser has better selectivity and far-reaching capabilities. Treatment can be conducted on an outpatient basis, and the method is quite simple. In many cases, local anesthetics are not required, and pain is minimal after treatment. Epithelialization is completed in 7 to 10 days. Pigmentation disappears completely, with no scarring.

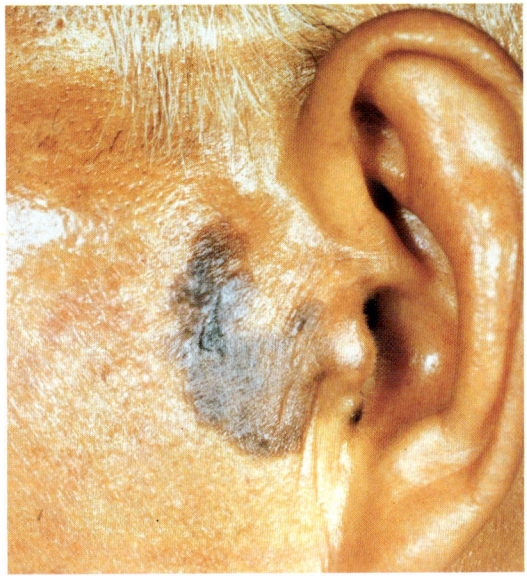

FIG. 8.31-A. Brownish-black pigmentation on the left frontal ear.

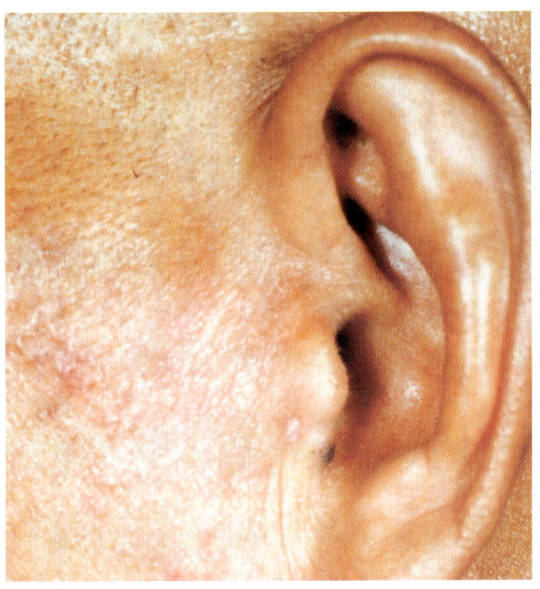

FIG. 8.31-B. One year after three ruby laser treatments (40 J/cm^2). No signs of recurrence or scarring are present.

Case courtesy of *Muneo Miyasaka*, M.D., *Ryuzaburo Tanino*, M.D., *Taichin Morita*, M.D., *Hiroto Yamada*, M.D., and *Mitsuhiro Osada*, M.D.

References

CASE 4.1

1. Apfelberg DB, Maser MR, Lash H. Review of usage of argon and carbon dioxide lasers for pediatric hemangiomas. *Ann Plast Surg* 1984; 12:353–361.

CASE 4.2

1. Ibid.

CASE 4.7

1. Stanley R, Roenigk RK. Actinic cheilitis: treatment with the carbon dioxide laser. *Mayo Clin Proc* 1988; 63:230–235.
2. Zelickson BD, Roenigk RK. Actinic cheilitis treated with the CO_2 laser. *Cancer* 1990; 65:1307–1311.

CASE 4.11

1. Wheeland RG, Bailin PL, Ratz J, Roenigk RK. CO_2 laser vaporization and currettage in the treatment of large or multiple superficial basal cell carcinomas. *J Dermatol Surg Oncol* 1987; 13:119–125.
2. Roenigk RK, Ratz JL, Bailin PL, Wheeland RG. Trends in the presentation and treatment of basal cell carcinomas. *J Dermatol Surg Oncol* 1986; 12(8):860–865.

CASE 4.32

1. Apfelberg DB, Maser MR, Lash H, White D, Flores JT. Comparison of argon and carbon dioxide laser treatment of decorative tattoos: a preliminary report. *Ann Plast Surg* 1985; 14:6–15.

CASE 4.34

1. Sunde D, Apfelberg DB, Sergott T. Traumatic tattoo removal: comparison of four treatment methods in an animal model with correlation to clinical experience. *Lasers Surg Med* 1990; 10:158–164.

CASE 4.45

1. Kantor GR, Wheeland RG, Bailin PL. et al. Treatment of earlobe keloids with carbon dioxide laser excision: a report of 16 cases. *J Dermatol Surg Oncol* 1985; 11:1063–1067.
2. Abergel RP, Meeker CA, Dwyer RM, et al. Non-thermal effects of Nd:YAG laser on biological function of human skin fibroblasts in culture. *Lasers Surg Med* 1984; 3:279–284.

CASE 4.57

1. Leshin B, Whitaker DC. Carbon dioxide laser matrixectomy. *J Dermatol Surg Oncol* 1988; 14:608–611.

CASE 4.61

1. Roenigk RK. CO_2 laser vaporization of rhinophyma. *Mayo Clin Proc* 1987; 62:676–680.

CASE 4.65

1. Wheeland RG, Bailin PL, Kronberg E. Carbon dioxide (CO_2) laser vaporization for the treatment of multiple trichoepithelioma. *J Dermatol Surg Oncol* 1984; 10:470–475.
2. Wheeland RG, Walker NPJ. Lasers—Twenty-five years later. *Int J Dermatol* 1986; 25:209–216.

CASE 4.68

1. Mittelman H, Apfelberg DB. Carbon dioxide laser blepharoplasty: advantages and disadvantages. *Ann Plast Surg* 1990; 24:1–6.

CASE 4.75

1. Hallock GG, Rice DC. In utero fetal surgery using a milliwatt carbon dioxide laser. *Lasers Surg Med* 1989; 9:482–484.

CASE 4.82

1. Apfelberg DB, Maser MR, Lash H, White DN. Treatment of xanthelasma palpebrarum with the carbon dioxide laser. *J Dermatol Surg Oncol* 1987; 13:149–151.

CASE 5.3

1. Pasyk KA, Argenta LC, Schelbert EB. Angiokeratoma circumscriptum: successful treatment with the argon laser. *Ann Plast Surg* 1988; 20:183–190.

CASE 5.4

1. Ibid.

CASE 5.5

1. Flores JT, Apfelberg DB, Maser MR, Lash H, White D. Angiokeratoma of Fordyce: successful treatment with the argon laser. *Plast Reconstr Surg* 1984; 74:835–838.

CASE 5.20

1. Apfelberg DB, Smith T, Maser MR, Lash H, White DN. Dot or pointillistic method for improvement in results of hypertrophic scarring in the argon laser treatment of port wine hemangiomas. *Lasers Surg Med* 1987; 5:539–552.

CASE 5.22

1. Achauer BM, Vander Kam VM. Capillary hemangioma (strawberry mark) of infancy: comparison of argon and Nd:YAG laser treatment. *Plast Reconstr Surg* 1989; 84(1):60–70.
2. Margileth AM, Museles M. Cutaneous hemangiomas in children, diagnosis, and conservative management. *JAMA* 1965; 194(5).

CASE 5.31

1. Apfelberg DB, Maser MR, Lash H, White D, Flores JT. Comparison of argon and carbon dioxide laser treatment of decorative tattoos: a preliminary report. *Ann Plast Surg* 1985; 14:6–15.

CASE 5.32

1. Apfelberg DB, Rivers J, Maser MR, Lash H. Update on laser usage in treatment of decorative tattoos. *Lasers Surg Med* 1982; 2:169–177.
2. Apfelberg DB, Maser MR, Lash H, White D, Flores JT. Comparison of argon and carbon dioxide laser treatment of decorative tattoos: a preliminary report. *Ann Plast Surg* 1985; 14:6–15.

CASE 5.34

1. Arndt KA. Adenoma sebaceum. Successful treatment with the argon laser. *Plast Reconst Surg* 1982; 70:91–93.
2. Janniger CK, Goldberg DJ. Angiofibromas in tuberous sclerosis: Comparison of treatment by carbon dioxide and argon laser. *J Dermatol Surg Oncol* 1990; 16:317–320.

CASE 5.35

1. Pasyk KA, Argenta LC, Schelbert EB. Angiokeratoma circumscriptum: successful treatment with the argon laser. *Ann Plast Surg* 1988; 20:183–190.

CASE 5.40

1. Cosman B, Apfelberg DB, Druker D. An effective cosmetic treatment for Ota's nevus. *Ann Plast Surg* 1989; 22:36–43.

CASE 6.18

1. Apfelberg DB, Maser MR, Lash H, White DN. Sapphire tip technology for YAG laser excisions in plastic surgery. *Plast Reconstr Surg* 1989; 84:273–280.

CASE 6.19

1. Apfelberg DB, Maser MR, White DN, Lash H. Preliminary study of the combined effect of neodymium:YAG laser photocoagulation and direct steroid instillation in the treatment of capillary/cavernous hemangiomas of infancy. *Ann Plast Surg* 1990; 22:94–104.
2. Apfelberg DB, Maser MR, White DN, et al. Benefits of contact and noncontact YAG laser for periorbital hemangiomas. *Ann Plast Surg* 1990; 24:397–409.

CASE 6.21

1. Hukki J, Harma M, Asko-Seljavaara S, Schroder T. Burn excision with contact Nd:YAG laser. *J Burn Care Rehabil* 1989; 10:402–405.
2. Kraemer MD, Jones T, Deitch EA. Burn contractures: incidence, predisposing factors, and results of surgical therapy. *J Burn Care Rehabil* 1988; 9:261–265.
3. Levine NS, Salisbury RD, Peterson HD, Pruitt BA. Clinical evaluation of the carbon dioxide laser for burn wound excisions: a comparison of the laser, scalpel and electrocautery. *J Trauma* 1975; 15:800–806.
4. Fidler JP, Law E, MacMillan BG, Fox SH, Rockwell RJ Jr. Comparison of carbon dioxide laser excision of burns with other thermal knives. *Ann NY Acad Sci* 1976; 267:254–262.
5. Jackson DM, Cason JS. Burn excision by a carbon dioxide laser. *Lancet* 1977; 1:1081–1084.
6. Heimbach DM, Neal GD, Doty JL, Colocousis J, Auth DC. The use of the argon laser-assisted quartz scalpel for burn wound excision to fascia. *J Trauma* 1980; 20:123–126.

CASE 6.22

1. Apfelberg DB, Maser MR, White DN, Lash H. A preliminary study of the combined effect of neodymium:YAG laser photocoagulation and direct steroid instillation in the treatment of capillary/cavernous hemangiomas of infancy. *Ann Plast Surg* 1989; 22:94–104.

CASE 6.23

1. Apfelberg DB, Maser MR, White DN, Lash H. A preliminary study of the combined effect of neodymium:YAG laser photocoagulation and direct steroid instillation in the treatment of capillary/cavernous hemangiomas of infancy. *Ann Plast Surg* 1989; 22:94–104.

CASE 7.29

1. Goldman MP. *Sclerotherapy treatment of varicose and telangiectatic leg veins.* St. Louis: Mosby-Year Book, 1991.
2. Goldman MP, Fitzpatrick RE. Pulsed-dye laser treatment of leg telangiectasia: with and without simultaneous sclerotherapy. *J Dermatol Surg Oncol* 1990; 16:338–344.
3. Goldman MP, Martin DE, Fitzpatrick RE, Ruiz-Esparza J. Pulsed dye laser treatment of telangiectases with and without sub-therapeutic sclerotherapy. Clinical and histologic examination in the rabbit ear model. *J Am Acad Dermatol* 1990; 23:23–30.

CASE 8.1

1. Apfelberg DB, Bailin P, Rosenberg H. Preliminary investigation of KTP/523 laser light in the treatment of hemangiomas and tattoos. *Lasers Surg Med* 1986; 6:38–43.

CASE 8.12

1. Apfelberg DB, Bailin P, Rosenberg H. Preliminary investigation of KTP/523 laser light in the treatment of hemangiomas and tattoos. *Lasers Surg Med* 1986; 6:38–43.

CASE 8.16

1. McCaughan JS Jr, Guy JT, Hicks W, Laufman L, Nims T, Walker J. Photodynamic therapy for cutaneous and subcutaneous malignant neoplasms. *Arch Surg* 1989; 124:211–216.

CASE 8.20

1. Apfelberg DB, Bailin P, Rosenberg H. Preliminary investigation of KTP/523 laser light in the treatment of hemangiomas and tattoos. *Lasers Surg Med* 1986; 6:38–43.

Glossary

Ablative Surgery removal of tissue (for example, tumor), vaporization.

Absorption action of a photon impinging on another photon with resultant energy transfer.

Absorption Coefficient wavelength's capability to be absorbed, i.e., in water, point at which maximum energy is absorbed.

Active Medium the pumped medium that supplies energy to the laser medium.

Argon Laser a visible light laser (488; 514 nm) in which argon gas is the active medium after ionization by an electric charge.

Attenuation the decrease in energy as a beam passes through an absorbing or scattering medium.

Beam a collection of rays that may be parallel, divergent or convergent.

Beam Diameter the distance between diametrically opposed points in the cross section of a beam where the power per unit area is 1/e times that of the peaks power unit area.

Beam Divergence increase in beam diameter with distance from the exit aperture of the laser.

Beam Spot Size radius or diameter of the laser beam or area of the beam cross-section.

Coagulation the irreversible denaturation that tissue proteins undergo when heated to between 50 and 100 degrees C.

Chromophore a light-absorbing compound.

CO_2 Laser 10.6 μm (far infrared), 99% absorbed in 90 μm.

Coherence all waves are in phase spatially and temporally.

Collimation all rays are parallel to each other.

Collision Pumping external power source that gets its energy by collision of particles.

Complicated Mode beam intensity profile that results in multiple spots.

Continuous Mode constant delivery of beam power density with time.

CW Laser produces a continuous laser beam without pulses.

Divergence the degree of spread of the beam as it travels. Laser light has a low degree of divergence.

Dye Laser a laser in which an organic dye is dissolved in a solvent serves as the active medium. These are "tunable" by adjusting the dye medium and the exciting radiation.

Electromagnetic Spectrum frequencies and wavelengths given off by atomic systems.

Energy watts $\times$ time (= joules).

Excited State atom with an electron in a high-energy state.

External Power Source a system outside the laser chamber that hyperexcites the atoms.

Fluence the energy per unit area measured in joules/cm^2.

Focal Length distance between focusing lens and focal point.

Focus (Focal Point) the exact point at which laser waves are at peak power.

Frequency the number of waves or cycles that pass a given point in a unit of time (seconds).

Gas Lasers lasers that contain gases as the laser medium.

Gaussian Curve the cross section of radiant power density.

Hand Piece that portion of the laser apparatus which contains the focusing lens system.

Helium-Neon Laser a visible light laser in which a mixture of helium and neon gases is the lasing medium. It is used as the red "aiming beam" for infrared lasers.

HpD hematoporphyrin derivative (used with tunable dye laser).

Ideal Mode a square wave of equal cross-sectional intensity.

Intensity the amount of power applied to a given area is known as intensity, irradiance, or power density.

Irradiance the power per unit area is measured in watts/cm^2. Power density, otherwise known as internal irradiance, determines the rate of tissue thermal effect.

Joule a unit of energy. One joule = one watt-second.

Laser *L*ight *A*mplification by *S*timulated *E*mission of *R*adiation.

Laser Beam beam of light emanating from the laser chamber.

Laser Cavity (Chamber) a resonator consisting of two reflecting mirrors on each end of a chamber which contains the active laser medium.

Laser Pumping a process that activates a laser medium by absorption of energy.

Micromanipulator ("Joystick") device that controls the direction of the laser beam when attached to a microscope.

Mode the geometric patterns of coherent radiation.

Mode Locked the phase or amplitude of the laser wave's output in locked in order to leave the cavity in a controlled train of extremely short pulses.

Monochromatic waves with exactly the same wave length (color).

Multi-mode laser emission at several closely spaced frequencies.

Neodymium: Yttrium Aluminum Garnet (Nd:YAG) Laser 1.06 μm, absorbed within 30 mm with moderate lateral scattering.

Optical Cavity laser cavity.

Optical Pumping method of imparting additional energy to the lasing medium in the chamber.

Photocoagulation use of laser beam to heat tissue below vaporization with the objective to stop bleeding and coagulate tissue.

Photon a discrete bundle of energy emitted in the form of light by excited atoms or molecules.

Plume smoke or vaporized tissue and debris liberated by the laser-tissue interaction.

Population Inversion when the number of excited atoms in a substance exceeds that of unexcited atoms.

Power Density power per unit area, watts/cm^2, equivalent to irradiance.

Pulsed Beam beam of energy produced in small durations of pulsed time.

Pulse Duration the time duration of a laser pulse.

Pumping the process of supplying energy to the laser medium.

Q Switched a laser that employs a "Q" switch or shutter to prevent laser emission until a desired time.

Resonant Cavity laser cavity.

Selective Photothermolysis selective thermal damage can be induced in tissue targets that absorb well focused emitted wavelength when the pulse duration or exposure time is shorter than the cooling time or thermal coagulation time of the target.

Semiconductor Laser lasing medium is a layer of semiconductor materials.

Single Mode laser emission at a single TEM mode, usually the smallest focused spot size available.

Spontaneous Emission release of photon of absorbed energy from a hyperexcited atom.

Stimulated Emission emission of electromagnetic energy from a higher energy state to a lower energy state in an activated laser medium.

Superpulse a pulsed laser emission which generated extremely high peak powers per pulse with extremely brief pulse widths with variable repetition.

TEM transverse electronic mode.

TEM$_{00}$ the lowest order mode possible, a bell-shaped distribution of light intensity across the laser beam cross section.

Thermal Effect CO_2 is absorbed in water and minimizes conductivity of heat.

Transmission the passage of electromagnetic radiation through a medium.

Tunable Laser a laser system that can be tuned to emit laser light over a continuous range of wavelengths or frequencies.

Vaporization conversion of a solid or liquid into a vapor.

Watt the unit of power or radiant flux.

Wavelength the distance from crest to crest in a periodice electromagnetic wave.

Bibliography

ARGON—VASCULAR

Achauer BM, Vander Kam VM. Argon laser treatment of strawberry hemangioma in infancy. *West J Med* 1985; 143:628–632.

Achauer BM, Vander Kam VM. Capillary hemangioma (strawberry mark) of infancy: comparison of argon and ND:YAG laser treatment. *Plast Reconstr Surg* 1989; 84:60–69.

Alderman DB. Therapy for essential cutaneous telangiectasia. *Post grad Med J* 1977; 61:91–95.

Apfelberg DB, Flores JT, Maser MR, Lash H. Analysis of complications of argon laser treatment for port wine hemangiomas with reference to stripe treatment. *Lasers Surg Med* 1983; 2:357–372.

Apfelberg DB, Greene RA, Maser MR, Lash H, Rivers JL, Laub DR. Results of argon laser exposure of capillary hemangiomas of infancy—Preliminary report. *Plast Reconstr Surg* 1981; 67:188–193.

Apfelberg DB, Kosek J, Maser MR, Laub D. Histology of port wine stains following argon laser treatment. *Br J Plast Surg* 1979; 32:232–237.

Apfelberg DB, Maser MR, Lash H. Review of usage of argon and carbon dioxide lasers for pediatric hemangiomas. *Ann Plast Surg* 1984; 12:353–361.

Apfelberg DB, Maser MR, Lash H. Argon laser management of cutaneous vascular abnormalitties. In: Lewis JR, ed. *The art of aesthetic plastic surgery*. Boston: Little Brown, 1989; 199–203.

Apfelberg DB, Maser MR, Lash H. Argon laser management of cutaneous vascular deformities: a preliminary report. *West J Med* 1976; 124:99.

Apfelberg DB, Maser MR, Lash H. Experience with the argon laser in the treatment of cutaneous lesions. In: Atsumi K, ed. *New frontiers in laser medicine and surgery*. Amsterdam: Excerpta Medica, 1983; 403–411.

Apfelberg DB, Maser MR, Lash H. In: Harahap M, ed. Experience with the argon laser in the treatment of cutaneous lesions in skin surgery. St. Louis: Warren H. Green, 1985.

Apfelberg DB, Maser MR, Lash H. Laser technology—Epitomes—Plastic surgery. *West J Med* 1982; 136(June):523–524.

Apfelberg DB, Maser MR, Lash H. Treatment of nevi aranei by means of an argon laser. *J Dermatol Surg Oncol* 1978; 4 (Feb):172–174.

Apfelberg DB, Maser MR, Lash H. Treatment of cutaneous vascular abnormalities with the argon laser—Progress report. *Ann Plast Surg* 1978; 1:14–19.

Apfelberg DB, Maser MR, Lash H, Rivers J. The argon laser for cutaneous lesions. *JAMA* 1981; 245:2073–2075.

Apfelberg DB, Maser MR, Lash H, Rivers J. The role of the argon laser in the management of hemangiomas. *Int J Dermatol* 1982; 21:579–589.

Apfelberg DB, Maser MR, Lash H, Rivers JL. Progress report on extended clinical use of the argon laser for cutaneous lesions. *Lasers Surg Med* 1980; 1:71–83.

Apfelberg DB, Maser MR, Lash H, White DN, Flores JT. Use of the argon and carbon dioxide lasers for treatment of superficial venous varicosities of the lower extremity. *Lasers Surg Med* 1984; 4:221–232.

Apfelberg DB, Smith T, White J. Preliminary study of the vascular dynamics of port wine hemangioma with therapeutic implications for argon laser treatment. *Plast Reconstr Surg* 1989; 83:820–828.

Apfelberg DB, Smith T, Maser MR, Lash H, White DN. Dot or pointilistic method for improvement of results in hypertrophic scarring in argon laser treatment of portwine hemangiomas. *Lasers Surg Med* 1987; 6:552–559.

Apfelberg DB. Argon laser treatment of port wine hemangiomas: summary of ten years experience. In: Williams HB, ed. *Symposium on malformations and melanotic lesions*. St. Louis: CV Mosby, 1983.

Apfelberg DB. Polka dot technique limits scarring in treatment of port wine stains. *Clin Laser Monthly* 1985; 3:4, 13.

Apfelberg DB. Summary of argon laser usage in plastic surgery. *Scand J Plast Surg* 1986; 20:13–18.

Apfelberg DB. Summary of the laser treatment of port wine hemangiomas. In: Brent B, ed. *The art of aesthetic surgery*. St. Louis: CV Mosby, 1987.

Arndt KA. Argon laser therapy of small cutaneous vascular lesions. *Arch Dermatol* 1982;118:220–224.

Barnes L, Estes SA. Laser treatment of hereditary malignant glomus tumors. *J Dermatol Surg Oncol* 1986; 12:912–915.

Barsky SH, Rosen S, et al. The nature and evolution of port wine stains. *J Invest Dermatol* 1980; 74:154–157.

Brauner G, Schliftman A. Laser surgery for children. *J Dermatol Surg Oncol* 1987; 13:178–187.

Buecker J, et al. Histology of port-wine stains treated with carbon dioxide laser. *J Am Acad Dermatol* 1984; 10:1014.

Carruth JAS. The establishment of precise physical parameters for the treatment of the port wine stain with the argon laser. *Lasers Surg Med* 1982; 2:37–42.

Cosman B. Clinical experience in the laser therapy of port wine stains. *Lasers Surg Med* 1980; 1:133–152.

Cosman B. Experience in the argon laser therapy of port wine stains. *Plast Reconstr Surg* 1980; 65:119–129.

Cosman B. Role of retreatment in minimal-power argon laser therapy for port wine stains. *Lasers Surg Med* 1982; 2:43.

Cotterill JA. Laser treatment of port wine stains. *Br Med J* 1982; 284:766.

Craig RDP, Purser JM, Lessells AM, Hufton AP. Argon laser therapy for cutaneous lesions. *Br J Plast Surg* 1985; 38:148–155.

Dicken CH. Argon laser treatment of red nose. *J Dermatol Surg Oncol* 1990; 16:33–37.

Dixon JA, Gilbertson JJ. Argon and neodymium YAG laser therapy of dark nodular port wine stains in older patients. *Lasers Surg Med* 1986; 6:5–11.

Dixon JA, Gilbertson JJ. Cutaneous laser therapy. *West J Med* 1985; 143:758–763.

Dixon JA, Davis RK, Gilbertson JJ. Laser photocoagulation of vascular malformations of the tongue. *Laryngoscope* 1986; 96:537–541.

Dixon JA, Huether S, Rotering R. Hypertrophic scarring in argon laser treatment of port-wine stains. *Plast Reconstr Surg* 1984; 73:771–777.

Dixon JA, Rotering RH, Huether SE. Patient's evaluation of argon laser therapy of port wine stain, decorative tattoo, and essential telangiectasia. *Lasers Surg Med* 1984; 4:181–190.

Finley J, Noe J, Arndt K, Rosen S. Port-wine stains. *Arch Dermatol* 1984; 120:1453–1455.

Finley J, et al. Healing of port wine stains after argon laser therapy. *Arch Dermatol* 1981; 117:486–489.

Flores JT, Apfelberg DB, Maser MR, Lash H, White D. Angiokeratoma of Fordyce: successful treatment with the argon laser. *Plast Reconstr Surg* 1984; 74:835–838.

Gilchrest B, Rosen S, Noe J. Chilling port wine stains improves the response to argon laser therapy. *Plast Reconstr Surg* 1982; 69:278–283.

Ginsbach G, et al. The treatment of hemangliomas, telangiectasia, radiodermatitis and tattoos with argon laser. In: Waidelich W, ed. *Laser 77 Opto-Electronics*. Guildford Surrey: IPC Science and Technology Press, 1977.

Ginsbach G, et al. Treatment of hemangiomas with argon laser [abstract]. *Plast Reconstr Surg* 1978; 62:145.

Goldman L, Dreffer R. Laser treatment of extensive mixed cavernous and port wine stain. *Arch Dermatol* 1977; 113:504–505.

Goldman L, et al. Histopathology of the laser treatment of port-wine lesions. *J Invest Dermatol* 1968; 2(50):141–146.

Goldman L, et al. Treatment of port wine marks by an argon laser. *J Dermatol Surg* 1976; 2:385–388.

Goldman L. The argon laser and port wine stain. *Plast Reconstr Surg* 1980; 65:137–139.

Greenwald J, Rosen S, et al. Comparative histological studies of the tunable dye (at 577 nm) laser and argon laser: the specific vascular effects of the dye laser. *J Invest Dermatol* 1981; 77:305–310.

Henning JP Hulsbergen, et al. Port wine stain coagulation experiments with a 540-nm continuous wave dye-laser. *Lasers Surg Med* 1983; 2:205–210.

Hobbs ER, Ratz JL. Argon laser treatment of angiokeratomas. *J Dermatol Surg Oncol* 1987; 13:1319–1320.

Hobby L. Treatment of port wine stains and other cutaneous lesions. *Contemp Surg* 1981; 18:22–45.

Hobby LW. Further evaluation of the potential of the argon laser in the treatment of strawberry hemangiomas. *Plast Reconstr Surg* 1983; 71:481.

Kalick SM, Goldwyn RM, Noe JM. Social issues and the body image concerns of port wine stain patients undergoing laser therapy. *Lasers Surg Med* 1981; 1:205–213.

Keller G, Doiron D, Weingarten C. Advances in laser skin surgery for vascular lesions. *Arch Otolaryngol* 1985; 111:437–440.

Kitzmiller K. Laser treatment of tattoos and angiomas. *J Med Assoc GA* 1970; 59:385–386.

Landthaler M, Haina D, Waidelich W, Braun-Falco O. Laser therapy of venous lakes (Bean-Walsh) and telangiectasias. *Plast Reconstr Surg* 1984; 73:78–83.

Larrow L, Noe J. Care of the patient with a port wine stain hemangioma. *Am J Nurs* 1982; 82:786–790.

Maillard G-F, Geinoz J. Argon laser photocoagulation of various angiomas. *Br J Plast Surg* 1985; 38:156–162.

Maser MR, Apfelberg DB, Lash H, Laub DR. Argon laser treatment of cutaneous vascular lesions—Epitomes of progress. *West J Med* 1980; 133:57–58.

McBurney E, Leonard G. Argon laser treatment of port-wine hemangiomas: clinical and histologic correlation. *South Med J* 1981; 74:925–930.

Noe J, Barsky S, et al. Port wine stains and the response to argon laser therapy: successful treatment and the predictive role of color, age, and biopsy. *Plast Reconstr Surg* 1980; 65:130–136.

Noe J, Finley J, Rosen S, Arndt K. Postrhinoplasty red nose: differential diagnosis and treatment by laser. *Plast Reconstr Surg* 1981; 67:661–664.

Ohmori S, et al. Recent progress in the treatment of port wine staining by argon laser. *Br J Plast Surg* 1981; 34:249.

Parkin J, Dixon J. Laser photocoagulation in hereditary hemorrhagic telangiectasia. *Otolaryngol Head Neck Surg* 1981; 98:204–208.

Pasyk KA, Argenta LC, Schelbert EB. Angiokeratoma circumscriptum: successful treatment with the argon laser. *Ann Plast Surg* 1988; 20:183–190.

Ratz JL, Goldman L, Baauman WE. Post-treatment complications of the argon laser. *Arch Dermatol* 1985; 121:714.

Scaglione R, Ceccolini E. The treatment of face telangiectasia and couperose with argon laser. *Biotecnologia Laser* 1987; 3:15–19.

Scheibner A, McCarthy WH. Argon laser treatment of superficial blood vessel malformations on the trunk and extremities in adults and on the face in children. *Lasers Surg Med* 1986; 6:244.

Silver L. Argon laser photocoagulation of port wine stain hemangiomas. *Lasers Surg Med* 1986; 6:24–28.

Solomon H, Goldman L, et al. Histopathology of the laser treatment of port wine lesions. *J Invest Dermatol* 1968; 50:141–146.

Solomon H, et al. Histopathology of the laser treatment of port wine lesions: biopsy studies of treated areas observed up to three years after laser impact. *J Invest Dermatol* 1968; 50:141.

Tan OT, Carney JM, Margolis R. Histologic responses of port wine stains treated by argon, carbon dioxide and tunable dye lasers. *Arch Dermatol* 1986; 122:1016–1022.

Tang S, Gilchrest B. Spectrophotometric analysis of normal, lesional, and treated skin of patients with port wine stains (PWS) [abstract]. *J Invest Dermatol* 1982; 78:340.

Touquet VLR, Carruth JAS. Review of the treatment of port wine stains with the argon laser. *Lasers Surg Med* 1984; 4:191–199.

Weston J, Apfelberg DB, Maser MR, Lash H. Laser treatment of hemangiomas and other cutaneous vascular lesions. *Vasc Diagn Ther* 1983; 4:17–33.

Yanai A, Fukuda O, Soyano S, Takayama O, Kataigi T. Argon laser therapy of port-wine stains: effects and limitations. *Plast Reconstr Surg* 1985; 75:520–525.

ARGON—MALIGNANT

Landthaler M, Haina D, Brunner R, Waidelich W, Braun-Falco O. Laser therapy of bowenoid papulosis and Bowen's disease. *J Dermatol Surg Oncol* 1986; 12:1253–1259.

McCarthy W, et al. Laser surgery for malignant melanoma and superficial malignancies. *Aust N Z J Surg* 1978; 48:656–661.

Roccia L, Fabrizio R, Gandolfo S. The treatment of leukoplakia simplex with argon laser. *Pratica Odontoiatrica* 1987; 1:28–35.

ARGON—INFLAMMATORY

Apfelberg DB, Druker D, Maser MR, Lash H, Spence B, Deneau D. Granuloma fasciale—Treatment with argon laser. *Arch Dermatol* 1983; 119:573–576.

Apfelberg DB. Discussion—Argon laser therapy of verrucous nevi. *Plast Reconstr Surg* 1984; 74:112–113.

Scaglione R, Cavenaghi R. Surgical treatment of warts with argon laser. *Biotecnologia Laser* 1986; 2:1–4.

Scaglione R, Ceccolini E. Treatment of giant condylomatosis of the lower genital tract with the argon laser. *Biotecnologia Laser* 1987; 3:7–11.

ARGON—TATTOO

Apfelberg DB, Manchester G. Current treatments of decorative and traumatic tattoo: pathophysiology and treatment. In: Stark RB, ed. *Plastic surgery of the head and neck*. New York: Churchill Livingstone, 1986; 171–181.

Apfelberg DB, Manchester GH. Decorative and traumatic tattoo biophysics and removal. In: Spira M, ed. *Clinics of plastic surgery, benign tumors and conditions of the skin and subcutaneous tissue*. 1987; 14:243–251.

Apfelberg DB, Maser MR. Argon laser treatment of decorative tattoos. *Br J Plast Surg* 1979; 32:141–144.

Apfelberg DB, Laub DR, Maser MR, Lash H. Pathophysiology and treatment of decorative tattoos with reference to argon laser treatment. In: *Clinics in Plastic Surgery*, vol. 7. Philadelphia: WB Saunders 1980, Chap IX.

Apfelberg DB, Maser MR, Lash H, White D, Flores JT. Comparison of argon and carbon dioxide laser treatment of decorative tattoos: a preliminary report. *Ann Plast Surg* 1985; 14:6–15.

Apfelberg DB, Rivers J, Maser MR, Lash H. Update on laser usage in treatment of decorative tattoos. *Lasers Surg Med* 1982; 2:169–177.

Arellano C, Leopold DA, Shafirof BB. Tattoo removal: comparative study of six methods in the pig. *Plast Reconstr Surg* 1982; 70:699.

Dixon JA, Rotering RH, Huether SE. Patient's evaluation of argon laser therapy of port wine stain, decorative tattoo, and essential telangiectasia. *Lasers Surg Med* 1984; 4:181–190.

Dixon JA. Laser treatment of decorative tattoos. In: Arndt KA, Noe JM, Rosen S, eds. *Cutaneous laser therapy: principles and methods*. New York: John Wiley 1983; 201–211.

Katalinic D. Elimination of tattoos with argon laser. *Investigacion Y Clinica Laser* 1987; 4:54–58.

ARGON—MISCELLANEOUS

Apfelberg DB, McBurney EI. Use of the argon laser in dermatologic surgery. In: Ratz JL, ed. *Lasers in cutaneous medicine and surgery*. Chicago: Year Book Medical, 1986; 31–71.

Apfelberg DB, Lash H, Maser MR, White DN. Comparison of the efficacy of argon and CO_2 lasers in the treatment of adenoma sebaceum in tuberous sclerosis. *Ann Plast Surg* 1985; 15:132–138.

Apfelberg DB, Maser MR, Lash H. Extended use of the argon laser for cutaneous lesions. *Arch Dermatol* 1979; 115:719–721.

Apfelberg DB, Maser MR, Lash H, Flores J. Expanded role of the argon laser in plastic surgery. *J Dermatol Surg Oncol* 1983; 9:145–151.

Apfelberg DB, Maser MR, Lash H, White D, Weston J. Preliminary results of argon and carbon dioxide laser treatment of keloid scars. *Lasers Surg Med* 1984; 4:283–290.

Arndt K. Adenoma sebaceum. Successful response to argon laser. *Plast Reconstr Surg* 1982; 70:91–93.

Arndt KA. Argon laser treatment of lentigo maligna. *J Am Acad Dermatol* 1984; 10:953–957.

Arndt KA. New pigmented macule appearing 4 years after argon laser treatment of lentigo maligna. *J Am Acad Dermatol* 1986; 14:1092.

Cosman B, Apfelberg DB, Druker D. An effective cosmetic treatment for Ota's nevus. *Ann Plast Surg* 1989; 22:36–43.

Flores JT, Apfelberg DB, Maser MR, Lash H. Trichoepithelioma: successful treatment with the argon laser. *Plast Reconstr Surg* 1984; 74:694–698.

Ginsbach G. New aspects in the management of benign cutaneous tumors. *Conference proceedings of the Laser 79 H Opto-Electronics*. 1979, 344–347.

Goldman L, et al. Long-term laser exposure of the senile freckle. *Arch Environ Health* 1971; 22:401–403.

Henderson D, Cromwell T, Mes L. Argon and carbon dioxide laser treatment of hypertrophic and keloid scars. *Lasers Surg Med* 1984; 3:271–277.

Henning JP Hulsbergen, van Gemert MJC. Rhinophyma treated by argon laser. *Lasers Surg Med* 1983; 2:211–215.

Landthaler M, Haina D, Waidelich W, Braun-Falco O. A three year experience with the argon laser in dermotherapy. *J Dermatol Surg Oncol* 1984; 10:456–461.

Landthaler M, Haina D, Waidelich W, Braun-Falco O. Argon laser therapy of verrucous nevi. *Plast Reconstr Surg* 1984; 74:108–111.

Olsen T. Laser surgery for blue rubber bleb nevus. *Arch Dermatol* 1979; 115.

Oshiro T. Treatment of pigmentation of the lips and oral mucosa in Peutz-Jegher's syndrome using ruby and argon lasers. *Br J Plast Surg* 1980; 33:345.

Pasyk KA, Argenta LC. Argon laser treatment of skin lesions in tuberous sclerosis. *Ann Plast Surg* 1988; 20:426–433.

ARGON—SURGICAL PROCEDURES

Krueger RR, Almquist EE. Argon laser coagulation for the anastamosis of small vessels. *Lasers Surg Med* 1985; 5:55.

CARBON DIOXIDE—VASCULAR

Apfelberg DB, Lash H, Maser MR, White DN. Benefits of the CO_2 laser for oral hemangioma excision. *Plast Reconstr Surg* 1985; 75:46–50.

Apfelberg DB, Maser MR, Lash H. Review of usage of argon and carbon dioxide lasers for pediatric hemangiomas. *Ann Plast Surg* 1984; 12:353–361.

Apfelberg DB, Maser MR, Lash H, White DN, Flores JT. Use of the argon and carbon dioxide lasers for treatment of superficial venous varicosities of the lower extremity. *Lasers Surg Med* 1984; 4:221–232.

Aronoff BL. The use of lasers in hemangiomas. *Lasers Surg Med* 1981; 1:323.

Bailin P, Kantor GR, Wheeland RG. Carbon dioxide laser vaporization of lymphangioma circumscriptum. *J Am Acad Dermatol* 1986; 14:257–262.

Barnes I, Estes SA. Laser treatment of hereditary multiple glomus tumors. *J Dermatol Surg Oncol* 1986; 12:912–917.

Ben-Bassat M, Kaplan I, Levy R. Treatment of hereditary haemorrhagic telangiectasia of the nasal mucosa with the carbon dioxide laser. *Br J Plast Surg* 1978; 31:157–158.

Choa DI, Smith MC, Evans JN, Bailey CM. Subglottic haemangioma in children. *J Laryngol Otol* 1986; 100:447–454.

Cotton RT, Tewfik TL. Laryngeal stenosis following carbon dioxide laser in subglottic hemangioma. Report of three cases. *Ann Otol Rhinol Laryngol* 1985; 94:494–497.

Crockett DM, Healy GB, McGill TJ, Friedman EM. Benign lesions of the nose, oral cavity, and oropharynx in children: excision by carbon dioxide laser. *Ann Otol Rhinol Laryngol* 1985; 94:489–493.

Dantow J, et al. Treatment of port wine stains with the CO_2 laser. *J Otolaryngol* 1986; 15:35.

Eliezri YD, Sklar JA. Lymphangioma circumscriptum: review and evaluation of carbon dioxide laser vaporization. *J Dermatol Surg Oncol* 1988; 14:357–364.

Healy G, et al. Carbon dioxide laser in subglottic hemangioma: an update. *Ann Otol Rhinol Laryngol* 1984; 93:370.

Kaplan I, Peled I. The carbon dioxide laser in the treatment of superficial telangiectases. *Br J Plast Surg* 1975; 28:214.

Levine HL, Bailin PL. CO_2 laser treatment of cutaneous tattoos and angiomas. *Arch Otolaryngol* 1982; 108:236–238.

Oshiro T. The CO_2 laser in the treatment of cavernous haemangioma of the lower lip: a case report. *Lasers Surg Med* 1981; 1:337.

Ratz J, et al. CO_2 laser treatment of port-wine stains: a preliminary report. *J Dermatol Surg Oncol* 1982; 8:1039.

Ratz JL, Bailin PL. The case for use of the carbon dioxide laser in the treatment of port-wine stains. *Arch Dermatol* 1987; 123:74–75.

Shafir R, Slutzki S, Bornstein LA. Excision of buccal hemangioma by carbon dioxide laser beam. *Oral Surg* 1977; 44:347.

Tan OT, Carney JM, Margolis R, et al. Histologic responses of port wine stains treated by argon, carbon dioxide and tunable dye lasers. *Arch Dermatol* 1986; 122:1016–1022.

van Gemert MJC, Welch AJ, Tan OT, Parrish JA. Limitations of carbon dioxide lasers for treatment of port-wine stains. *Arch Dermatol* 1987; 123:71–73.

CARBON DIOXIDE—MALIGNANT

Adams EL, et al. Treatment of basal cell carcinomas with a carbon dioxide laser. *J Dermatol Surg Oncol* 1979; 5:803–806.

Adams GL, Griebie MS. Role of the CO_2 laser in the management of localized carcinoma of the oral cavity. Emphasis on second primary malignancies. *Minn Med* 1985; 684:285–289.

Bailin PL, Ratz JL, Lutz-Nagey L. CO_2 laser modifications of Mohs surgery. *J Dermatol Surg Oncol* 1981; 7:623.

Bailin PL. Use of the CO_2 laser in microscopically controlled excision (Moh's surgery). In: Epstein E, ed. *Controversies in dermatology*. Philadelphia: WB Saunders, 1984; 170–173.

Carruth JAS. Resection of the tongue with the carbon dioxide laser: report of 100 cases. *J Laryngol Otol* 1985; 99:887–889.

Chiesa F, Sala L, Costa L, et al. Excision of oral leukoplakias by CO_2 laser on an out-patient basis: a useful procedure for prevention and early detection of oral carcinomas. *Tumori* 1986; 723:307–312.

Chiesa F, et al. Excision of oral leukoplakias by CO_2 laser on an out-patient basis: a useful procedure for prevention and early detection of oral carcinoma. *Tumori* 1986; 72:307.

Chu FW, Silverman S, Dedo HH. CO_2 laser treatment of oral leukoplakia. *Laryngoscope* 1988; 98:125–129.

Dufrense RG, Garrett AB, Bailin PL, Ratz JL. Carbon dioxide laser treatment of chronic actinic cheilitis. *J Am Acad Dermatol* 1988; 19:876–878.

Duncavage JA, Ossoff RH. Use of the CO_2 laser for malignant disease of the oral cavity. *Lasers Surg Med* 1986; 6:442–445.

Friedman E. The use of the CO_2 laser for tumors of the head and neck, breast and soft tissues. *New York* 1983; 3:146.

Gamaleya N, et al. Treatment of skin tumors by pulsed neodymium and continuous wave carbon dioxide lasers. *Dermatol Dig* 1977; 43–50.

Giler S, Ben-Bassat M, Kaplan I. The use of the Sharplan CO_2 laser for lymph node dissection in cases of malignant melanoma. *Lasers Surg Med* 1980; 3:100–106.

Goldman L. The laser in the current cancer program. *Ann NY Acad Sci* 1976; 267:324–328.

Hirano M, et al. CO_2 laser in treating carcinoma of the tongue. *Auris Nasus Larynx* 1985; 12:510.

Hirano M, Ohkubo H, Durita S, et al. CO_2 laser in treating carcinoma of the tongue. *Auris Nasus Larynx* 1985; 12:10–14.

Horch HH, Gerlach KL, Schaefer HE. CO_2 laser surgery of oral premalignant lesions. *IJO* 1986; 15:19–24.

Horch HH, et al. CO_2 laser treatment of oral dysplastic precancerous lesions: a preliminary report. *Lasers Surg Med* 1982; 2:179.

Kaplan I, Ger R. Partial mastectomy and mammoplasty performed with CO_2 surgical laser: a comparative report. *Br J Plast Surg* 1973; 26:189.

Lanzafame RJ, Rogers DW, Naim JO, Herrera HR, DeFranco C, Hinshaw JR. The effects of CO_2 laser excision on local tumor recurrence. *Lasers Med Surg* 1986; 6:103–106.

Sacchini V, Lovo GF, Arioli N, Nave M, Vandieramonte G. Carbon dioxide laser in scalp tumor surgery. *Lasers Surg Med* 1984; 4:261–266.

Slutzki S, et al. Use of the carbon dioxide laser for large excision with minimal blood loss. *Plast Reconstr Surg* 1977; 60:250–255.

Stanley RJ, Roenigk RK. Actinic cheilitis: treatment with the carbon dioxide laser. *Mayo Clin Proc* 1988; 63:230–235.

Walker NPJ. Carbon dioxide laser treatments of basal cell epitheliomas. *Br J Dermatol* 1983; 109:17–18.

Wheeland RG, Bailin PL, Kanton GR, Walker NPJ, Ratz JL. Treatment of actinic cheilitis by carbon dioxide laser, an examination of post laser histology. *J Surg Oncol* 1984; 10:792.

Wheeland RG, Bailin PL, Ratz JL, Roenigk RK. Carbon dioxide laser vaporization and currettage in the treatment of large or multiple superficial basal cell carcinomas. *J Dermatol Surg Oncol* 1987; 13:119–127.

Whitaker DC. Microscopically proven cure of actinic cheilitis by CO_2 laser. *Lasers Surg Med* 1987; 7:520–523.

CARBON DIOXIDE—INFLAMMATORY

Apfelberg DB, Druker D, Maser MR, Lash H, White DN. Benefits of the CO_2 laser for verruca resistant to other modalities of treatment. *J Dermatol Surg Oncol* 1989; 15:371–379.

Apfelberg DB, Maser MR, Lash H, Druker D. CO_2 laser resection for giant perineal condyloma and verrucous carcinoma. *Ann Plast Surg* 1983; 11:417–423.

Baggish MS. Carbon dioxide laser treatment for condylomata acuminata venereal infections. *Obstet Gynecol* 1980; 55:711.

Baggish MS. Improved laser techniques for the elimination of genital and extragenital warts. *Am J Obstet Gynecol* 1985; 153:545–550.

Baggish MS. Treating venereal infections with the CO_2 laser. *J Reprod Med* 1987; 27:737.

Baldwin HE, Geronomus RG. Lasers: the treatment of Zoon's balanitis with the carbon dioxide laser. *J Dermatol Surg Oncol* 1989; 15:491–498.

Bellina JH. The use of the CO_2 laser in management of condyloma acuminata with eight year follow-up. *Am J Obstet Gynecol* 1983; 147:375–378.

Borovay M. CO_2 laser vaporization of multiple resistant recurrent recalcitrant plantar verrucae, *Bull Sinai Hosp Detroit* 1984; 3:366.

Cacciaglia GB, Reigelhaupt RW. Effectiveness of lasers on plantar papillomas: a preliminary study. *J Foot Surg* 1985; 74:71–75.

Calkins JW, Masterson BJ, Magrina JF, Capen CV. Management of condylomata acuminata with the carbon dioxide laser. *Obstet Gynecol* 1982; 59:105–108.

Calkins MP, et al. Management of condylomata acuminata with the carbon dioxide laser. *Obstet Gynecol* 1982; 59:105.

Chegin VM, Skobelkin OK, Bredhov EII. Laser surgery for soft tissue purulent diseases. *Lasers Surg Med* 1984; 4:279–282.

Evans AS, Monaghan JM, Beattie AS. Carbon dioxide laser treatment of cervical warty atypias. *Gynecol Oncl* 1984; 17:296–300.

Ferenczy A, Mitas M, Nagai N, et al. Latent papillomavirus and recurring genital warts. *N Eng J Med* 1985; 313:784–788.

Ferenczy A. Laser therapy of genital condylomata acuminata. *Obstet Gynecol* 1984; 63:703–707.

Ferenczy A. Treating genital condyloma during pregnancy with the carbon dioxide laser. *Am J Obstet Gynecol* 1984; 148:9–12.

Fidler J, et al. Carbon dioxide laser excision of acute burns with immediate autografting. *J Surg Res* 1974; 17:1–11.

Fidler J, et al. Comparison of carbon dioxide laser excision of burns with other thermal knives. *Ann NY Acad Sci* 1976; 167:254–262.

Fuselier HA, et al. Treatment of condylomata acuminata with carbon dioxide laser. *Urology* 1980; 15:265–266.

Fuselier HA, McBurney EI, Brannan W, Randrup ER. Treatment of condylomata acuminata with carbon dioxide laser. *Urology* 1980; 115:265–266.

Giler S, Ben-Bassat M, Taube E, Kaplan I. The surgery of pilonidal sinus with the CO_2 laser. *Lasers Surg Med* 1980; 3:201–203.

Glass LF, Berman B, Llaub D. Treatment of perifolliculitis capitis abscedens et suffodiens with the carbon dioxide laser. *J Dermatol Surg Oncol* 1989; 15:673–679.

Grundsell H, Larsson G, Bekassy Z. Treatment of condylomata acuminata with the carbon dioxide laser. *Br J Obstet Gynaecol* 1984; 91:193–196.

Hahn GA. Carbon dioxide laser surgery in treatment of condyloma. *Am J Obstet Gynecol* 1981; 141:1000–1008.

Hinshaw JR, Herrera HR, Lanzafame RJ, Pennino RP. The use of the carbon dioxide laser permits primary closure of contaminated and purulent lesions and wounds. *J Dermatol Surg Oncol* 1987; 13:581–584.

Jackson DM, Cason JS. Burn excision by a carbon dioxide laser. *Lancet* 1977; 5:1081–1084.

Kantor G, Roenigk RK, Bailin PL, Bergfeld W, Bass J. Cutaneous blastomycosis: report of a case presumably acquired by direct inoculation and treated with carbon dioxide laser vaporization. *Cleve Clin J Med* 1987; 54:121–124.

Kaplan I, Ralf J. The Sharplan carbon dioxide laser in clinical surgery: seven years' experience. In: Goldman L, ed. *The biomedical laser*. New York: Springer-Verlag, 1981; 89–98.

Kaufman RH, Friedrich EGJ. The carbon dioxide laser in the treatment of vulvar disease. *Clin Obstet Gynecol* 1985; 28:220–229.

Krebs HB, Wheelock JB. The CO_2 laser for recurrent and therapy-resistant condylomata acuminata. *J Reprod Med* 1985; 30:489–492.

Krebs HB. Combination of laser plus 5-fluorouracil for the treatment of extensive genital condylomata acuminata. *Lasers Surg Med* 1988; 8:135–138.

Kuttner BJ, Siegle RJ. Treatment of chromomycosis with CO_2 laser. *J Dermatol Surg Oncol* 1986; 12:965–972.

Leffel DJ, Brown MD, Swanson NA. Laser vaporization—A novel treatment of botryomycosis. *J Dermatol Surg Oncol* 1989; 15:703–710.

Levine N, et al. Clinical evaluation of the carbon dioxide laser for burn wound excisions. A comparison of the laser, scalpel, and electrocautery. *J Trauma* 1975; 15:800–807.

Levine N, et al. Use of a carbon dioxide laser for the debridement of third degree burns. *Ann Surg* 1974; 179:246–252.

Malfetano JH Sr, Marin AC, Malfetano JHJ. Carbon dioxide laser treatment of condylomata acuminata. *Ariz Med* 1983; 40:467–469.

McBurney E, Rosen DA. Carbon dioxide laser treatment of verrucae vulgares. *J Dermatol Surg Oncol* 1984; 10:45–48.

Mueller TJ, Carlson BA, Lindy MP. The use of the carbon dioxide surgical laser for the treatment of verrucae. *J Am Podiatr Med Assoc* 1980; 70:136.

Perksy MS. Carbon dioxide laser treatment of oral florid papillomatosis. *J Dermatol Surg Oncol* 1984; 10:64–66.

Ratz JL. CO_2 laser for the treatment of balanitis xerotica obliterans. *J Am Acad Dermatol* 1984; 10:925–928.

Rayhan S. CO_2 excision method preferred to vaporization for difficult warts. *Clin Laser Monthly* 1986; 4(Aug):4S.

Rayhan S. CO_2 laser treatment of choice in recalcitrant wart. *Lasers Med Surg* 1986; 6:250.

Rosenberg SK, Fuller T, Jacobs H. Rapid superpulse carbon dioxide laser treatment of urethral condylomata. *Urology* 1981; 17:149–151.

Rosenberg SK, Jacobs H, Fuller T. Some guidelines in the treatment of urethral condylomata with carbon dioxide laser. *J Urol* 1982; 127:906–908.

Scott RS, Castro DJ. Treatment of condyloma acuminata with carbon dioxide laser: a prospective study. *Lasers Surg Med* 1984; 4:157–162.

Stein S. CO_2 laser surgery of the cervix, vagina, and vulva. *Surg Clin North Am* 1984; 64:885–897.

Stellar S, et al. Carbon dioxide laser debridement of decubitus ulcers followed immediately by immediate rotation flap or skin graft closure. *Ann Surg* 1974; 179:230–237.

Stellar S, et al. Carbon dioxide laser excision of burn eschars. *J Trauma* 1973; 13:45.

Stellar S, et al. Carbon dioxide laser for excision of burn eschars. *Lancet* 1971; 1(706):945.

Stellar S, et al. Laser excision of acute third-degree burns followed by immediate autograft replacement: an experimental study in the pig. *J Trauma* 1973; 13:45–53.

Stellar S. The CO_2 surgical lasers in neurological surgery, decubitus ulcers and burns. *Lasers Surg Med* 1980; 1:15.

Wheeland RG, Ashley JR, Smith DA, et al. Carbon dioxide laser treatment of granuloma faciale. *J Dermatol Surg Oncol* 1984; 10:730–733.

CARBON DIOXIDE—TATTOO

Apfelberg DB, Manchester G. Current treatments of decorative and traumatic tattoo: pathophysiology and treatment. In: Stark RB, ed. *Plastic surgery of the head and neck.* New York: Churchill Livingstone, 1981; 171–181.

Apfelberg DB, Manchester GH. Decorative and traumatic tattoo biophysics and removal. *Clin Plast Surg* 1987; 4:2243–2251.

Apfelberg DB, Manchester GH. Decorative and traumatic tattoo biophysics and removal. In: Spira M, ed. *Clinics of plastic surgery benign tumors and conditions of the skin and subcutaneous tissue.* 1987; 14:243–251.

Apfelberg DB, Maser MR, Lash H, White D, Flores JT. Comparison of argon and carbon dioxide laser treatment of decorative tattoos: a preliminary report. *Ann Plast Surg* 1985; 14:6–15.

Arellano C, Leopold DA, Shafirof BB. Tattoo removal: comparative study of six methods in the pig. *Plast Reconstr Surg* 1982; 70:699.

Bailin P, Ratz J, Levine H. Removal of tattoos by CO_2 laser. *J Dermatol Surg Oncol* 1980; 6:997–1001.

Beacon JP, Ellis H. Surgical removal of tattoos by carbon dioxide laser. *J R Soc Med* 1980; 73:298.

Brady SC, Blokmanis A, Jewett L. Tattoo removal with the carbon dioxide laser. *Ann Plast Surg* 1979; 2:482–490.

Dufrense RG, Garrett AV, Bailin PL, Ratz JL. CO_2 laser treatment of traumatic tattoos [letter]. *J Am Acad Dermatol* 1989; 20:137–138.

James SE, Venn GE, Russell RC. Experience using the carbon dioxide laser in the removal of cutaneous tattoos. *Br J Surg* 1985; 72:265–266.

Koranda FC, Norris CW, Diestelmeier MF. Carbon dioxide laser treatment of granulomatous reactions in tattoos. *Otolaryngol Head Neck Surg* 1986; 943:384–387.

Kyanko ME, Pontasch MJ, Brodell RD. Red tattoo reactions: treatment with the carbon dioxide laser. *J Dermatol Surg Oncol* 1989; 15:652–658.

Levine H, Bailin P. Carbon dioxide laser treatment of cutaneous hemangiomas and tattoos. *Arch Otolaryngol* 1982; 108:236–238.

Reid R, Muller S. Tattoo removal by CO_2 laser dermabrasion. *Plast Reconstr Surg* 1980; 65:717.

Ruiz-Esparza J, Goldman MP, Fitzpatrick RE. Tattoo removal with minimal scarring: the chemo-laser technique. *J Dermatol Surg Oncol* 1988; 14:1372–1376.

Sunde D, Apfelberg DB, Sergott T. Traumatic tattoo removal: comparison of four treatment methods in an animal model with correlation to clinical experience. *Lasers Surg Med* 1990; 10:158–164.

CARBON DIOXIDE—MISCELLANEOUS

Ali KM, Callari RH, Mobley DL. Resection of rhinophyma with CO_2 laser. *Laryngoscope* 1989; 99:453–455.

Apfelberg DB, Lash H, Maser MR, Rothermel ED, Witfeldt A. Preliminary results of carbon dioxide laser treatment of nail disorders. *Foot Ankle* 1983.

Apfelberg DB, Lash H, Maser MR, White DN. Comparison of the efficacy of argon and CO_2 lasers in the treatment of adenoma sebaceum in tuberous sclerosis. *Ann Plast Surg* 1985; 15:132–138.

Apfelberg DB, Maser MR, Lash H, White DN, Efficacy of the carbon dioxide laser in hand surgery. *Ann Plast Surg* 1984; 13:320–327.

Apfelberg DB, Maser MR, Lash H, White DN. Treatment of xanthelasma palpebrarum with the carbon dioxide laser. *J Dermatol Surg Oncol* 1987; 13:149–156.

Apfelberg DB, Maser MR, Lash H, White D, Weston J. Preliminary results of argon and carbon dioxide laser treatment of keloid scars. *Lasers Surg Med* 1984; 4:283–290.

Apfelberg DB, Maser MR, Lash H, White DN, Cosman B. Superpulse CO_2 laser treatment of facial syringomata. *Lasers Surg Med* 1987; 7:533–539.

Apfelberg DB, Maser MR, White DN, Lash H. Failure of carbon dioxide laser excision of keloids. *Lasers Surg Med* 1989; 9:382–388.

Apfelberg DB, Rathermel E, Widtfeldt A, Maser MR, Lash H. Progress report on use of carbon dioxide laser for nail disorders. *Current Podiatry* 1983; 32:29–32.

Apfelberg DB, Rathermel E, Widtfeldt A, Maser MR, Lash H. Preliminary report on the use of carbon dioxide laser in podiatry. *J Am Podiatr Med Assoc* 1984; 74:509–513.

Apfelberg DB. Summary of carbon dioxide laser usage in plastic surgery. *Scand J Plast Reconstr Surg* 1986; 20:19–24.

Bailin P. Use of the CO_2 laser for non-PWS cutaneous lesions. In: Arndt KA, Noe JM, Rosen S, eds. *Cutaneous laser therapy: principles and methods.* New York: John Wiley 1983; 187–200.

Bailin PL, Ratz JL, Wheeland RG. Carbon dioxide (CO_2) laser perforation of exposed cranial bone to stimulate granulation tissue. *Plast Reconstr Surg* 1985; 75:898–902.

Bellack GS, Shapshay SM. Management of facial angiofibromas in tuberous sclerosis: use of the carbon dioxide laser. *Otolaryngol Head Neck Surg* 1986; 94:37.

Ben-Bassat M, et al. The CO_2 laser in surgery of the tongue. *Br J Plast Surg* 1978; 31:155–156.

Bickley LK, Goldberg DJ, Imaeda S, Lambert WC, Schwartz RA. Lasers: treatment of multiple apocrine hidrocystomas with the carbon dioxide laser. *J Dermatol Surg Oncol* 1989; 15:599–605.

Bohigian RK, Shapshay SM, Hybels RL. Management of rhinophyma with carbon dioxide laser: Lahey Clinic experience. *Lasers Surg Med* 1988; 8:397–401.

Carruth JAS. Resection of the tongue with the carbon dioxide laser: report of 100 cases. *J Laryngol Oto* 1985; 99:887–889.

Dover JS, Smoller BR, Stern RS, Rosen S, Arndt KA. Low-fluence carbon dioxide laser irradiation of lentigines. *Arch Dermatol* 1989; 124:1219–1225.

Frame JW. Removal of oral soft tissue pathology with the CO_2 laser. *J Oral Maxillofac Surg* 1985; 43:850.

Frame JW. Treatment of sublingual dermatosis with CO_2 laser. *Br J Dermatol* 1984; 156:243.

Fukutake T, Yamashita T, Tomoda K, Kumazawa T. Laser surgery for allergic rhinitis. *Arch Otolaryngol Head Neck Surg* 1986; 112:1280–1282.

Gladstone GJ, Bachman H, Elson LM. CO_2 laser excision of xanthelasma lesions. *Arch Ophthalmol* 1985; 103:440–442.

Goldman L, Perry E, Stevanovsky D. A flexible sealed tube transverse radio frequency excited CO_2 laser for dermatologic surgery. *Lasers Surg Med* 1983; 2:317–332.

Greenbaum SS, Glogau R, Stegman SJ, Tromovitch TA. Carbon dioxide laser in the treatment of erythroplasia of Queyrat. *J Dermatol Surg Oncol* 1989; 15:747–754.

Greenbaum SS, Krull EA, Watnick K. Comparison of CO_2 laser and electrosurgery in the treatment of rhinophyma. *J Am Acad Dermatol* 1988; 18:363–368.

Groot DW, Jognston PA. Carbon dioxide treatment of porokeratosis of Mibelli. *Lasers Surg Med* 1985; 5:603.

Hallock GG. Laser treatment of rhinophyma. *Aesthetic Plast Surg* 1988; 12:171–174.

Hassard AD, Carbon dioxide laser treatment of acne rosacea and rhinophyma: How I do it. *J Otolaryngol* 1988; 17:336–337.

Henderson D, Cromwell T, Mes L. Argon and carbon dioxide laser treatment of hypertrophic and keloid scars. *Lasers Surg Med* 1984; 3:271–277.

Huerter CJ, Wheeland RG, Bailin PL, Ratz JL. Lasers: treatment of myxoid cysts with carbon dioxide laser vaporization. *J Dermatol Surg Oncol* 1987; 13:723–727.

Huerter CJ, Wheeland RG. Laser corner: multiple eruptive vellus cysts treated with carbon dioxide laser vaporization. *J Dermatol Surg Oncol* 1987; 13:260–265.

Huerter CJ, Wheeland RG, Bailin PL, Ratz JL. Lasers: treatment of myxoid cysts with carbon dioxide laser vaporization. *J Dermatol Surg Oncol* 1987; 13:723–729.

Hylton RP. Use of CO_2 laser for gingivectomy in a patient with Sturge-Weber disease complicated by Dilantin hyperplasia. *J Oral Maxillofac Surg* 1986; 448:646–648.

Kantor GR, Ratz JL, Wheeland RG. Treatment of acne keloidalis nuchae with carbon dioxide laser. *J Am Acad Dermatol* 1986; 14:263–267.

Kantor GR, Wheeland RG, Bailin PL, Walker NPJ, Ratz JL. Treatment of earlobe keloids with carbon dioxide laser excision: a report of 16 cases. *J Dermatol Surg Oncol* 1985; 11:1063–1067.

Kaplan I, Labandter H. Onychogryphosis treated with the CO_2 surgical laser. *Br J Plast Surg* 1976; 29:102.

Kaymen AH, Nasr A, Grekin RC. The use of the carbon dioxide laser in lichen myxedematous. *J Dermatol Surg Oncol* 1989; 15:862–868.

Labandter H, Kaplan I. Experience with a "continuous" laser in the treatment of suitable cutaneous conditions: preliminary report. *J Dermatol Surg Oncol* 1977; 5:527–530.

Leshin B, Whitaker DC. Carbon dioxide laser matrixectomy. *J Dermatol Surg Oncol* 1988; 14:608–611.

McBurney E. Carbon dioxide laser treatment of dermatologic lesions. *South Med J* 1978; 71:795–797.

Melcher J, Chaumette MT, Melcer F, et al. Treatment of dental decay by CO_2 laser beam: preliminary results. *Lasers Surg Med* 1984; 4:311–321.

Olbricht SM, Arndt KA. Carbon dioxide laser treatment of cutaneous disorders. *Mayo Clin Proc* 1988; 63:297–300.

Olbricht SM, Stern RS, Arndt KA. CO_2 laser and cold steel surgical treatment of keloids give comparable results. *Lasers Surg Med* 1988; 8:187.

Pick RM, Pecaro BC, Silberman CJ. The laser gingivectomy. The use of the CO_2 laser for the removal of phenytoin hyperplasia. *J Periodontol* 1985; 568:492–496.

Ratz JL, Bailin PL, Wheeland RG. Carbon dioxide laser treatment of epidermal nevi. *J Dermatol Surg Oncol* 1986; 12:567–570.

Rayhan S. Combination of CO_2 laser abrasion with collagen implant in treatment of acne scar. *J Am Soc Laser* April, 1989.

Robinson JK, Garden JM, Taute PM, Leibovich SJ, Lautenschlager EP, Hartz RS. Wound healing in porcine skin following low-output carbon dioxide laser irradiation of the incision. *Ann Plast Surg* 1987; 18:499–506.

Roenigk RK, Ratz JL. CO_2 laser treatment of cutaneous neurofibromas. *J Dermatol Surg Oncol* 1987; 13:187–190.

Roenigk RK. CO_2 laser vaporization for treatment of rhinophyma. *Mayo Clin Proc* 1987; 62:676–680.

Rosenberg SK, et al. Continuous wave CO_2 laser dermabrasion. *Urology* 1983; 19:539–541.

Rothermel E, Apfelberg DB. Carbon dioxide laser use for certain diseases of the toenails. In: Fryberg RG, ed. *Clinics in podiatric medicine and surgery*. Philadelphia: WB Saunders, 1983; 809–823.

Sacchini V, Lovo GF, Arioli N, Nava S, Bandieramonter G. Carbon dioxide laser in scalp tumor surgery. *Lasers Surg Med* 1984; 4:279–282.

Sawchuk WS, Heald PW. CO_2 laser treatment of trichoepithelioma with focused and defocused beam. *J Dermatol Surg Oncol* 1984; 10:905–907.

Shapshay SM, Strong MS, Anastasi GW, Vaughan CW. Removal of rhinophyma with the carbon dioxide laser. *Arch Otolaryngol* 1980; 106:257–259.

Spenler CW, Achauer BM, Vander Kam VM. Treatment of extensive adenoma sebaceum with a carbon dioxide laser. *Ann Plast Surg* 1988; 20:586–589.

Stoner MF, Hobbs ER. Treatment of multiple dermal cylindromas with the carbon dioxide laser. *J Dermatol Surg Oncol* 1984; 14:1263–1267.

Tra Mi Thi Luu S. Treatment of rhinophyma with CO_2 laser. *Cleveland Clinic Foundation* 1984; 3:336.

Trau H, Orenstein A, Schewach-Miller M, Tsur H. Pseudomelanoma following laser therapy for congenital nevus. *J Dermatol Surg Oncol* 1986; 12:984–994.

Truhan AP, Garden JM, Roenigk HH. Nodular primary localized cutaneous amyloidosis: immunohistochemical evaluation and treatment with carbon dioxide laser. *J Am Acad Dermatol* 1986; 146:58–62.

Weston J, Apfelberg DB, Maser MR, Lash H, White D. Carbon dioxide laserbrasion for treatment of adenoma sebaceum in tuberous sclerosis. *Ann Plast Surg* 1985; 15:132–137.

Wheeland RG, McGillis ST. Lasers: Cowden's disease—treatment of cutaneous lesions using carbon dioxide laser vaporization. *J Dermatol Surg Oncol* 1989; 15:1055–1063.

Wheeland RG, Bailin PL, Ratz JL. Combined carbon dioxide laser excision and vaporization in the treatment of rhinophyma. *J Dermatol Surg Oncol* 1987; 13:172–177.

Wheeland RG, Bailin PL, Kantor GR, Walker NPJ, Ratz JL. Treatment of adenoma sebaceum with carbon dioxide laser vaporization. *J Dermatol Surg Oncol* 1985; 11:861–864.

Wheeland RG, Bailin PL, Reynolds OD, Ratz JL. Carbon dioxide laser vaporization of multiple facial syringomas. *J Dermatol Surg Oncol* 1986; 12:225–227.

Wheeland RG, Bailin PL, Kronberg E. Carbon dioxide laser vaporization for the treatment of multiple trichoepithelioma. *J Dermatol Surg Oncol* 1984; 10:470–475.

Wheeland RG. Excisional surgery performed with the carbon dioxide laser. In: Wheeland R, ed. *Lasers in skin disease*. New York: Thieme Medical, 1988; 105–137.

CARBON DIOXIDE—SURGICAL PROCEDURES

Abergel RP, David LM. Aging hands: a technique of hand rejuvenation by laser resurfacing and autologous fat transfer. *J Dermatol Surg Oncol* 1989; 15:725–731.

Bergman RS, Murphy BJ, Foglietti MA. Clinical experience with the CO_2 laser during carpal tunnel compression. *Plast Reconstr Surg* 1988; 81:933–939.

David LM, Abergel RP. Carbon dioxide laser blepharoplasty: conjunctival temperature during surgery. *J Dermatol Surg Oncol* 1989; 15:421–424.

David LM, Sanders G. CO_2 laser blepharoplasty: a comparison to cold steel and electrocautery. *J Dermatol Surg Oncol* 1987; 13:110–119.

David LM, Lask GP, Glassberg E, Jacoby R, Abergel RP. CO_2 laserbrasion for cosmetic and therapeutic treatment of facial actinic damage. *Cutis* 1989; 43:583–587.

Giler S, Kaplan I. The use of the CO_2 laser for the treatment of cutaneous lesions in an outpatient clinic. In: Atsumi K, Nimsakal N, eds. *Proceedings of the fourth congress of the International Society for Laser Surgery*. Tokyo: Intergroup, 1981.

Hallock GG, Rice DC. Skin deepithelialization using the carbon dioxide laser. *Ann Plast Surg* 1987; 18:283.

Hallock GG. Extended applications of the carbon dioxide laser for skin deepithelialization. *Plast Reconstr Surg* 1988; 83:717–722.

Kaplan I, Ger R. The carbon dioxide laser in clinical surgery. *J Med Sci* 1973; 9:79–83.

Kaplan I, Sharon U. Current laser surgery. *Ann N Y Acad Sci* 1976; 267:247–253.

Kaplan I, et al. The carbon dioxide laser in plastic surgery. *Br J Plast Surg* 1973; 16:359–362.

Kirschner RA. Cutaneous plastic surgery with the CO_2 laser. *Surg Clin North Am* 1984; 64:871–883.

Klein D. The use of the carbon dioxide laser in plastic surgery. *South Med J* 1977; 70:429–431.

Leshin B, Whitaker DC. Carbon dioxide laser matrixectomy. *J Dermatol Surg Oncol* 1988; 14:608–611.

Mittelman H, Apfelberg DB. Carbon dioxide laser blepharoplasty—Advantages and disadvantages. *Ann Plast Surg* 1990; 24:1–6.

Negro AG, Rogers DW, Naim JO, Perry FW. Rapid communication: comparison of microsurgical suture and CO_2 laser welded anastomosis of rabbit uterine cornua. *Lasers Surg Med* 1987; 6:533–536.

Oosterhuis JW, et al. Experimental surgery on the Cloudman S91 melanoma with the carbon dioxide laser. *Acta Chir Belg* 1975; 74:422–429.

Oosterhuis JW. Tumor surgery with the CO_2 laser, studies with the Cloudman S91 mouse melanoma. *Oude Kijk In't Jatstraat* 1977; 69.

Pariente R. Role of laser in hand surgery. In: Atsumi K, ed. *New frontiers in laser medicine and surgery*. Amsterdam: Excerpta Medica, 1983; 429–436.

Pfefferman R, Merhav H, Rothstein H, Simon D. The use of laser in rectal surgery. *Lasers Surg Med* 1986; 6:467–470.

Quigley MR, Bailes JE, Kwaan HC, Cerullo LJ, Lastre CL, Monma D. Microvascular anastomosis using the milliwatt CO_2 laser. *Lasers Surg Med* 1985; 5:357–365.

Selkin SG. Laser turbinectomy as an adjunct to rhinoseptoplasty. *Arch Otolaryngol* 1985; 111:446.

Serure A, Withers EH, Thomsen S, Morris J. Comparison of carbon dioxide laser-assisted microvascular anastomosis and conventional microvascular sutured anastomosis. *Surg Forum* 1983; 34:634–636.

Vale HV, Frenkel A, Trenka-Benthin S, Matlaga BF. Microsurgical anastomosis of rat carotid arteries with the CO_2 laser. *Plast Reconstr Surg* 1986; 77:759–766.

Wheeland RG, Bailin PL. Scalp reduction surgery with the carbon dioxide laser. *J Dermatol Surg Oncol* 1984; 10:565–569.

Wheeland RG. Revision of full thickness skin graft using the carbon dioxide laser. *J Dermatol Surg Oncol* 1988; 14:130–134.

Nd:YAG—VASCULAR

Achauer BM, Vander Kam VM. Capillary hemangioma (strawberry mark) of infancy: comparison of argon and Nd:YAG laser treatment. *Plast Reconstr Surg* 1989; 84:60–69.

Apfelberg DB, Maser MR, Lash H, White DN. Sapphire tip technology for YAG laser excisions in plastic surgery. *Plast Reconstr Surg* 1989; 84:273–280.

Apfelberg DB, Maser MR, White DN, Lash H. A preliminary study of the combined effect of neodymium:YAG laser photocoagulation and direct steroid instillation in the treatment of capillary cavernous hemangiomas of infancy. *Ann Plast Surg* 1989; 22:92–104.

Apfelberg DB, Maser MR, White DN, Lash H. High and low technology solutions for massive cavernous hemangiomas of the face: lasers and leeches to the rescue. *Ann Plast Surg* 1989; 23:341–349.

Apfelberg DB, Maser MR, White DN, Lash H, Lane B, Marks MP. Benefits of contact and noncontact YAG laser for periorbital hemangiomas. *Ann Plast Surg* 1990; 24:398–408.

Apfelberg DB, Maser MR, White DN, Lash H, Lane B, Marks MP. Combination treatment for massive cavernous hemangioma of the face: YAG laser photocoagulation plus direct steroid injection followed by YAG laser resection with sapphire scalpel tips, aided by superselective embolization. *Lasers Surg Med* 1990; 10:217–223.

Apfelberg DB. Nd:YAG laser, direct steroid instillation used to treat hemangiomas. *Clin Laser Monthly* 1989; 7:32–42.

Dixon JA, Gilbertson JJ. Argon and neodymium YAG laser therapy of dark nodular port wine stains in older patients. *Lasers Surg Med* 1986; 6:5–11.

Landthaler M, Haina D, Brunner R, et al. Neodymium-YAG laser therapy for vascular lesions. *J Am Acad Dermatol* 1986; 14:107–117.

Landthaler M, Haina D, Brunner R, Waidelich W, Braun-Falco O. Neodymium-YAG laser therapy for vascular lesions. *J Am Acad Dermatol* 1986; 14:107–117.

Rosenfeld H, Sherman R. Treatment of cutaneous and deep vascular lesions with the Nd:YAG laser. *Lasers Surg Med* 1986; 6:20–24.

Rosenfeld H, Wellisz T, Reinisch JF, Sherman R. The treatment of cutaneous vascular lesions with the Nd:YAG laser. *Ann Plast Surg* 1988; 21:223–231.

Shapshay SM, David LM, Zeitels S. Neodymium-YAG laser photocoagulation of hemangiomas of the head and neck. *Laryngoscope* 1987; 97:323–330.

YAG—MALIGNANT

Brunner R, Landthaler M, Haina D, Waidelich W, Braun-Falco O. Treatment of benign, semimalignant, and malignant skin tumors with the Nd:YAG laser. *Lasers Surg Med* 1985; 5:105–111.

Gamaleya N, et al. Treatment of skin tumors by pulsed neodymium and continuous wave carbon dioxide lasers. *Dermatol Dig* 1977; 11:43–50.

Nd:YAG—MISCELLANEOUS

Abergel RP, Dwyer R, Meeker C, Lask G, Kelly P, Uitto J. Laser treatment of keloids: a clinical trial and an in vitro study with Nd:YAG laser. *Lasers Surg Med* 1984; 4:291–295.

Abergel RP, Meeker CA, Dwyer RM, Lesavoy MA, Uitto J. Nonthermal effects of Nd:YAG laser on biological functions of human skin fibroblasts in culture. *Lasers Surg Med* 1984; 3:279–284.

Apfelberg DB, Smith T. Study of the benefits of the Nd:YAG laser in plastic surgery. In: Ogura Y, Joffee S, eds. *Advances in Nd:YAG laser surgery*. New York: Springer-Verlag, 1988.

Apfelberg DB, Smith T, Lash H, Maser MR, White DN. Preliminary report on use of the neodymium:YAG laser in plastic surgery lasers. *Lasers Surg Med* 1987; 7:189–198.

Castro DJ, Abergel RP, Meeker CA, Dwyer RM, Lesavoy MA, Uitto J. Effects of the Nd:YAG laser on DNA synthesis and collagen production in human skin fibroblast cultures. *Ann Plast Surg* 1983; 11:214–222.

Castro DJ, et al. Wound healing: biological effects of Nd:YAG laser on collagen metabolism in pig skin in comparison to thermal burn. *Ann Plast Surg* 1983; 11:131–140.

Goldman L, Nath G, Schindler G, Fidler J, Rockwell RJJ. High power Nd:YAG laser surgery. *Acta Derm Venereol* 1973; 53:45–49.

Landthaler M, Brunner R, Haina D, Frank F, Waidelich W, Braun-Falco O. First experiences with the Nd:YAG laser in dermatology. In Joffe SN, ed. *Neodymium-YAG lasers in medicine and surgery*. New York: Elsevier, 1983; 176–183.

Sherman R, Rosenfeld H. Experience with the neodymium:YAG laser in the treatment of keloid scars. *Ann Plast Surg* 1988; 21:231–236.

Zimmerman I, Stern J, Frank F, Keiditsch E, Hofstetter A. Interception of lymphatic drainage by Nd:YAG laser irradiation in rat urinary bladder. *Lasers Surg Med* 1984; 4:167–172.

Zimmerman I, Stern J, Frank F, Keiditsch E, Hofstetter A. Drainage by Nd:YAG laser irradiation in rat urinary bladder. *Lasers Surg Med* 1984; 4:167.

Nd:YAG—SURGICAL PROCEDURES

Abergel RP, Lyons RF, White RA, Lask G, Matsuoko LY, Dwyer RM, Uitto J. Skin closure by Nd:YAG laser welding. *J Am Acad Dermatol* 1986; 14:810–814.

Apfelberg DB, Smith T. Study of the benefits of the Nd:YAG laser in plastic surgery. In: Joffee SN, Oguro Y, eds. *Advances in neodymium:YAG laser surgery*. New York: Springer-Verlag, 1988; 214–226.

Daikuzono N. Contact delivery systems and accessories. In: Joffee SN, Ogura Y, eds. *Advances in Nd:YAG laser surgery*. New York: Springer-Verlag, 1988; 19–29.

Hukki J, Krogerus L, Castren M, et al. Effects of different contact laser scalpels on skin and subcutaneous fat. *Lasers Surg Med* 1988; 8:276.

Jain KK, Gorisch W. Repair of small blood vessels with the neodymium:YAG laser; a preliminary report. *Surgery* 1979; 85:684.

Jain KK. Sutureless end-to-side microvascular anastomoses using neodymium:YAG laser. *Vasc Surg* 1983; 17:240.

Ohyama M, Yamashita K, Furuta S, et al. Applications of the Nd:YAG laser in otorhinolaryngology. In: Joffee SN, Ogura Y, eds. *Advances in Nd:YAG laser surgery*. New York: Springer-Verlag, 1988; 156–179.

Sankar MY. Laser hemorrhoidectomy. In: Joffee SN, Ogura Y, eds. *Advances in Nd:YAG laser surgery*. New York: Springer-Verlag, 1988; 247–256.

Sasako M, Iwasaki M, Konishi T, Maruyama Y, Wada O. Clinical application of the Nd:YAG laser in endoscopy. *Lasers Surg Med* 1982; 2:137–147.

Welch AJ, Motamedi M, Gonzales A. Evaluation of cooling techniques for the protection of the epidermis during Nd:YAG laser radiation of the skin. In: Joffee SN, ed. *Neodymium-YAG lasers in medicine and surgery*. New York: Elsevier, 1983.

TUNABLE DYE—VASCULAR

Anderson R, Parrish J. Selective photothermolysis: precise microsurgery by selective absorption of pulsed radiation. *Science* 1983; 220:524.

Cotterill JA. Preliminary results following treatment of vascular lesions of the skin using a continuous wave tunable dye laser. *Clin Exp Dermatol* 1986; 11:628–635.

Garden JM, Polla LL, Tan OT. The treatment of port-wine stains by the pulsed dye laser. *Arch Dermatol* 1988; 124:889–896.

Garden JM, Tan OT, Kerschmann R, et al. Effect of dye laser pulse duration on selective cutaneous vascular injury. *J Invest Dermatol* 1988; 87:653–657.

Garden JM, Tan OT, Parrish JA. The pulsed dye laser: It's use at 577 nm wavelength. *J Dermatol Surg Oncol* 1987; 13:134–149.

Garden JM, et al. Effect of dye laser pulse duration on selective cutaneous vascular injury. *J Invest Dermatol* 1986; 87:653.

Garden JM, et al. The instrument of port wine stains by the pulsed dye laser: analysis of pulse duration and long-term therapy. *Arch Dermatol* 1988; 124:889.

Glassberg EE, Lask G, Rabinowitz LG, Tunnessen WW. Capillary hemangiomas: case study of a novel laser treatment and a review of therapeutic options. *J Dermatol Surg Oncol* 1989; 15:1214–1226.

Glassberg E, Lask GP, Tan EML, et al. The flashlamp-pumped 577-nm pulsed tunable dye laser: clinical efficacy and in vitro studies. *J Dermatol Surg Oncol* 1988; 14:1200–1208.

Goldman MP, Fitzpatrick RE. Pulsed-dye laser treatment of leg telangiectasia: with and without simultaneous sclerotherapy. *J Dermatol Surg Oncol* 1990; 16:4, 338–344.

Greenwald J, Rosen S, et al. Comparative histological studies of the tunable dye (at 577 nm) laser and argon laser: the specific vascular effects of the dye laser. *J Invest Dermatol* 1981; 77:305–310.

Henning JP, Hulsbergen, van Gemert M, Lahaye C. Clinical and histological evaluation of port-wine stain treatment with a microsecond-pulsed dye-laser at 577 nm. *Lasers Surg Med* 1984; 4:375–380.

Keller GS, Doiron DR, Keller RS. Treatment of vascular lesions with a CW yellow dye laser: initial trials. *Otolaryngol Head Neck Surg* 1986; 95:527–530.

Morelli JG, Tan OT, Garden J, Margolis R, Seki Y, Boll J, Carney JM, Anderson RR, Furumoto H, Parrish JA. Tunable dye laser (577 nm) treatment of port wine stains. *Lasers Surg Med* 1986; 6:94–99.

Nakagawa H, Tan OT, Parrish JA. Ultrastructural changes in human skin after exposure to a pulsed laser. *J Invest Dermatol* 1985; 84:396–400.

Orenstein A, Nelson JS. Treatment of facial vascular lesions with a 100-micron spot 577-nm pulsed continuous wave dye laser. *Ann Plast Surg* 1989; 23:310–317.

Parrish J, et al. Selective thermal effects with pulsed irradiation from lasers: from organ to organelle. *J Invest Dermatol* 1983; 80:75.

Polla LL, Tan OT, Garden JM, Parrish JA. Tunable pulsed dye laser for the treatment of benign cutaneous vascular ectasia. *Dermatology* 1986; 174:11–17.

Rogalla C. Treating benign vascular lesions using the new theory selective photothermolysis. *Laser Nursing* 1989; 3:16–23.

Scearbo M. Pediatric nursing interventions during tunable pulsed dye laser therapy. *Laser Nursing* 1989; 3:4–7.

Scheibner A, Wheeland RG. Argon-pumped tunable dye laser therapy of facial port-wine stain hemangiomas in adults—A new technique using small spot size and minimal power. *J Dermatol Surg Oncol* 1989; 15:277–281.

Sherwood KA, Tan OT. Treatment of a capillary hemangioma with the flashlamp pumped dye laser. *J Am Acad Dermatol* 1990; 22:136–137.

Tan OT, Gilchrest BA. Laser therapy for selected cutaneous lesions in a pediatric population: a review. *Pediatrics* 1988; 82:652–662.

Tan OT, Gilchrest BA. Laser therapy for selected cutaneous vascular lesions in the pediatric population: a review. *Pediatrics* 1988; 82:71.

Tan OT, Morelli JG. Lasers in dermatology. *Curr Prob Derm* 1989; 1:1–27.

Tan OT, Stafford TJ. Treatment of port wine stains at 577 nm: clinical results. *Med Instrum* 1987; 21:218–221.

Tan OT, Carney JM, Margolis R, Seki Y, Boll J, Anderson RR, Parrish J. Histologic responses of port-wine stains treated by argon, carbon dioxide, and tunable dye lasers. *Arch Dermatol* 1986; 122:1016–1022.

Tan OT, Sherwood K, Gilchrest BA. Treatment of children with port-wine stains using the flashlamp-pulsed tunable dye laser. *N Engl J Med* 1989; 320:416–421.

Tan OT, et al. Action spectrum of vascular specific injury using pulsed irradiation. *J Invest Dermatol* 1989; 92:868.

Tan OT, et al. Histologic responses of port wine stains treated by argon, carbon dioxide and tunable dye lasers. *Arch Dermatol* 1986; 122:1016.

Tan OT, et al. Pulsed dye laser (577 nm) treatment of port wine stains: ultrastructural evidence of neovascularization and mass cell degranulation in healed lesions. *Soc Invest Derm* 1988; 90:395.

Tan OT, et al. Ultrastructural changes in red blood cells following pulsed irradiation in vitro. *Soc Invest Derm* 1989; 92:100.

TUNABLE DYE—MISCELLANEOUS

Tan OT, Kerschmann R, Parrish JA. Effect of epidermal pigmentation on selective vascular effects of pulsed laser. *Lasers Surg Med* 1984; 4:365–374.

Tong AK, Tan OT, Boll J, Parrish JA, Murphy GF. Ultrastructure: effects of melanin pigment on target specificity using a pulsed dye laser (577 nm). *J Invest Dermatol* 1987; 88:747–752.

Wheeland RG, Applebaum J. Flashlamp-pumped pulsed dye laser therapy for poikiloderma of civatte. *J Dermatol Surg Oncol* 1990; 16:1, 12–16.

NEW TECHNOLOGY

Apfelberg DB, Bailin P, Rosenberg H. Preliminary investigation of KTP/532 laser light in the treatment of hemangiomas and tattoos. *Lasers Surg Med* 1986; 6:38–43.

Goldman L, Rockwell J, Meyer R, et al. Laser treatment of tattoos, a preliminary survey of three year's clinical experience. *JAMA* 1967; 201:841–844.

Laub D, Yules R, Arras M, et al. Preliminary histopathological observation of Q-switched ruby laser radiation on dermal tattoo pigment in man. *J Surg Res* 1968; 8:220–224.

Reid WH, McLeod PJ, Ritchie A, Ferguson-Pell M. Switched ruby laser treatment of black tattoos. *Br J Plast Surg* 1983; 36:455–459.

GENERAL

Abergel RP, Lam TS, Lask G, Dwyer RA, Castel JC, Uitto J. Biological effects of lasers. *Invest Clin Laser* 1986; 3:7–14.

Abergel RP, Lyons R, Dwyer R, White RR, Uitto J. Use of lasers for closure of cutaneous wounds: experience with Nd:YAG, argon, and CO_2 lasers. *J Dermatol Surg Oncol* 1986; 12:1181–1185.

Abergel RP, Lyons RF, Castel JC, Dwyer RM, Uitto J. Biostimulation of wound healing by lasers: experimental approaches in animal models and in fibroblast cultures. *J Dermatol Surg Oncol* 1987; 13:127–134.

Abergel RP, Meeker CA, Lam TS, Dwyer RM, Lesavoy MA, Uitto J. Control of connective tissue metabolism in the skin by lasers: recent developments and future prospects. *J Am Acad Dermatol* 1984; 11:1142–1150.

Abergel RP, Zaragoza EJ, Uitto J. Differential effects of Nd:YAG laser on collagen and elastin production by chick embryo aortae in vitro. *Biochem Biophys Res Commun* 1985; 131:462–468.

Albright SD. Ten commandments of dermatologic laser surgery. *Laser Med Surg News* 1985; 3:1.

Andrews AH. The use of the CO_2 laser in otolaryngology: ten years of experience. *Lasers Surg Med* 1984; 4:305–310.

Apfelberg DB, Vistnes LM. Treatment of hemangioma and lymphangioma. In: Georgiade N, Riefkohl R, Barwick WJ, eds. *Essentials in Plastic, Maxillofacial, and Reconstructive Surgery.* Baltimore: Williams & Wilkins, 1986; 187–194.

Apfelberg DB, Maser M, Lash H. The role of lasers in current surgical practice. *Plastic Surgery Nursing* 1986; 6:10–21.

Apfelberg DB, Maser MR, Lash H. Summary of clinical use of lasers. In: McCarthy J, ed. *Converse textbook of plastic surgery.* New York: WB Saunders, 1989.

Apfelberg DB, Maser MR, Lash H. Use of argon and CO_2 lasers in clinical plastic surgery practice. In: Aston S, ed. *Plastic Surgery.* Boston: Little Brown, 1990.

Apfelberg DB, Maser MR, Lash H, White DN, Smith T. Past, present, and future usages of lasers in plastic surgery, dermatology, and podiatry. In: Apfelberg DB, ed. *Evaluation and Instillation of Surgical Laser Systems.* New York: Springer-Verlag, 1986; 210–228.

Apfelberg DB. A comprehensive laser center. *Perioperative Nursing Quart* 1985; 57–63.

Apfelberg DB. Applications of lasers in plastic surgery and dermatology. In: Joffee SN, ed. *Lasers in general surgery.* Baltimore: Williams & Wilkins 1989; 238–250.

Apfelberg DB. Biophysics, advantages, and installation of surgical laser systems. In: Apfelberg DB, ed. *Evaluation and installation of surgical laser.* New York: Springer-Verlag, 1986; 1–17.

Arendt-Nielsen L, Bjerring P. Laser-induced pain for evaluation of local analgesia: a comparison of topical application (EMLA) and local injection (lidocaine). *Anesth Analg* 1988; 67:115–123.

Arndt KA. Treatment techniques in argon laser therapy: comparison of pulsed and continuous exposure. *J Am Acad Dermatol* 1984; 11:90–97.

Arndt KA, Noe JM. Lasers in dermatology. *Arch Dermatology* 1982; 118:293–295.

Arndt KA, Noe JM, Northam DBC, Itzkan I. Laser therapy: Basic concepts and nomenclature. *J Am Acad Dermatol* 1981; 5:649–654.

Bailin P, Ratz J. Use of the CO_2 laser in dermatologic surgery. In: Ratz J, ed. *Lasers in cutaneous medicine and surgery.* Chicago: Year Book, 1986.

Bailin P. Lasers in dermatology—1985. *J Dermatol Surg Oncol* 1985; 11:328–334.

Bailin PL, Ratz JL. Argon laser. In: Roenigk RK, Roenigk HH, eds. *Dermatologic surgery: principles and practice.* New York: Marcel Dekker, 1988; 881–896.

Bailin PL, Ratz JL, Wheeland RG, eds. *Dermatologic clinics.* Philadelphia: WB Saunders, 1987.

Bailin PL, Ratz JL, Wheeland RG. Laser therapy of the skin. *Dermatol Clin* 1987; 5:259–285.

Bailin PL, Ratz JL, Wheeland RG. Lasers in dermatology. *J Dermatol Surg Oncol* 1987; 13:109.

Bailin PL, Ratz JL, Wheeland RG. Laser therapy of the skin: a review of principles and applications. In: Bailin PL, Ratz JL, Wheeland RG, eds. *Dermatologic clinics.* Philadelphia: WB Saunders, 1987; 5:259–285.

Bailin PL. Laser therapy: Its mechanisms and applications to clinical practice. *Mod Med* 1988; 56:52–59.

Bailin PL. Lasers in dermatology—Principles and clinical applications. *Prog Dermatol* 1987; 21:1–8.

Bailin PL. The CO_2 laser in dermatology. *Cleve Clin J Med* 1989; 56:118.

Bandieramonte G, Chiesa A, Andreola S. The use of CO_2 laser in microsurgical oncology. *National Cancer Institute* (Milano, Italy) 1984; 3:364.

Benke RA, Clark JW, Wisoff PJ, et al. Comparative study of suture and laser-assisted anastomoses in rat sciatic nerves. *Lasers Med Surg* 1989; 9:602–615.

Brody NI. Lasers in dermatology. *Drug Update* 1986; 5:21–30.

Buell BR, Schuller DE. Comparison of tensile strength in CO_2 laser and scalpel skin incisions. *Arch Otolaryngol* 1983; 109:465.

Carruth JA. Lasers in medicine and surgery. *J Med Eng Technol* 1984; 84:161–167.

Dixon JA. Lasers in surgery. *Curr Probl Surg* 1984; 21:1.

Eastern J. Lasers in private dermatologic practice. *Cutis* 1986; 293.

Evans PH, Frame JW, Brandrick J. A review of carbon dioxide laser surgery in the oral cavity and pharynx. *J Laryngol Otol* 1986; 100:69–78.

Fasano VA, Ponzio RM, Benech F, Sicuro M. Effects of laser sources (argon, Nd:YAG, CO_2) on the elastic resistance of the vessel wall: histological and physical study. *Lasers Surg Med* 1983; 2:45–54.

Fischer JD. The power density of a surgical laser beam: Its meaning and measurement. *Lasers Surg Med* 1983; 2:1.

Fischer SE, Frame JW. The effects of the carbon dioxide surgical laser on oral tissues. *Br J Oral Maxillofac Surg* 1984; 226:414–425.

Frame JW. Carbon dioxide laser surgery for benign oral lesions. *Br Dent J* 1985; 158:125–128.

Frame JW. Removal of oral soft tissue pathology with the CO_2 laser. *J Oral Maxillofac Surg* 1985; 43:850–855.

Frame JW. CO_2 laser surgery in the mouth. *Dent Update* 1984; 118:465–466, 468, 470 passim.

Fry TL, et al. Effects of laser, scalpel, and electrosurgical excision on wound contracture and graft take. *Plast Reconstr Surg* 1980; 65:729–731.

Fuller T. Fundamentals of lasers in surgical medicine. In: Dixon J, ed. *Surgical applications of lasers.* Chicago: Year Book, 1983; 11–28.

Garden JM, Geronemus RG. Dermatologic laser surgery. *J Dermatol Surg Oncol* 1990; 16:156–168.

Garden JM. Dye laser in dermatologic surgery: principles and practice. Polnigk RK, Roenigk HH, eds. New York: Marcel Dekker, 1989; 897–906.

Giorgini RJ. *Podiatric applications of laser surgery.* NY Coll Podiatr Med 1983; 3:184.

Goldman L, Dreffer R. Microwaves magnetic iron particles and lasers as a combined test model for investigation of hyperthermia treatment of cancer. *Arch Dermatol Res* 1976; 257:227–232.

Goldman L. Current developments in laser dermatologic surgery. *Dermatol Clin* 1981; 2:293–302.

Goldman L. Effects of new laser systems on the skin. *Arch Dermatol* 1973; 108:385–390.

Goldman L. Laser instrumentation in dermatology: diagnosis and treatment. In: Goldman L, ed. *Biomedical laser technology and clinical applications.* New York: Springer-Verlag, 1981.

Goldman L. Laser surgery for skin cancer. *NY State J Med* 1977; 77:1897–1902.

Goldman L. Surgery by laser for malignant melanoma. *J Dermatol Surg Oncol* 1979; 5(2):141–144.

Goldman L. Laser surgery in cosmetic dermatology. *Cutis* 1976; 17(1):38.

Goldman L. The laser in skin cancer. *Int Adv Surg Oncol* 1978; 1:217–225.

Goldman L, et al. Resecting vulvar lesions with CO_2 laser. *Contemp Ob/Gyn* 1975; 6:35.

Hall R, et al. A carbon dioxide surgical laser. *Ann R Coll Surg Engl* 1971; 48:181.

Hornblass A, Heischorn BJ. CO_2 laser surgery in hemophilia. *Am J Ophthalmol* 1983; 96:689.

Hukki J, Lipasti J, Castren M, Puolakkainen P, Schroder T. Lactate dehydrogenase in laser incisions: a comparative analysis of skin wounds made with steel scalpel, electrocautery, superpulse-continuous wave mode carbon-dioxide lasers, and contact Nd:YAG laser. *Lasers Med Surg* 1989; 9:589–594.

Kamat BR, Tang SV, Arndt KA, Stern RS, Noe JM, Rosen R. Low influence CO_2 laser irradiation: selective epidermal damage to human skin. *J Invest Dermatol* 1985; 853:274–278.

Kaplan I. Current CO_2 laser surgery. *Plast Reconstr Surg* 1982; 69:552.

Kaplan I, Sharon U. Current laser surgery. *Ann NY Acad Sci* 1976; 267:247.

Keijzer M, Jacques SL, Prahl SA, Welch AG. Light distribution in artery tissue: Monte Carlo simulations for finite-diameter laser beams. *Lasers Surg Med* 1989; 9:148–154.

Kirschner RA. Introduction to laser surgery. *Surg Clin North Am* 1984; 64:839–841.

Kirschner RA. Cutaneous plastic surgery with the CO_2 laser. *Surg Clin North Am* 1984; 645:871–883.

Koranda FC, Grande DJ, Whitaker DC, Lee RD. Laser surgery in the medically compromised patient. *J Dermatol Surg Oncol* 1982; 8:471–474.

Kubasova T, Kovacs L, Somosy Z, Unk P, Kokai A. Biological effect of He-Ne laser: investigations on functional and micromorphological alterations of cell membranes in vitro. *Lasers Surg Med* 1984; 4:381–388.

Landthaler M, Haina D, Brunner R, Waidelich W, Braun-Falco O. A 5 year experience with laser therapy in dermatology. *Curr Probl Dermatol* 1986; 15:272–281.

Lanzafame RJ, Rogers DW, Naim JO, DeFranco CA, Ochej H, Hinshaw R. Rapid communication: reduction of local tumor recurrence by excision with the CO_2 laser. *Lasers Surg Med* 1986; 6:439–442.

Lanzafame RJ, Rogers DW, Naim JO, Herrera HR, DeFranco C, Hinshaw JR. The effect of CO_2 laser excision on local tumor recurrence. *Lasers Surg Med* 1986; 6:103–105.

Loertscher H, Rol P. Basic physics of Nd:YAG laser. *Int Ophthalmol Clin* 1985; 25:1.

Lyons Rf, Abergel RP, White RA, Dwyer RM, Castel JC, Uitto J. Biostimulation of wound healing in vivo by a helium-neon laser. *Ann Plast Surg* 1987; 18:47–50.

Maser MR, Apfelberg DB, Lash H. Clinical applications of the argon and carbon dioxide lasers in dermatology and plastic surgery. *World J Surg* 1983; 7:684–691.

McBurney E. Carbon dioxide laser treatment of dermatology lesions. *South Med J* 1978; 71:795–798.

McKenzie AC, Carruth JA. Lasers in surgery and medicine. *Phys Med Biol* 1984; 29:619.

Oshiro T. The CO_2 laser as an ideal microsurgical tool. *Lasers Surg Med* 1986; 6:29–37.

Olbricht SM, Arndt KA. In: Fuller T, ed. *Lasers in cutaneous surgery in surgical lasers: a clinical guide.* New York: Macmillan, 1987; 113–146.

Olbricht SM, Stern RS, Tang SV, Noe JM, Arndt KA. Complications of laser surgery. *Arch Dermatol* 1987; 123:345–349.

Ossoff RH. The use of modern technology in head and neck cancer. *Otolaryngol Clin North Am* 1985; 18:515.

Polanyi TG. Physics of surgery with lasers. *Clin Chest Med* 1985; 6:179.

Ratz JL, Bailin PL. CO_2 laser. In: Roenigk RK, Roenigk HH, eds. *Dermatologic surgery: principles and practice.* New York: Marcel Dekker, 1988; 865–879.

Ratz JL. Laser update. In: Callen JC, ed. Current issues in dermatology, Boston: Hall Medical, 1984; 2:244–252.

Ratz JL. Laser applications dermatology and plastic surgery. In: Dixon JA, ed. *Surgical application of lasers*, 2nd ed. Chicago: Yearbook Medical, 1987; 160–182.

Rhys-Evans PH, Frame JW, Brandrick J. A review of carbon dioxide laser surgery in the oral cavity and pharynx. *J Laryngol Otol* 1986; 100:69–77.

Schnizer W, Erdl R, Schops R, Seichert N. The effects of external CO_2 application of human skin microcirculation investigated by laser doppler flowmetry. *Int J Microcirc Clin Exp* 1985; 44:343–350.

Tan OT, et al. Spot size effects on guinea pig skin following pulsed radiation. *Soc Invest Derm* 1988; 90:877.

Tennino R, et al. Applications of the CO_2 laser in general surgery. *Cont Surg* 1986; 28:13.

Walsh J, et al. Laser tissue interactions and their clinical applications. *Curr Probl Dermatol* 1986; 115:94.

Wheeland R, Bailin PL. Dermatologic applications of the argon and CO_2 lasers. *Current Concepts in Skin Disorders* 1984; 5.

Wheeland RG, Walker NP. Lasers—25 years later. *Int J Derm* 1986; 25:209–216.

van Gemert MJC, Welch AJ. Treatment of port wine stains: analysis. *Med Instrum* 1987; 21:213–217.

van Gemert MJC, Welch AJ, Amin AP. Is there an optimal laser treatment for port wine stains? *Lasers Surg Med* 1986; 6:76–83.

PHYSIOLOGY

Abergel RP, Lyons RF, Glassberg E, et al. Wound repair by laser welding. *Proc Soc Photo-Opt Inst Eng* 1986; 605:37–41.

Ben-Baruch G, Fidler J, Wessler T, et al. Comparison of wound healing between chopped mode-superpulse mode CO_2 laser and steel knife incision. *Lasers Surg Med* 1988; 8:596–599.

Ben-Bassat M, et al. A study of the ultrastructural features of the cut margin of skin and mucous membrane specimens excised by carbon dioxide laser. *J Surg Res* 1976; 21:77.

Finsterbush A, Rousso M, Ashur H. Healing and tensile strength of CO_2 laser incisions and scalpel wounds in rabbits. *Plast Reconstr Surg* 1982; 70:360.

Fisher J. The power density of a surgical laser beam: Its meaning and measurement. *Lasers Surg Med* 1983; 2:301–315.

Fuller TA. The physics of surgical lasers. *Lasers Surg Med* 1980; 1:5.

Haina D, Landthaler M, Braun-Falco O, Waidelich W. Comparison of the maximum coagulation depth in human skin for different types of medical lasers. *Lasers Surg Med* 1987; 7:355–362.

Hobbs EH, Bailin PL, Wheeland RG, Ratz JI. Superpulsed lasers: minimizing thermal damage with short duration, high irradiance pulses. *J Dermatol Surg Oncol* 1987; 13:955–964.

Kamat BR, Carney JM, Arndt KA, et al. Cutaneous tissue repair following CO_2 laser irradiation. *J Invest Dermatol* 1986; 87:268–271.

Lahaye CT, van Gemert MJ. Optimal laser parameters for port wine stain therapy. a theoretical approach. *Phys Med Biol* 1985; 6:573–587.

Landthaler M, Haina D, Brunner H, et al. Effects of argon, dye, and Nd:YAG lasers on epidermis, dermis and venous vessels. *Lasers Surg Med* 1986; 6:87–93.

Lane RJ, Llnsker R, Wynne JJ, et al. Ultraviolet laser ablation of skin. *Arch Dermatol* 1985; 121:609–617.

Lanzafame RJ, Naim JO, Rogers DW, Hinshaw JR. Comparison of continuous-wave, chop-wave, and super-pulse laser wounds. *Lasers Surg Med* 1988; 8:119–124.

Maiman TH. Stimulated optical radiation in ruby. *Nature* 1960; 187:493–494.

Moreno RA, Hebda PA, Zitelli JA, Abell E. Epidermal cell outgrowth from CO_2 laser and scalpel-cut explants: implications for wound healing. *J Dermatol Surg Oncol* 1984; 10:863–868.

Oosterhuis JW. *Tumor surgery with the CO_2 laser: studies with the Cloudman 591 mouse melanoma* [Thesis]. Netherlands: University of Groningen, 1978.

Padilla RS, Pennino RP. Carbon dioxide laser vaporization: relationship of scar formation to power density. *J Dermatol Surg Oncol* 1989; 15:232.

Rayhan S. Comparison of scar produced in skin with argon and CO_2 laser with scar produced by cold scalpel. *Lasers Surg Med* 1987; 7:95.

Walsh JT, Flotte TJ, Anderson RR, Deutsch TF. Pulsed CO_2 laser tissue ablation: effect of tissue type and pulse duration on thermal damage. *Lasers Surg Med* 1988; 8:108–118.

SURGICAL PROCEDURES

Neblett CR, Morris JR, Thomsen S. Laser assisted microvascular anastomosis. *Neurosurgery* 1986; 19:914–934.

Oshiro T. *Laser treatment for nevi.* Tokyo: Medical Research Lab, 1980.

Ward H. Laser recanalization of atheromatous vessels using fiber optics. *Lasers Surg Med* 1984; 4:353–363.

White RA, Abergel RP, Lyons R, Klein SR, Kopchok G, Dwyer RM, Uitto J. Biological effects of laser welding on vascular healing. *Lasers Med Surg* 1986; 6:137–141.

White RA, Kopchok G, Donayre C, Lyons R, White G, Klein SR, Abergel RP, Uitto J. Laser welding of large diameter arteries and veins. *Trans Am Soc Artif Intern Organs* 1986; 32:181–183.

SAFETY

Apfelberg DB, Chadi B, Maser MR, Lash H. Study of carcinogenic effects of in vitro argon laser exposure of fibroblasts. *Plast Reconstr Surg* 1983; 71:93–97.

Apfelberg DB, Mittelman H, Chadi B, Maser MR, Lash H. Innovations: investigations of carcinogenic effects of in vitro argon and CO_2 laser exposure of fibroblasts. *Lasers Surg Med* 1984; 4:73–181.

Apfelberg DB, et al. Carcinogenic potential of in vitro carbon dioxide laser exposure of fibroblast. *Obstet Gynecol* 1983; 61:493–496.

Baggish MS. Complications associated with carbon dioxide laser surgery in gynecology. *Am J Obstet Gynecol* 1981; 139:568–574.

Bellina JH, Stjerholm RL, Kurpel JE. Analysis of plume emissions after papovavirus irradiation with the carbon dioxide laser. *J Reprod Med* 1982; 27:268–270.

Forrest DA. Laser Plume—Is it an operating room environmental contaminate? *Laser Nursing* 1988; 2:10–12.

Garden JM, O'Banion K, Shelnitz LS, et al. Papilloma virus in the vapor of carbon dioxide laser treated verrucae. *JAMA* 1988(Feb 26); 1199–1202.

Goldman L. Some concerns about current laser surgery of condyloma acuminata. *J Am Acad Dermatol* 1988; 4:744–745.

Huton J, Oswal VH. Metal tube anaesthesia for ear, nose and throat carbon dioxide laser surgery. *Anesthesia* 1985; 40:1210–1212.

Lanzafame RJ, Pennino R, Herrera HP, Hinshaw JR. Inexpensive retractors for laser operations. *Surg Gynecol Obstet* 1985; 161:392–393.

Lundergan DL. Practical laser safety. In: Dixon JA, ed. *Surgical application of lasers*, 2nd ed. Chicago: Year Book Medical, 1987; 79–94.

Milstein HG. A simple solution to decreasing the hazards of carbon dioxide laser plume in the operating room. *J Am Acad Dermatol* 1989; 20:708.

Mullarky MB, Norris CN, Goldberg ID. The efficacy of the CO_2 laser in the sterilization of skin seeded with batgeria: survival at the skin surface and in the plume emissions. *Laryngoscope* 1985; 95:186–187.

Nezhat C, Winer WK, Nezhat F, et al. Smoke from laser surgery: Is there a health hazard? *Lasers Surg Med* 1987; 7:376–382.

Ossoff RH, Karlan MS. Instrumentation for CO_2 laser surgery of the larynx and tracheobronchial tree. *Surg Clin North Am* 1984; 645:973–980.

Smith JP, Moss E, Bryant CJ, et al. Evaluation of a smoke evacuator used for laser surgery. *Lasers Surg Med* 1989; 9:276–281.

Walker NP, Matthews J, Newsonm SWB. Possible hazards from irradiation with the carbon dioxide laser. *Lasers Surg Med* 1986; 6:84–86.

Wheeland RG, Bailin PL, Ratz JL, Schreffler DE. Use of scleral shields for periorbital surgery. *J Dermatol Surg Oncol* 1987; 13:156–163.

Wong KC, Dykman PF. Anesthesia for laser surgery. In: Dixon JA, ed. *Surgical applications of lasers*. Chicago: Year Book Medical, 1983; 29–39.

ADDITIONAL BOOKS

Advances in Nd:YAG Laser Surgery. Joffee SN, Ogura Y, eds. New York: Springer-Verlag, 1988.

Evaluation and installation of surgical laser systems. Apfelberg DB, New York: Springer-Verlag, 1987.

Atlas of CO_2 laser techniques. Lanzafame RJ, Hinshaw JR, eds. St. Louis: Ishiyaku-Euro America, 1988.

CO_2 laser surgery. Berlin L, Kaplan I, Giler S, eds. New York: Springer-Verlag, 1984.

Cutaneous laser surgery. Arndt KA, Noe JM, Rosen S, eds. New York: John Wiley, 1983.

Surgical application of lasers, 2nd ed. Dixon JA, ed. Chicago: Year Book Medical, 1987.

Surgical lasers: a clinical guide. Fuller TA, ed. New York: Macmillan, 1987.

Lasers and hematoporphyrin derivative in cancer. Hayata Y, Dougherty TJ, eds. Tokyo: Igaku-Shoin, 1983.

Illustrated cutaneous laser surgery. Dover JS, Arndt KA, Geronemus NG, Olbricht SM, Noe JM, Stern RS, eds. Norwalk, CT: Appleton and Lange, 1990.

Laser treatment for nevi. Oshiro T, ed. Tokyo: Medical Laser Research, 1980.

Lasers in cutaneous medicine and surgery. Ratz JL, ed. Chicago: Year Book Medical, 1986.

Lasers in general surgery. Joffee SN, ed. Baltimore: Williams & Wilkins, 1989.

Lasers in skin disease. Wheeland RG, ed. New York: Thieme Medical, 1988.

Medical lasers: science and clinical practice. Carruth J, McKinzie A. Boston: Adam Hilger, 1986.

Microscopic and endoscopic surgery with the CO_2 laser. Andrews A, Polanyi T, eds. Boston: John Wright, 1982.

Neodymium-YAG laser in medicine and surgery. Joffee SN, Muckerheide MC, Goldman L, eds. New York: Elsevier, 1983.

Perioperative laser nursing. Mackety CJ, ed. Thorofave, NJ: NM Slack, 1984.

Photosensitization-molecular, cellular and medical aspects. Morenok G, Pottier NH, Truscott TG, eds. *NATO ASI series H: Cell Biology*. New York: Springer-Verlag, 1987.

The biomedical laser. Goldman L, ed. New York: Springer-Verlag, 1981.

Vascular birthmarks: hemangiomas and malformations. Muliken JB, ed. Philadelphia: WB Saunders, 1988.

Subject Index

A
Abdomen, neurofibromatosis of, 130–131
Acne rosacea
  argon laser treatment of, 210–211
  facial, 210–211
  post-treatment care, 210
Acne scarring
  CO_2 laser ablation of, 106–108
  CO_2 laserbrasion of, 191–192
  facial, 106–108,191–192
  keloids and, 106–108
Actinic cheilitis
  CO_2 laser treatment of, 33–34,35–36,37–38,39–41
  epithelial dysplasia and, 37–38
  histopathology of, 35
  post-treatment care, 35,36,37
  squamous cell carcinoma and, 33–34,39–41
Adenoma sebaceum
  argon laser treatment of, 266–267
  facial, 266–267
Adnexal neoplasm
  CO_2 laser excision of, 96
  facial, 96
Angiofibroma
  anesthesia for, 212
  argon laser treatment of, 212–213,266–267,268
  facial, 266–267,268
Angiokeratoma
  argon laser treatment of, 214–215,216–217,218–219,416
  of chest/arm, 345–346
  circumscriptum, 214–215,216–217
  diffuse, 345
  of Fordyce, 218–219
  hexascan use in, 416–418
  port wine hemangioma and, 416–417
  post-treatment care, 214,216,218,345
  tunable dye laser use in, 345–346
Argon laser
  CO_2 laser comparison, 260–261,270
  description of, 11
  disadvantages of, 363
  hexascan use with, 406,408,412,414,421,445
  indications for, 209,445
  krypton laser and, 428
  KTP laser comparison, 424–425,443–444
  Nd:YAG laser comparison, 304,310
  pigmentation effects, 217,239,267
  properties of, 8,210,212,218
  scarring and, 242,244
  schematic of, 10
  thermal effects of, 6,242
  tunable dye laser comparison, 361,363,382
  wavelength of, 3,4,210
Argon/copper laser, gated, indications for use, 419
Arteriovenous malformation
  of finger, 292–293
  Nd:YAG laser treatment of, 292–293

B
Basal cell carcinoma
  argon dye laser use in, 428–430,431–432
  CO_2 laser excision of, 42–43,44–45,46–47,162–163
  invasive, 42–43
  of lip, 42–43
  Moh's micrographic technique for, 44–45
  of nose, 428–430,431–432
  of parotid area, 162–163
  PDT of, 428–430,431–432
  photofrin uptake by, 428,431,432
  recurrent, 44–45
  skin graft and, 163
  superficial, 46–47
  of temple, 44–45
  of trunk, 46–47
Blepharoplasty
  in blepharochalasia, 164–166
  CO_2 laser use in, 164–166
  scalpel technique comparison, 164–166
Bowen's disease
  CO_2 laser excision in, 48–49
  of finger, 48–49
  of toe, 48–49
Breast ductal carcinoma
  axillary dissection in, 339–340
  infiltrating, 339–340
  Nd:YAG laser dissection of, 339–340
Buccal mucosa
  argon laser treatment of, 230,258
  cavernous hemangioma of, 296

475

Buccal mucosa (*contd.*)
   CO_2 laser treatment of, 103–105,122–124,137–138
   irrational fibroma of, 103–105
   lichen planus of, 122–124
   lymphangioma of, 230
   Nd:YAG laser treatment of, 296
   periapical granuloma of, 137–138
   post-treatment appearance of, 105–125
   venous malformation of, 258
Burns
   argon laser treatment of, 270
   bleeding and, 143,331,332
   of buttock, 334
   CO_2 laser treatment of, 143–145,270
   of face, 144
   fatty tissue in, 331,332
   hypertrophic scar in, 143–145,270
   laser treatment related, 270
   Nd:YAG contact laser excision in, 331–334
   nonsequential complete incision of, 331–334
   ruby laser treatment of, 447
   steel scalpel treatment comparison, 331,333–334
   of thigh, 333

C

Cafe-au-lait lesion
   argon dye laser and hexascan use in, 445
   epidermal melanosis and, 448
   ruby laser use in, 448
Carbon dioxide (CO_2) laser
   advantages of, 44,50,63,103,122
   applications, 23–24
   argon laser comparison, 260–261,270
   biopsy use, 63–64
   char layer formation, 64,105,124
   coagulation effects, 7,25,27,29,44,78
   description of, 10
   dissection with, 25,26,29
   eye protection for, 25,27
   in fetal rat surgery, 182–183
   lymphatics and, 31,42,44,96
   Nd:YAG laser comparison, 7,111,296,339
   schematic of, 10
   test treatment and, 133
   thermal effects of, 6
   tissue effects of, 7
   wavelength of, 3,4
Carbon dioxide superpulse laser
   advantages of, 109,143,153
   in facial syringoma removal, 153–155
   in hypertrophic scar treatment, 143
   properties of, 109
Cherry angioma
   Candela flashed-pump dye laser use in, 347–348
   of forehead, 347–348
   post-treatment care, 347
Cherry hemangioma
   of calf, 349
   tunable dye laser use in, 349
Chondrodermatitis nodularis
   of ear, 91
   CO_2 laser vaporization of, 91
Coagulation
   CO_2 laser effects, 7,25,27,29,44
   Nd:YAG laser effects, 296,300,302,320,322,329,331,335
Comedones
   CO_2 laser excision of, 92–93
   cyst sac removal, 92,93
   facial, 93
Compound nevus
   biopsy of, 94
   CO_2 laser excision of, 94–95
   of face, 94–95
Condyloma
   acetic acid visualization of, 53
   acuminata, 51–52,55
   biopsy of, 51
   CO_2 laser treatment of, 51–52,53–54,55,56,57
   HPV typing of, 53
   of labia, 51–52
   penile, 53–54
   perianal, 56
   post-treatment care, 54
   prognosis in, 51,55
   rectal, 51,53
   urethral, 57
   of vagina, 51–52
Copper vapor laser, properties of, 404

D

Debridement
   CO_2 laser use in, 187–188,189–190,205–207
   of heel ulcer, 187–188
   of ischemic foot ulcer, 189–190
   of squamous cell carcinoma, 205–207
De-epithelialization
   CO_2 laser use in, 178–179
   in reduction mammaplasty, 178–179
Dupuytren's contracture
   of finger and palm, 180–181
   CO_2 laser excision in, 180–181
   skin flap design in, 181

E

Ear
   ruby laser treatment of, 458
   seborrheic keratosis of, 458
Earlobe
   anesthesia for, 272
   argon laser treatment of, 272–274
   CO_2 laser treatment of, 109–110,111–113
   keloid removal, 109–110,111–113,272–274
Ectrodactyly-ectodermal dysplasia-clefting (EEC) syndrome, papillomatosis of lip, 284–285
Electromagnetic spectrum, wavelengths of, 4
Epithelial dysplasia
   CO_2 laser treatment of, 37–38
   histology of, 38

of lip, 37–38
post-treatment care, 37
Eye
cornea of, 21
laser injury of, 14–15,21–22
laser shields, 22
protection of, 15–16,21–22,25,198,312,328,335,356, 364,369
retina of, 22
Eyelid
argon laser use on, 226–227,238–239,246–247,278–279
capillary/cavernous hemangioma of, 326–327
CO_2 laser use on, 151–152,153–155,156–157,161,198–199
divided nevus of, 446
eyeliner tattoo removal, 167–168
hemangioma of, 226–227,238–239,246–247,306–309
of infant, 246–247,306–308
Kaposi's sarcoma of, 312–313
Nd:YAG laser treatment of, 306–308,312–313,326–327
nevus of Ota of, 278–279
port wine hemangioma of, 372–373
ruby laser use on, 446
seborrheic keratosis of, 151–152
superpulsed CO_2 laser use on, 167–168
syringoma removal, 153–155,156–157
tunable dye laser use on, 372–373
xanthelasma of, 161,198–199

F

Face
acne rosacea of, 210–211
acne scarring of, 106–108,191–192
adnexal neoplasm of, 96
anesthesia for, 158,234,378
angiofibroma of, 266–267
argon laser treatment of, 210–211,234–235,236–237, 238–239,246–247,252,266–267,278,279,280–281, 287,426–427
basal cell carcinoma of, 445
cavernous hemangioma of, 320–321,324–325
cherry angioma of, 347–348
CO_2 laser treatment of, 25–26,27–28,89–90,93,96, 99–101,106–108,116–118,119–121,129–131, 153–155,191–192
comedones of, 93
compound nexus of, 94–95
copper vapor laser treatment of, 404–405
epidermal melanosis of, 447,448
hemangioma of, 25–26,27–28,342–344
hexascan use for, 406–407,408–409,426–427
hypertrophic scar of, 143–145
of infant, 246–247,381
keloids of, 106–108,116–118,119–121
lentigo senilis of, 449
lupus erythematosis dermabrasion of, 99–101
Nd:YAG laser treatment of, 300–301,302–303,304–305, 320–321,324–325
neurofibromatosis of, 129–131

nevocellular nevus of, 128
nevus araneus of, 359–360
nevus of Ota of, 278–279
nevus sebaceum of, 280–281
perinasal tricoepithelioma of, 158–160
port wine hemangioma of, 234–235,236–237,238–239, 287–289,302–303,304–305,361–362,363–364, 365–366,367,368–369,371,372,376–377,425–426
port wine stain of, 404–405,406–407,408–409,410–411
post-treatment care of, 89,116,119,191,234,236,359
ruby laser treatment of, 447,448,455
seborrheic keratosis of, 286
spider angioma of, 378–379
strawberry hemangioma of, 246–247
syringoma of, 153–155
tattoo removal from, 89–90
telangiectasia of, 252,354–355,356–358,381–383,386–387, 388–389,426–427
tunable dye laser treatment of, 342–344,347–348, 356–358,359–360,381–383,384–385,386,387,406,408
Fetal surgery, rat
CO_2 laser use in, 182–183
hysterotomy in, 182–183
of upper lip, 183
Fibroblast growth
CO_2 laser use and, 143
Nd:YAG laser use and, 111
Fibroma
of buccal mucosa, 103–105
CO_2 laser excision of, 103–105
irritation induced, 103–105
Finger
anesthesia of, 67,68,97,126
argon laser treatment of, 259
arteriovenous malformation of, 292–293
Bowen's disease of, 48–49
CO_2 laser use on, 48–49,62,66–67,68–69,97–98,126–127, 180–181,200–201
in Dupuytren's contracture, 180–181
mucous cyst of, 200–201
myxoid cysts of, 97–98
nail excision, 126–127
Nd:YAG laser treatment of, 292–293
periungual wart of, 68–69
pyogenic granuloma of, 62
squamous cell carcinoma of, 48–49
tattoo removal, 439–440
verruca vulgaris of, 259
wart removal, 66–67
Flashlamp excited dye (FED) laser, properties of, 356–357,358,376,378,398
Foot
anesthesia of, 184,190,215
angiokeratoma of, 214–215
argon laser treatment of, 214–215
CO_2 laser treatment of, 184–186,187–188,189–190
ganglion cyst excision, 184–186
heel ulcers, 187–188
ischemic ulcers of, 189–190

G

Gallium-arsenide laser, semiconducting elements of, 3
Ganglion cyst
   CO_2 laser excision, 184–186
   of upper foot, 184–186

H

Hemangiolymphangioma
   A-V fistula and, 29–30
   of chest wall, 29–30
   CO_2 laser resection of, 29–30
Hemangioma
   angiogenital and or perineal, 220–222
   argon laser treatment of, 220–222,228–229,287–289
   capillary
      argon laser treatment of, 223,224,226–227,229–230
      characteristics of, 342
      of eyelid, 226–227
      of face, 342–344
      of hand, 350
      of infant, 223,226–227,342–344,350,402–403
      or lip, 224,229–230,342–344
      of nose area, 223,402–403
      post-treatment care, 224,226,229,342,402
      superficial, 350
      tunable dye laser use in, 342–344,350
   capillary/cavernous
      of cheek, 328–330
      CO_2 laser treatment of, 25–26,27–28
      of eyelid, 326–327
      of infant, 294–295,328–330,337–338
      of lip, 337–338
      Nd:YAG laser treatment of, 294–295,320–321, 326–327,328–330,337–338
      of neck, 294–295
      of nose, 25–26
      post-treatment care, 294,326,328,337
      ulcerated, 337–338
   cavernous
      arteriography in 320,322
      of buccal mucosa, 296
      of chest, 322–323
      of face, 320–321,324
      healing problems of, 322
      of lip, 297
      Nd:YAG laser treatment of, 296,297,320–321, 322–323,324–325
      resection of, 320,322
      sapphire scalpel use in, 322–323
   cherry, 349
   dot/pointillistic technique for, 287–289
   hypertrophic, 236–237
   in infant, 220–221,294–295,335–336
   in lip, 250–251,287–289
   of nose, 380
   of perineum, 335–336
   periorbital/conjunctival, 226–227
   port wine. See also Port wine stain.
      anesthetic for, 298,369,372
      argon laser use in, 234–235,236–237,238–239,240–241, 242–243,244–245,372,424–425
      argon pumped tunable laser use in, 365–366
      Candela flashlamp tunable dye laser use in, 368–369
      of chest, 370
      CW dye laser use in, 372–373
      of eyelid, 239,372–373
      of face, 234–235,236–237,238–239,242–243,298–299, 302–303,304–305,361–362,363–364,365–366,367, 368–369,371,421–423,424–425
      hexascan use in, 420
      incomplete removal of, 366,372,374
      in infant, 363,364,368
      KTP laser use in, 424–425
      of lip, 238–239,240–241,242–243,244–245,304–305
      Nd:YAG laser use in, 298–299,302–303,304–305
      of neck, 234–235,421–423,424–425
      of nose, 287–289
      patient age and, 363,368
      "polka dot" treatment of, 302,305,375
      post-treatment care, 234,236,298,302,361,363,367,368, 371,425
      scarring and, 242,244,372,423
      treatment interval for, 370,371
      tunable dye laser use in, 342,361–362,363–364,367, 370,420
      wavelength of choice for, 367,374
   skin flap development in, 26,27,28
   spider type, 380
   strawberry
      anesthesia for, 226,248
      of anogenital region, 248–249
      argon laser treatment of, 225,226–227,246–247, 248–249,250–251
      argon-Nd:YAG laser comparison for, 310
      on buttock, 225
      conjunctival, 226–227
      of eyelid, 227,246,306–309
      of face, 294–295
      of flank, 310–311
      in growth phase, 225,250
      in infant, 225,246–247,248–249,250–251,294–295, 306–309,310–311
      of lip, 250–251
      of medial canthus, 246–247
      Nd:YAG laser treatment of, 294–295, 306–309,310–311
      post-treatment care of, 226,246,248,250,310
      slide-compression treatment of, 307
      ulcerated, 310–311
   tunable dye laser use in, 349,350,380
   ulceration of, 249,335–336
   of vermilion, 228–229
   of vulva/perineum, 335–336
Heterotopic gastric mucosa
   CO_2 laser resection of, 102
   of tongue, 102
Hexascan
   argon laser and, 406,408,412,414,416,421,426,445
   copper vapor laser nad, 404–405
   description of, 406,407,408,410,414,421,445

indications for use, 406,408,410,412,414,416,420,421,
426,445
for infants, 408,410
pain and, 404,406,408,410,412,414,416
scarring and, 404,405,407,410,421,423,427
tunable dye laser and, 406,408,410,412,416,420
Hyperkeratotic nevus
argon laser treatment of, 276–277
post-treatment care, 276
Hypertrophic scar
argon laser treatment of, 270–271
of cheek, 143–145
CO_2 laser treatment of, 143–145,270
fibroblasts and, 143
icing of, 270,271
paresthesias relief in, 143
post-treatment care of, 270
of sternotomy, 270–271
thermal burn induced, 143–145,270
Hysterotomy
CO_2 laser use in, 182–183
for fetal rat surgery, 182–183

I
Infants
argon laser treatment of, 220–222,223,246–247,248–249,
250–251,363
capillary hemangiomas in, 223,402–403
hexascan use on, 408,410,412
KTP laser use on, 402–403
Nd:YAG laser use on, 294–295,306–309,310–311
port wine hemangioma in, 363–364,368
strawberry hemangioma in, 220–222,246–247,248–249,
250–251,294–295,306–309,310–311
tunable dye laser advantage for, 363
tunable dye laser use in, 363–364,368

K
Kaposi's sarcoma
of eyelid, 312–313
Nd:YAG laser treatment of, 312–313
Keloids
acne related, 106–108,318–319
anatomic location and recurrence, 116
argon laser treatment of, 272–274,275
on chin, 119–121
CO_2 laser ablation of, 106–108,109–110,111–113,
114–115,116–118,119–121
CO_2 superpulse laser ablation of, 109–110
of earlobe, 109–110,111–113,272–274
on face, 106–108,116–118
fibroblast growth and, 111,272
follicular infection related, 116–118
of forearm vortex, 316–317
icing of, 272,273
Nd:YAG laser treatment of, 111,316–317,318–319
on neck, 114–115,116–118,119–121
post-traumatic, 316–317
on pubic area, 275

recurrence of, 109,110,113,116,118,272,274
sebaceous cyst related, 114–115
tension and, 111,116
two stage removal of, 111–113
Krypton laser
argon laser comparison, 428
in PDT, 428–429
photofrin excitation and, 428

L
Laser absorptive dose (LAD), unit in laser dosimetry, 9
Lasers. *See also specific laser types.*
absorption vs wavelength, 8
aiming device for, 7
categories of, 3
characteristics of, 1–2
coagulation effects of, 7,25,27,29,44,296,300,302,320,335
coherence of light and, 5
concepts in, 2–3
continuous wave (CW), 6
delivery systems of, 5–6
dosimetry in, 8–9
dye type, 3,11
energy absorption from, 7–8
energy delivery rate, 6
energy levels of, 2–3
excimer types, 3
gas type, 3
hexascan use with, 406,407–408,410
liquid type, 3
medical history of, 1
mode of operation, 6–7
myocotic organism destruction, 58
population inversion and, 2,3
pulsed, 6
Q-switched, 6,7
safety classification of, 14
stimulated emission, 2,3
TEM of, 6–7
thermal effects of, 6,7–8
tissue interactions, 7–8
types of, 3,6,9–11
wavelengths of, 3–4
Laser safety
check list use in, 14
documentation in, 14
education in, 13,14,16,19
electrical systems in, 17
equipment maintenance and, 19
eye injury and, 14–15,21–22
eye protection and, 15–16,198,312,328,335,356,364,402
FDA role in, 14
fire protection and, 17–18
guidelines for, 13–14,21
laser classification in, 14
laser operator and, 17
policies for, 20
safety officer and, 19–20
teeth and, 33,102
smoke evacuation systems and, 18

Laser safety (contd.)
   smoke, protection from, 68,198
   viral particles and, 68
   warning signs for, 16
   windows and, 16
Leg
   angiofibroma of, 212–213
   angiokeratoma of, 216–217
Lentigo maligna
   of auricular area, 50
   CO_2 laser excision of, 50
Lentigo senilis
   of cheek, 449
   ruby laser treatment of, 449
Lichen planus
   biopsy of, 122,123,124
   of buccal mucosa, 122–125
   CO_2 laser excision, 122–125
   recurrence of, 125
Lip
   actinic cheilitis of, 33–34,35–36,37–38,39–41
   anesthetic for, 33,35,39,224,228,250,297,400
   argon/copper gated laser use on, 419
   argon laser treatment of, 224,228–229,238–239,240–241,
      242–243,250–251,255,256–257,258,284–285,287–289
   basal cell carcinoma of, 42–43
   capillary/venous malformation of, 224
   CO_2 laser treatment of, 33–34,35–36,37–38,39–41,42–43
   CW tunable dye laser use on, 374–375
   epithelial dysplasia of, 37–38
   FED laser use on, 398
   hemangioma of, 238–239,240–241,242–243,244–245,
      250–251,287–289,297,304–305
   of infant, 250–251
   ND:YAG laser use on, 297,304–305
   papillomatosis of, 284–285
   port wine stain of, 374–375,412–413
   resurfacing of, 33,37–38
   squamous cell carcinoma of, 33–34,39–41
   tunable dye laser use on, 400
   venous lake of, 255,256–257,398–399,400
   venous malformation of, 258
   vermilion of, 36,39–41,228–229
Lipoma
   of back, 193
   of chest, 193–195
   CO_2 laser excision of, 193–195
Lupus erythematosis
   biopsy of, 99
   CO_2 laser dermabrasion of, 99–101
   discoid, 99–101
   hypopigmentation and, 99,101
Lymphangiohemangioma
   CO_2 laser resection of, 31–32
   of tongue, 31–32
Lymphangioma
   argon laser treatment of, 230,231
   of buccal mucosa, 230
   of tongue, 231

M

Mammaplasty
   CO_2 laser de-epithelialization in, 178–179
   in macromastia, 178–179
Maxillary plate
   CO_2 laser biopsy of, 63–65
   pyogenic granuloma of, 63–65
Mohs' micrographic technique
   for basal cell carcinoma excision, 44–45
   CO_2 laser modification of, 44–45
Mucous cyst
   CO_2 laser excision of, 200–201
   of finger DIP joint, 200–201
Myocutaneous flap
   CO_2 laser dissection of, 175,177
   of latissimus dorsi, 175,177
Myxoid cysts
   CO_2 laser excision of, 97–98
   of finger nail bed, 97–98
   recurrence of, 97

N

Neck
   argon laser treatment of, 234–235
   CO_2 laser use on, 116–118,119–121
   hexascan use and, 410–411
   keloid removal, 116–118,119–121
   port wine hemangioma of, 234–235,425–426
   port wine stain of, 410–411
   tunable dye laser use on, 411–412
Neodymium:yttrium-aluminum garnet (Nd:YAG) laser
   argon laser comparison, 304,310
   coagulation effects of, 7,296,300,302,322,329,331,335
   CO_2 laser comparison, 7,111,296,339
   description of, 9–10
   eye protection for, 312
   fibroblast growth and, 111,316,318
   properties of, 292,294,296,298,300,302,306,322,328
   sapphire scalpel use and, 320,339–340
   schematic diagram of, 9
   thermal effects of, 6,320,322,324
   tissue effects of, 7
   wavelength of, 3,7
Neurofibromata
   anesthesia for, 133
   CO_2 laser excision of, 132–133
   forms of, 132
Neurofibromatosis
   on abdomen, 130–131
   anesthesia for removal, 130
   CO_2 laser excision of, 129–131
   of face, 129–131
Nevocellular nevus
   CO_2 laser excision of, 128
   of nasolabial fold, 128
Nevus. See also specific forms of.
   araneus, 359–360
   argon laser treatment of, 278–279,280–281,282–283

compound, 94-95
cryosurgery of, 278,279,281,282
divided, 446
on eyelid, 446,453-454
on face, 278-279,300-301,359-360,455
hyperkeratotic, 276-277
on knee, 456-457
on leg, 450-451
Nd:YAG laser treatment of, 300-301
nevus cell, 450-451,452
of Ota, 278-279,453-454
port wine, 300-301
post-treatment care, 276,280,282,359
ruby laser use on, 450-451,452,453,455,456,457
sebaceum, 280-281
on shoulder, 452
spilus, 455,456-457
tunable dye laser use on, 359-360
unilateralis, 282-283
Nose
acne rosacea of, 210-211
anesthesia of, 232
argon laser treatment of, 135,210-211,223,232-233,252, 253,287-289
basal cell carcinoma of, 428-430
capillary hemangioma of, 223,402-403
CO_2 laser treatment of, 25-26,135-136,146-147,148-150
columella of, 396-397
debulking of, 146-147
hemangioma of, 25-26,287-289
infants, 223
post-rhinoplasty red blush of, 232-233
red nose syndrome of, 135
rhinophyma and, 146-147,148-150
sebaceous gland hypertrophy of, 148-150
spider hemangioma of, 380
telangiectasia of, 252,253,351-353,390,396-397
tunable dye laser use on, 351-353,390,396-397
vascular discolorization of, 135-136

O

Onychocryptosis
CO_2 laser excision in, 134,139-140
nail plate narrowing in, 134
pincer nail deformity, 139-140
Onychomycosis
CO_2 laser vaporization of, 58-59,60-61
fungal culture in, 60-61
post-treatment care, 58
prognosis in, 60

P

Papillomatosis
argon laser treatment of, 284-285
EEC syndrome and, 284
of lip, 284-285
Paresthesias relief, in CO_2 laser treatment, 143
Penis

CO_2 laser treatment of, 53-54
condyloma of, 53-54
Periapical granuloma
canine tooth associated, 137-138
CO_2 laser treatment of, 137-138
Periungal warts
bleeding control and, 69,70
CO_2 laser excision, 68-69,70-71
histology of, 71
prognosis in, 68,69,71
Photodynamic therapy (PDT)
apparatus for, 434
argon dye laser use in, 428-430,431-432
in basal cell carcinoma, 428-430,431-432
cylinder implantation in, 429
dihematoporphyrin use in, 433
photofrin photosensitizer use in, 428,431,432
post-treatment care in, 428
squamous cell carcinoma treatment by, 433-435
treatment protocol, 428-429
treatment results in, 433
Pigmentation
in argon laser use, 217,239
in CO_2 laser use, 54,55,99,101,158
hexascan use and, 406,408,410,414
hyper, 54,58,217,366,395
hypo, 54,55,99,239,299,406,408,410,436
of lentigo senilis, 449
in Nd:YAG laser use, 299
post-traumatic, 447
in pulsed tunable dye laser use, 366
in ruby laser use, 436,447,448,450-451,452,453
sunlight exposure and, 158
in tunable dye laser use, 395
Pilar cyst
CO_2 laser excision of, 141-142
of scalp, 141-142
Port wine stain
angiokeratomas and, 416-417
argon/copper gated laser use in, 419
argon laser use in, 404,410,416
Candela flashlamp-pulsed dye laser use in, 368-369
copper vapor laser use in, 404-405
CW dye laser use in, 372-373
facial, 368-369,372-373,376-377,404-405,406-407, 408-409,410-411,419
FED laser use in, 376-377
hexascan use in, 404-405,406-407,408-409,410-411, 412-413,414-415,416-418
on leg, 414-415,416-418,420
on lip, 374-375,412-413,419
post-treatment care, 405
residual in, 405
tunable dye laser use in, 406,408,410,412,414,420
Potassium titanyl phosphate (KTP) laser
argon laser comparison, 424-425,443-444
blanching effects, 403
eye protection for, 402
properties of, 402,443
wavelength of, 3,424,425,443

Pyogenic granuloma
  CO_2 laser treatment, 62,63–65
  of finger, 62
  as intraoral lesion, 63–65
  lesion size and, 62
  Sturge-Weber syndrome and, 63

R

Rhinophyma
  CO_2 laser excision, 146–147,148–150
  sebaceous gland hypertrophy and, 148–150
Ruby laser
  applications, 436,439,440,447,448,449,450–451,452,453, 456,458
  energy densities of, 436,440,441,446,449,454
  Q-switched pulsed, 436–438,439–440,447,448
  wavelength of, 436

S

Scalp
  CO_2 laser treatment, 141–142,196–197
  pilar cyst of, 141–142
  squamous cell carcinoma of, 196–197
Sebaceous cyst
  anesthetic for, 202
  CO_2 laser excision of, 114,202–204
  keloid development and, 114
  of trunk area, 202–204
Sebaceous gland
  CO_2 laser treatment of, 148–150
  hypertrophy of, 148–150
  in rhinophyma, 148–150
Seborrheic keratosis
  argon laser excision of, 286
  CO_2 laser excision of, 151–152
  of ear, 458
  of eyelid, 151–152
  of forehead, 286
  ruby laser use in, 458
Skin graft, CO_2 laser treatment and, 162–163
Spider angioma
  anesthetic for, 378
  CW tunable dye laser use in, 378–379
  facial, 378–379
  FED laser use in, 378
  of nose, 380
  tunable dye laser use in, 380
Squamous cell carcinoma
  actinic cheilitis and, 39–40
  argon laser use in, 433–435
  CO_2 laser debridement of, 205–207
  CO_2 laser excision of, 33–34,39–40,48–49,196–197
  CT scan of, 196
  of eyelid, 433–435
  of finger, 48–49
  in situ, 48–49
  of lip, 33–34,39–40
  PDT use in, 433–435
  of preauricular area, 205–207

  recurrence of, 207
  of scalp, 196–197
  of toe, 48–49
Surgical scar. *See* Hypertrophic scar and Keloids.
Syringomas
  CO_2 laser excision of, 153–155,156–157
  of eyelid, 153–155,156–157
  recurrence of, 153

T

Tattoo removal
  of amateurs tattoo, 87,436–438,439–440,441,442
  anesthetic for, 80,168,314,437
  argon laser/CO_2 laser comparison for, 260–261
  argon laser use in, 86,260–261,262–263
  on arm, 87–88,260–261,262–263,264–265,438,443–444
  on back, 78–79
  on breast, 80–82
  char removal in, 260,262
  CO_2 laser use in, 78–79,80–82,83–84,85–86,87–88, 89–90,169–171,172–174,260
  on deltoid area, 83–84,85–86,169–171,260–261
  on face, 89–90
  FED laser use in, 376–377
  on fingers, 439–440
  on hand, 436–438,441–442
  heat removal during, 80,81
  KTP laser use in, 443–444
  mechanical debridement in, 83,85
  Nd:YAG laser use in, 314,315
  operating microscope use in, 80,88
  pigment depth and, 87,436
  post-treatment care, 78,81,85,88,89,167,169–171,172,260, 262,264,314,443
  pulsed ruby laser use in, 436–438,439–440,441–442
  residual scars in, 78,79,80,81,82,84,172
  sequential treatment of, 315
  on shoulder, 315
  superpulsed CO_2 laser use in, 167–168
  tattoo age and, 87
  of upper eyelid liner, 168–169
  urea ointment use in, 169,170,172
  on wrist, 172–174
Teeth, laser injury protection of, 33,102
Telangiectasia
  adult onset, 381–383
  argon laser treatment of, 252,253,382,426–427
  Candela tunable dye laser use in, 384–385,393–395
  congenital, 391–392
  copper vapor laser use in, 404
  CRST syndrome and, 354
  erythema and, 426–427
  essential, 384–385,386
  fair complexion and, 384
  of face, 252,354–355,356–358,381–383,384–385,386,387, 388–389,426–427
  FED laser use in, 356–358
  of leg veins, 393–395
  matted, 354–355,356–358,393–395
  nasal venous, 390

of nose, 252,253,351–353,396–397
post-treatment care of, 354,357,384,388,390,394
purpura and, 351,354,355,358,384
retreatment of, 386,387,390,392,396
sclerotherapy in, 391,393
on thigh, 392–392
tunable CW dye laser use in, 351–353,354–355,356–358, 381–383,386
tunable dye laser use in, 387,388–389,390,391–392

Toe
anesthesia of, 140
CO_2 laser treatment of, 48–49,134,139–140
onychomycotic buildup and, 58–59
post-treatment care, 139
squamous cell carcinoma of, 48–49

Tongue
argon laser treatment of, 231
CO_2 laser resection of, 31–32,102
heterotopic gastric mucosa of, 102
lymphangiohemangioma of, 31–32
lymphangioma of, 231

Transverse electromagnetic wave mode (TEM), of lasers, 6–7

Trichoepithelioma
CO_2 laser excision of, 158–160
of perinasal area, 158–160
post-treatment care, 159

Tuberous sclerosis, angiofibroma treatment in, 266–267,268

Tunable dye laser
advantages of, 342,351,356,381
argon laser comparison, 361,363,382
argon pumped, 365–366
Candela type, 342,346,347–348,354,359,368,384–385, 393–395,396
CW, 351,372,374,378,386
description of, 11,351
eye protection for, 356,364,369
FED type, 356–357,358,376,378,398
flashpump, 347
painless nature of, 342,349,356,367,369,386,388
power settings for, 356–357,358,359,362,363,368,369, 372,374,376,380,381,384
schematic of, 11
sclerotherapy and, 391,393
wavelengths of, 3,349,351,356

U

Ulcer
of chest wall, 175–177
CO_2 laser excision of, 175–177
CO_2 laser debridement of, 187–188,189–190
of heel, 187–188
ischemic, of foot, 189–190
myocutaneous flap repair of, 175,177
post-radiation, 175

Urea ointment, use in post-treatment care, 169,170,172

Urethra
condyloma of, 57
CO_2 laser treatment of, 57

Urticaria pigmentosa, argon laser treatment of, 254

V

Venous lake
argon laser treatment of, 255,256–257
diascopy technique for, 398,399
FED laser use in, 398
of lip, 255,256–257,398–399,400
post-treatment care, 398

Vulva/perineum
capillary hemangioma of, 335–336
Nd:YAG laser treatment of, 335–336

W

Warts
anesthetic for removal, 67,72
argon laser treatment of, 259
CO_2 laser excision of, 66–67,68–69,70–71,72–74, 75–76,77
histology of, 71
of index finger, 66–67
non-healing planter, 75
pathology of, 66
periungual, 68–69,70–71
planter, 72–74,75–76,77
post-treatment care, 72,75
recurrence, absence of, 67,68,69,72,74,76
treatment end point, 66

X

Xanthelasma palpebrarum
CO_2 laser treatment of, 161,198–199
laser eye protection and, 198